Optometric Management of
Learning-Related
Vision Problems

OPTOMETRIC MANAGEMENT OF LEARNING-RELATED VISION PROBLEMS

Mitchell M. Scheiman, O.D.

Chief, Pediatric/Binocular Vision Service,
Pennsylvania College of Optometry,
Philadelphia, Pennsylvania

Michael W. Rouse, O.D., M.S.Ed.

Chief, Vision Therapy Service,
Southern California College of Optometry,
Fullerton, California

with **129** illustrations

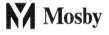 Mosby

St. Louis Baltimore Berlin Boston Carlsbad Chicago London Madrid
Naples New York Philadelphia Sydney Tokyo Toronto

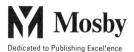
Dedicated to Publishing Excel!ence

Editor: Martha Sasser
Developmental Editor: Kellie F. White
Project Manager: Mark Spann
Production Editor: Carl Masthay
Designer: David Zielinski
Manufacturing Supervisor: Theresa Fuchs

Printed in the United States of America
Composition by Clarinda
Printing/binding by Maple Vail

Mosby–Year Book, Inc.
11830 Westline Industrial Drive
St. Louis, Missouri 63146

Library of Congress Cataloging in Publication Data

ISBN 0-8151-6385-7   94-3010
94 95 96 97 / 9 8 7 6 5 4 3 2 1

Contributors

Penni Blaskey, Ph.D.
Assistant Professor
Licensed, School Certified Psychologist,
Pennsylvania College of Optometry,
The Learning Center,
Philadelphia, Pennsylvania

Eric Borsting, O.D., N.S.
Assistant Professor,
Southern California College of
   Optometry,
Fullerton, California

Michael Cron, O.D.
Professor and Associate Dean,
College of Optometry,
Ferris State University,
Big Rapids, Michigan

Susan A. Cotter, O.D.
Associate Professor,
Illinois College of Optometry,
Chicago, Illinois

Nathan Flax, O.D., M.S.
Professor Emeritus,
College of Optometry,
State University of New York,
New York, New York

Michael Gallaway, O.D.
Associate Professor,
Pennsylvania College of Optometry,
Philadelphia, Pennsylvania

Ralph P. Garzia, O.D.
Professor,
University of Missouri—St. Louis,
School of Optometry,
St. Louis, Missouri

Sidney Groffman, O.D.
Associate Clinical Professor,
College of Optometry,
Director, Learning Disabilities Unit,
State University of New York,
New York, New York

Louis G. Hoffman, O.D., M.S.
Professor,
Southern California College of
   Optometry (Retired),
Fullerton, California

Michael W. Rouse, O.D., M.S.Ed.
Professor,
Chief, Vision Therapy Service,
Southern California College of
   Optometry,
Fullerton, California

Janice Emigh Scharre, O.D., M.A.
Professor of Optometry,
Chief, Pediatric/Binocular Vision Service,
Illinois College of Optometry,
Chicago, Illinois

Mitchell M. Scheiman, O.D.
Associate Professor,
Chief, Pediatric/Binocular Vision
   Service,
Pennsylvania College of Optometry,
Philadelphia, Pennsylvania

Richard Selznick, Ph.D.
Director of the Learning Center,
The Eye Institute,
Pennsylvania College of Optometry,
Philadelphia, Pennsylvania

Harold Solan, O.D., M.A.
Professor,
State College of Optometry,
State University of New York,
New York, New York

To Maxine, Ariella, Eliyahu and Daniel for their love and understanding.

Mitchell Scheiman

To Janet, Kayla, and my parents for their love and support.

Michael Rouse

Acknowledgments

My thanks to the following persons who have had such a strong influence on my professional development:

Dr. Jerome Rosner, who was instrumental in teaching me how to teach. Drs. Nathan Flax, Irwin Suchoff, Jack Richman, Martin Birnbaum, and Arnold Sherman, who inspired me to devote my professional career to the areas of vision therapy, pediatrics, and vision and learning.

My special thanks to my family for showing so much patience with me during the many months of writing and editing.

Mitchell Scheiman

My special thanks to Louis Hoffman for his professional mentorship that began in my residency and for his continuing friendship and support. He has had an enormous impact on this area of optometry through his teachings and sharing his clinical wisdom and experience. I would also like to thank Eric Borsting for his help in, not only writing chapters, but also reviewing many other chapters of this text. My thanks also goes to Richard L. Hopping and my clinical colleagues at the Southern California College of Optometry for supporting academic and clinical programs dedicated to the diagnosis and treatment of learning-related vision problems. Many thanks to Albert Garcia for his expert photographic and illustrative assistance. My thanks also to Patricia Carlson for her invaluable library assistance and expertise in checking chapter references.

Michael Rouse

We would like to thank all of the contributing authors for helping to make this book a reality.

Preface

Optometry has a long history of involvement in the area of vision and learning. Much of this interest has been generated by parental concern and the referrals of teachers, psychologists, and other professionals who often turn to us for answers about whether a child has a vision problem that is contributing to or responsible for poor school performance.

Optometry's effort for a better understanding of the relationship between vision and learning has led to a considerable body of professional literature. In addition, courses covering the diagnosis and management of learning-related vision problems are part of the curriculum of every school and college of optometry in the United States. Pediatric and vision therapy residency programs have also been developed in many of our schools of optometry to prepare a core of optometrists specialized in this area.

Despite of all of this involvement and activity there is currently no comprehensive textbook for optometrists entirely devoted to the subject of vision and learning. There are chapters in several textbooks that cover specific related topics, and there are several books that are compilations of articles about vision and learning. Missing, however, is a book that provides comprehensive information and an organized clinical model for both assessment and treatment of learning-related vision problems. Optometric educators teaching this topical area have long been frustrated by the lack of such a book. We have undertaken this project to try to fill this void.

One of our primary concerns in taking on this task is the difference in opinion within our profession about the relationship between vision and learning and the management of these problems. Very different approaches have been advocated by various authors. At one extreme are those who believe that there is little relationship between vision and learning and optometry's role is simply to ensure that the child sees clearly and has healthy eyes. At the other extreme are optometrists who believe that inadequate vision development (in a broad sense) is generally the main reason for school failure. Proponents of this philosophy suggest that treatment of the underlying vision problem leads directly to better school performance without any other intervention. A more reasonable approach, the one we will use for this text, is that vision can contribute to learning difficulties but that it is generally not the primary etiological factor. Rather, vision disorders represent factors that can interfere with a child's school performance and make it difficult for a child to perform up to potential.

The model that we present in this book is based on this last concept. We believe that there is a strong relationship between vision and learning and that every child that is experiencing problems in school requires an appropriate optometric evaluation. To consider the relationship between vision and learning the model we are presenting proposes dividing vision into three dimensions. The first, which every optometrist routinely evaluates, includes visual acuity, refractive status, and eye health. The second is visual efficiency and includes an evaluation of accommodation, binocular vision, and oculomotor skills. The third is visual information processing skills and incorporates various aspects of visual perception and motor integration. The first two dimensions of this model are relatively easy to explain, and there is general agreement in the profession about optometry's role in the assessment and management of these conditions. The third dimension, visual information processing skills, is more controversial. Although optometry has been involved for many years with visual perception, other professions such as special education, psychology, and occupational therapy also evaluate and treat visual perceptual problems. Some optometrists question whether the evaluation and treatment of visual perceptual skills is truly an appropriate concern for optometrists. Even among those optometrists who believe that we should be testing and treating visual perceptual anomalies, there is no general agreement about how this should be done.

Our model is based on the work of Hoffman, Richman, Solan, and others who have suggested the use of a broad array of standardized tests to assess visual perceptual skills. This approach allows the examiner to develop a profile of a child's visual perceptual development, identifying sub-skill areas of strength and weakness. The areas of weakness are then correlated with entering signs and symptoms to determine if there is a relationship.

Perhaps the most important concept in our model is that optometrists evaluate and *treat vision problems* that may be interfering with school performance. We do not directly treat the reading or learning problem. A key element in our philosophy is the recognition of the multifactorial nature of learning disorders and we will stress the importance of an interdisciplinary approach in this book. Children will generally need a variety of services such as educational remediation, psychological counseling, and speech-language therapy to deal with the actual learning disorder. This is a critical concept and represents the key to why optometry has been criticized by other professionals. They perceive that we are or have been suggesting that optometric treatment leads directly to improved reading or learning. Although this may occur in some instances, we understand and stress that in most cases our goal is to eliminate vision problems as an interfering factor. Once a reliable and efficient visual system is established the child has the necessary readiness skills to be more available to the educator and other professionals.

We will present a model that will provide students and practicing optometrists with an understandable and clinically applicable approach for managing children presenting with learning problems. The book begins with four chapters that cover important background information including an overview of normal child development, visual and visual motor development, the normal learning process, and an overview of the topical area of learning disabilities. The next section discusses the relationship between vision and learning with specific chapters exploring the relationship between visual efficiency problems and learning, and visual perceptual problems and learning. The third section of the text covers the rationale for the role of the optometrist and the assessment process, including case history, evaluation of visual efficiency and visual processing skills, a description of psychoeducational testing and arriving at a final assessment. The final section is devoted to establishing an overall management strategy and then the specific treatment of visual efficiency and visual information processing problems with a final chapter on case studies that highlight the types of patients optometrists will most often encounter.

Although we understand that the approach we have taken is only one among several possible available models, in our experience it will provide the student or practitioner with a solid and rational approach to the diagnosis and management of learning-related vision disorders. It is our hope that this book will help to create some uniformity in approach within our profession and a new interest in research leading to the development of even better assessment and treatment tools.

Contents

PART IV   TREATMENT

APPENDICES

Optometric Management
of Learning-Related
Vision Problems

PART ONE

BACKGROUND INFORMATION

CHAPTER **1**

Overview of Normal Child Development

MICHAEL CRON

KEY TERMS

maturational theory
psychoanalytic theory
organismic theory
behavioral theory
Apgar
creeping
crawling
pincer grasp
Piaget
sensorimotor
preoperational

concrete operations
formal operations
pivot open class
attachment
basic trust versus mistrust
separation anxiety
autonomy versus shame and doubt
fear
anger
initiative versus guilt
self-esteem

From the moment when that one successful sperm penetrates the surface of an ovum somewhere in the fallopian tube of the female abdomen, a miraculous sequence of events is initiated. The orchestration of these events is carried out by the unique arrangement of proteins that constitute the genetic material of that particular individual. Although each evolves into his or her own person, the process of development and the stages and phases through which they progress are remarkably similar. Developmental psychologists have spent years attempting to unravel the secrets of this process. In this initial chapter, we will overview developmental theory and then take a look at the normal developmental sequence in the prenatal period, as well as the young child's acquisition of motor, cognitive, and language skills and emotions before puberty.

CONCEPT OF CHILD DEVELOPMENT

The systematic analysis of changes throughout childhood is called "child development"—the scientific study of children. Any aspect of progress children make and their interaction with their environment and the significant people in it is open to investigation. The questions raised are of considerable importance, both in understanding how children feel and think and behave as well as in the development of policies, laws, and programs that affect our youth.

In the history of this still emerging field, studies of child development have taken differing approaches. The earliest studies concentrated on physical change and motor skill acquisition. Developmental norms were established. Arnold Gesell (1880-1961) founded the Clinic of Child Development at Yale University in 1911, where he catalogued developmental changes in children from birth to 10 years of age. As an outgrowth of his investigations, he proposed what has become a fundamental concept in developmental thinking; that stages in development follow a universal and nonvarying sequence.[1] Thus Gesell touted a maturational theory of child development, one that asserts that biological maturation is the principle force in development.

Several other theoretical systems have emerged over the years to explain child behavior. Sigmund Freud and followers, notably Erik Erikson, concentrated on psychosocial development of early childhood. Freud believed that personality developed just as physical characteristics develop and that stages needed to be achieved for a normal personality to emerge. Of particular note was Freud's psychosexual theory, which described the emergence of sexuality in stages of development. Both Freud and Erikson asserted that each new stage of development was built upon and incorporated the outcome of earlier stages.[2]

Cognitive development means how children obtain and use knowledge and the thinking processes they acquire, including memory, creativity, problem solving, and abstract thought. Jean Piaget (1896-1980), a Swiss psychologist, observed that children did not merely know less than adults (quantitatively), but that their thinking differed qualitatively as well. Piaget postulated a sequence of stages of the development of levels of mental reasoning, detailing the many developmental changes children undergo in the methods used to construct knowledge.[3]

In contrast to these theories of Gesell and Freud and Piaget, which consider biology and maturation to be critical factors in paving the road for child development, B.F. Skinner and others promote a behaviorist philosophy. Behaviorism explains child development as the sum of learned responses, based on experiences. For behaviorists, the key element is how the environment is structured and not how the child is constructed or understands what it experiences. Thus gradual change is the rule as, through standard mechanisms of learning, the person has more experiences. Learning occurs through classical conditioning, as described by the behaviorist

Pavlov,[4] and through operant conditioning used in Skinner's research.[5] A relatively recent variant of behaviorism, called "social learning theory," takes the nature of the being into account in describing learning. For example, the social learning theorists allow for vicarious reinforcement, where learning can take place through observation of the modeling of others without actually having had exposure to direct reinforcement.[6]

So several theoretical approaches to the study of child development exist. By the nature of their diverse perspectives, the types of research designs and theoretical questions that are constructed differ widely. There is a lack of agreement even on a common set of problems to be studied. Each theory remains true to its arena, and little competition exists. As long as each theory remains helpful in explaining and aiding our understanding of behavior, each will persist with a following. These theories are summarized in Table 1-1.

NORMAL PREGNANCY AND THE BIRTH PROCESS
Ovum stage

Within the female ovary, eggs are formed. On what is for most young women a regular and recurring cycle, an egg is released into the fallopian tube near the ovary. If sperm are present at this time, one of them may eventually penetrate the ovum or egg. At this point, with the fusion of the nuclear material from each cell, a zygote is formed. This new cell has the full complement of 46 chromosomes, the normal number in humans. Both the egg and the sperm carried 23 chromosomes each to the mating.

After less than 2 days this new zygote begins to divide and is moving down the fallopian tube toward the uterus. All the newly forming cells are duplicates of the initial cell. As they multiply, living off the yolk of the ovum, they form a hallow sphere called the "blastocyst." These first 10 to 14 days after conception are called the "ovum stage."

During the second week of the ovum stage, the blastocyst starts to embed itself into the uterine wall. The blastocyst is singly layered on one side, where the placenta, umbilical cord, and amniotic sac will develop, and doubly layered on the other side, where the embryo will eventually emerge. Under normal conditions the blastocyst will be embedded fully in the wall of the uterus 2 weeks after conception. When this occurs, the embryo stage begins.

Embryo stage

One of the hallmarks of the embryo stage is cell differentiation. No longer do all the cells continue to look identical to the initial cell. Important and distinct body systems begin to emerge. Three layers of cells differentiate into their own systems. The ectoderm, or outermost layer, forms into skin, the nervous system, and sensory cells. Muscles, blood, and the excretory system emerge from the middle layer called the "mesoderm." The inner layer, or endoderm, forms the lungs, digestive systems, and thyroid gland.

TABLE 1.1   Different approaches to development

	Maturational	Psychoanalytic	Organismic	Behavioral
Theorist	Gesell	Freud	Piaget	Skinner
Basic assumptions	Development is guided by maturation	Development is the result of resolving different social and instinctual needs	Development reflects changes in the way children acquire knowledge about the world	Development is the result of the effects of learning
Focus of study	Biological systems growth	Effects of instinctual needs	Stage-related transformations	Frequency of behavior
Method of study	Case studies	Examination of conflicts	Understanding transformations between stages	Conditioning and modeling processes
Areas of greatest impact	Child-rearing	Personality development	Understanding cognitive development	Behavior management and change

From Salkind NJ, Ambron SR: *Child development*, New York, 1987, CBS College Publishing.

Another significant event occurring during this embryo stage is the development of the protective chamber and nutritional supply for this rapidly changing organism. Nutrition and oxygen come to the embryo, and waste products leave the embryo through the two arteries and one vein contained within the umbilical cord. This supply route connects to the placenta, which is a large, disk-shaped tissue attached to the inner wall of the uterus. It develops to approximately 8 inches in length and 1 pound in weight and serves as a juncture with the circulatory system of the mother. While in proximity within the placenta, the embryonic and maternal blood never come into contact. All exchanges take place through cell boundaries, which limit the type and size of materials that may be passed through in either direction. These boundaries are unable to discriminate beneficial from harmful substances and thus allow a whole host of chemicals that may harm the developing embryo to pass freely.

The protective chamber completely surrounds the embryo by the end of the eighth week. This amniotic sac with its layer of protective fluid embracing the embryo keeps it at a constant temperature and buffers it against jolts or blows that the mother may experience.

The embryo itself begins to appear human and approaches 1 inch in length by the end of this stage. About half of this is the head, which contains distinguishable mouth, eyes, and nose. Arms and legs are seen. After 2 months of development, the major body organs are all present, including a heart that is beating, a liver producing blood cells, and kidneys that are filtering waste products from the blood.

Fetal stage

The third and final stage of the pregnancy is called the "fetal stage" and lasts from the ninth week until the thirty-eighth week, the usual time for the birth of the baby. An intricate series of developmental refinements continues throughout this period, as well as substantial increases in size and weight of the fetus. The fourth month sees the fastest growth spurt for the fetus when it almost doubles in length. During the fourth and fifth months the mother may begin to feel movement from the fetus. The fetus becomes able to open and close its mouth, suck its thumb, swallow, and make head movements. The skin becomes fully developed in the fifth month and has hair and nails.

In the sixth month of pregnancy the eyelids are open and the fetus weighs on the average 670 g (24 ounces). Periods of sleep and wakefulness are exhibited. From month 7 on to the end of the pregnancy the fetus has a good chance of survival if it is delivered. It is gaining about 8 ounces per week during these last 8 weeks.

THE BIRTH PROCESS

The birth process begins for many with the first contraction of labor. An initial contraction may lead quickly to stronger ones and be accompanied by other signs, or may precede the actual delivery by days, weeks, or even months. These early and mild contractions can be distinguished from real labor contractions by the significant discomfort, greater regularity, and increasing frequency of the latter. While in the early stages, labor can also be indicated by back pain and by "water breaking," or discharge of fluid from the vagina. When some blood-tinged mucus has emerged from the vagina and contractions become regular with escalating strength, labor is certainly underway.

The time frame for the birth process varies substantially from one pregnancy to another and one person to another. The average length of labor is about 15 hours. Labor lasts longer for initial children than for subsequent ones and takes longer for male than for female offspring.[7]

The process of a normal labor is described in three stages: dilatation, expulsion, and placental. There is an enormous range of potential variability between women and between different pregnancies in the timetable that labor may follow. The dilatation stage may take as long as 20 hours or more, or may be only 2 hours. At the onset of labor a woman's cervix may be dilated very little, or opened as much as 3 to 4 cm. As the involuntary contractions of labor begin, their initial purpose is to open the cervix to at least 10 cm to allow passage of the baby. These early contractions are typically spaced 15 to 20 minutes apart and last about half a minute.

During the expulsion stage the mother begins to feel the need to bear down during contractions. The cervix has opened around the baby's head, the top of which may begin to appear during some contractions. This is called "crowning" and occurs as the mother sweats and becomes flushed during each succeeding spasm. Eventually the entire head makes its way through the cervix and is free. The shoulders and the rest of the body follow easily afterward, and the baby is completely delivered.

Once the head is free, or when the entire baby has emerged, the infant gasps for breath and starts to cry its first cry. The delivering doctor will usually aspirate mucus and fluid from the baby's mouth and nose as soon as the head is reachable to assist in the breathing process. The doctor will also clamp and cut the umbilical cord immediately after the baby is delivered.

At this point the infant's health is evaluated, including instillation of prophylactic eye drops in most hospitals. Many locations still use silver nitrate as the medication of choice for ophthalmia neonatorum prevention, whereas others use erythromycin ointment as the preferable treatment. An overall assessment of viability such as the Apgar rating[8] is performed. This system was devised by Virginia Apgar in 1953 and quickly addresses the five areas of color, heart rate, reflexive activity, muscular tone, and respiration on a scale of 0, 1, or 2. Thus the maximum score is 10, and a doctor or nurse can quickly establish if problems exist and indicate such with a lower Apgar rating (Table 1-2). The score is usually given at 1 minute and

TABLE 1.2 Apgar scoring

Factor	0	1	2
Heart rate	Absent	<100	>100
Respiration effort	Absent	Irregular (hypoventilation)	Regular
Muscle tone	Limp	Some flexion of extremities	Well flexed
Reflex irritability	No response	Some motion; grimace	Cry, cough, sneeze
Circulation	Blue (or pale)	Body pink, extremities blue	Completely pink

again at 5 minutes post partum, with a score of 5 or be low being of significant concern. Ninety percent of children score 7 or higher.[9]

The final stage of labor and delivery is brief and is composed of expulsion of the remainder of the umbilical cord and the placenta. The delivering physician will examine the placenta carefully to ensure that it has entirely emerged, and then this placental stage is complete.

CHARACTERISTICS OF THE NEONATE

So what does this new package look like? With what characteristics does the newborn infant enter the world? Let us address these questions by looking at various bodily systems and see how they are functioning at birth.

From the standpoint of appearance, a newborn baby is often someone only a father and mother could love. The infant's head, composed of soft and incompletely formed skull bones, has been distorted or molded during its passage through the cervix. The nose has often been flattened or compressed as well. Although the head soon recovers its normal shape, the initial appearance can be disturbing. This is coupled with skin that is reddish, wrinkled, and thin and is easily irritated after months of soaking in the amniotic fluid. If deficient in a specific liver enzyme, the infant may appear jaundiced or yellow until the level of bilirubin is controlled by the liver. Many babies are bald, whereas others have a full head of dark hair. Some are born with a fine downlike hair on their shoulders and back, ears, and other areas.

It is essential that the respiratory system begin functioning immediately. The loss of oxygen supply from the mother's blood circulation once the umbilical cord is clamped and severed should result in reflex breathing on the part of the infant as carbon dioxide begins to build up in its system. The first gasp and cry should start lung expansion as air rushes into the alveoli, which are filled with fluid or compressed. At first, the baby's breathing may be somewhat irregular and noisy until residual fluid is absorbed and control of the larynx and the diaphragm is developed. The capillaries in the lungs open and receive a greater blood supply from the heart as breathing continues.

The circulatory system, particularly as it relates to respiration, has some significant changing to do once the baby has been delivered. The umbilical system now must shut down. The foramen ovale, an opening between the two auricles in the heart that is present at birth, must gradually seal up so that oxygenated and nonoxygenated blood is not mixed and system efficiency improves. Additionally, a shunt vessel between the aorta and pulmonary artery, which allows blood from the two ventricles to mingle, must close. This ductus arteriosus does seal up and allow for complete isolation of the blood flow. The heart beats rapidly for the young infant, up to 120 to 140 beats per minute.

At birth the baby has a strong sucking reflex and is ready to begin ingesting liquid by mouth to complete the transfer away from the umbilical feeding it has been dependent on for months. The baby is fed initially about 12 hours after birth and then on a regular schedule it acquires. If the child is to be breast fed, the mother's milk starts to flow the second or third day after birth, beginning with colostrum. This supplies antibodies to the young child. After the initial feedings are processed by the digestive system, the child passes its first stool. The makeup of this stool is a dark green substance called "meconium." Once passed, usually within the first day, the stools switch to a characteristic lighter, golden brown color and occur often associated with feedings. During the first few days it is typical for the newborn to lose a little weight until the processes of digestion and absorption of nutrients begin to work effectively. This loss is usually about a half a pound.

Skeletally the newborn has all the necessary parts, but they are very underdeveloped. Many bones are still mainly cartilage or connective tissue. The skull is moldable, as previously described, and has large soft spots called "fontanelles," which allow for compression and growth until they gradually solidify by the end of the first year of life. The skin layer of the newborn has little fat, and sweat glands are not developed. These factors, combined with the fact that the muscle system for shivering is also not functional, make temperature regulation very difficult for the newborn. The youngster is dependent to a significant extent on others to protect it from temperature extremes.

NORMAL MOTOR DEVELOPMENT

As we look at the normal acquisition of motor skills of various types throughout childhood, we must continually be cognizant of the fact that physical maturation of the anatomical systems that serve as substrates for motor activity must also be noted. Without the sequential evolving and emerging of the equipment to work with, the child would be unable to develop the motor skills we will discuss.

An infant's life is often chronicled by a recording of the achievement of motor milestones in the early years. Yet growth changes are important indicators as well and can foretell normal or potentially abnormal conditions. During the first 2 or 3 years the child grows at a faster rate than he or she ever will again. All systems are acquiring more sophisticated levels of functioning.

Pediatricians have developed some rules of thumb to assist in determining "normal" development in children. Birth weight should double in the first 5 months of life, triple by the end of the first year, and quadruple by 30 months of age. In the height category, the baby should gain 20% by 3 months, and a 50% increase in length can be expected by the end of the first year. What is of importance to monitor is the rate of change in these features, with steady progress preferable to sudden increases and then periods of no change. Normative tables of height and weight with percentiles for each age level are used for plotting these physical changes. One other key indicator is head circumference, which can be plotted as well.

The proportions of the infant's body change as it ages. When born, the body is 20% muscle, 15% internal organs, and 15% nervous system. By adulthood these have shifted to 45% muscle, 10% internal organs, and only 3% nervous system. The baby's body is 75% water, and this declines to 60% by 12 years of age. The infant's skin acquires substantial amounts of fat during the first 9 months of life, and then this baby fat thins out again through 5 years of age. The skeleton begins to move from flexible cartilage to calcified bone. Born with all the muscle fibers they will need, the child's muscles increase in length and bulk or thickness.

Activities of the young child emerge as if headed toward two objectives, motion and manipulation. The ability to get from place to place, particularly standing upright, and the skill to handle and use objects with the hands are two major goals of motor development.

The sequential nature of the acquisition of fine-motor control by the hands has been well documented.[10] It involves the integration of several components. Some reflexes that are present at birth, such as the grasping reflex, serve temporary purposes. By 1 month of age, this tight grip when the palm is touched starts to lessen, and by 4 months it is gone. However, at about this time the child starts to reach for objects. By about 6 months of age, the baby shows grasp and manipulation skill and may even be able to transfer from one hand to the other. This release ability is at first accidental, and then the 8-month-old has learned to let go on purpose, picking objects up, holding them, and then dropping them. Opposition between the thumb and forefinger is emerging, and the 1-year-old can skillfully pick up small objects, whether it be food, candy, a toy, or pieces of fuzz and dirt on the floor.

One major motor accomplishment parents anticipate is the first time a child rolls over. This may occur as early as 4 months but does not come until the infant has learned to coordinate several movements together. Rolling over involves head, shoulder, trunk, and leg teamwork. Once this has been achieved, however, the child will roll over both for the enjoyment of the movement and to accomplish an objective such as reaching an object.

Sitting up alone is another milepost in motor-skill acquisition and has its own prerequisites. The infant must acquire sufficient strength in the muscles of the back and neck to maintain head control. Early on, the child suffers from head lag as it either droops into the chest or flops backward when the infant is picked up or held. But by an average of 7 months, the infant has sufficient neck strength to sit propped on its hands. The back muscles improve to the point that in another month or two the child is able to sit unsupported for long periods and may even be able to get to a sitting position on its own.

Seven months of age is also a time when babies are beginning to get around by creeping. This may start out as sideways or backwards motion before the child figures out how to get where it wants to go. Lying on its front, the child makes reflex arm movements that eventually become coordinated and purposeful actions. This pulling forward with the arms or creeping varies in extent from child to child.[11] Creeping becomes more directed and for many develops into effective crawling, the use of all fours. Most children creep before they learn to walk, but some do not, and so creeping may not be a stage that is necessary for normal motor development. Crawling has its own developmental pattern, from one limb at a time to the efficient synchrony of contralateral and simultaneous movement of the extremities, that is, right arm and left leg in the same direction at the same time. However, about 20% of crawlers move the ipsilateral leg and arm together.[11] At this same time, infants can also pull themselves up to a standing position alongside an object such as a piece of furniture. As time progresses, the child who has developed good crawling skill may not be the earliest walker, because it already has a locomotion system that meets most of its needs.

As the second year of life is beginning, the child's body has made substantial changes. Ossification and calcification of the skeleton are strengthening its ability to serve as support for the toddler. The height and weight have increased substantially, and the proportions of the body have altered as well, with the head representing an ever-decreasing percentage of overall body length. The central nervous system matures rapidly. All these coordinated anatomical changes serve to enable the child to make further adaptive and motor-skill acquisitions.

Although there is significant variation from child to child, the average toddler is walking unassisted by 12 months of age. This is a major accomplishment in a child's life that parents eagerly anticipate and reward. It opens up even more opportunities for the child to explore its environment. Although occasional setbacks may occur from illness or injury, progress from the first independent steps to skillful walking is steady. It is not long after those first few wide-gaited steps before the toddler begins spreading out the feet and using the arms for balance. Frequent falling is the rule but does not daunt the practice, which leads to more flat-footed walking and eventually to adventures like short bursts of running and balancing on one foot.

In the period around 18 months and 2 years, the toddler bears close watching. The newfound freedom of mobility brings dangers with it, both for the safety of the child and to items in the household, such as tabletop treasures, objects on counters and in cupboards, and so forth. Each opportunity for exploration is a new adventure, and full of energy and improving motor abilities, the child may break or mess up a parent's favorite trinket or project from work. By 2 years of age the child can jump, go up and down stairs fairly well, and run easily.

The remainder of the preschool years affords the opportunity for increasing size. The trunk and legs are increasing in their contribution to overall size, and by 6 years of age the legs are half of the overall height, a proportion that remains throughout life. Boys enter school age on the average slightly taller and heavier than girls. Boys have more muscle, and girls more fatty tissue as this development progresses. Muscle development represents most of the weight that boys and girls acquire during these years. As the larger body muscles develop, gross motor skills emerge. With time, smaller muscle groups become refined and with practice acquire more specific and fine movement patterns, which require precise coordination. Some of the improvements in coordination of both large and small muscle groups are the direct result of maturation in the nervous system, as more and more cells become myelinated and mature and their dendritic connections become established.

Size, speed, strength, and coordination are some of the clearly identifiable advances of the preschool years. The 3-year-old loves to incorporate sudden starts, turns, and stops in his or her running. Jumping is added to the repertoire of the 4-year-old, and by the time they reach school age children can throw, balance, climb, and skip. From 6 years on, though fairly even to that point, boys develop more strength than girls, a difference that becomes particularly exaggerated after puberty. Most children participate in competitive activities with each other, often focused on motor skills such as strength or speed. The level of coordination of voluntary motor action that a child possesses becomes increasingly important to them socially, beyond the need for skill in a particular motor act. They develop skills necessary both in rivalry and in cooperation. An increasing portion of the individualization of the development of motor skills comes from environmental influences as the child ages.

The progression of fine motor and manipulative skills is a rapid one as well. As previously mentioned, the 1-year-old becomes capable of utilizing what is termed the "pincer grasp," holding objects between a finger and opposing thumb. Independent control of each of the fingers is also achieved, delighting and entertaining toddlers for hours as they explore the infinite variety of combinations of movements possible with their 10 digits. The child begins to hold objects in one hand and manipulate them with the other and begins to develop a preference for use of the right or left hand. The walking 15-month-old has new vistas to explore with new items to fondle and inspect as it ventures beyond the limits imposed on the crawler.

An 18-month-old at play with its toys loves to stack, only to watch them fall, and to pick up its toys and run around with them. There is some potential for danger to the child from this practice because falling is still common. By 2 years the child will look at books and can turn the pages and can begin to scribble with pencil or crayon, though the results are primitive.

One area where children are eager to test and use their fine-motor skills is when eating. Around 1 year of age children begin to seek food actively. They acquire the ability to hold a cup with two hands and to begin to manipulate a spoon. Although inefficient at first, the young child is also determined to learn these skills and will stubbornly keep trying as the size of the mess on the child, high chair, parent, and floor increases. The independence of self-feeding takes on great importance for the child, and by 3 years they master the skills necessary to be accomplished eaters. In the interim parents have to observe and encourage patiently all the practice that is required to develop dexterity with a spoon and later fork and knife.

As coordination of small muscle groups continues, many forms of manipulative skill emerge. A 2-year-old may be able to build a tower of six or seven blocks. By 3 the tower might be as high as 10 blocks before it topples. Activities such as finger painting become exciting. At 5 the child can cut with scissors, reproduce simple shapes on paper, paint with a brush, and occasionally catch a small ball.

Entrance into elementary school provides structure and organization within which a child's motor skills continue to develop and are displayed for peers and adults to judge. The growth rate for both boys and girls is steady but much slower than it was as an infant. Although occasional spurts do occur, often between 6 and 8 years of age, nothing spectacular will happen again until adolescence begins. The trends of growth through the elementary years do serve to change body proportions somewhat, as limbs continue to elongate and the trunk slims down. The head now represents the one-eighth portion of overall height that is typical of the adult, and permanent teeth replace the 20 deciduous, or baby, teeth. General motor coordination improves, just as strength and endurance do. Fine-motor manipulative skills, particularly as they relate to use of writing implements, make significant strides. The complexity of small muscle movements that are possible expands, and children begin many avocational activities such as musical instrument lessons. The uniqueness of each individual becomes more evident as the child, with his or her own personal talents and skills, reaches puberty.

Table 1-3 summarizes early motor development.

TABLE 1.3   Summary of early motor milestones

Approximate age (months)	Event
4	Rolls over
5	Two times birth weight
6	Grasping and manipulating
7	Sits alone
	Creeping
12	Three times birth weight
	50% increase in height
	Walking
	Pincer grasp
24	Jumps crudely, runs, climbs stairs
	Scribbling
	6-block tower
	Throws a small ball 4 to 5 feet
30	Four times birth weight
36	Hops 2 or 3 steps
	Throws a ball 10 feet
	Draws a simple cross

NORMAL COGNITIVE DEVELOPMENT

As described previously, cognitive development is about the thinking process and how children acquire knowledge. Although many people have made contributions to this area, all are dwarfed by the influence of the writings of Jean Piaget. His descriptions and theories are used as the bases for most discussion in cognitive development, and a good understanding of this area can be gained from an overview of Piaget's concepts in the organization of cognitive development.

Piaget stated that children passed through a series of stages from infancy to adolescence. This passage was the result of biological pressures to adapt to the environment and to organize ways of thinking.[12] His descriptions of thought were qualitative in nature, rather than quantitative, as would result from a standardized intelligence test. Although described in regard to stages of development, no child is an exact sample of any particular stage because some aspects of behavior advance at rates different from that of others. Also, although ages are given, they are not exact either because a good deal of individual variation exists as a result of environment and physiological factors. However, each stage is necessary preparation for the succeeding ones, and the sequence does not vary from child to child—the order is essential.

As his theory evolved, Piaget described four distinct stages or levels of mental reasoning that children progressed through: sensorimotor stage, preoperational stage, concrete operational stage, and formal operational stage. The sensorimotor stage lasts from birth to about 2 years. In this stage, thinking is merely associated with the immediate sensory experiences and motor behaviors. It is very "hands-on," or in many cases "mouth-on," thinking concerned only in terms of the direct actions with objects. When the child is not interacting, the object does not exist—"out of sight, out of mind."[13] Infants and toddlers in this stage do not have the ability to create symbols, such as an image, to represent an object or an activity. Thus, if a bottle is taken from an 8-month-old and placed under a nearby blanket in full view of the child, he or she will make no attempt to reach for it, for it has no independent existence.

During this sensorimotor period, infants acquire organized patterns of perception and behavior called "schemas" (Greek "schemata"), which become the basic building blocks of mental organization. The primitive schemas become modified and expanded by two processes that occur to some extent at all stages of development—assimilation and accommodation. Assimilation is the incorporation of new experiences into already established schemas, and accommodation is the adaptation of existing schemas to meet the demands of new experiences.

Within this sensorimotor period, Piaget described six stages of development, summarized as follows:

> **Stage 1** = Reflex activity (birth to 1 month)
> Cannot distinguish between self and other objects; reflex activity.
> **Stage 2** = Primary circular reactions (1-4 months)
> Displays curiosity and some primitive anticipations. Some hand-mouth coordination.
> **Stage 3** = Secondary circular reactions (4-10 months)
> Increased manipulation; some imitation; development of eye-hand coordination.
> **Stage 4** = Coordinating secondary schemas (10-12 months)
> Anticipates and imitates more often and accurately. Uses learned responses in new situations.
> **Stage 5** = Tertiary circular reactions (12-18 months)
> Experimentation with objects to learn more about the environment through trial and error.
> **Stage 6** = Symbolic representation (18-24 months)
> Imitates in the absence of a model.
> Beginnings of thought; early problem solving.
> Can imagine, that is, develop symbolic representation.

Another classic example of how Piaget discovered this evolution is in descriptions of the concept of object permanence. As children progress through the six sensorimotor stages, they emerge from the dependence on only what is immediate to the point at approximately 18 months when they can locate an object even if it is hidden or has been moved.

The second, or preoperational, stage lasts from approximately 2 to 7 years of age. Symbol formation now comes into being for children in an ever-increasing fashion. Many different types of symbol systems evolve, one of the most useful being language. Although useful, the preoperational level symbol systems still are limited because the child cannot conceive of transformations, or changes from one state of being to another. Several important basic concepts begin to develop in this preoperational stage, including concepts of time, space, and quantity, including both conservation and one-to-one correspondence, necessary for counting. Children also develop the ability to classify, to organize ideas and things into usable categories. In the concrete operational stage, children can conceive of how objects change, not just how they appear at different times. From 7 years to early adolescence, concrete operations are refined. In his classic experiment of conservation of mass, Piaget distinguished concrete operational thinking from preoperational thinking. Two identical glasses filled to the same level with liquid were agreed to contain like amounts of drink. The contents of one glass were then poured into a taller and thinner glass. Preoperational thinking would allow children only to perceive that now the taller glass had more drink, whereas concrete operational thinkers were able to understand that the amount of liquid had not changed. Concrete operation also allows children to be able to reverse their thinking, as in trying to sort rods from smallest to longest. The ability to shift to another perspective or to see things from a view other than one's own is called "decentration" and is developed in this stage. It permits the child to acquire some social conscience and to be able to function socially.

The fourth and final stage is the stage of formal operations. This is the stage of abstract thought. According to Piaget,[14] this stage may be achieved as early as 11 or 12 years of age, though some people reach it much later in adolescence, and some not at all. The stage of formal operations differs from that of concrete operations in that, in addition to being able to think about things, that is, actual objects or events, the person can also think about thoughts. The individual is now able to consider several alternative explanations for the same event, to deal with proposals or ideas that are contrary to fact, and to deal with metaphors, or symbols of symbols.

Table 1-4 summarizes early cognitive development.

TABLE 1.4   Summary of cognitive development

Approximate age	Stage

Birth to 24 months	Sensorimotor period
	    Stage 1: Reflex activity (birth to 1 month)
	    Stage 2: Primary circular reactions (1-4 months)
	    Stage 3: Secondary circular reactions (4-10 months)
	    Stage 4: Coordinating secondary schema (10-12 months)
	    Stage 5: Tertiary circular reactions (12-18 months)
	    Stage 6: Symbolic representation (18-24 months)

2-7 years	Preoperational period
7-11 years	Period of concrete operations
11 years on	Period of formal operations

NORMAL LANGUAGE DEVELOPMENT

Any discussion of normal language acquisition and use must incorporate a discussion of hearing, for it is with this nonvisual sensory process that the infant learns of the existence of language. In utero the fetus is able to hear sound.[15] Shortly after being delivered, infants can discriminate between low-pitched and high-pitched sounds[16] and respond preferentially to a pitch within the range of a human voice.[17] Most children appear to be attuned to respond to speech in a unique fashion, even including which side of the head is turned up when the infant is sleeping on its stomach.[18]

Language quickly becomes important to a child. Interactions between an infant's sounds, gestures, and facial expressions and the behaviors of their caregivers, particularly when the child feels good afterwards, result in reinforcement of the behaviors that were effective. Babies begin babbling and cooing before having an understanding of language or an ability to speak. However, by the end of their first year they are able to use a few words. In addition to gestures such as pointing, the toddler may associate a word that is fairly clear and recognizable. This pattern is particularly likely when the child desires something, like a favorite toy or a bottle.

Infants initially communicate through crying. All their various needs and feelings, whether it be hunger or thirst or pain or discomfort, become expressed by crying. Each baby's cry becomes distinctive and can be recognized by the parents as different from other babies' cries at a young age.[19] Although often left with the feeling that they are being manipulated, parents must be careful not to ignore the cry of an infant. Doing so may possibly mean missing an important warning sign. An infant's cry when ill may even be slightly different from normal to help reduce the odds of being ignored.

Observations by those who study language development, called "psycholinguists," have shown that there are many universals in the human race with respect to the acquisition of language processing skills, regardless of the particular language that is involved. Although the initial sound production of the infant is a precursor to language, this screaming and crying and gurgling is not considered real language by most psycholinguists.[20] At approximately 6 months, babbling, which characterizes the playful imitation of sounds, becomes an attempt at language. The infant is beginning to understand some of the common spoken words used in its life as well. But regardless of the language being used or the socioeconomic level, children go through the same stages in moving from baby talk or babbling to adult-level communication.[21]

The imitative aspect of early language leads the infant to mimic some of the intonations in sounds they hear from adults. Babies do spend time observing facial expressions, which they often attempt to duplicate, as well as speech production. Early syllables such as *ma-ma* and *da-da* are short sequences of sounds and not single entities. The development of more of these sounds as the child continues to listen to and watch adults and other models helps prepare the child for more refined communication with adults.[22]

The understanding of language precedes the ability to produce it, and thus toddlers have a significant receptive vocabulary as they begin to try to use words. This difference between comprehension and performance will continue to exist. The 1-year-old child begins to acquire some control over its environment by the use of new language like *bye-bye* or *night-night* or *no*. The toddler starts associating each of the new words it acquires with some object or feeling or action. In addition to expanding the vocabulary, this process also facilitates memory by providing a verbal label for each feeling or experience. The absence of this ability to label and thus appropriately to file away the information prevents us from remembering events from our very early life.

As the toddler progresses toward full-fledged language use, its language development for the rest of its lifetime could be described by the level of skill development in four areas of language. These include the use of phonemes, which are the smallest units of sound in basic speech; the understanding of semantics, or the definitions or meanings of words; a grasp of syntax, the rules about how words can be associated with each other or combined; and the use of pragmatics, or understanding how to use language effectively for a purpose.

Although the 1-year-old starts with single-word utterances, the meaning the child is attempting to convey can be much more than the single word. Unable to yet manipulate syntax effectively, the toddler is left with this holophrastic speech, where one word must do the job of an entire sentence.[23] The 18-month-old develops duophrastic speech, as two words become joined together. This opens up many new vistas for communication for the child. The use of duophrastic speech has also been described as pivot open-class language, where one word of the pair serves as an anchor around which a collection of other words may pivot.[24] For example, the pivot *my* could be associated with many words such as *ma-ma* or *cup* or *doll* or *cookie*. The pivot could also function as the second word, such as *bye-bye* in *da-da bye-bye* or *doggy bye-bye* or *grandma bye-bye*. Any other words in the child's vocabulary could cycle around the pivot word.

In the beginning, pivots are usually not nouns, and the associated words are all nouns. As the child becomes more sophisticated in language usage, nouns may occupy both positions in the duophrastic units. The child is developing a language that is concise in that it does not yet contain any modifiers, articles, or prepositions. Children become fairly proficient at the use of these two-word sentences by 2 years of age.

The basic sound components, or phonemes, in a language have no inherent meaning and need to be grouped together. The smallest portion of a word that does convey a meaning is called a "morpheme." A morpheme cannot be broken up further without losing its meaning, and so many morphemes are words, such as *car* or *cat*. Since they can stand alone these are termed "free morphemes." Bound morphemes are word parts that are not meaningful unless attached to a free morpheme, such as the *-s* that turns *car* into *cars*. Usually the early words of the child are free morphemes. They learn to improve the accuracy of their speech as time moves on by making use of bound morphemes. There are indications that there is a regular pattern that varies very little between children in the order of acquisition of morphemes.[25]

Beyond this point, children gradually acquire the ability to form complete, grammatical sentences. There is no uniformity of opinion as to the learning process that eventually results in that skill. Different theorists have analyzed how language develops in the context of overall cognitive development. But, whether language develops as the result of reinforcement of primitive attempts at sentences and elaboration by the parent, or by trial and error after observation of adults and others, grammatical accuracy improves. This is the foundation of a language, the ability to use the rules by which words are arranged.

As has been noted in the investigation of many skills with developmental patterns, there have been changes with time in the approach to the study of language acquisition. Early reportings were journalistic records of individual researchers' notes. Later, developmental psychologists looked for patterns and discovered some language milestones, which become apparent to them after looking at large groups of children. Researchers noted, for example, when children typically moved from two-word speech to three-word sentences. What got missed in the documentary nature of these studies, however, was a look towards the increasing level of complexity of grammar, syntax, and pragmatics employed by the children. It became evident that a sophisticated look at language development would necessitate trying to answer questions about what children knew about language; we could not settle merely for observational descriptions of when they acquired which skill.

It was for these reasons that psycholinguists became intimately involved in studies of cognitive development. Various aspects of language became subjected to research. Word meanings for children can vary with age, and developmental trends are evident. As children begin to master comparative terms like *long* or *more* and studies around those concepts, the depth of cognitive understanding a child has about them can begin. Children may experience confusion for a long time when dealing with relational words. Until they acquire a set of rules of how specific words are used and which ones are appropriate for a given circumstance, children's language will lack precision and clarity but may indeed be humorous.

Piaget[26] spent time describing the development of language during the stages of cognitive development and specifically addressed the preschoolers egocentric speech. It was delineated in three forms: repetition or repeating of someone else's speech, monolog or out-loud speech to no particular person, and collective monolog, in which a child will be with others and speak aloud without needing to be understood. Young toddlers are basically egocentric; their speech is not necessarily intended to serve as anything other than a form of play and a way to rehearse language. As they get slightly older and begin to try to communicate with others, they have initial difficulty because they have not learned to see the world through other people's eyes. This skill is necessary before they can develop effective language and communication. As Piaget describes this evolution, it is social pressure that forces the transition from egocentric thought into language.

Piaget's hypotheses are not uniformly accepted as descriptions of language progression during cognitive development. Vygotsky[27] similarly spent time observing the behavior of young children and developed his schema for language evolution. He believes that the toddler's egocentric speech is not a distinct kind of language but merely a transition stage between the youngster's vocal and later inner speech. He believes that the child is attempting to communicate from the time they first learn to speak.

One other aspect of the development of the use of language is the acquisition of skill in written language. As youngsters approach school age, they develop an ability to distinguish and discriminate graphemes, or geometric forms such as letters. The more mature children are able to notice even subtle differences in letter formation, as between *M* and *W*, or *U* and *V*. When children enter school, they have already developed the ability to recognize letters of their language as distinguished from other shapes. Learning the significance of the different letters, their names, and the associated sounds are all skills taught to them once formal schooling begins.

Tables 1-5 and 1-6 summarize early language development.

NORMAL EMOTIONAL DEVELOPMENT

The most striking feature of the emotional development of young children is the dependence on the care and attention the children receive as infants. They acquire their sense of self from the actions and reactions of others. This sense includes both their physical self, that is, arms, legs, and so forth, and their emotional self, that is, sense of worth.

TABLE 1.5 Summary of early language milestones

Approximate age (months)	Event
0	Crying
6	Babbling
12	Single words
18	Duophrastic speech
24	Two-word sentences

TABLE 1.6 Change in size of the child's vocabulary from 8 months to 6 years of age

Years/months	Number of words	Change
0/8	0	0
0/10	1	+1
1/0	3	+2
1/3	19	+16
1/6	22	+3
1/9	118	+96
2/0	272	+154
2/6	446	+174
3/0	896	+450
3/6	1222	+326
4/0	1540	+318
4/6	1870	+330
5/0	2072	+202
5/6	2289	+219
6/0	2562	+273

From Smith ME: An investigation of the development of the sentence and the extent of vocabulary in young children, *University of Iowa Studies, Child Welfare* 3(5):218, 1926.

The development of a bond between an infant and a caregiver is called "attachment." These emotional ties have been extensively studied as they are necessary for the baby's growth and survival. Attachment takes on particular significance beginning at about 6 to 7 months of age. Before that, the child requires only that its needs be met by someone, and substitutes for parents are allowed. At around 7 months, however, they acquire a special attachment, and by 10 months 90% of infants have formed these attachments, usually to parents. As a result of this development, they cry when the parent leaves, they do not accept substitutes willingly, and they need parental reinforcement, either in the form of the parent's presence, or a glance, a voice, or a touch.

As described by Ainsworth[28], some of the bases of attachment are pre-programmed in our human species, but the importance of feedback is also emphasized. She describes the different stages of attachment. Initially, the infant relates well to everyone, but then a special relationship is developed with the primary caregiver. This happens at around 6 months of age. At around 1 year, strangers are recognized and withdrawn from as the child enthusiastically greets the caregiver. Finally, in the last stage, we see the development of a very strong bond with the primary caregiver, who becomes responsible for the child's feelings of security.

There has been a great deal of research on bonding and attachment in certain animal species. Noted examples include Konrad Lorenz,[29] who had goslings bond to himself and to mechanical decoys, and Harry Harlow,[30] who presented infant monkeys with two substitute mothers made of chicken wire and soft cloth.

Although there are some similarities, the development of attachment in the human species is more complex. In most, the emergence of attachment comes when the youngster first begins to be mobile. At that point the infant needs to have its basic needs met, as in previous months, but also demands tactile and social stimulation from the caregiver. An opportunity for a relationship to develop while the parent is giving a bottle to a child may be missed if the bottle is propped up in a holder while the parent leaves the room.

The roles of both sexes of parents are important in the normal emotional development of a child. Only recently has the important role of the father been identified and more clearly described. Infants become attached to fathers in the same time frame as to their mothers.[31] This attachment can be strengthened by early and extended contact, whether it be in play or in feeding. Fathers have been shown to be successful in both of these activities if the will is present.[32] The type of activities often engaged in by fathers with their infants are unique and provide a diversity of stimulation for the child. For example, fathers are more apt to toss a child in the air, wrestle on the floor, and playfully mimic or tease.

So, parenting is not a responsibility solely laid at the feet of the mother. In families where the father and mother cooperatively spend time with the child, an enhancing effect takes place.[33] In families where the mother is working outside the home, or in single-parent father-only families, it is normal for children to acquire additional attachments to other relatives, such as grandparents, aunts, and uncles, and to other caregivers, such as baby-sitters. In circumstances where the father becomes the primary caregiver, the behaviors of the father differ very little from a mother in the interactions with the child.

A child's normal emotional development requires some basic activities. One is physical contact. Infants need contact and a caregiver who supplies and even promotes this contact for periods of time. Although a significant degree of individual difference will exist between children in the amount of cuddling they seek or will tolerate, each infant needs a certain amount to remain content.[34] Another behavior that is important to the infant is smiling. As a form of communication, a smile can be very effective. As an infant gets positive feedback from smiles, including smiles in return from caregivers, they begin to use them purposefully.

Noted psychoanalyst Erik Erikson[35] has developed a schema of crises that individuals must deal with throughout a lifetime. Of his 8 psychosocial stages, three of them occur in the preschool years. The first one he outlines in an infant's life is basic trust versus basic mistrust. A child has to have consistent sensations and experiences so as to feel comfortable in life and trust itself. A set of expectations about the world is acquired. As long as the basic needs of the child are met by the world (through the infant's caregivers), the trust with its inherent positive feelings toward both itself and the world is maintained by the child. Fear and insecurity can result, however, if the child's needs are not always cared for in a predictable manner. If stability is not present, a basic mistrust will emerge.

If a pattern of basic mistrust is felt by an infant, it all too often becomes reinforced by the parents or caregivers. They are inclined to ignore the cries of the child more often, and the infant will be labeled as cranky or irritable. The parents are seen to yell at the child more often, and when physical contact does occur, it is usually out of a feeling of desperation, rather than affection. This is sensed by the infant, and the mistrust continues to be reinforced. In addition, very little smiling between child and caregiver occurs. The basic mistrust pattern eventually leads to self-defeating behaviors, reduced feelings of self-worth, and problems dealing effectively with others.

Another topic that parents must deal with in their infants is anxiety produced by the presence of strangers. This feeling is a direct result of the child's attachment to the parents and thus emerges at about 7 or 8 months of age, on the average. The visibility of an unfamiliar adult, particularly in the parents' absence, results in a fear response from the child, such as squirming, screaming, or crying. If the parent is present, the child will hang on for dear life and often bury its head to avoid eye contact with the stranger. These reactions are the strongest among children with the greatest parental attachment.[36] They are reacting negatively to foreign stimuli, stimuli that are not consistent with the parental face, voice, and mannerism.

Information detailing the extreme effects of lack of any kind of attachment on infant emotional development has come from studies of institutionalized children.[37] Although infants who must be cared for in an institution cry for prolonged periods when very young, the absence of regular and quickly responsive caregivers results in a reduction in their crying. They become quietly indifferent and unresponsive. As a result, motor and cognitive skills, as well as social and emotional development, become delayed. The effects can be noted as early as 3 or 4 months of life and increase as the length of deprivation continues.[38]

It is conceivable that, given a stimulatory environment and responsive caregivers, institutionalized children could develop without serious emotional retardation, but it would take significant effort on the part of the staff.[39] One way to break the pattern described is for the child to get foster home placement. Although far from perfect as a system, infants placed in foster homes generally receive more responsive care and show fewer personality disturbances.[40]

As a normally developing child ages, the previously described fear of strangers fades around the end of the first year. An equally normal and customary fear, itself also the direct result of attachment, becomes manifest and persists. This fear is separation anxiety, the fear of abandonment. It is a fear of being out of contact with the important people who anchor the child's world. The environment is often not crucial, for 10- to 12-month-old children will be content even in unfamiliar surroundings if a parent is accessible. The child who has established a trusting attachment will touch base with the parent and feel at ease exploring. Should separation occur, normal children even up to 18 months of age will cry and attempt to get to or locate a parent and will then hover closer once the parent returns, showing a need for reassurance. Thus, as a toddler ages, he or she needs to be allowed some freedom to explore with the understanding that support and care will be available from a loving caregiver when it is needed. This form of healthy relationship will develop as long as the caregiver has provided comfort and assistance during the crucial first 2 years of the child's life when quality attachments are built.

Separation anxiety is present throughout childhood, and it bears addressing in less pleasant contexts. During times in family life when there is upset or instability, significant fears can result for a child, and emotional disturbances can be the result. A child, separated for whatever reason from the attached parent for a significant period of time, goes through a predictable sequence of first protest, then despair, and finally detachment in response to the separation.[41] Preschoolers are not capable of understanding the expected duration of a separation and sometimes significant behavioral changes occur. One example of this is regression to earlier behavior patterns such as baby talking or loss of bowel or bladder control.[41]

Should contact with the parent be renewed after days or weeks of separation, the initial response of the child is to continue the feeling of detachment for some period. The child will treat its parent like a stranger for at least a few hours if not a few days. Eventually, however, the trust appears to become reestablished. If, on the other hand, this pattern is repeated and parental absence or separation for prolonged periods recurs while the child is 3 years of age or less, the child's detachment may persist in some form for many years. Although seemingly comfortable with the substitute caregivers they encounter, such as nurses, nannies, or other relatives, the child avoids making a significant emotional investment in anyone. The effects of this type of prolonged separation are most profound if they occur during the second 6 months of an infant's life.[42]

A child's emotional development is shaped by several factors, which include the expectations of its social circle. A process of socialization or learning how to fit in with others develops as the toddler has more and more opportunities for interactions with others. The learning occurs in many ways and on many fronts. Some of the learning is within the confines of home with parents and siblings; other learning occurs in a relative's lap or on a playground. Some is from negative reinforcement such as being scolded for an infraction, but much of socialization also is learned from positive feelings after good behavior. A child observes parental behavior, and from these examples and the guidance of its own activities the child begins to acquire appropriate behavior controls. The toddler realizes more and more that other people must be taken into account when planning actions.

As the process of socialization occurs, the parents are providing the child with their interpretation of the values, customs, and beliefs to be incorporated into their lives.[43] The version that each child receives is filtered and affected by the personal characteristics of the parents. Eventually, however, many commonalties still exist in American families. Most parents hope that by 3 years of age their children are toilet trained and can feed themselves without making an embarrassing mess. They expect them to be able to control their voices in public places, leave their clothes on, be nice to relatives and friends, and kiss mom and dad good night.

A mixed blessing for parents that comes early in the socialization process is a measure of autonomy for the child—some level of independent behavior. When children learn to walk and achieve that level of independence, the ability to move from place to place, they begin to meet their own needs. This can set up crises and conflicts for the child, and this is the second of Erikson's crises in psychological development—autonomy versus shame and doubt. This is encountered in the second year of life. Along with the muscle control of ambulation comes some measure of control over their own bladder and bowels. As children gradually learn these controls, a variety of physical and emotional rewards and sensations can be produced.

The ability to control the anal sphincter muscles, which restrain elimination, follows a developmental course. As with developmental skills, individual variations certainly exist, but most children are toilet trained by age 2.[44,45] The ability to relax the anal sphincter willingly once positioned on a toilet develops before control of the bladder. Delaying toilet training makes acquiring the skill easier for the child and reduces bed-wetting and soiling complications. The quality of the parental relationship with the child ultimately has the greatest influence on success. Strictness or coercion may be met by resistance as autonomy is still being sought. In good relationships the child will conform without feeling a loss of autonomy, coming away with the gratification of pleasing its parents with a free-will choice to do so. With final control the child eventually gains more autonomy and a sense of personal pride. It has met the autonomy-versus-shame crisis and come away without doubt of self or shame but rather a sense of self-control.

This feeling of positive encouragement and support that the child receives from parents during the development of autonomy in toilet training needs to spill over into many other areas of exploration and learning. Unfortunately for many children, parents often find less to gain in these other adventures and restrict the child. Children need words of encouragement from parents when acquiring other new skills and also need to be afforded the chance to safely fail. This applies to such endeavors as self-feeding, dressing and undressing, and stair climbing. In an effort to minimize the stress on the parent, sharp and potentially harmful objects should be placed out of reach, as well as breakables and heirlooms. The child will require nearly constant supervision.

Socialization for a toddler as emotional development progresses means learning to deal with two significant emotions—fear and anger. Both of these conditions do occur in young children, and they need to find a socially acceptable way for expression. The two earliest fears of infants and toddlers we have already addressed—fear of strangers and separation. As children grow, other fears are noted as well. Newborns are startled by loud noises and by falling, but since both are usually unanticipated, they are not typical fears. Life's experiences result in some fears as events with strongly negative outcomes result in apprehension when a similar circumstance arises. This might range from a sock in the arm from a naughty cousin to a shot in the behind from a nurse, or a scratch on the face from the neighbor's cat.

Other common fears develop, some a result of observing a reaction in parents. A child becomes tense during thunderstorms or shies from spiders. But parents can also help in overcoming fears or preventing their initiation. The naturally exploratory nature of the child can be turned to controlled exposures that reduce fears. With a combination of prompt comfort and gradual encouragement, the child can confront the problem when ready to face it and can resolve the fear.[46]

Anger, and its expression through aggression, may be to a significant degree innate in the human species.[47] However, we expect children to learn to control this emotion and not attack parents, siblings, or other children, playmates, or pets. By the end of their second year, children have difficulty at times with complete control and occasionally lose it. These expressions of anger are called "temper tantrums" and result in attracting some attention. Whether the result of strict behavioral expectations of the child, or if elicited by feelings of jealousy, parents are alarmed by the often wild, noisy, or violent display. Since it usually happens in view of other people, the outburst cannot be ignored. Parents also fear that giving children what they want or providing immediate affection will reinforce this tantrum behavior and make it likely to be repeated in similar circumstances in the future.

Parents usually do give in to stop temper displays. Although isolation or ignoring would occasionally be effective, the most successful way to quiet children appears to be to give them what they want or remove whatever was irritating them. This approach often creates conflict for the parent, however. In a longitudinal study of tantrum behavior, Goodenough[48] concluded that parents would be most successful if they viewed expressions of anger from their children with "serenity and tolerance."

After the second year, the aggressive behaviors of the child are very dependent on the examples they have experienced. Anger and aggression are more often displayed in children who have been conditioned by inconsistent parents and by occasional violent outbursts.[50] Parents who disapprove of aggression but who discipline children with physical acts such as spanking are likely to produce feelings of aggression in their children.[44]

An area that is receiving increasing attention in the study of emotional and social development in preschool children is the effect of the day care environment. Whether the child is in a center type of day care facility or a private home, either its own or someone else's, the experience of interactions with different caregivers and peers can have lasting effects. In general, the children become more peer oriented and play at an elevated developmental level. Both ends of the interactive behavior spectrum are increased; day care children share more and they fight more.[50] As day care is a relatively recent cultural phenomenon, longitudinal research to help us understand all its ramifications has not yet been completed and is sorely needed.

Preschool children have to start wrestling with some emotional questions that may remain with them the rest of their lives. They are dealing not only with control of anger, but with other identity issues as well. Who am I? Am I a girl or a boy, and why does that matter? Of what should I be afraid, and how do I control this fear?

One source of conflict that emerges is the desire for independency. Although we are all dependent on others to some degree, the relationships differ in preschoolers. Young children are not nearly as reciprocal in their nurturing as adults become. Rather, they demand attention and affection when "performing," or they require assistance in some new or difficult task. They often have trouble expressing inner emotional needs and feelings because of underdeveloped language skills. The child's independence and associated feelings of self-worth become intimately related to the way in which its parents handle the early strivings for independence. The level of protectiveness adopted by the parents will have lifelong implications.

During the evolution of increasing amounts of independence, another of Erikson's crises is encountered by preschoolers; this one termed "initiative versus guilt."[35] As children acquire a multitude of new skills, they become increasingly confident in their ability to effect change in their world. With each encountered problem that they successfully resolve comes an increase in feelings of energy and power. Simultaneously, however, they become aware that there are requirements placed upon them that restrict their behaviors in certain ways. They learn that parents and other adults will not tolerate their always doing what they are now capable or desirous of doing. Thus the crises occur—the resolution between feeling more powerful than ever but knowing that they must control their actions or feel guilty when they are unable to do so.

The control over expressions of aggression continues its development during the preschool years. A balance must ultimately be reached. Adults do not want their children to appear to be overly aggressive or act the bully, and yet they desire a level of assertiveness, a willingness to promote and protect self-interest. Hostile aggression for the purpose of injury needs to be controlled to a greater extent than instrumental aggression, which may be aimed only at achieving a nonaggressive goal.[51] This can come about only through control over the cause or provocation for hostile aggression—frustration.

Preschool children face frustration regularly, both from external sources such as invasions of privacy and from inner conflicts like initiative versus guilt. When attempts to remove the cause of frustration prove unsuccessful, getting even becomes the next action. If that is not possible, displaced hostile aggression is the result.

Punishment, in the long run, will not deter this type of aggression because it will not serve to remove the cause—the frustration. In fact, aggressive punishment may actually heighten both the likelihood and the level of future outbursts. Rather, diversion to healthy, nondestructive outlets, like athletics and exercise, and learning strategies for dealing with frustration will serve these children far greater.

As children continue to age, the level of physical aggression that is displayed is reduced. This is often replaced with verbal aggression, that is, name-calling and insults. This may be largely in response to a change in the way the parents are controlling the child, from previous physical force to more verbal controls.

During the years of middle childhood, youngsters develop an understanding of who they are and what makes others who they are. Comparisons are common as children judge others and are judged as well. The concept of one's own skills, attributes, and limitations—self-esteem—is highly influenced by others.[52] These influences and the strength of a child's self-esteem have substantial effects on behavior. The range of activities a child will attempt is expanded or restricted, as is the level of originality and imagination displayed. Children with higher self-esteem spend more time talking to others, show initiative, and display more leadership skills.[53] The parents of children with high self-esteem tend to have high self-esteem also. Additionally, children with close relationships with their parents, especially the parent of the same sex, have higher self-esteem.[54,55]

Self-esteem has separate components, such that a child feels confident in cognitive skills, social skills, physical feats, and general self-worth.[56] These four areas are distinct in that a child could feel differently about one aspect of his or her competency compared to another. Children with high self-esteem are more likely to have a close friend. They are also more successful in academics.

The effect of fears on emotional development changes as a child matures throughout the preschool and middle childhood years. Fortunately for the child, they begin to rely on an ever-increasing scope of people for comfort, reaching beyond parents to caregivers, family, and peers and also within themselves.

Preschoolers suffer stress and thus develop fears in unfamiliar social settings. They withdraw and become shy as a defense that fortunately should be only occasional, especially if they are supported and encouraged by their parents. Fears of a specific nature can be learned, too. Traumatic personal experiences or events witnessed on television or in movies or stories can produce "irrational" fears. A child's own imagination may be the source of terrifying fears as well, such as the monsters in the shadows at night. With age, these fears normally shift from ugly and scary monsters to more realistic fears of physical danger or harm to loved ones or themselves. Experience in life determined by such factors as social status also affects the type of fears that may be felt.

Fortunately, most children, regardless of the intensity of their fears, overcome them. This resolution occurs more quickly in younger children, but eventually the irrational fears are overcome and those with some basis in reality are dealt with and controlled.[57]

Another emotional response that is quite commonly seen in children is anxiety. This feeling differs from fear in that it is not focused on a particular object or circumstance, though it is a response to a perceived danger, which may or may not exist. Anxious children are not aware of what is worrying them. In elementary school, the body's response to the anxiety may produce such symptoms as insomnia, headaches, or stomachaches. These symptoms can be manifest when the conflict that prompts the anxiety is encountered.

A small percentage of children may develop more serious emotional problems because of their fears and anxiety. A phobia is a serious and excessive fear manifest as an extreme desire to avoid the situation or object that prompts the fear. Some children develop school phobia, a concern to parents, teachers, and all who deal with the child. Luckily, most phobias can be cured by gradual and controlled exposure to the feared object with comforting reassurance.

An obsession is a preoccupation that the child cannot get out of his or her mind. The anxiety and worry of an obsession usually comes from a phobia. Most normal children show certain measures of obsessive behavior, especially around 7 and 8 years of age when rule-governed games and play are commonplace. The disturbed child, however, has compulsions peculiar to them. Unlike the games, they get no pleasure or benefit from the compulsive activity.

Hysteria can also be seen in children who have serious anxiety responses. These can be manifest as a loss of function, such as becoming deaf or mute, or in the development of a tic. Tics, whose incidence peaks at age 6 in girls and 7 in boys, can be distracting to observers.[58] Common tics include face, head, and neck muscles and are manifest as repetitive yawning, shoulder shrugs, throat clearing, or blinking. Excessive and forceful blinking is a common reason for presentation to a vision care specialist for examination. Fortunately, most tics will disappear if they are ignored. If this does not work, behavioral therapies are effective.[59]

The underlying cause of many cases of significant emotional disturbance in childhood including hostility, aggression, delinquency, and psy-

TABLE 1.7   Summary of early emotional development

Approximate Age	Event
7 months	Attachments formed
	Anxiety about strangers
12 months	Separation anxiety
24 months	Toilet trained
	Temper tantrums
6 years	Females may develop tics
7 years	Males may develop tics
7-8 years	Obsessive behavior

chosomatic illness has been found to be depression.[60] Depression in children is manifest differently from that in adults. It is often a response to a significant loss, such as loss of a parent.[61] Hostility and anger, which may accompany the depression and loss, will often alienate adults and compound the problem for the child. Negative feelings become more internalized, and the child feels evil, loses self-esteem, and may eventually become suicidal.[62] Several different types of depression have been identified in children. Once such depressions are recognized, professionals and parents can focus on the restoration of the child's feeling of self-worth, elimination of the sadness and despair, and fortification of the will to live.

Table 1-7 summarizes early emotional development.

SUMMARY

The human development process is an intricate and complex one. Child development study has ranged from the collecting of normative data regarding growth and behaviors to theoretical models of the reason for behaviors. Within the models are the concepts of stages of development through which we all pass in a systematic order. Whether describing the pregnancy, labor, and delivery process, the acquisition of motor skills, the development of language, or the emergence of emotions, orderly progress is the rule. A basic understanding of these normal processes is a necessary backdrop for the investigation of problems in development.

CHAPTER REVIEW

1. Describe fundamental differences among the four general theories of child development outlined.
2. List the three stages of pregnancy and the three stages of labor and delivery with their defining events.
3. List and briefly describe Piaget's four periods of cognitive development.
4. Describe some important aspects of attachment.
5. List and briefly describe Erikson's three crises preschoolers must deal with in their lives and their psychosocial stages of development.

REFERENCES

1. Gesell A, Amatruda CS: *Developmental diagnosis: normal and abnormal child development*, New York, 1941, Hoeber.
2. Erikson E: *Childhood and society*, New York, 1950, Norton.
3. Piaget J: *The psychology of intelligence*, New York, 1950, Harcourt.
4. Pavlov IP: *Conditioned reflexes* (GV Anrep, translator and editor), New York, 1927, Dover.
5. Skinner BF: *The behavior of organisms: an experimental analysis*, New York, 1938, Appleton.
6. Bandura A, Walters RH: *Social learning and personality development*, New York, 1963, Holt, Rinehart & Winston.
7. Maccoby EE, Jacklin CN: *The psychology of sex differences*, Stanford, Calif., 1974, Stanford University Press.
8. Apgar V: A proposal for a new method of evaluation in the newborn infant, *Anesth Anal* 52:260-267, 1953.
9. Self P, Horowitz F: Olfaction in newborn infants, *Dev Psychol* 7:349-363, 1972.
10. Erhardt RP: *Developmental hand dysfunction*, Laural, MD, 1982, RAMSCO Publishing.
11. Cratty BJ: *Perceptual and motor development in infants and children*, Englewood Cliffs, NJ, 1979, Prentice Hall, Inc.
12. Piaget J: *The construction of reality in the child*, New York, 1954, Basic Books.
13. Piaget J: *The origins of intelligence in children*, New York, 1952, International Universities Press.
14. Piaget J: Intellectual evolution from adolescence to adulthood, *Hum Dev* 15:1-12, 1972.
15. MacFarlane A: What a baby knows, *Hum Nature*, Feb 1978.
16. Schneider B, Trehub SE, Bull D: High frequency sensitivity in infants, *Science* 207:1003-1004, 1980.
17. Webster RL, Steinhardt MH, Senter MG: Changes in infants' vocalization as a function of differential acoustical stimulation, *Dev Psychol* 7:39-43, 1972.
18. Saling M: Lateral differentiation of the neonatal head turning response: a replication, *J Genet Psychol* 135(2):307-308, 1979.
19. Morsback G, Bunting C: Maternal recognition of their neonates' cries, *Dev Med Child Neurol* 21:178-185, 1979.
20. Engel W: The development from sound to phoneme in child language. In Ferguson CA, Slobin, DI, editors: *Studies of child language development*, New York, 1973, Holt, Rinehart & Winston.
21. Brown R: The first sentences of child and chimpanzee. In *Psycholinguistics: selected papers*, Glencoe, IL., 1970, The Free Press.
22. Salkind NJ, Ambron SR: *Child development*, New York, 1987, CBS College Publishing.
23. Dore J: What's so conceptual about the acquisition of linguistic structures? *J Child Lang* 6:129-138, 1979.
24. Braine MDS: The ontogeny of English phrase structure: the first phase, *Language* 39:1-13, 1963.
25. Brown R: *A first language: the early stages*, Cambridge, Mass., 1973, Harvard University Press.
26. Piaget J: *Language and thought of the child*, London, 1926, Routledge, Kegan Paul.
27. Vygotsky L: *Thought and language*, Cambridge, Mass., 1962, MIT Press.
28. Ainsworth M, Blehar MC, Waters E, Wall S: *Patterns of attachment*. Hillsdale, N.J., 1978, Erlbaum.
29. Lorenz K: *Evolution and modification of behavior*, Chicago, 1965, University of Chicago Press.
30. Harlow HF, Harlow MK: Learning to love, *Am Scientist* 54:244-272, 1966.
31. Lamb ME: Father-infant and mother-infant interaction in the first year of life, *Child Dev* 48:167-181, 1977.
32. Parke R, Sawin DB: The family in early infancy. In Pederson F, editor: *One father-infant relationship: observational studies in a family context*, New York, 1980, Praeger.
33. Parke RD, O'Leary SE: Father-mother-infant interaction in the

newborn period: some findings, some observations and some unresolved issues. In Riegel K, Meachem J, editors: *The developing individual in a changing world*, The Hague, 1976, Mouton.

34. Ainsworth M, Bell SM, Slayton DJ: Individual differences in the development of some attachment behaviors, *Merrill-Palmer Q* 18:123-143, 1972.

35. Erikson E: *Childhood and society*, New York, 1963, Norton.

36. Schaffer H, Emerson PE: The development of social attachments in infancy, *Monographs of the Society for Research in Child Development*, no. 94, 1964.

37. Spitz RA: Hospitalization: an inquiry into the genesis of psychiatric conditions of early childhood. In Freud A, et al, editors: *The psychoanalytic study of the child*, New York, 1945, International Universities Press.

38. Provence S, Lipton RC: *Infants in institutions: a comparison of their development with family-reared infants during the first year of life*, New York, 1962, International Universities Press.

39. Skeels HM: Adult status of children with contrasting early life experience, *Monographs of the Society for Research in Child Development* 31:1-65, 1966.

40. Fanshel D, Shinn EG: *Children in foster care: a longitudinal investigation*, New York, 1978, Columbia University Press.

41. Bowlby J: *Attachment and loss: separation*, vol 2, New York, 1973, Basic Books.

42. Campbell JD, Yarrow MR: Perceptual and behavioral correlates of social effectivenes, *Sociometry* 24:1-20, 1961.

43. Baumrind D: Parental disciplinary patterns and social competence in children, *Youth & Society* 9:239-276, 1978.

44. Sears RR, Maccoby EE, Levin H: *Patterns of child rearing*, Evanston, Ill., 1957, Row, Peterson.

45. Heinstein M: *Child rearing in California*, Berkeley, 1966, Bureau of Maternal and Child Health, State Department of Public Health.

46. Ritter B: Treatment of a dissection phobia (unpublished manuscript), St. John's, Nfld., Canada, 1965, Queens College.

47. Suomi SJ: Development of attachment and other social behaviors in rhesus monkeys. In Alloway T, Pliner P, Drames L, editors: *Attachment behavior*, New York, 1977, Plenum.

48. Goodenough FL: *Anger in young children*, Minneapolis, 1931, University of Minnesota Press.

49. Bandura A, Huston AC: Identification as a process of incidental learning, *J Abnormal and Social Psychol* 63:311-318, 1961.

50. Belsky J: Infant day care and child development. Testimony before the U.S. House of Representatives, Sept 5, 1984.

51. Hartup WW: Aggression in childhood: developmental perspectives, *Am Psychol* 29:336-341, 1974.

52. Sullivan HS: *The interpersonal theory of psychiatry*, New York, 1953, Norton.

53. Coopersmith S: *The antecedents of self-esteem*, San Francisco, 1967, Freeman.

54. Dickstein E, Posner JM: Self-esteem and relationship with parents, *J Genet Psychol* 133:273-276, 1978.

55. Elrod MM, Crase SJ: Sex differences in self-esteem and parental behavior, *Psychol Rep* 46:719-727, 1980.

56. Harter S: The perceived competence scale for children, *Child Dev* 53:87-97, 1982.

57. Graziano AM, DeGiovanni IS, Garcia KA: Behavioral treatment of children's fears: a review, *Psychol Bull* 86:804-830, 1979.

58. MacFarlane JW, Allen L, Honzik MP: *A developmental study of the behavior problems of normal children*, Berkeley, 1954, University of California Press.

59. Baer DM: The control of the developmental process: Why wait? In Nesselroade JR, Reese HW, editors: *Life-span developmental psychology: methodological issues*, New York: 1973, Academic Press.

---

60. Toolan JM: Therapy of depressed and suicidal children, *Am J Psychother* 32:243-251, 1978.

61. Bradley SJ: The relationship of early maternal separation to borderline personality in children and adolescents: a pilot study, *Am J Psychiatry* 136:424-426, 1979.

62. Suicide surveillance, Atlanta, Ga., 1985, Centers for Disease Control.

CHAPTER **2**

Overview of Visual and Visual Processing Development

ERIC BORSTING

KEY TERMS

visual information processing
perceptual
accommodation
vergence
fixations
pursuit eye movements
saccadic eye movements

visual-spatial
reversals
visual-analysis
form perception
visual-attention
visual-memory
visual-motor integration

Optometrists working with children who have learning-related vision problems are faced with clinical issues that require an understanding of vision and visual information processing development. For example, are reversal errors at 8 years of age normal? Will a 6-year-old use similar strategies to remember when they are compared to an 8-year-old's? Should a 5-year-old be able to draw a diamond? To address these and other issues adequately the clinician needs to have a general understanding of specific developmental sequences.

Optometry has historically been concerned with developmental visual problems from a clinical perspective. The clinician is providing care for children with visual dysfunctions such as accommodation, saccadic eye movements, visual-motor integration, or other visual areas that are evaluated in an optometric examination. As a result, this review provides an overview of the developmental characteristics of vision and visual information processing from a clinical perspective. This is not intended to be an exhaustive or critical review of the vast literature in these areas. In-

35

stead, concepts that are directly related to the clinical model that is developed later in the text are highlighted.

In the vision model developed in the text the visual system is separated into three areas, visual acuity, vision efficiency and visual information processing, to match the clinical evaluation. However, one should remember that all three processes are interrelated and do not function in isolation. The first category, visual acuity, which includes refractive status, was excluded from this review, but there are several comprehensive reviews on this topic for the interested reader.[1-3] The second category is vision efficiency, which refers to accommodation, vergence, and oculomotor skills. The final category, visual information processing, refers to a group of visual cognitive skills used for extracting and organizing visual information from the environment and coordinating this information with other sensory modalities and higher cognitive functions. Visual information processing is separated into three broad categories; visual-spatial, visual-analysis, and visual-motor.

VISION EFFICIENCY DEVELOPMENT

Investigation of the developmental characteristics of accommodation, vergence, and oculomotor skills has focused extensively on the infant. During this period the rapid development of sensory and motor processing results in considerable improvement in vision skills.[4] In fact, during the first 6 months of life accommodation, vergence, and oculomotor skills all emerge and improve rapidly. Investigation of developmental changes beyond this period is sparse but accommodative, and vergence skills are qualitatively adultlike by the end of the first year of life. However, there is evidence that oculomotor skills do not reach adultlike ability until adolescence.[5] This is not surprising because oculomotor skills are more closely linked to attentional and cognitive factors than are accommodative and vergence abilities.

Accommodation

The amplitude and accuracy of accommodative responses improve rapidly during the first 3 months of life.[6,7] The newborn infant does not utilize its capacity to accommodate because its depth of focus is large.[6] That is, large changes in target distance do not produce changes in perceived blur, and because blur, is the primary stimulus for accommodation, little if any accommodative responses will be produced. One consequence of inaccurate accommodation in infants is that they can accommodate incorrectly without blur being noticed. This is seen in the 1-month-old who accommodates to a distance of 20 cm when viewing distant targets.[8] The inaccuracies in accommodation disappear by the end of the third month of life.

The pronounced changes in accommodative accuracy during the first 3 months can be measured by an accommodative response curve having the accommodative response plotted versus the stimulus. If the accommodative response equals the stimulus, a slope of 1.0 would be seen. If no accommodative response was elicited, the slope would be 0. During the first 3 postnatal months the depth of focus decreases and the accommodative response improves. The response function has a slope of 0.5 in the 1-month-old, improves to 0.75 in the 2-month-old, and to about 0.8 in the 3-month-old.[6] The adult slope is 0.95. As long as there is not a significant uncorrected refractive error the infant can accommodate to a broad range of target distances at the end of 3 months of age.

Accommodative responses to changes in dioptric power are almost adultlike by 6 months of age. However, clinical evaluation of accommodative responses in the school-aged child, including amplitude, lag, and facility, are influenced by developmental factors. The amplitude of accommodation does decrease in a predictable course during the school-aged years because of sclerosis of the lens.[9] The lag of accommodation appears to increase slightly during this period. A study by Rouse et al.[10] evaluated the lag of accommodation in elementary school children and found that the average lag increased from first grade (+0.21) to sixth grade (+0.45). This difference may be attributed to younger children not using the chromatic aberration interval to help establish the lag of accommodation.[11] The ability of the child to respond to subjective tests may be influenced by verbal and cognitive development. This has been observed in accommodative facility testing of school-aged children. Children that are 6 years of age exhibit fewer cycles per minute on average than 10- to 12-year-old children.[12] Scheiman et al.[12] cited automatic digit naming ability (speed of letter or number recognition) as a factor that contributes to slower performance observed in children at different ages.

Vergence

The vergence system has motor and sensory components that are responsible for maintaining ocular alignment. At birth cosmetically acceptable binocular alignment may be present, but it is uncertain if bifoveal fixation exists.[13] In the subsequent months the vergence system goes through an unstable period until 4 to 6 months of age when stable bifixation is established. This is seen by the clinical finding that over 50% of infants at 1 month of age exhibit an intermittent or constant exotropia.[14] The presence of esotropia is under 5%. By the end of the sixth postnatal month most of the exotropic infants are no longer manifesting the ocular deviation. In esotropia the manifestation of the deviation beyond 2 months of age usually indicates the presence of infantile esotropia.

The ability to change vergence to view near targets undergoes rapid improvement during the first 3 to 4 postnatal months. This requires several vergence components (accommodative, proximal, and disparity) to work in accord with each other. Infants in the first 2 postnatal months do not consistently change vergence response with sufficient magnitude to maintain accurate bifoveal fixation at near distances.[15,16] However, the direction of the vergence change is typically appropriate for the change in target distance. By the end of the third postnatal month changes in the vergence angle more closely match the changes in target distance. However, individual components of the vergence system do not have the same developmental course. Accommodative vergence responses, which indicate a linkage between the accommodative and vergence system, have been demonstrated at 2 to 3 months.[17] On the other hand, disparity fusional vergence responses appear later, between 4 to 6 months of age.[16]

The binocular sensory component of the vergence system relies on retinal image disparity for stereopsis. Behavioral methods (such as preferential looking) indicate that stereopsis emerges from 4 to 6 months of age, a time that parallels the development of disparity vergence responses.[18,19] Measurement using the visual evoked potential (VEP) signal indicates positive responses to stereoscopic disparity between 3 to 5 months of age.[20] Although the emergence of stereopsis appears quite early in life, improvements in stereoacuity thresholds occur later in the preschool years. A recent study by Ciner et al.[21] used an operant conditioning technique with random-dot stereo targets to determine stereoacuity measurement in children from 18 to 65 months of age. The results of the study indicated improvements in stereoacuity from 250 seconds of arc in the youngest children to 60 seconds of arc on the oldest group. This indicates that stereoacuity probably does not reach adult levels until the end of the preschool years.

Oculomotor

A clinical evaluation of the oculomotor system usually assesses three types of eye movements: fixation, pursuits, and saccades. Eye movements are essential for effective visual processing.[22] For example, the saccadic system shifts the fovea to an area of interest so that detailed information can be processed. Another example of the importance of eye movements for visual processing is reading, where the individual will make a series of small saccades and short fixation pauses. Investigation of the dynamics of oculomotor skills (such as latency) has focused on the infant, and very little research has been done to evaluate preschool and school-aged children. In the school-aged years investigation of oculomotor skills has centered on eye-movement patterns during reading.

Fixations. The newborn's foveal immaturity and poor visual acuity indicate that fixations may be poorer than adults during the first 2 to 3 postnatal months.[23] The central retinal region is probably equally sensitive over a 5-degree area during the first 2 postnatal months.[4] As a result, a specific central site where fixation preference would be advantageous may not exist during this period. Direct evidence of this supposition is not available because of the uncertainty of measuring the kappa angle early in life.[4] However, newborns will steadily fixate on an object and infrequently shift fixation to another object. The tendency to fixate on new objects does increase during the first 3 months of life.[24]

In adults, fixational movements are composed of slow drifts, fixation saccades, and rapid micromovements. By 2 to 3 months of age drifts and saccades have been observed in infants, but the fixations are of shorter duration and have a higher drift rate than those of adults.[4,23] Measurements of fixations in a small sample of preschool and 10-year-old children have found less precise fixation control than that of adults.[22,25] The difference between these children and adults is the intrusion of large saccades and the presence of higher drift rates during fixation. This indicates that children may have poorer oculomotor control when compared to adults. However, the large saccadic intrusions have been attributed to attentional factors rather than to poor oculomotor control.[26]

Pursuit eye movements. Pursuit eye movements enable continuous clear vision of moving objects within a stable visual environment.[27] These eye movements would appear to be susceptible to postnatal foveal development and corresponding reduction in visual acuity.[4] This may account for the finding that infants under 8 weeks of age do not show smooth pursuit eye movements when tracking pendular target motion at varying velocities.[5,28] Instead, tracking responses consist of saccades, which act to catch the eye up to the moving target. At 2 to 3 months of age the infant is capable of generating a smooth pursuit eye movement to track a moving target. However, the eye movements are still not adultlike, and fixation tends to lag behind the target.[5,28] There is evidence that pursuit eye movements continue to improve during childhood.[22,25,29,30] For example, children tended to wait longer than adults to change the direction when tracking a target with a predictable path.[22,25]

Saccadic eye movements. Saccadic eye movements are rapid shifts in fixation from one part of the visual field to another in order to place a new image on the fovea. These eye movements are easily observed in newborns but tend to be infrequent. During the first 3 postnatal months the frequency of changing fixation to new visual objects increases.[24] Accurate saccades depends on coordinating the locus of retinal stimulation with a neuromotor command.[13] That is, a peripheral target at 10 degrees should result in a saccade of approximately the same amount. At 1 to 2 months the infant has difficulty generating an accurate saccade. He will change fixation to a new target with a series of small saccades that rarely exceed 50% of the target distance.[24,31] The saccades are in the right direction but are grossly hypometric. There is a systematic improvement during infancy with a decrease in the number of saccades needed to reach the target and an increase in the amplitude of the primary saccade.[31] By 7 months of age the hypometric responses are reduced, but accuracy is still not adultlike.[31]

The latency of a saccadic response is also different in the infant. Latencies are typically much longer than those found in adults but during some saccades can approach adult levels.[24] Although infants show a significant improvement in their saccadic eye movements early in life, there is a continuation of improvement into childhood. Children from 4 to 10 years of age tend to have longer latencies when making saccades to targets under a variety of conditions as compared to adults.[22,25,32] Based on current research, it is unclear exactly when saccades reach adultlike levels.

Upon entering school the child is faced with different demands on the eye movement system. In preschool the visually based activities include building puzzles, coloring, and block play. In elementary school, learning to read requires smaller and more accurate saccadic eye movements than tasks in the preschool years do.[33] An illustration of saccadic eye movement when reading is shown in Figure 2.1. Eye movements during reading are characterized by a series of rightward saccades, which are called "forward fixations." When the end of the line is reached, a large leftward saccade, or return sweep, of about 10 degrees returns the eye to the beginning of the line. This may be accompanied by a small corrective saccade if the return sweep was not accurate. A small leftward movement of the eye is a regression that occurs approximately 5% to 20% of the time.[34] On each fixation, or pause, the fovea processes the linguistic information while the retinal periphery directs future saccadic eye movements. The length of time that the eye pauses during a fixation is called the "duration of fixation." The amount of reading material that is processed during a fixation pause is the span of recognition.

In the elementary school years reading eye movements show a steady improvement.[35] The number of forward fixations and regression show a sharp reduction from grades 1 to 4. After this point, the decrease is more gradual (Table 2.1). There is also an accompanying increase in the span of recognition and reading rate during this period. Why do young children show an increased number of fixations and regressions when read-

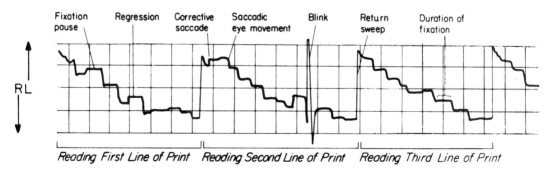

FIGURE 2.1 Recording of reading eye-movement patterns taken from a photoelectric Eye Track. This illustrates the characteristics of eye movement patterns during reading.

From Grisham D, Simons H: Perspectives on reading disabilities. In Rosenbloom AA, Morgan MW, editors: *Pediatric optometry*, Philadelphia, 1989, Lippincott.

TABLE 2.1 Developmental trends in reading eye movements

Grade	1	2	3	4	5	6	7	8	9	10	11	12	Collimation
Fixations (including regressions) per 100 words	224	174	155	139	129	120	114	109	105	101	96	94	90
Regressions per 100 words	52	40	35	31	28	25	23	21	20	19	18	17	15
Average span of recognition (in words)	0.45	0.57	0.65	0.72	0.78	0.83	0.88	0.92	0.95	0.99	1.04	1.06	1.11
Average duration of fixation (in seconds)	0.33	0.30	0.28	0.27	0.27	0.27	0.27	0.27	0.27	0.26	0.26	0.25	0.24
Rate with comprehension (in words per minute)	80	115	138	158	173	185	195	204	214	224	237	250	280

From Taylor EA: *The fundamental reading skill*, Springfield, Ill, 1966, Charles C Thomas.

ing? There are probably two principle factors: underdeveloped oculomotor control and limited linguistic processing skills. Before starting school, children have little experience generating the types of eye movements that reading requires. Therefore young children would be expected to have difficulty programming a sequence of small saccades. To test this hypothesis would require measuring eye movement patterns to targets that simulate eye movement patterns made when reading. In this approach the child does not have to comprehend specific text but simply scans a series of targets. Gilbert[33] investigated the ability of children in grades 1 through 9 to fixate on a series of digits. The results indicate that fixation and regression patterns in this task are similar to those found in reading. Younger children showed an increased number of fixations and regressions, both of which declined with age.

The ability to process semantic and syntactic information is also a factor that contributes to poorer eye movements in younger children.[34] Improvement in linguistic processing would result in a reduced number of fixations and regressions because the child is better able to process the meaning of the text. That is, eye movement patterns during reading, to a large extent, reflect the ability to understand the reading material. However, this theory does not account for the developmental changes in oculomotor control found by studies having children scan a series of letters or numbers that simulate reading.[33,36]

The general developmental trends indicate that all three vision-efficiency skills emerge and improve rapidly in the first 6 postnatal months. Development beyond this period is minor for accommodation and vergence ability. However, oculomotor skills appear to show significant improvement in the preschool and school-aged years. This may be the result of later developing oculomotor control skills or the influence of attentional and cognitive factors. Probably both factors affect performance on eye movement evaluations. Further research is needed to determine the contribution of each factor to the normal development of eye movement skills.

DEVELOPMENT OF VISUAL INFORMATION PROCESSING

Visual information processing refers to a group of visual cognitive skills used for extracting and organizing visual information from the environment and integrating this information with other sensory modalities and higher cognitive functions. When catching a ball, writing letters or numbers, or trying to picture problems in your head, you are using visual processing skills. Other terms such as "perception," "perceptual-motor," and "visual-spatial" have been used to describe similar skills. In this text the term "visual information processing" is used to cover a broad group of skills that are evaluated by the optometric practitioner. Before proceeding to the specific developmental trends in visual-spatial, visual-analysis, and visual-motor it is important to review some general concepts of visual processing.

Visual processing, or perception, involves the ability to extract and select information from the environment. Gibson and Levine[37] have defined perception as the process of extracting information from stimulation emanating from objects, places, and events in the world around us. However, the information that strikes the retina is vast, and the visual system cannot process all the potential visual stimuli. The individual must select the information that is most important for the task that he is performing, and therefore certain information is chosen for processing whereas other information is ignored. As a result the visual system must be selective while extracting relevant information.

The selection of information from the environment depends on several factors including motivation, prior experience, and development.[38] Motivation plays a key role because the individual in part sees what he or she wants to see (see Chapter 3). Information that is relevant to the task at hand or makes things easier to perform is more likely to be attended to. Prior experiences and the current needs of the individual also determine the motivation of the individual to respond to some visual stimuli and ignore others. Past experiences build memory traces of similar events and aid in processing the visual information that is relevant to the current task. Finally, the developmental level of the child places limits on the type of information that is processed. For example, in the infant, reduced visual acuity and contrast sensitivity restrict accommodative skills.

Once information is extracted or selected from the environment, meaning has to be attached to the visual stimuli.[38] The individual needs to understand what is seen. This process involves a complex interaction between visual processing and cognitive factors that are influenced by past experiences, motivation, and development. Visually based tasks require recognition, analysis, and manipulation of information. The distinction between perception and cognition has created some confusion for the student learning about visual processing development. In this model, perception and cognition are considered overlapping concepts that influence each other in the processing of information and are not seen as distinct and separable entities. Essentially, perception provides visual cognitive information that is used in higher-order cognitive functions. As a result, the term "visual information processing" is used to describe the visual processing skills evaluated by the clinician. This is in agreement with Richman et al.[39] who use the term "perceptuo/cognitive" to describe similar aspects of visual processing.

Visual information is also integrated with other sensory systems, but the optometrist is primarily concerned with the ability to integrate the visual and motor systems. Visual-motor integration is used in many activities such as block building, handwriting, and catching a ball. One method

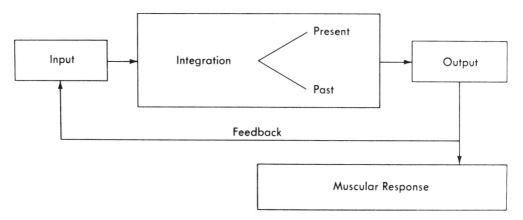

FIGURE 2.2 Diagram of a closed-loop system.

From Kephardt NC: *The slow learner in the classroom,* Columbus, Ohio, 1971, Charles E. Merrill.

to analyze the interaction between visual and motor processing is a closed-loop system (Figure 2.2).[40] This model consists of four components: input, central processor or integration, output, and feedback. In such a system the output influences the input through a feedback system, and the central processor is responsible for programming motor actions. The goal of most visual-motor tasks is to reduce or minimize the discrepancy between the visual input and the motor output. An example of how this model works would be catching a ball. The input would be the trajectory of the ball along with prevailing environmental conditions such as wind. The central processing would make the decision on where to move and where to put the hand to catch the ball based on past experiences and the visual input. The output is the actual motor response or where the hand is actually placed. Feedback relates to the discrepancy between the output and the input, and if a discrepancy is seen, changes are made in the position of the hand in relation to the ball. When visual-motor behavior during copying skills is analyzed, a more detailed model will be presented.

The rate of development of visual processing skills is not uniform during infancy, preschool, and school-aged years. We can illustrate this concept by viewing visual processing development as a curvilinear function with a decreasing slope with increasing age (Figure 2.3). In the early years the rate of development is more rapid than that seen in the later years. The difference between a 4-year-old and a 5-year-old is much greater than the difference between a 12-year-old and a 13-year-old. This becomes important when one is comparing performance among different age groups because a 1-year delay can cause an overestimation or underestimation of the actual performance deficit of the child.[41]

The development of visual information processing skills with age is considered an active process. The child or infant is exploring and searching for information in the environment, and it does not rely on passive absorption of information.[37,42] In a sense we possess an internal drive or mo-

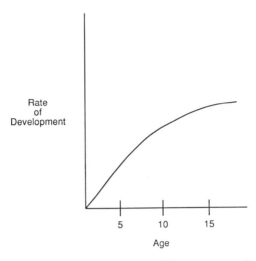

FIGURE 2.3 Example of a hypothetical rate of development for a visual processing skill.

tivation to actively learn more about our world. One consequence of the active nature of development is that visual processing skills are learned, though recent research in visual processing development has revealed that the infant's development is far more advanced than previously believed. However, their level of processing and conceptualization is still primitive and primarily reflexive in nature. During development there is an elaboration of exploration and processing strategies that allow the child to perform more complex visual processing tasks.

PREVIOUS APPROACHES TO VISUAL-MOTOR DEVELOPMENT

Theories of visual-motor development have been proposed by investigators interested in the effect of visual-motor performance on learning disabilities (see Chapter 7 for a more detailed description).[40,42] These models proposed that early motor development laid the foundation for later developing visual perceptual and cognitive skills. However, research in visual perceptual abilities in infants clearly calls into question the theory that motor development is critical for the development of perceptual skills. Many of the basic visual-perceptual skills have emerged by 6 to 8 months of age. As a result visual-perceptual development is not entirely dependent on motor development. This is especially true during the first 6 months of life when many visual skills are emerging. After this period visual-motor skills are important for exploring and extracting information from the environment. This aids in the development of efficient visual processing.

In contrast to some previous approaches, a clinically based model of visual processing development must recognize that global theories cannot account for the diverse functions performed by visual processing skills. Therefore, visual processing skills are treated as separate abilities that are used to perform specific skills.[43] Each of the three components, visual-spatial, visual-analysis, and visual-motor, would relate to specific skills that an individual would perform. For example, poor visual-motor integration would be expected to affect tasks where eye-hand coordination is important as in handwriting.

VISUAL-SPATIAL SKILLS

Visual-spatial skills refer to the ability to understand directional concepts that organize external visual space. These skills relate to understanding the difference between the concepts of up and down, front and back, and right and left as they relate to the body and to objects in space. The individual develops an awareness of his position in space as well as the relationship of objects to himself.[44] Spatial abilities are important for many skills including navigating through the world (such as right and left turns), understanding directions (such as: Put your name on the top right-hand side of the page.), recognizing the orientation and sequence of linguistic symbols (such as *b* versus *d*), and manipulating visual information.

One method used to evaluate visual-spatial ability is to ask the child to identify the position of body parts (such as: Show me your right ear.) or objects in space (such as: Is the pencil to the right or left of the coin?). One result of this verbal assessment method is that visual-spatial development is difficult to evaluate in children under 2 years of age. Even the preschooler may have difficulty understanding certain spatial directions because of limited receptive language skills. Despite these limitations, it is clear that children understand the difference between front and back and up and down before they can consistently differentiate between right and left.[45] Preschool children, 3 to 4 years of age, can correctly identify front and back and up and down on themselves and on objects.[45,46] The correct identification of right and left on self is usually seen at 6 to 7 years of age.[45,47,48] The identification of right and left directions on objects in space develops between 7 and 12 years of age.[45,47,48]

Practitioners working with learning-disabled children will frequently encounter children who have difficulty with right and left concepts but not up and down and front and back directions. For the purposes of this text an awareness of the right and left sides of the body is referred to as "laterality." The ability to use directions to understand and organize external visual space is called "directionality." This section concentrates on the specific developmental characteristics of laterality and directionality.

The specific developmental sequence of right and left knowledge using verbal labels was extensively investigated by Laurendeau and Pinard.[48] They assessed laterality and directionality using a test of right and left knowledge that measures three separate but interrelated concepts (see the box). The first problem is the assessment of laterality, or the ability to identify the right and left sides of individual body parts. The second problem is an evaluation of one aspect of directionality. This relates to developing

Test of Right and Left Knowledge

Problem 1 (designation of subject's body parts)

Show me your right hand.
Show me your left leg.
Show me your right ear.
Show me your left hand.
Show me your right leg.
Show me your left ear.

Problem 2 (designation of parts of the examiner)

Show me my left hand.
Show me my right ear.
Show me my left leg.
Show me my right hand.
Show me my left ear.
Show me my right leg.

Problem 3 (relative position of three objects*)

Is the pencil to the left or to the right of the plate?
Is the plate to the left or to the right of the block?
Is the block to the left or to the right of the pencil?
Is the pencil to the left or to the right of the block?
Is the plate to the left or to the right of the pencil?
Is the block to the left or to the right of the plate?

From Laurendeau M, *Pinard A: The development of the concept of space in the child,* New York, 1970, International Universities Press, pp 450-451.
*The block, the plate, and the pencil are placed in front of the child from left to right.

an understanding that right and left positions on another person change depending on his orientation. For example, a child needs to realize that the right and left sides of someone sitting across from him are opposite to his own right and left. The final problem assesses the ability to understand the directional relationship objects have in space. They described four stages of development, stages 0, 1, 2, and 3, of right and left knowledge in children from 5 to 12 years of age. This becomes important because two children may be unable to solve the same problem in an assessment of right and left knowledge but their understanding of these concepts may be very different.

The first stage (stage 0) is a state of "total incomprehension" of right and left knowledge. The child's responses to questions on the assessment do not show an awareness that the right and left sides of the body are different. However, the responses are not entirely random and the child typically attempts to use a particular strategy to "figure out" the problem. For example, a child may point to his or her body parts correctly but always point to the right or left side. These types of responses are typical for children under 6 years of age.

In stage 1 the child begins to understand that the right and left sides of the body are different. Typically, children will develop this awareness on themselves first and then on other people. In this investigation the researchers also considered a systematic reversal of right and left labels on themselves as a correct response. There are two substages within stage one (substage 1A and substage 1B). Substage 1A is a "transitional phase" where the child is aware of the difference between the right and left sides of the body. However, the application of this knowledge to solve the first two problems is unstable. This is characterized by the child's inability to apply an appropriate strategy in both the first and second problems. The child will solve the first or second problem correctly but will show chance responses when asked to solve the other problem. Therefore one of four possible responses is observed. In response to the first problem the child will answer all questions correctly or show systematic reversals. When asked questions about the examiner's right and left the child will revert to chance responses that characterized stage 0. The child may also give chance responses to the first set of questions but will correctly identify the examiner's right and left or systematically reverse the directions. The median age of children at substage 1A is 5.10 years of age.

In substage 1B the concept of right and left as representing different sides of the body becomes solidified, and this is an advancement in right and left knowledge over substage 1A. The child will accurately identify right and left on himself, or systematically reverse the two, but has difficulty understanding the examiner's right and left. In contrast to substage 1A, responses to both problems one and two show an understanding of right and left as different sides of the body. Two paths are typically taken by the child in an attempt to answer the questions regarding right and left on the examiner. First, the child will project his or her right and left onto the examiner's right and left and produce a systematic reversal response or a correct response (depending if he or she systematically reversed to begin with). Second, the child may realize that a different method is required to identify the examiner's right and left, but the child is only partially successful in this attempt. The child will quickly revert to using his or her own right and left to make this judgment. In both substages the child will have difficulty solving the problem of three objects in a table. He or she may be able to identify the two end items correctly but is unable to grasp the relation of the middle item. The median age for stage 1B is 7.2 years of age.

In stage 2 the child understands the role of perspective in making right and left judgments. The child understands that when the examiner is facing him that right side and left side become reversed in relation to his own body. This represents an advancement in right and left knowledge, but the child is unable to respond accurately to questions in problem 3. This stage of development occurs at a median age of 7.9 years.

In stage 3 the child is able to identify the relationship of the three objects to each other. In this stage the child is able to coordinate his own perspective of right and left judgments (such as judging the position of the end items on problem 3) with the realizations that the objects themselves constitute a separate component of visual space. Essentially, objects occupy their own space where the middle object's right and left position depends not on the viewer's perspective but on the arrangements of the items on the table. This is the last step in right and left development and occurs at a median age of 10.11 years.

Reversal of symbols

The reversal of letters and numbers is a common entering complaint of parents of learning-disabled children. The most common errors are reversals around the vertical, or *y*-axis, such as *b* and *d*, whereas reversals around the horizontal axis are much less frequent. Reversal errors of individual letters and numbers is a normal finding as children enter school. However, a steady decline in the frequency of reversals should occur as the child proceeds through the primary grades. By 8 years of age or beyond second grade most children will cease making these errors when reading and writing.[49-51]

Why do many children reverse letters and numbers when they enter school? One likely explanation is that children tend to ignore orientation as one of the important features that is necessary for correct recognition of linguistic symbols. This is expected given that recognition and identification of nonlinguistic objects and forms usually does not depend on their orientation. For example, identification of a chair does not depend on whether it is pointing to the right or the left. However, when orientations of certain letters are changed, the meaning is altered (such as a *b* becoming a *d*), or reversal of other letters results in an incorrect response. This explanation is supported by the experimental work of Gibson et al.[52] who found that children at 5 years of age were significantly more likely to make confusions of forms that were rotated or reversed than children at 8 years of age, who rarely made these types of errors. When the child enters school, he must learn to be aware of orientation as an important feature for correct identification of letters and numbers.[37] This learning process is part of normal development for children in the early grades.

Another factor that may affect the child's ability to discriminate the orientation of forms is an understanding of laterality and directionality concepts.[49,53] Reversal errors have been associated with right and left confusions.[54] However, a cause-and-effect relationship have not been established between the two skills. As discussed previously, children's understanding of right and left concepts develops rapidly from 5 to 8 years of age. This probably becomes important for identifying reversal errors around the vertical axis. The child needs to identify the correct right and left orientations of certain letters. As a result a poor understanding of directionality may interfere with the child's ability to become aware of the role of orientation in recognizing letters and numbers.

Reversal errors that persist beyond second grade are considered abnormal and are usually associated with reading disabilities.[49,53,55] The specific causes of these errors remain controversial. Several possible factors have been identified and include visual-memory, laterality and directionality, form perception, visual-motor integration, and language.[49,53,56,57]

VISUAL-ANALYSIS SKILLS

Visual-analysis skills are a group of abilities used for recognition, recall, and manipulation of visual information. These skills are an important part of many activities including judging similarities or differences among forms and symbols, remembering forms and symbols, and visualization. Visual-analysis skills are subdivided into the following general categories: form perception, visual-attention, and visual-memory. Visual-attention is placed in this section because clinical evaluation of attention is in many cases very similar to tests used for assessing visual-analysis skills. However, visual attention is a function that is important for all visual processing tasks. For each set of skills the general developmental characteristics are described.

Form perception

The recognition of your car in a parking lot is an example of form perception. The incoming perceptual information has to be organized and compared to an internal representation of your car for similarities and differences until a match is made. This task illustrates three process that are involved in form perception: feature analysis, comparison, and memory. Feature analysis involves the extraction of specific features of forms including size, shape, and color.[58] Certain visual information is selected so that appropriate judgments regarding similarities and differences with other objects can be made. The process of comparison and memory can be illustrated in three types of form perception tasks: discrimination, recognition, and identification.[58] In a *discrimination task,* two or more forms are compared simultaneously or in close succession to find similarities or differences. This type of task places minimal demand on memory because the visual information is readily available for review. In a recognition task a comparison between a form that is present and an internal representation that is stored in memory of that pattern is required, for example, recognizing a person you met at a party the previous week. In this case the comparison depends, in part, on storing an accurate internal representation of the form, which places more demand on memory skills. In an *identification task* the form must be compared to an internal representation first and then more detailed processing places the form in a conceptual category in order to arrive at the appropriate label.

The development of form-perception skills in infancy has received considerable attention by researchers. This research clearly indicates that infants are able to discriminate and recognize visual forms. The use of preferential looking and habituation techniques have yielded evidence that infants possess the ability to recognize specific features of a form (such as line versus curve) and are able to integrate features into an identifiable whole by 6 months of age (such as recognition of a face).[58,59] Two additional form-perception skills, size and shape consistency, allow the perception of an object to remain fairly constant despite large changes in the retinal image. These skills appear to be present by 6 to 8 months of age.[60,61] Therefore it appears that by 7 to 8 months of age the infant has acquired many of the basic form-perception skills. However, this does not mean that form-perception development has ended. As the child matures, there are important changes in visual and cognitive development that enrich visual processing. The older child is able to process more information and has a greater understanding of the meaning of visual forms and objects.

Many clinical evaluations of form perception require the individual to compare similarities and differences between two or more targets. The process chosen by the individual to make the comparison is reflected in a strategy of visual search and exploration.[62] Strategies are voluntary actions by the individual to aid or enhance visual processing in a particular context and depend on the developmental level of the individual, his or her motivation, and prior experience. In form-perception tasks the individual will visually search or explore objects or forms for specific items or features depending on the demands of the task. An example of this process is illustrated in a form-perception test of visual discrimination that consists of five figures where one figure matches the target and the other figures differ by orientation (Figure 2.4). The optimal strategy would be to identify the distinctive feature (orientation) and make a systematic comparison between the target figure and the possible choices until a match is

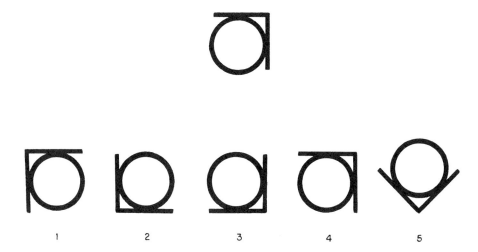

FIGURE 2.4 Example of a visual discrimination task.

From Gardner M: *The Test of Visual Perceptual Skills*, Burlingame, Calif., 1985, Psychological and Educational Publications, Inc.

made. If a comparison is not made or a certain feature is ignored, errors may result. In the above task, if the individual looked at only two of the four possible targets and then guessed the wrong answer, his or her strategy would not reflect a systematic search for the distinctive feature of the target stimulus.

As the child matures, there is a progressive change in the ability to use organized and efficient search strategies to solve a visual form–perception problem. Two overall developmental trends in strategies were described by Rosinski[58] in relation to visual discrimination tasks. First, the ability to make comparisons among objects and figures become more efficient; that is, more features can be compared in a given time period. Second, the comparison between objects and figures becomes more systematic. There is a progression from a random comparison of objects to a more systematic comparison method.

Several investigations of perceptual discrimination in children have confirmed these trends, and one representative experiment by Vurpillot is used to illustrate developmental changes in visual strategies.[52,63,64] In this experiment, two houses, each of which had six windows, were presented to children between 2 and 9.5 years (Figure 2.5). The children were asked to identify whether the contents of the windows in the two houses were identical. To measure the visual search patterns used by the subjects, eye movements were recorded. The windows in the houses were either identical or differed by one, three, or five paired windows. In the example (Figure 2.5) one house is identical, and the other has three different windows. Therefore, recognizing that the houses are not identical could be made with a different number of comparisons depending on the number of nonidentical windows between the two houses. Two identical houses would require six comparisons, whereas two houses with five different windows would require at most two comparisons.

The results of the experiment indicated that children under 5 years of age had search patterns that were incomplete and unsystematic. With increasing age there were changes in the scanning behavior and accuracy of performance (Figure 2.6). The preschool child may identify the houses as identical without comparing all six of the windows. They tended to scan the same number of windows regardless of the number of differences (Figure 2.6, **b**). This resulted in a higher number of errors when compared to older children especially for houses that differed by only one or three windows (Figure 2.6, **a**). The younger children also tended not to use a pair-by-pair comparison method (Figure 2.6, **c**). In contrast, older children (6 years of age and older) tended to use a complete and systematic visual search pattern that was influenced by the number of differences between the two houses. In houses with fewer differences they made more comparisons (Figure 2.6, **b**). This resulted in a similar number of correct responses regardless of the number of differences between the houses

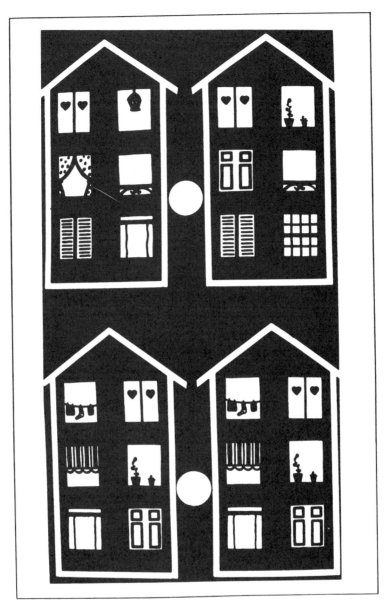

FIGURE 2.5 Examples of the houses used in the Vurpillot experiment: a pair of different houses and a pair of identical houses.

From Rosinski RR: *The development of visual perception*, Santa Monica, Calif., 1977, Goodyear Publishing Co.

(Figure 2.6, **a**). The older children also used a paired-comparison method by comparing matching windows in the two houses (Figure 2.6, **c**).

Even though infants possess many of the basic form-perception skills, they are unable to use them efficiently. During the preschool and school-aged years the ability to make feature comparisons and to search and explore patterns in a complete and systematic way become the crucial com-

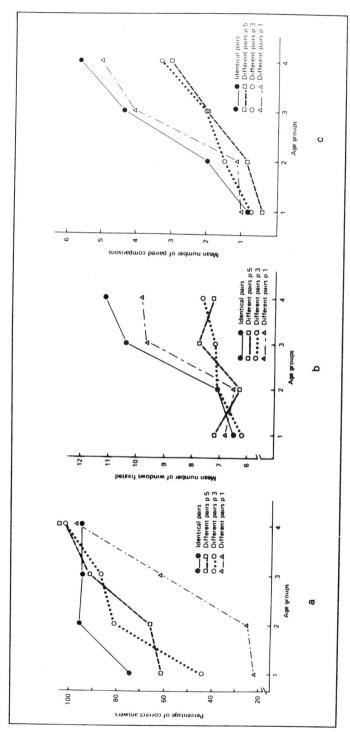

FIGURE 2.6 Development changes in discrimination performance when comparing houses: **a**, percentage of correct responses; **b**, number of windows fixated, and **c**, number of paired comparisons. The average age for group 1 was 3.1 years; group 2, 5.0 years; group 3, 6.6 years; group 4, 8.9 years.

From Rosinski RR: *The development of visual perception,* Santa Monica, Calif., 1977, Goodyear Publishing Co.

ponents of form-perception development. The ability to efficiently use these form-perception skills probably does not reach adultlike ability until early adolescence.

Clinical evaluations of form-perception skills usually involve discrimination, recognition, or identification as part of the test. Furthermore they are usually divided into several subskills, which include visual discrimination, visual figure ground, and visual closure.[65] Visual discrimination is the ability to analyze the distinctive features of form, including size, shape, color, orientation, and position, to determine similarities and differences among forms. Visual figure ground is the ability to attend to a specific feature or form while maintaining an awareness of the relationship of this form to the background information. Finally, visual closure is the ability of the individual to be aware of clues in the visual array that allow him to determine the final percept without the necessity of all the details being present. A more detailed description of these form-perception tasks is given in the chapters on diagnosis and remediation of visual information processing deficits (see Chapters 11 and 16).

Visual-attention and cognitive style

When a child engages in a test of visual discrimination or other visual processing tasks, he will attend to certain parts of the form and ignore others. How the child approaches such tasks relates to his visual-attention and cognitive style. Attention is the ability to focus consciousness on a task and is essential for all information-processing tasks.[66] Cognitive style relates to how the child solves problems. There are several clinical and theoretical models of how attention and cognitive style develop in children.[67,68] One clinical model of attention is highlighted because it represents those aspects of attention and cognitive style that would be of most concern for the optometrist working with children who have learning-related vision problems. Furthermore the effects of poor attention on visual processing is emphasized, but similar factors also affect auditory processing.

Attention consists in three separate but interrelated components: coming to attention, decision making, and sustaining attention.[69-71] Coming to attention is the ability to analyze, organize, and determine salient features of a visual target. In other words, it is the ability to focus attention on the requirements of the task and allows the individual to get appropriately involved in the activity. This component of attention has been measured by the use of the Children's Embedded Figures Test.[69,70] In this test the child has to extract the salient feature (such as a triangle) that is embedded within a picture. There is a definite trend in the school-aged years toward improved ability to analyze more complex visual stimuli and extract the salient features that will be used for decision making.[72]

Decision making refers most closely to the cognitive style of the child. This represents a continuum from the child who is impulsive (a fast and inaccurate decision maker) to the one who is reflective (a thoughtful problem solver).[69-71] The Matching Familiar Figure Test (MFFT) allows one to assess the speed and accuracy of the visual response in a visual discrimination task.[73] In this test the child has to find an exact match of a target figure from several alternative choices while the response time or the latency is recorded. The child's response gives an index of the tradeoff that the child may make between the speed and accuracy of the visual response. A child who responds quickly but is incorrect is impulsive. On the other hand, the reflective child takes more time to respond and is more accurate. Preschool children tend to be very impulsive, but as they become older, they also become more reflective. Up to 10 years of age, school-aged children show an increase in the latency of the visual response and a decrease in errors as measured by the MFFT.[74] After 10 years of age the number of errors stabilizes, and the latencies tend to decrease.

Finally, sustaining attention is the ability to maintain attention once the task is started. One can usually measure this ability by having the child perform a repetitive task, such as crossing out certain numbers from a visual display, and then assess omissions or errors. Certain items are missed or omitted or the wrong item is crossed out. This results from the child not attending consistently to the requirements of the task. That is, the child is able to perform the task successfully at certain times, but his or her attention wanders during the activity. The ability to maintain attention improves with age.[75] The younger child has difficulty holding his attention on certain visual tasks for the same length of time that the older child can.

Visual-memory

Visual-memory is the ability to recall visually presented material. An example of a memory test is shown in Figure 2.7. Look at the picture for 5 seconds, close the book, and draw the figures. To help remember the figures you probably used a strategy such as visualizing the figures in your head. Identifying what strategy or lack of strategy is used is the key to understanding how children perform on standardized tests of memory.

Researchers in visual information processing have delineated three types of memory: sensory information store, short-term memory, and long-term memory.[76] The sensory information store, or iconic store, is a short-lived type of memory where visual information is maintained for only fractions of a second after the stimulus has disappeared. This type of memory causes a sensation of the image to persist beyond the initial presentation of the stimulus. Information is held for less than a second in the sensory store, and therefore this is not considered a permanent memory storage system. It is not clear if processing in this stage is essential for the next stage of memory.[77]

Short-term memory allows the individual to retain information for several seconds or longer if the information is actively rehearsed or attended to in some way. The active attention to the stimulus keeps the information refreshed. An example of a short-term memory task occurs when you

FIGURE 2.7 Example taken from the Monroe Visual Three Test of visual memory. From Ilg FL, Ames LB: *School readiness,* New York, 1972, Harper & Row.

are told a new telephone number. You might repeatedly say it to yourself before writing the number down on a piece of paper. Unless you actively rehearse the number the memory trace begins to fade, and you may have difficulty recording the new number. This type of memory does have a limited storage capacity, with approximately 7 chunks of information being stored at one time. However, chunks of information can consist of more than one item. For example, a familiar home telephone number typically consists of only two chunks of information.

Long-term memory is where permanent records of objects, events, scenes, and abstract knowledge are stored. In contrast to short-term memory no active rehearsal is necessary to maintain items in long-term memory, and it appears to have unlimited storage capacity. Standardized tests of memory ability usually assess only short-term memory, and this section will concentrate on the specific developmental trends in this area.

It is generally accepted that older children have a greater memory capacity than younger children have.[78] However, anyone who has worked with children in the preschool years realizes that their memory skills for certain events or objects is almost adultlike. Young children will remember a story after only a few readings and may even point out any errors that the reader of the story makes. These events or experiences take place in a context that is meaningful and easily understandable for the child. As a result this type of memory involves the simple recognition of previous events or objects.[78,79] The individual is not making a conscious effort to remember but the act of memory just happens. This type of memory probably shows very little improvement with age and is present in infancy.[78,79]

In contrast, tasks such as remembering a series of symbols or objects that are typically used in standardized testing present difficulties for the younger child. These tasks are usually not part of a meaningful context where simple recognition memory occurs. The child is now faced with doing something to remember the items. This something is termed a "strategy," which is a method or systematic attempt by the individual to aid or enhance memory.[78,79] The child now has to make a voluntary effort to use a particular strategy in a given context. An example of a memory strategy would be tying a string around your finger to remember to go to the grocery store.

As the child matures, there are clear changes in the types of strategies that are used for remembering. In one type of experiment, children of several different ages were given a series of pictures to remember. The experimenter then observed whether children verbally rehearse by observing any movement of their mouths. Children at 5 years of age tend not to use this type of strategy, but at 7 years of age more children will verbally rehearse, and by 10 years the majority of children will use a verbal rehearsal method.[80] In a similar experiment, researchers were able to train younger children (those who did not rehearse) to name the objects or pictures that resulted in an improvement in memory capacity. This indicates that younger children are capable of using verbal rehearsal to aid memory, but they will not spontaneously generate this type of strategy.[81] This has been termed a "production deficit."[79] That is, younger children possess the ability to use memory strategies but are deficient in knowing when, where, and how to use them effectively.

Even after the child is likely to generate a memory strategy there is a continued refinement in how they are used.[78] As children mature, they are able to pick the method that would be best suited for the particular task. They are able to use a broader range of strategies and are aware of when to utilize each method. For example, older children maybe more likely to use imagery or making a picture in their head when the presented items are similar to the ones in Figure 2.7. However, when given a series of letters to remember, they would supplement the visual imagery with verbal rehearsal to enhance their memory.

VISUAL-MOTOR INTEGRATION

Visual-motor integration is the general ability to coordinate visual information processing skills with motor skills. In this section one component of visual-motor integration, which is the ability to integrate form-perception skills with the fine-motor system in order to reproduce complex visual patterns, is emphasized.[65] The integration between the eye and the hand is necessary to perform a broad range of tasks including building puzzles, coloring, and writing. Furthermore, when the child enters school, copying skills are important for successful achievement. Children suffering from a visual-motor dysfunction or delay will often have difficulty copying written work accurately and efficiently.

Early visual-motor development

Early in life visual-motor responses are used to explore and investigate objects in the world. Initially, the infant is faced with the task of coordinating visually guided motor movements. A systematic investigation of the visually directed responses was conducted by White, who described a specific sequence of development.[82] In the first postnatal month the infant will regard visual targets but will not attempt to reach for them. At approximately 2 to 3 months the infant attempts to swipe at objects with a closed fist, but the infant does not attempt to grasp the object. From 3 to 4 months the hands often meet at the body's midline and grasp each other. At approximately 5 months the infant is able to integrate the eye and the hand. The infant will successfully reach for objects and will monitor the position of his hand in relation to the object that he is reaching for.[58,82] Once the child successfully grasps an object he will typically place it in his mouth. In subsequent months there is a refinement of the visual-motor response, and the accuracy while reaching for objects improves.

During the preschool years the child's ability to use underlying visual-motor integration skills to reproduce visual forms emerges. The ability to reproduce visual forms is commonly evaluated by the use of puzzles or paper and pencil tasks. A developmental sequence of reproducing block designs using 1-inch cubes is one method to assess reproduction skills.[83] At approximately 3.0 years the child is able to build a train, at 3.5 years a bridge, and at 4.5 years a gate. These tasks not only require more accurate eye-hand coordination, but also demonstrate the ability to reproduce specific forms. The first attempts to draw are seen at 1.5 to 2.0 years of age when the child starts to scribble lines. There are specific development milestones for when the average child can accurately draw certain geometric forms. At 3 years of age a child can draw a circle, at 4.5 of age a square, at 5 to 5.5 years of age a triangle, and at 8 years of age a diamond.[84]

Visual-motor integration and copying skills

One usually evaluates visual-motor integration in the school-aged years by having the child copy a series of geometric designs using paper and pencil. The most common tests are the Developmental Test of Visual Motor Integration and the Bender Gestalt Test.[84,85] Three primary components contribute to performance on these tests; visual form perception, fine-motor coordination, and integration of visual and motor systems.[39]

The relationship between form perception and visual-motor integration has been researched by correlating nonmotor tests of perception (such as Motor Free Visual Perception Test and the Test of Visual Perceptual Skills) with the Developmental Tests of Visual Motor Integration. Most studies find a correlation on the order of 0.4.[86,87] This indicates that form perception is only moderately correlated with visual-motor integration and that the two tasks measure largely different functions. This is further illustrated by the fact that children can recognize and discriminate forms before they are able to reproduce them.[88] For example, a 3-year-old may recognize a triangle but is unable to copy this figure. However, a certain degree of form-perception ability is probably necessary for performing adequately on tests of visual-motor integration. The relationship between motor skills, both gross and fine, and performance on tests of visual-motor integration has been assessed by correlation of motor-based tests with the Developmental Test of Visual Motor Integration. These studies have found low correlations between the two tasks.[86,87] Motor skills do contribute to performance on tests of visual-motor integration but do not play a major role in the final outcome of the visual-motor integration task. The results of these studies indicate that the integration of the visual and motor systems appears to be the primary factor that determines performance on copying tests and not visual-form perception or fine-motor coordination.

The ability to control and manipulate the writing tool requires adequate fine-motor ability and is one component of performance on visual-motor tests. One of the simplest ways to assess this ability is to observe the child's pencil grip. Gardner[49] assessed the frequency of three commonly seen pencil grips in children from 5 to 15 years of age. The first type was the simian grip, where the pencil or crayon is held with a closed fist. The thumb is often covering the index finger and two or more fingers are wrapped around the pencil (Figure 2.8, *A*). Children using this type of grip usually do not use their finger, wrist, or forearm to control movement. Instead, motion comes from above the elbow, and it is primarily a gross motor movement. This grip is commonly seen in preschool children who are drawing or coloring.

The second type is the intermediate grip, which is a transition from the simian grip to a normal adult pencil grip. This is essentially a three-

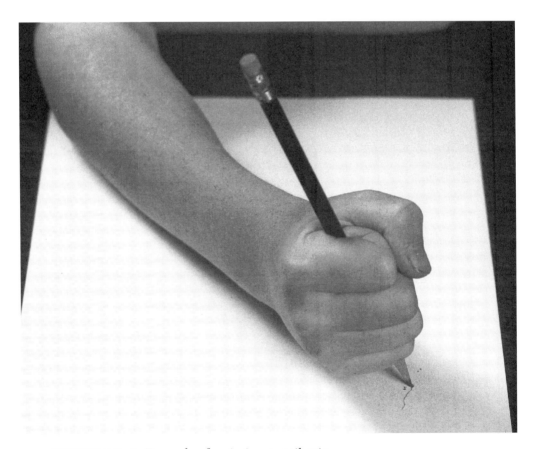

FIGURE 2.8 A, Example of a simian pencil grip.

fingered grip where the pencil is held between the thumb, index, and third finger (Figure 2.8, *B*). The distinctive feature of this grip is that the index and third fingers are hyperextended rather than flexed as in the case with adultlike grips. As a result the pencil is usually rigidly held and control comes primarily from the forearm rather than the fingers and hand.

The third grip is a pincer or tripod grasp, which is considered an adultlike grip (Figure 2.8, *C*). The thumb, index, and third finger are used to hold the pencil, but the fingers are flexed rather than hyperextended. The pencil makes contacts at the tips of the fingers where the pencil rests between the first and index finger. With this grip the pencil is loosely held and can be easily wiggled by the examiner. The primary movement comes from the first three fingers and not the hand or forearm. This indicates that sophisticated fine-motor movements are utilized to control the pencil instead of the less precise movements that characterized the simian and intermediate grips.

A normative study by Gardner[49] assessed the frequency of the three types of pencil grips in children ages 5 through 15. Children who used a pencil grip that did not fit into one of the three categories were excluded from the study (5%). At 5 years of age, when children are entering school, 57% used a tripod grip, 30% used an intermediate grip, and 13% used a simian grip. By 7 years of age 70% used a tripod grip, but 11% were still using a simian grip. At 9 years of age 85% of children used a tripod grip and beyond this age over 90% of children used a tripod grip. These re-

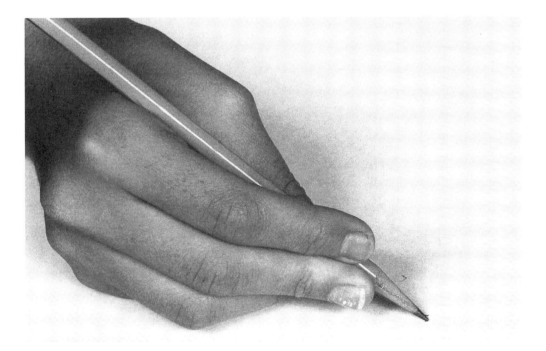

FIGURE 2.8 B, Example of an intermediate pencil grip.

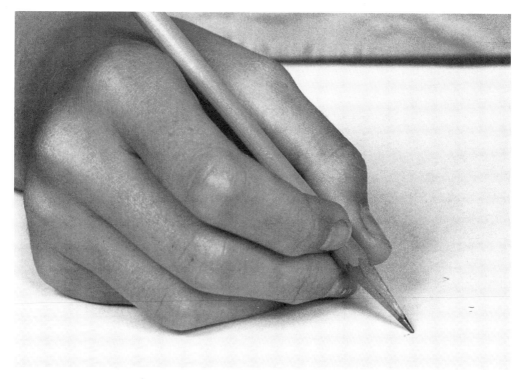

FIGURE 2.8 C, Example of a tripod pencil grip.

sults indicate that a significant number children in the early school years will use a simian or intermediate pencil grip.

Closed-loop system and visual-motor integration

Visual-motor responses can be analyzed within the framework of closed-loop theory. In this approach the motor output influences the visual input through a feedback system. A closed-loop model consists of four interconnected components: input, central processing units (the standard and motor programming unit), output, and feedback loops. A specific model of visual-motor integration using closed-loop theory has been developed by Laszlo and Bairstow[89] to describe visual-motor responses when figures were copied (Figure 2.9).

Input relates to information the subjects receives before copying. Information about the environmental conditions would relate to visual observation about the shapes of the geometric figures and the instrument used for writing. A kinesthetic awareness of body and limb position are necessary to assume the correct position when they are copying. Finally, instructions about the tasks can influence a child's performance. For example, the child may emphasize speed more than accuracy if an instructional set emphasizes this aspect of the task. The instructions should include information about the necessity of reproducing the model figure in size or shape and whether the subject should concentrate on performing the task rapidly or on accuracy.

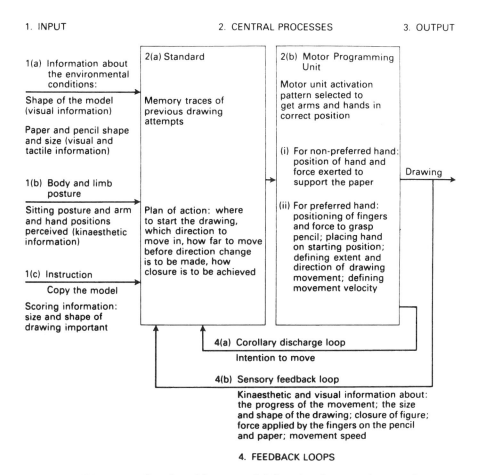

FIGURE 2.9 Diagram of a closed-loop model for visual-motor integration.

From Laszlo JI, Bairstow PJ: *Perceptual-motor behavior: developmental assessment and therapy,* London, 1985, Holt, Rinehart & Winston.

The information from the input system is processed by the *standard* which is the first step of the central processing component. The standard stores memory traces from previous attempts to copy similar figures and sets the level of motivation to perform the task. Based on all the above information, the standard will form a plan of action, which includes the following: the starting point, the direction of movement, where to change direction, and how closure is to be achieved. Once the plan of action is formed, the standard relays the information to the *motor programming unit,* which is the second component of the central processing system. In the motor programming unit the activation of motor units for the dominant and nondominant hand are carried out.

The output is the motor movement made when the child is copying. As part of the closed-loop system two feedback loops carry information back to the standard. The corollary discharge loop is a motor trace of the signal sent to the muscles. The sensory-feedback loop provides ongoing information about the motor movements, which is monitored by the standard. There are two types of sensory information. The kinesthetic information is generated by the muscle receptors and transmits information about static position of limbs and the movement of the limbs including extent, direction, velocity, and force. The visual-feedback loop works in accord with the kinesthetic-feedback system in detecting errors.

What develops in the ability to draw figures? Laszlo and her colleagues have investigated changes in copying behavior as children develop.[90] Specifically they looked at the accuracy for drawing a square and a diamond. These were chosen because oblique lines are more difficult to draw than horizontal or vertical lines. In one experiment they measured the area discrepancy between the drawn figure and the target figure in children 5 to 12 years of age and adults. There was a significant improvement with age in the ability to copy the figures more accurately. The diamonds were especially difficult for the children at 5 to 6 years of age who were largely unsuccessful in their attempts to replicate this figure. The mean percent error improved from 48 in 5-year-olds to 15% for adults.

The younger child may have difficulty drawing a diamond because they are deficient in the ability to draw oblique lines. One can test this hypothesis by having children trace a diamond and compare this performance to the drawing. In tracing and drawing the identical motor movements are required. However, during tracing the demands on planning motor movements are minimized. The children even at 5 years of age were able to trace a recognizable diamond successfully.[90] They tended to deviate from the line more than an older child (indicating poorer fine-motor ability), but they were able to successfully complete the diamond before an age when this would be expected developmentally. These results indicate that the spatial programming and planning ability is a source of difficulty in the younger children and these skills improve with age. Younger children would need external visual cues. which help them organize an appropriate visual-motor plan, to draw complex forms.[91] In contrast, older children would be able to use spatial programming and motor planning skills that are internally generated to draw more complex forms. Another contributing factor to visual-motor development is improvements in the ability to use kinesthetic and visual feedback to monitor and update ongoing performance in drawing. As children mature, they are better able to use feedback information to alter ongoing performance.

SUMMARY

This overview of the developmental characteristics of vision and visual information processing was intended to provide the clinician with an understanding of the normal developmental characteristics of visual skills that are diagnosed and managed by the optometrist. It is important for the clinician to have a solid foundation in the normal developmental pattern of visual skills in order to better understand how deviations in development affect the child. This is especially true for visual processing skills because there are significant changes in performance during the school-aged years. In contrast, accommodation and vergence appears close to adultlike levels by the end of infancy. However, oculomotor skills appear to continue to develop in the preschool and school-aged years.

CHAPTER REVIEW

1. How are developmental trends different when comparing accommodation and vergence ability to oculomotor ability?
2. What are laterally and directionality? When does each ability develop?
3. Why do most children reverse letters and numbers when they enter school? At what age do most children stop making reversal errors?
4. Why do young children remember stories very well but have difficulty remembering a sequence of numbers?
5. What are the components of the closed-loop model for copying figures?

REFERENCES

1. Baldwin WR. Refractive status of infants and children. In Rosenbloom AA, Morgan MW, editors: *Principles and practices of pediatric optometry*, Philadelphia, 1989, JB Lippincott.
2. Banks MS, Dannemiller JL: Infant visual psychophysics. In Salapatek P, Cohen L, editors: *Handbook of infant perception*, vol 1: *From sensation to perception*, New York, 1987, Academic Press.
3. Ciner EB: Management of refractive error in infants, toddlers, and preschool children. In Scheiman MW, editor: *Problems in optometry*, Philadelphia, 1990, JB Lippincott, vol 2.
4. Schor C: Visuomotor development. In Rosenbloom AA, Morgan MW, editors: *Principles and practices of pediatric optometry*, Philadelphia, 1989, JB Lippincott.
5. Shea SL: Eye movements: developmental aspects. In Chekaluk E, Llewellyn K, editors: *The role of eye movements in perceptual processes* (Advances in psychology, 88), Amsterdam and New York, 1992, North-Holland Publishing Co.
6. Banks MS: The development of visual accommodation during early infancy, *Child Dev* 51:646-666, 1980.
7. Brookman KE: Ocular accommodation in human infants, *Am J Optom Physiol Opt* 60:91-99, 1983.
8. Haynes H, White BL, Held R: Visual accommodation in human infants, *Science* 148:528, 1965.
9. Hofstetter HW: Useful age-amplitude formula, *Opt World* 38:42, 1950.
10. Rouse MW, Hutter RF, Schiftlett R: A normative study of the accommodative lag in elementary school children, *Am J Optom Physiol Opt* 61:693-697, 1984.
11. Sivak JG, Bobier CW: Accommodation and chromatic aberration in young children, *Invest Ophthal Vis Sci* 17:705-708, 1978.
12. Scheiman M, Herzberg H, Frantz K, Margolies M: Normative study of accommodative facility in elementary schoolchildren, *Am J Optom Physiol Opt* 65:127-34, 1988.
13. Aslin RN: Motor aspects of visual development in infancy. In Salapatek P, Cohen L, editors: *Handbook of infant perception*, vol 1: From sensation to perception, New York, 1987, Academic Press, Inc.
14. Sondhi N, Archer S, Helveston EM: Development of normal ocular alignment, *J Pediatr Ophthalmol Strabismus* 25:210-211, 1988.

15. Slater AM, Findlay JM: Binocular fixation in the newborn baby, *J Exp Child Psychol* 20:248-273, 1975.
16. Aslin RN: Development of binocular fixation in human infants, *J Exp Child Psychol* 23:133-150, 1977.
17. Aslin RN, Jackson RW: Accommodative convergence in young infants: development of a synergistic sensory-motor system, *Can J Psychol* 33:222-231, 1979.
18. Birch EE, Gwiazda J, Held R: Stereoacuity development for crossed and uncrossed disparities in human infants, *Vision Res* 22:507, 1982.
19. Fox R, Aslin RN, Shea SL, Dumais ST: Stereopsis in human infants, *Science* 207:323-324, 1980.
20. Braddick OJ, Atkinson J: Some recent findings on the development of human binocularity: a review, *Behav Brain Res* 10:71-80, 1983.
21. Ciner EB, Schanel-Klitsch E, Scheiman M: Stereoacuity development in young children, *Optom Vis Sci* 68:533-536, 1991.
22. Kowler E, Martins A: Eye movements of preschool children, *Science* 215:997-999, 1982.
23. Harris CM, Hainline L, Lemerise E, Abramov I: Infant eye movements: quality of fixations, *Invest Ophthalmol Vis Sci* (ARVO suppl) 26:252, 1985.
24. Aslin RN, Salapatek P: Saccadic localization of visual targets by the very young human infant, *Percept and Psychophysics* 17(3):292-302, 1975.
25. Kowler E, Fachiano DM: Kids' poor tracking means habits are lacking, *Invest Ophthalmol Vis Sci* (ARVO Suppl) 22:103, 1982.
26. Aslin RN, Ciuffreda K: Eye movements of preschool children, *Science* 222:74-75, 1983.
27. Leigh RJ, Zee DS: *The neurology of eye movements*, Philadelphia, 1983, FA Davis Co, p 69.
28. Aslin RN: Development of smooth pursuit in human infants. In Fisher DF, Monty RA, Sender JW, editors: *Eye movements: cognition and visual perception*, Hillsdale, NJ, 1981, Lawrence Erlbaum.
29. Maples WC, Atchley J, Ficklin T: Northeastern State University College of Optometry oculomotor norms, *J Behav Optom* 3:143-150, 1992.
30. Palmer LL, Macdonald JE: Monocular and binocular measurements of smooth eye pursuit by rural children in kindergarten and grade two, *Percept Mot Skills* 70:608-610, 1990.
31. Harris CM, Jacobs M, Shawket F, Taylor D: The development of saccadic accuracy in the first seven months, *Clin Vis Sci* 8(1):85-96, 1990.
32. Ross SM, Ross LE: Children's and adults' predictive saccades to square wave targets, *Vision Res* 27:2177-2180, 1987.
33. Gilbert LC: Functional motor efficiency of the eyes and its relationship to reading, *Univ. of Calif Publications in Education* 11(3):159-232, 1953.
34. Grisham D, Simons H: Perspectives on reading disabilities. In Rosenbloom AA, Morgan MW, editors: *Principles and practices of pediatric optometry*, Philadelphia, 1989, JB Lippincott.
35. Taylor EA: *The fundamental reading skill*, ed 2, Springfield, Ill, 1966, Charles C Thomas.
36. Vurpillot E: *The visual world of the child*, New York, 1976. International Universities Press, pp 249-251.
37. Gibson EJ, Levin H: *The psychology of reading*, Cambridge, Mass., 1975, MIT Press, 12-45.
38. Blankenship E: A first primer on visual perception, *J Learn Disabl* 10:39-42, 1971.
39. Richman JE, Cron MT, Garzia RP: Perceptual cognitive development: topical review, *J Optom Vis Dev* 15:4-29, 1984.
40. Kephardt NC: *The slow learner in the classroom*, Columbus, Ohio, 1971, Charles E. Merrill, pp 107-114.
41. Solan HA, Suchoff IB: *Tests and measurements for the behavioral optometrist*, Santa Ana, Calif, Optometric Extension Program, pp 22-27, 1991.
42. Getman GN: *How to develop your child's intelligence*, White Plains, Md, 1984, Research Publication.

43. Cratty BJ: Sensory-motor and perceptual-motor theories and practice: an overview and evaluation. In Walk RD, Pick HL, editors: *Intersensory perception and sensory integration;* New York, 1981, Plenum Press.
44. Suchoff IB: *The visual-spatial development in the child,* New York, 1981, State University of New York Print Shop.
45. Ilg FL, Ames LB: *School readiness,* New York, 1972, Harper & Row, pp 159-189.
46. Kuczaj SA, Maratsos MP: On the acquisition of front, back and side, *Child Dev* 46:202-210, 1975.
47. Piaget J: *Judgement and reasoning in the child,* London, 1928, Routledge & Kegan Paul, pp 96-134.
48. Laurendeau M, Pinard A: *The development of the concept of space in the child,* New York, 1970, International Universities Press, pp 278-309.
49. Gardner RA: *The objective diagnosis of minimal brain dysfunction,* Cresskill, NJ, 1979, Creative Therapeutics.
50. Davidson HP: A study of confusing letters b, d, p, and q, *J Genet Psychol* 47:458-468, 1935.
51. Ilg EL, Ames LB: Developmental trends in reading behavior, *J Genet Psychol* 76:291-312, 1950.
52. Gibson EJ, Gibson J, Pick A, Osser H: A developmental study of the discrimination of letter like forms, *J Comp Physiol Psychol* 55:897-906, 1962.
53. Kaufman NL: Review of research on reversal errors, *Percept Mot Skills* 51:55-79, 1980.
54. Ginsburg GP, Hartwick A: Directional confusion as a sign of dyslexia, *Percept Mot Skills* 32:535-543, 1971.
55. Boone HC: Relationship of left-right reversals to academic achievement, *Percept Mot Skills* 62:27-33, 1986.
56. Kurihara J, Borsting E, Winklestein A: Reversal errors and perceptual ability: a retrospective study, *Optom Vis Sci* (Suppl), 75, 1990.
57. Vellutino FR: Dyslexia, *Sci Am* 256(3):34-41, 1987.
58. Rosinski RR: *The development of visual perception,* Santa Monica, Calif, 1977, Goodyear Publishing.
59. Fantz RL, Fagen JF, Miranda SB: Early visual selectivity. In Cohen LB, Salapatek P, editors: *Infant perception: from sensation to cognition,* New York, 1975, Academic Press.
60. Fagen JF: Infant's recognition of invariant features of faces, *Child Dev* 47:627-638, 1976.
61. Goldstein EB: *Sensation and perception,* Belmont, Calif, 1989, Wadsworth Publishing, pp 333-337.
62. Rogow SM, Rathwell D: Seeing and knowing: an investigation of visual perception among children with severe visual impairments, *J Vis Rehab* 3:55-66, 1989.
63. von Michwitz M: The effect of type and amount of familiarization training on pattern recognition, doctoral dissertation, University of Pittsburgh, 1973.
64. Vurpillot E: The development of scanning strategies and their relation to visual differentiation, *J Exp Child Psychol* 6:632-650, 1968.
65. Solan HA, Groffman S: Understanding and treating developmental and perceptual motor disabilities. In Solan HA, editor: *Treatment and management of children with learning disabilities,* Springfield, Ill, 1982, Charles C Thomas.
66. Goldstein EB: *Sensation and perception,* Belmont, Calif, 1984, Wadsworth Publishing. p 201.
67. Richman JE: Use of sustained attention task to determine children at risk for learning problems, *J Am Optom Assoc* 57:20-26, 1986.
68. Richards GP, Samuels J, Turnure JE, Ysseldyke JE: Sustained and selective attention in children with learning disabilities, *J Learn Disabil* 23:129-136, 1990.
69. Borsting E: Measures of visual attention in children with and without visual efficiency problems, *J Behav Optom* 6:151-156, 1991.
70. Brown RT, Wynne ME: An analysis of attentional components in hyperactive and normal boys, *J Learn Disabil* 17:162-166, 1984.
71. Keogh BK, Margolis J: Learn to labor and to wait: attentional prob-

lems of children with learning disorders, *J Learn Disabil* 9:276-286, 1976.

72. Witkin HA, Oltman P, Karp S: Manual for the Children's Embedded Figures Test, Palo Alto, Calif, 1971, Consulting Psychological Press.

73. Kagan J, Rosman BL, Kay D, Albert J, Phillips W: Information processing in the child: significance of analytical and reflective attitudes, *Psychological Monographs, General and Applied* 78:578, 1964.

74. Salkind NJ, Nelson CF: A note on the developmental nature of reflection-impulsivity, *Dev Psychol* 6:237-238, 1980.

75. Brown RT: A developmental analysis of visual and auditory sustained attention and reflection-impulsivity in hyperactive and normal children, *J Learn Disabil* 15:614-618, 1982.

76. Spoehr KT, Lehmkuhle SW: *Visual information processing*, San Francisco, 1982, WH Freeman & Co, pp 6-7.

77. Haber RN: The impending demise of the icon: a critique of the concept of iconic storage in visual information processing, *Behav Brain Sci* 6:1-54, 1983.

78. Miller PH: *Theories of developmental psychology*, New York, 1989, WH Freeman & Co, pp 289-304.

79. Flavall JH: *Cognitive development*, Englewood Cliffs, NJ, 1977, Prentice-Hall, pp 183-218.

80. Flavell JH, Beach DR, Chinsky JM: Spontaneous verbal rehearsal in a memory task as a function of age, *Child Dev* 37:283-299, 1966.

81. Keeney TJ, Cannizzo SR, Flavell JH: Spontaneous and induced verbal rehearsal in a recall task, *Child Dev* 38:953-966, 1967.

82. White BL, Held R: Observations on the development of visually-directed reaching. In Hellmuth J, editor: *Exceptional infant*, Seattle, 1967, Special Child Publications.

83. Ames LB, Gillespie C, Haines J, Ilg FL: *The child from one to six*, London, 1980, Hamish Hamilton, pp 66-73.

84. Beery KE: *The developmental test of visual motor integration*, Cleveland, 1982, Modern Curriculum Press.

85. Bender L: *A visual motor gestalt test and its clinical use*, Research Monograph 3, New York, 1938, Am Orthopsychiatric Assoc.

86. Erickson G, Borsting E, Motomeni M: The contributions of visual and motor factors to performance on a visual motor integration task: a retrospective study, *Optom Vis Sci* (Suppl), p 103, 1992.

87. Leonard P, Foxcroft C, Kroukamp T: Are visual-perceptual and visual-motor skills separate abilities? *Percept Mot Skills* 67:423-426, 1988.

88. Bee HL, Walker RS: Experimental modification of the lag between perceiving and performing, *Psychonomic Science* 2:127-128, 1968.

89. Laszlo JI, Bairstow PJ: *Perceptual-motor behavior: developmental assessment and therapy*, London, 1985, Holt, Rinehart & Winston.

90. Laszio JI, Broderick PA: The perceptual-motor skill of drawing. In Freman NH, editor: *Visual order of the nature and development of pictorial representation*, New York, 1985, Cambridge University Press.

91. Broderick P, Laszlo JI: The effects of varying planning demands on drawing components of squares and diamonds, *J Exp Child Psychol* 45:18-27, 1988.

CHAPTER 3

Overview of the Normal Learning Process

LOUIS G. HOFFMAN

KEY TERMS

learning	**developmental readiness**
attention	**reinforcement**
cognition	**motivation**
metacognition	**generalization**
strategies	**transferability**
behavior	**anxiety**

With the recognition that behavior can indeed be changed, the learning principles governing the modification of behavior and the larger question of how the organism adapts to its environment have become central issues of twentieth-century psychology.[1]

A general knowledge of the basic principles of learning is extremely important and useful to health care providers, especially those in optometric practice. The primary care optometric practitioner educates patients on a daily basis anticipating that changes in behavior will occur when learning takes place. For example, routine patient education might include explaining the importance of regular vision care; the application, removal, and care of contact lenses; the procedures for home or in-office vision therapy; the care and use of spectacles or a low vision device; or the appropriate dosage and scheduling of medications to prevent or treat ocular disease. How effectively the optometrist understands the basic principles of learning and communicates the information will determine if learning takes place and behavioral changes occur.

A background foundation in learning principles is critical for the optometrist involved in the diagnosis and management of the vision problems of children and adults manifesting learning problems.

THEORIES OF LEARNING

There are many theories of learning, with each theory having it supporters.[2] This chapter is not designed to discuss these theories in depth but rather to give you a brief overview of some of the major theories and their underlying concepts. The goal is to acquire a basic understanding of learning theory and an appreciation of the complexity and importance of learning. This knowledge is significant not only in an educational setting, but also in optometric practice. As noted above, this is especially true if the practitioner is involved in the diagnosis and management of vision deficiencies of patients manifesting difficulties in the learning situation.

The association theories of learning promoted by James[3] and Dewey[4] were concerned with how complex ideas were learned in the first place. The proponents of this theory generally agreed that acquiring a new idea required consistency. What the individual took in through his sensory organs had to be consistent. It could not look, smell, or sound one way one time and another way another time. Attention was another important component of this theory and was called "mental concentration."[5] Also, repetition of the original stimulus or learning situation was critical. Therefore there were three significant components: consistency of the sensory input, attention, and repetition. They also stressed that complex ideas were derived from combining simple ideas. In this theory, learning occurred when sensory impressions were consistent, attention was directed toward the stimuli, and their associations resulted in the formation of simple ideas, which were then combined to form more complex ideas. Repetition then helped to strengthen the associations.

Thorndike's theory of trial and error[6] was the result of experiments performed with animals and observation of the animal's resultant behavior. Thorndike theorized that when confronted with a new situation the motivated learner uses trial and error to obtain satisfaction. A basic premise of this theory is that everything we do as human beings is done to reach some goal we have set or that will satisfy us in some way. There are many different motives or reasons for our behavior in any given situation. Sooner or later, by chance, the individual responds with a set of responses that results in motive satisfaction. Eventually, other less-satisfying responses cease to exist and only the motive-satisfying response remains. Thorndike called this the "law of effect." Skinner[7] expanded the work of Thorndike and used the term "reinforcement" for the term "law of effect." Skinner's concept of learning is that reinforcement is a particular arrangement of stimulus-and-response conditions that bring about new learning.[8] Repetition of the learning situation and its appropriate response is necessary for automaticity. This theory has been called the "contingency of reinforcement theory."

Cognitive psychologists consider the individual an integral part of the learning act. The individual is considered to be an active information processor who actively interacts with the environment and does not passively react to impinging stimuli.[9-11] Cognitive psychologists conceptualize two systems of internal organization: the representational system and the executive system.[9] The representational system deals with how information input is selectively organized, attended to, and meaningfully interpreted. The executive system explains the control processes manifested in the planning, monitoring, checking, and evaluating of our actions. It is these control processes that direct and edit our behavior.[12]

In this approach to learning, the individual must first attend to the task at hand, then selectively organize the sensory input, and then interpret this organized input in a meaningful way that could lead to some action. The individual must then plan and carry out some form of action. Unless this is done, there is no way to ascertain if attention, organization, and meaningful interpretation have occurred. This planned action will be monitored, and the feedback from this monitoring process will be evaluated to ensure accuracy. Any alterations that occur in the original plan of action will be the result of monitoring and evaluating the feedback occurring as a result of the action process.

An education approach for learning-disabled students based on these principles advocates that, first, these students must actively participate in their learning and must assume control of the learning situation.[13,14] Second, teachers must instill in these children the ability to plan, self-monitor, and self-evaluate.[15] Unfortunately, many children who are unsuccessful in the academic situation often develop a passive, maladaptive learning style and acquire maladaptive traits typical of learning "helpless" children.[16,17]

An outgrowth of cognitive psychology and learning theory has resulted in the field of metacognition. Metacognition can be defined as an awareness and regulation of cognitive activity.[18] Two components have been described in defining metacognition.[19,20] The first component is the stable knowledge one possesses about his or her own cognitive processes, referred to as "metacognitive knowledge." An example might be the person who is aware that one would prepare differently for a job interview than for a meeting with friends. The second component is referred to as the "regulation of cognitive activity." For example, the same person who plans an approach to the job interview, monitors the effectiveness of the approach, and evaluates the outcome is engaging in the regulation of cognition.

An important metacognitive concept that has direct application in optometric vision therapy is the use of strategies that allow the individual to go from covert to overt actions. Flavell[21] originated the concept of metacognition and proposed that children failed to generalize learned strategies because they were not aware of the parameters governing the outcome of their performance. Adults, on the other hand, are aware of these parameters. Metacognition enables us to use suitable strategies to deal effectively with task demands.[21,22] Flavell described strategies as a series of steps . . . through which students proceed in order to solve a problem. These steps can be abstracted as general plans for any task, or they can be very task specific. Strategies impose structure by controlling the organization and sequencing of information and the timing and rate of response demand. They can be visible behaviors or internalized cognitive habits.[23]

Metacognitive theories have led to metacognitive instructional methods. The focus of metacognitive instruction is to assist students to identify and enlist strategies to promote and monitor learning. The features of such instruction include (1) careful analysis of the task at hand, (2) the identification of strategies that will promote successful task completion, (3) the explicit instruction of these strategies accompanied by metacognitive information regarding their application, (4) the provision of feedback regarding the usefulness of the strategies and the success with which they are being acquired, and (5) instruction regarding the generalized use of the strategies.[19] It is easily recognizable that this instructional method includes one of the most significant underlying concepts of cognitive psychology—that the student or learner is involved in active participation.[24,13]

By focusing on metacognitive learning we may run the risk of ignoring the need for an adequate knowledge base. Because of the interdependence between knowledge and strategy, we cannot afford to overlook the important educational task of also increasing the content knowledge in the domain upon which metacognitive strategy is to be applied.[25]

WHAT IS LEARNING?

Webster's dictionary defines learning as the acquisition of knowledge or skill. This can be acquired by study, experience, or instruction.[26] Kendel and Hawkins stated that learning is the process by which we acquire new knowledge and memory is the process by which we retain that knowledge over time.[27] The observer of the learning event anticipates that a change in behavior will occur when learning takes place. Therefore behavior can be compared before and after the learning situation to assess whether learning has actually occurred. An increased capability for some type of performance would be expected. There are two additional requirements to be met before learning can be said to have occurred. The change in capability cannot be attributed to growth, and it has to be capable of being retained for some concrete period of time.

A more comprehensive definition and description of learning that combines the above concepts was presented by Gagne.[28] He defined learning as a change in human disposition or capability, that can be retained and that is not simply attributed to the process of growth. He went on to describe the kind of change called learning as one that exhibits itself as a change in behavior, and the inference of learning is made when one compares what type of behavior was possible before the individual was placed in a "learning situation" and what behavior was exhibited after such treatment.

TYPES OF LEARNING

Learning is considered to have occurred when there is a change in performance or behavior as a result of the individual being placed in a learning environment. I will be presenting a model of the learning event that embodies the common characteristics and elements from several different types of learning, but first I would like to review briefly the major types of learning that have been described in the literature.

The conditioned response of Pavlov[29] is well known. In classical conditioning, a stimulus called the "conditioned stimulus" (or more correctly, the "to-be-conditioned stimulus") is repeatedly paired with a highly effective stimulus called the "unconditioned stimulus." The conditioned stimulus initially produces only a small response or no response at all, whereas the unconditioned stimulus elicits a powerful response without requiring any prior conditioning. As a result of conditioning (or learning) the conditioned stimulus becomes capable of producing either a larger response or a completely new response. For conditioning to occur, the conditioned stimulus generally must be correlated with the unconditioned stimulus and precede it by a certain critical time period.[27]

An extension of classical conditioning is operant conditioning or operant learning in which the overt response that is being connected with the new stimulus is not a reflex.[2] Also, in operant conditioning, it is not the presentation of a preceding stimulus that evokes or controls the response. Often, no preceding stimulus can be identified. On the contrary, it is the consequences of the behavior that determine whether it will occur again. Another difference between operant and classical conditioning is that in operant conditioning, the individual must "operate" on the environment before reinforcement takes place.[1] To put it another way, the individual must first do something before reinforcement occurs.

Two other significant types of learning are modeling, or observational, learning[30] and discovery learning.[28] Modeling, or observational, learning takes place through watching or listening to a more experienced individual perform a task. Reinforcement for good performance is also part of this process. As with all types of learning, attention to relevant stimuli that are present in the learning situation is a requirement. Another term that is frequently used for observational learning is imitation learning.

Discovery learning[28] occurs as a result of continued practice of a task, or as a result of experience, with a sudden insight occurring on the part of the learner. This would be comparable to the formation of a *Gestalt*, which could be defined as the sudden reorganization of a field of experience or the discovery of the solution to a problem.[31-33]

BASIC ELEMENTS OF LEARNING EVENTS

In every type of learning event, there are three basic elements. First, there has to be a learner. Second, there must be an event or a stimulus situation. Through the learner's senses and muscles, the stimulus situation in the learner's environment starts a chain of nervous impulses that are organized by the central nervous system. Third, there must be a measurable or observable response to the stimulus, which is the action that results from the stimulus and subsequent nervous system activity. Generally, we refer to these responses as performances or behaviors.[28]

BASIC CONDITIONS OF LEARNING

There are several basic conditions of learning. Rarely do individuals come to any learning situation without some prior knowledge that may be related to the task at hand. Some level of knowledge or experience functions as a prerequisite to the learning event. As an example, an individual may be attempting to learn to take an automobile engine apart. Generally, he or she would know where the engine is located and have some knowledge as to how it functions. These initial capabilities of the learner play an important part in determining the conditions or modifications that may be required if subsequent learning is to take place.

Also, there may be independent external or environmental situations that can have a positive or negative effect in the learning situation.[28] An example of a positive effect might be that it is much easier to learn and remember a foreign language when learned in the country in which that language is spoken compared to a classroom in the United States. An example of the negative effect might be the effects upon learning that may occur during an extremely stressful situation, such as being ridiculed by the teacher while reading aloud in the classroom.

FACTORS AFFECTING THE LEARNING PROCESS

There are two very important factors that have an enormous effect on the learning process: developmental readiness, and cognitive development. The developmental skills the child brings to the classroom can have a significant impact on the success of early learning.

Developmental readiness

Limitations in the performance of human beings can often be directly related to processes of growth. A certain amount of neurological growth must occur before, for example, an infant can take that first step or say that first word. If we attempt to have the infant learn to perform these activities before he or she is maturationally ready, it is generally impossible. The concept of developmental readiness and the associated notion of "stages of development" are the direct result of these observations.[28] If you try to teach something to an individual before that person is developmentally ready to learn it, learning will not occur in a reasonable amount of time and, in some cases, will not occur at all.

The differences in intellectual performance in tasks at different ages, according to Piaget, are reflections of differences in the intellectual skills of logical thinking.[34] In other words, is the child at the necessary cognitive level to be able to deal with materials presented in specific ways? An alternative view is that differences in developmental readiness are primarily attributable to differences in the number and kind of previously learned intellectual skills.[28] In effect, limitations in the learning process may be the result of inadequate developmental readiness, both physically and intellectually.

Individuals require a readiness for learning that includes several factors that must effectively precede the learning event. There must be attention, motivation, and an appropriate level of developmental readiness, both physical and intellectual before learning can occur.

Cognitive development

Another type of developmental process that is significant in learning is cognitive development. The two persons most known for their cognitive theories are Piaget and Werner.

Unlike intelligence or achievement tests, which can tell us a great deal about what a child has learned, Piaget's descriptions of the sequential changes in cognitive ability tell us much more about how a person thinks and learns. Piaget described the sequences in levels of thinking through which children progress and demonstrated the ways in which the thinking process is significantly different in each of the stages of cognitive development.[35] Piaget's stage theory of cognitive development involved four phases of intellectual development.[35]

The first stage is the sensorimotor stage, or stage of sensorimotor intelligence (birth to 2 years). An important point is that Piaget, as have others after him, viewed the infant not as a passive, receptive organism soaking up knowledge like a sponge but rather as an active and interactive organism that operates on his or her environment, seeks new experiences, seeks stimulation, and learns that his or her actions have causal effects on the environment. There are two main tasks in this stage. First, the child establishes a primitive notion of causal thinking. For example, a child learns that by touching the mobile in his or her crib, he or she can make it move. And second, the child establishes object permanence, or constancy.[34] As an example, the child learns that just because his or her mother left the room it does not mean that she is gone forever. In this stage, the child develops internal representations of real objects in his or her surroundings, as well as an internal representation of his or her own body.

During the second stage, the preoperational stage (2 to 7 years of age), the child develops symbolic function. This is the time when a name stands for an object. Egocentrism, the regarding of the self as the center of all things or the inability to take another person's perspective, also occurs in this stage. In the early preoperational stage, the child does not easily understand verbal descriptions but can follow drawings, pictures, or other visual representations of events or concepts.[34]

The concrete operations stage (7 to 11 years of age) is the stage where children are able to reason using factual verbal propositions. They can solve "Who is taller?" problems, they can conserve volume, length, and area and are able to maintain the idea of constancy over apparent change. They can also mentally reverse processes.[9] Not only are they aware that someone is their brother, but they also know that they are this person's brother.

The last stage is the formal operations stage (11 years of age and older). In this stage, adolescents can reflect on their own thinking. They are also able to use deductive reasoning and are extremely concerned about themselves, both from the standpoint of how they look and how their performance is evaluated by others.[34]

Without going into further details about these stages, we should note that although Piaget gave time periods for these stages the significant issue was that they always occurred in the above noted sequence. On the other hand, Werner looked for general principles that applied to cognitive growth.[36] He believed that cognitive development proceeded from syncretic or global undifferentiated functioning to a differentiated and articulated functioning.[37] He, like Piaget, felt that cognitive development proceeded from egocentrism to relativism and from rigidity to flexibility. Werner is not as tied to specific sequences as is Piaget.[37] Where Piaget appears to include the interaction of maturation and experience, which combines nature and nurture, Werner is more attached to nurture.[38]

THE LEARNING-EVENT SEQUENCE

All learning takes place over a finite period of time, and the sequence of events or phases for any of the types of learning is similar (see the box). Initially, we have the presentation of a stimulus situation. An important aspect of this phase is that the presenter should always be aware of the type of stimulus situation that would be most likely to lead to the subsequent phase. Next is the apprehending phase, which involves selective at-

---

An Overview of the Learning-Event Sequence

- Stimulus situation
- Apprehending phase (attending, perceiving, coding)
- Acquisition phase (acquiring)

Result in learning

- Storage phase (retention, memory, storage)
- Retrieval phase (recognition, recall of verbal information, reinstatement and transfer of intellectual skills)
- Observed performance

Result in remembering

tention to the stimulus, perceiving (perception) of the stimulus, and cat-agorizing or coding of the stimulus. This is followed by an acquisition phase, which involves the step of actually acquiring the information. It is at this point that we are able to act upon this new information. The three phases, the stimulus phase, the apprehending phase and the acquisition phase, result in learning. Some internal activity then "puts it into memory store" so that it can be retained over time. This storage phase includes retention and memory storage and leads to the retrieval phase. The retrieval phase includes recognition, recall of verbal information, reinstatement, and transfer of intellectual skills. We can now observe the performance of remembering.[28] It is at this point that we can see the person remember either by recognition or recall, take this information and use it directly in a specific situation, or transfer it to other relevant situations. For example, a child may have learned that ovens are hot and that he can burn himself if he touches or gets too close to the oven. The stimulus situation may have included a picture of an oven or the actual event of getting burned in the past. The child then goes home and sees the oven at home, which may look different from the picture that he was shown, but he understands that it is similar and may also be hot.

Individuals manifesting learning problems in the academic situation may have difficulties in either the apprehending phase of learning or in the retrieval phase. If the apprehending phase is deficient, the individual may have difficulty attending to the stimulus situation. This may result from the inability or difficulty of bringing the stimuli-gathering equipment (such as vision) to bear on the stimulus. As an example, the child may have difficulty aiming his eyes at and maintaining fixation on the object of regard long enough to "apprehend" the stimuli. Deficiencies in the visual system may interfere with an individual's ability to attend to the stimulus situation for the period of time necessary for apprehending. This may be attributable to symptoms of discomfort, which then may result in termination of attention or even complete avoidance of the task. Other health problems, such as allergies, eczemas, or emotional problems may interfere with the ability to attend in the same manner.

Attention is an important prerequisite for perception, occurring during the apprehending phase, and later for cognition. Attentional sets appear to be part of a much larger group of intellectual strategies known as "self-management behaviors."[39] They tend to direct the individual's information-gathering activities and are frequently referred to as "cognitive strategies."[28] Therefore lack of attention can have an enormous effect on perception.

How effectively an individual attends and what he or she perceives is dependent on the individual's mental set. This mental set can be stimulated by verbal instructions or the creation of a specific environment.[40] Most learning situations require specific instructional sets to create an appropriate mental set. As an example, if you were going to teach a specific mathematical concept such as fractions, you might have a picture of a pie divided up into fractional parts to assist in the explanation. Birnbaum[41] describes the significance of communications skills in establishing such mental sets during vision therapy. An accurate perception of the stimulus involves the discrimination of stimuli or parts of stimuli from each other. How effectively the individual can do this is dependent on previous discrimination learning, known as "perceptual learning."[42] At the conclusion of the apprehending phase the individual must then finally code this newly acquired perception. The coding of the information is an important step in the subsequent acquisition phase.

The acquisition phase is difficult to measure. Generally one evaluates it by ascertaining if a target or expected type of performance or behavior that was not present before the learning event is now present. As an example, we might be interested in determining if a child can solve a simple arithmetic problem after we have attempted to teach him or her the concept underlying a similar problem. Even though the child may say he can solve the problem, we would not be certain that the acquisition phase has occurred until the child actually solves the problem. Upon solving the problem we can say that the acquisition phase has occurred and that learning has actually taken place.

If learning is to be considered truly to have occurred, the individual should be able to use the information at a later date to solve a problem. This ability will depend on how effectively the information is stored in memory. There are two types of storage or memory. First, short-term memory, which has a limited capacity and has a duration of up to only approximately 30 seconds. Second, long-term memory, which has unlimited capacity and may persist indefinitely.[28] Long-term memory is of greatest relevance to instruction in educational settings.[28]

The retrieval of information is a major requirement of the learning situation. The retrieval of information may take several forms, such as the retrieval of verbal information, the ability to do some action, or the transfer of learning. Gagne[28] referred to the latter as the reinstatement and transfer of intellectual skills, which requires the individual use his learned capabilities in a new situation. Again, this is significant concept because in the academic situation new information is constantly added to previously learned concepts.

The instructor has the ability to prepare the individual for the learning event by the use of communication skills, the use of specific materials, or the appropriate sequencing of learning events. These conditions generally precede learning and assist in the probability and possibility that it will occur in any given situation.[43] These conditions have a direct effect on the individual's readiness to learn and may be considered the "preconditions" of learning. They are also the most important factors that can be influenced by an instructor. They all relate to an internal state of the learner that can be managed by manipulation of the external environment of the learner. Thus the instructor can facilitate or hinder the learning process by his or her actions.

The apprehending phase, which is the initial stage of every learning act, requires a high level of attention to the stimulus so that perception can occur. By arranging the stimulus presentations to contain, for example, movement, novelty, change, noise, and intensity, we can assist in heightening the individual's level of attention. For example, the noise of a rattle and pleasant verbal sounds are very effective in gaining the attention of an infant. In addition, rather than the parent simply holding the rattle stationary, the parent would move (increased visual stimulus) and shake the rattle (auditory stimulus) to capture the infant's attention. As an individual develops, the ability to control attention internally occurs, and this allows him or her to select the stimuli to be attended to at the appropriate time. This internal set is known as an "attentional set."[40] The individual must learn to direct the sense organs toward the source of the stimulus, discriminate the essential cues within the stimulus, maintain the internal cues that determine sequences of action, and continue the activity that has been begun despite distractions, some of which may be internal. All these events fall within the category of attentional set.[28]

Another factor that may effect the quality of attention is the child's ability to extract the "necessary cues" from the presented stimuli for learning to take place. The child may not even have learned which stimuli to attend to in a particular situation. He or she might not be ready in that he or she does not have the prerequisite knowledge or experience for the presented learning situation. An example might be the individual who wishes to learn how to repair an automobile engine but has absolutely no idea how it works. When the symptoms of the engine problem are described or the damaged parts of the engine are placed before this person, he or she does not have any idea which "necessary clues" might be significant or even where to direct his or her attention.

OTHER FACTORS AFFECTING THE LEARNING PROCESS

There are several other important factors that can affect (positively or negatively) either the individual's learning readiness or the actual learning process just described. Reinforcement, motivation, anxiety, generalization and transferability, response extinction and regression, and anticipatory responses are just a few of these factors that we believe you should have a general knowledge of.

Reinforcement

Another term associated with learning is "reinforcement." Thorndike's "law of effect" stated that learning was believed to be positively influenced when an animal attained through its activity a satisfying state of affairs.[10] Other authors were more direct and suggested that reinforcement was said to have occurred when a motive was directly satisfied, as when the drive for hunger was satisfied, or when there was a reduction in intensity.[35,44,45] Reinforcement serves to strengthen a learned association, its recall, or both. To Skinner[8] the term referred to the particular arrangement of stimulus-and-response conditions to bring about the learning of a new association.

There are different methods of reinforcement that use either positive or negative reinforcement. The "pat on the back" for a job well done and the "slap on the backside" for an objectionable action are respective examples. A cookie, other favors, or a smile may serve as reinforcement. Social reinforcements are rewards derived from social experiences. Social reinforcements are sometimes difficult to ascertain and also tend to change with the times. For example, the changing role of men and women in society has significantly changed the structure of previous social reinforcements.

The schedule of reinforcement will also have an effect on behavior. Animal and human studies have demonstrated that learned behavior that is periodically reinforced persists longer than behavior that is constantly reinforced.[24] In life, partial reinforcement is the rule rather than the exception. This is easily demonstrated by the success of Las Vegas, Atlantic City, and state lotteries across the United States. The gamblers keep coming back even after long periods of losing.

The immediacy of the reinforcement may also have an effect on the learning event. As a rule, the more immediate the reinforcement follows the response, the stronger the association between the two will be; therefore the more likely there will be a repetition of this behavior.

Motivation

Motivation is another significant aspect of human behavior and learning. Much study has gone into this complex subject, and there are several excellent books on the topic.[46-48] Individuals may have many sets of motives. Each may wish to be a member of a specific group, to learn to read, to learn to play certain sports, to be loved, to earn a great deal of money, to maintain his or her health, all at the same time. Many individual's goals may be internally driven, such as the desire for food, warmth and oxygen. These may be considered biological needs, since they are necessary for survival. Secondly, many goals are acquired desires for particular rewards, such as grades, money, power, and acceptance by friends.

The individual must learn an appropriate set of responses to satisfy his or her needs or motives. What may be deemed appropriate in one segment of society may be inappropriate in another. As an example, stealing to acquire money may be acceptable for one segment of the population but not in another. When we have a need or motive and no methods of satisfying this need or motive, tension and frustration occur.

There is a relationship and at times interestingly a lack of relationship between motives and behavior. We expect, for example, that the student who wishes to get good grades will study the appropriate materials for the necessary amount of time to attain this goal. This would demonstrate a positive relationship between motivation and behavior. There are others who claim to want to achieve good grades but do not study. The student who claims to want good grades but does not study may actually have other goals or priorities that take precedence over achieving good grades. What determines whether a motive will produce goal-related behavior? First, the individual must have learned appropriate responses that can effectively satisfy the motive. For example, the child who wants good grades but does not appear to study the necessary amount of time may never have learned appropriate study techniques and habits. Thus we can see the importance of teachers, other role models, books, television, movies, magazines, and newspapers in shaping appropriate responses in our society. Second, the individual must expect that the chosen response in any situation will be successful in reaching the desired goal. The child who studies and fails to get good grades eventually stops studying. The child in the foster home who asks for affection and receives none will stop asking and possibly even withdraw or act out in other ways. The lower the expectancy of gratifying a motive, the less chance the child will behave in a way directed at achieving the goal. There are several critical motives that need to be satisfied for normal child development (see the box).

If the individual has a motive to achieve a goal, we should expect that deprivation of that goal should result in some possible behavioral consequences. Behavior should change after such deprivation, and new behavior should be exhibited that is goal oriented. We can also expect that a new response that results in obtaining the goal should be learned more effectively after, rather than before, deprivation of the goal. The goal may even be used as "bait" or as a reward for learning new behavior. Achieve-

---

Motives of Crucial Importance to a Child's Development

1. Motive for physical contact.
2. Motive for positive evaluation from others.
3. Motive for instrumental aid or assistance from others. (Aid in solving problems or overcoming obstacles.)
4. Motive to reduce uncertainty.
5. Motive for autonomy. (The desire to control one's destiny.)
6. Motive to dominate others.
7. Motive to cause harm or anxiety to others (usually called "hostility").
8. Motive for genital stimulation.
9. Motive for competence.
10. Motive to maximize congruence between one's behavior, motives, or thoughts, and previously acquired standards.

From Flavell JH: In Resnick LB, editor: *The nature of intelligence,* Hillsdale, NJ, 1976, Lawrence Erlbaum, pp 231-235.

ment of the goal may therefore be a form of reinforcement. Presentation of the goal itself may produce a change in behavior. As an example, the offer of tickets to a popular sporting event might significantly change the behavior of a 12-year-old but would have little effect on changing the behavior of a 2-year-old.

Differences among members of our society in the strength and occurrence of various motives are, generally, the result of different value systems of parents and friends and the behaviors they reward. Factors, such as social class, ethnic background, religious affiliations, and even position in the family may affect motives. In real life, many motives may be combined, and such combinations may make it difficult to define the initial motives. As an example, an individual may be highly motivated to acquire money, but the initial motive may be social recognition. In turn, this person may have many material possessions, and the money may allow the domination of others. Motivation is an extremely important factor in learning.

Motivation may be intrinsic or extrinsic. Intrinsic motivation is not dependent on external circumstances; it is inherent in the individual. Intrinsic motivation is generally directed at some goal the individual wants independent of what others may think. In effect, it satisfies the individual. As an example, some individuals strive for good grades even though their home environment may not be conducive to studying. Family and friends may not be interested in becoming educated, thus providing little extrinsic motivation for the individual to study and learn. Extrinsic motivation is not inherent in the individual and generally requires someone else setting the goals for the individual. Unfortunately, in some cases the individual doing the work has to wait for the goal setter to inform him or her if the goal has been achieved. This delays the reinforcement that accompanies successful achievement of a goal. It's much like the puppy looking up to the master or waiting for a pat on the head to ascertain if the action taken by the puppy was what was wanted.

Generalization and transferability

In new situations, the principle of stimulus generalization may be involved in the individual's response to a new stimulus. This principle states that when a response to one cue or stimulus has been learned it is likely to occur to similar stimuli.[28] Very young children overgeneralize and, for example, call all males "Daddy." The developmental or learned correction for this is to develop discrimination of similarities and differences. Again, as the aforementioned young child learns to better discriminate, only the father is called "Daddy." Transferability refers to the use of a particular response in a similar but not exactly the same situation in which the response was learned.[28] An example might be the use of something learned in school and then being applied to a practical situation outside of school. The greater the degree of similarity between the original stimuli and those in the new situation, the greater is the likelihood that the response will occur. Generalization and transferability, as is all learning, are affected by intelligence.

Response extinction and regression

Learned responses do not always continue to remain strong. If responses are not followed by reinforcement, the association between stimulus and response becomes weak and eventually no response occurs. This is referred to as "response extinction."[49] Lack of reward is not the only reason for lack of response. There is a response hierarchy that changes depending on many variables, for example, an individual's age. The change from drinking from a bottle to drinking from a glass occurs because of changing reinforcement from the parents as the child ages.[50] A return to older, more primitive forms of responding is called "regression"; for example, when a new baby is brought home from the hospital, the 3-year-old sibling who has learned to drink from a glass may regress and want a bottle.

Anticipatory responses

Anticipatory responses are common in learning. Responses associated in time with reward or pain may occur earlier in a behavior sequence and affect the efficiency of future behavior.[49] Examples might be the expectation of failure resulting in failure, the child who closes his eyes when the ball is hit to him because he has been hit before, or the child who is laughed at when reading in class refusing to read again.

Anxiety

The emotion of anxiety may have a strong effect in a learning situation. "Anxiety" is a psychological term for that state characterized by an unpleasant feeling tone and either anticipation of an unwanted event or uncertainty about the future.[49] There are several conditions that are most likely to produce anxiety in children (3 years and older): anticipation of loss of nurturance or affection, or physical harm, or the lack of consistency between a rule or socialization the child has learned and his evaluation of his current beliefs or behaviors.

The results of anxiety are the unpleasant effects of helplessness, depression, guilt, and shame. These tend to be present during preschool and early school years.[49] The child who has a history of failure in the learning situation will tend to be anxious in any situation that resembles the original situation.

HIGHER ORDER LEARNING

The learning of complex abilities and content such as ideas, concepts, rules, and principles involves associations between internal processes, as well as the principles of generalization or transfer and discrimination. Gagne proposed a cumulative learning theory or model that attempts to

---

The Eight Types of Learning Proposed by Gagne

1. *Signal learning* (learning a response to a signal, as in classical conditioning)
2. *Stimulus response learning* (learning a connection between a response and a discriminated stimulus)
3. *Chains* (chains of two or more response connections)
4. *Verbal associations* (learning of chains that are verbal)
5. *Multiple discrimination* (in which the individual learns to make different identifying responses to as many different stimuli)
6. *Concept learning* (the acquisition of a capability of making a common response to a class of stimuli that may differ from each other widely in physical appearance)
7. *Principle learning* (a chain of two or more concepts)
8. *Problem solving* (a kind of learning that requires the internal events usually called "thinking")

---

account for such learning. He stated that there are eight types of learning, with the more simple type of learning being a prerequisite for each successive kind of "higher-order" learning (see the box). In thinking, two or more previously acquired principles must be combined to produce a new capability.[28]

STRUCTURING THE LEARNING SITUATION

Inherent in any discussion of learning is how to structure a learning situation to maximize the potential for learning to take place. This is valid both in the classroom and in optometric practice. Control of the external events in the learning situation is what is typically meant by "instruction." It is the teacher or doctor who controls and manipulates these components of instruction. Gagne[3] listed nine steps for controlling and manipulating instruction (see the box). We have found that this a helpful checklist to follow when preparing instruction sets for routine patient education. It may be especially helpful in situations where the patient's behavior has not changed as a result of the doctor's initial instruction. The doctor may be able to identify one or more steps that were not addressed adequately in the case presentation and to use this knowledge to reemphasize important components during follow-up visits.

SUMMARY

This discussion of learning can be synthesized down to four basic learning steps: (1) There must be an awareness on the part of the learner as to what is to be learned. (2) Initially, external feedback must be provided. The instructor (teacher or doctor) must inform the patient if his or her performance is acceptable and why it is or is not acceptable. (3) At some point, the patient must learn to evaluate his or her own performance and should be encouraged to assume this responsibility. (4) Repetition is necessary before knowledge, a skill, or a strategy becomes automatic. The pa-

---

Gagne's Nine Steps for Controlling and Manipulating Instruction

1. *Gaining and controlling attention* (an external stimulus arouses the appropriate attentional set)
2. *Informing the learner of expected outcomes* (communication, usually verbal, tells the learner about the kind of performance he will be able to do after he has learned)
3. *Stimulating recall of relevant prerequisite capabilities* (the learner is reminded of the relevant intellectual skills and also verbal knowledge he has previously learned)
4. *Presenting the stimuli inherent to the learning task*
5. *Offering guidance for learning* (using prompts and hints, usually verbal, the learner's thinking guided)
6. *Providing feedback* (the learner is provided feedback relative to performance)
7. *Appraising performance* (opportunity is given for the learner to verify his achievement)
8. *Making provisions for transferability* (additional examples are used to establish increased generalizability of newly acquired capability)
9. *Ensuring retention* (provisions are made for practice in the new capabilities)

---

tient must be placed in different situations that allow for repetition of the learned capability. This assists in the process of developing automaticity as well as transferability of this new capability. In all learning situations, there must be attention, developmental readiness, and motivation. The learner should be as anxiety free as possible, and, as progress in the learning situation occurs, appropriate reinforcement, repetition, and variety should be provided.

CHAPTER REVIEW

1. Define the term "learning" and describe the sequential steps in a learning event including remembering.
2. Describe the sequential process of metacognitive instruction.
3. Describe the role of the instructor in the learning event.
4. Describe the motives that appear to be most significant to a child's development.
5. Describe Gagne's nine steps for controlling and manipulating instruction.
6. Describe the process of generalization and transferability.

REFERENCES

1. Stoyva J: Learning principles, biofeedback, and behavioral medicine. Simons RC, Pardes H, editors: *Understanding human behavior*, ed 2, Baltimore/London, 1981, Williams & Wilkins.
2. Hilgard ER, Bower GH: *Theories of learning*, New York, 1954, Appleton-Century-Crofts, Educational Division, Meredith Corp.
3. James W: *Principles of psychology*, New York, 1890, Holt, Rinehart & Winston.

4. Dewey J: *How we think,* Boston, 1910, Heath.
5. Mill J: *Analysis of the phenomena of the human mind,* London, 1869, Longmans, Green, Reader and Oyer.
6. Thorndike EL: Animal intelligence: an expermental study of the associative processes in animals, *Psychol Rev Monogr* (Suppl), 2, no 4, 1898.
7. Skinner BF: *The behavior of organisms; an experimental analysis,* New York, 1938, Appleton-Century-Crofts.
8. Skinner BF: *The technology of teaching,* New York, 1968, Appleton-Century-Crofts.
9. Anderson JR: *Cognitive psychology and its implications,* San Francisco, 1975, Freeman.
10. Mandler G: What's cognitive psychology? What isn't? Invitational address, Division of Philosophical Psychology, American Psychological Association Convention, Los Angeles, August 1981.
11. Reeves RA, Brown AL: Metacognition reconsidered: implications for instructional research, *J Abnorm Psychol* 13:343-356, 1985.
12. Miller GA, Galanter E, Pribram KH: *Plans and the structure of behavior,* New York, 1960, Holt, Rinehart & Winston.
13. Brown AL: Metacognitive development and readiness. In Spiro RJ, Bruce BB, Brewer WF, editors: *Theoretical issues in reading comprehension,* Hillsdale, NJ, 1980, Lawrence Erlbaum.
14. Reid DK, Hresko WP: *A cognitive approach to learning disabilities,* New York, 1981, McGraw-Hill.
15. Wong BYL: Metacognition and learning disabilities. In Waller TG, Forrest-Pressley D, McKinnon E, editors: *Metacognition, cognition and human performance,* New York, 1985, Academic Press.
16. McKinney JD, McClure S, Feagans L: Classroom behavior of learning disabled children, *Learning Disability Q 5:45-52, 1982.*
17. Torgeson JK: The role of nonspe-cific factors in task performance of learning-disabled children: a theoretical assessment, *J Learning Disabilities* 10:27-34, 1977.
18. Palincsar AS, Brown DA: Enhancing instructional time through attention to metacognition, *J Learning Disabilities* 20:66-75, 1987.
19. Brown AL: The development of memory: knowing about knowing, and knowing how to know. In Reese HW, editor: *Advances in child development and behavior,* vol 10, New York, 1975, Academic Press.
20. Brown AL: Knowing when, where and how to remember: a problem of metacognition. In Glasser R, editor: *Advances in instructional psychology,* vol 1, Hillsdale, NJ, 1978, Lawrence Erlbaum.
21. Flavell JH: Metacognitive aspects of problem solving. In Resnick LB, editor: *The nature of intelligence,* Hillsdale, NJ, 1976, Lawrence Erlbaum.
22. Wong BYL: Cognitive methods. In Kavale KA, Forness SR, Bender M, editors: *Handbook of learning disabilities,* vol 2: *Methods and interventions,* Boston/Toronto/San Diego, 1988, College Hill Publications, Little, Brown & Co.
23. Lloyd J: Academic instruction and cognitive behavior modification: the need for attack strategy training, *Except Child Q* 1:53-63, 1980.
24. Wittrock MC: The cognitive movement in instruction, *Educational Psychologist* 13:15-30, 1978.
25. Wong BYL: Potential means of enhancing content skills acquisition in learning-disabled adolescents, *Focus on Exceptional Children* 17:1-8, 1985.
26. Neufeldt V, Guralnik DB: *Webster's new world dictionary of American english,* third college edition, Webster's New World, New York, 1988, Simon & Schuster, Inc.
27. Kendel ER, Hawkins RD: The biological basis of learning and individuality, *Sci Am,* special edition, *Mind and Brain,* vol 267, no 3, Sept 1992.
28. Gagne RM: The conditions of

learning, ed 2, New York, 1960, Holt, Rinehart & Winston.

29. Pavlov IP: *Controlled reflexes* (translated by GV Anrep), London, 1927, Oxford University Press.

30. Bandura A, Walters RH: *Social learning and personality development*, New York, 1963, Holt, Rinehart & Winston.

31. Wertheimer M: *Productive thinking*, New York, 1945, Harper & Row.

32. Kohler W: *The mentality of apes*, New York, 1927, Harcourt, Brace & World.

33. Koffka K: *The growth of the mind*, ed 2, New York, 1929, Harcourt, Brace & World.

34. Farley GK: Cognitive development. In Simons RC, Pardes H, editors: *Understanding human behavior*, ed 2, Baltimore/London, 1981, Williams & Wilkins.

35. Piaget J: *The origins of intelligence in children*, New York, 1952, International University Press.

36. Werner H: *Comparative psychology of mental development*, New York, 1973 (originally 1943), International University Press.

37. Werner H: The concept of development from a comparative and organismic point of view. In Harris D, editor: *The concept of development*, Minneapolis, 1957, University of Minnesota Press.

38. Stone LJ, Church J: *Childhood and adolescence, a psychology of the growing person*, ed 4, New York, 1979, Random House.

39. Christ AE: An overview of child and adolescent behavior. In Simons, RC, Pardes H, editors: *Understanding human behavior*, ed 2, Baltimore/London, 1981, Williams & Wilkins.

40. Hebb DO: *A textbook of psychology*, ed 2, Philadelphia, 1966, WB Saunders.

41. Birnbaum MH: The role of the trainer in visual training, *J Am Optom Assoc* 48:1035-1039, 1977.

42. Gibson EJ: Perceptual learning. In Gagne RM, Gephart WR, editors: *Learning research and school subjects*, Itaska, Ill, 1968, Peacock.

43. Gagne RM, Bolles RC: A review of factors in learning efficiency. In Galanter E, editor: *Automatic teaching: the state of the art*, New York, 1959, Wiley.

44. Hull CL: *Principles of behavior*, New York, 1943, Appleton-Century-Crofts.

45. Spence KW: *Behavior theory and conditioning*, New Haven, Conn, 1956, Yale University Press.

46. McClelland DC, Atkinson JW, Clark RA, Lowell EL: *The achievement motive*, New York, 1953, Appleton-Century-Crofts.

47. Hall JF: *Psychology of instruction*, Philadelphia, 1961, Lippincott.

48. Cofer CN, Appley MH: *Motivation: theory and research*, New York, 1964, Wiley.

49. Mussen PH, Conger JJ, Kagan J: *Child development and personality*, ed 3, New York, 1969, Harper & Row.

50. Miller NE: Liberalization of basic S-R concepts: extensions to conflict, behavior, motivation and social learning. In Koch S, editor: *Psychology, a study of a science*, vol 2, New York, 1959, McGraw-Hill.

CHAPTER **4**

Overview of Learning Disabilities

HAROLD A. SOLAN

KEY TERMS

sensory integration	impulsivity
prevalence	attention deficit disorder
genetics	psychostimulants
nutrition	dyslexia
etiology	Irlen filters
low birth weight	eye movements
psychological status	transient/sustained processing
socioeconomic status	PL 94-142

The concept of learning disabilities (LD) has evolved over the past 50 years. Although there were some serious attempts to create a neuropsychological theory before the twentieth century,[1] around the year 1900 two events took place that encouraged psychologists to develop a better understanding of the emerging problem. First, compulsory education laws became effective, resulting in an increased population of school children some of whom displayed limitations in intellectual development. Second, Binet and Simon developed the intelligence test, a milestone that would contribute to providing a means of distinguishing among the normal, the mentally defective, and the "ill balanced." According to Binet and Simon, the "ill-balanced" child was characterized by "unruliness, talkativeness, lack of attention, and sometimes wickedness," a description that appears to resemble some aspects of the learning-disabled child.[2]

Before discussing the characteristics of the learning-disabled child, we should acknowledge that learning is not a single, unitary process. Not only does one kind of learning differ from another, but there are also different kinds of learners. Although the major issues in learning theory have not yet been resolved, it is evident that we are dealing with a heterogeneous population. Not only are their different subtypes of learning-disabled children, but also the subtypes may vary at different age levels.

DEFINITIONS AND THEORIES

As we shall see, a comprehensive testable definition of learning disabilities has eluded the educational community for several decades. Initially I shall attempt to define learning disabilities in terms of the hypotheses and clinical experiences of several respected theorists. The cumulative efforts of these scholars have provided optometry with a philosophical basis to establish the developmental strengths and weaknesses of children who have been identified as learning disabled.

More than 50 years ago Strauss differentiated between the child with hereditary mental retardation and the child whose history was suggestive of the presence of an acquired neurological disorder. That is, he distinguished the endogenously affected child with a familial history of mental retardation from the child who had parents and siblings with normal mentality but whose history revealed evidence of exogenous disorders. Etiological factors included pre-, intra-, and post-natal abnormalities and slight (soft) neurological signs without conspicuous motor impairment. Behavioral signs showed hyperactivity, distractibility, impulsivity, perceptual disorders such as dissociation, perseveration, and catastrophic reactions, all of which came to be known as the "Strauss syndrome,"[3] the predecessor of "learning disabilities." Strauss was probably the first to implicate the central nervous system as a primary cause of learning disorders.

Subsequently, other theorists enhanced Strauss's clinical observations of the peculiarities in thinking, reasoning, and concept formation in these children. For example, Werner[4] stressed that development in the normal child proceeds from a state of relative globality and lack of differentiation to a state of increasing differentiation, articulation, and hierarchical integration. He pointed out that true development in the learning-disabled child must reveal evidence of an increase in complexity of behavior to distinguish it from simple growth. Developmental or ordinal theories of learning, as espoused by Werner, are especially appealing to the developmental optometrist because they provide a "road map" for therapy.

According to Piaget,[5] learning is a function of an individual's biological maturation, especially of the nervous system and of mental functions. He linked normal learning to an individual's development. He postulated that development is not the sum of discrete learning experiences, but rather a total and spontaneous process in which each element of learning occurs as a function of total development. Learning can be a limited process, sometimes limited to a single structure or didactic point. Learning in the absence of suitable developmental structures precludes assimilation and internalization. Although the stimulus is processed and stored, it remains *undigested,* and the ensuing associative learning does not result in generalization. For example, a 3-year-old may be taught to recognize visually the words *bat* and *fig* and to associate the words with a picture of each object. Possibly, albeit not likely, the child may also learn the verbal sub-skills: /b/,/ba/,/at/,/t/, /f/,/fi/,/ig/,/g/. It is not probable, however, that the child will be able to generalize the subskills spontaneously to read the words *big* and *fat* before 5 or 6 years of age when the appropriate developmental structures in the brain become available. That is, without the prior development of an operational framework, the learning disabled child is dependent on external reinforcement, and learning is more likely to be temporary.

Jensen[6] defined readiness to learn as the ability to integrate subskills into a cognitive whole and to generalize and transfer previous learning to new learning. This explanation of learning, in effect, complements Piaget's biological maturation postulate and delineates for the optometrist an orderly three step therapeutic sequence—integrate, generalize, transfer. Jensen also stressed the need for the child to develop his own perception of his increasing mastery of the skills he is trying to acquire. Piaget suggested that this secondary reinforcement results in *intrinsic motivation*.

Birch related learning and reading disorders to the hierarchical integration of the sensory systems. He defined sensory development as an orderly ontogenesis of sensory dominance from the proximoceptive input (gustatory, somatic, and tactual) of the infant and toddler to the telereceptor control system (auditory and visual) of a 7-year-old child. Specifically, Birch[7] concluded: "Reading disability may stem from the inadequate development of appropriate hierarchical organization of sensory systems and so, at least in part, be the product of the failure of the visual system's hierarchical dominance. Failure for such dominance to occur will result in a pattern of functioning which is inappropriate for the development of reading skills." It is probable that Birch's conceptualization of intersensory integration was influenced by Sherrington,[8] who observed that the essential strategy in the evolution of the nervous system has not been the evolution of new avenues of sense, but rather the development of increased liaison among the existing major sensory input systems. The investigations of Birch and Belmont[9] almost three decades ago and Solan et al.,[10] more recently, substantiated that the ability to equate a temporally distributed auditory stimulus to a spatially distributed visual response is one of the characteristics that differentiates good from poor readers in the primary and elementary grades.

Modern definitions

One of the first formal definitions of learning disabilities was developed in 1967 by the National Advisory Committee on Handicapped Children and later incorporated into legislation in Public Law 94-142.[11] This definition has been the standard applied in determining eligibility for services under that law. It reads as follows:

> "Specific learning disability" means a disorder in one or more of the basic psychological processes involved in understanding or in using language, spoken or written, which may manifest itself in an imperfect ability to listen, think, speak, read, write, spell, or do mathematical calculations. The term includes such conditions as perceptual handicaps, brain injury, minimal brain dysfunction, dyslexia, and developmental aphasia. The term does not include children who have learning problems which are primarily the result of visual, hearing or motor handicaps, of mental retardation, of emotional disturbance, or of environmental, cultural, or economic disadvantage.

Combining the theoretical constructs with the operational definitions of learning and reading disabilities into a single coherent statement is a formidable task. This is the problem that the Interagency Committee on Learning Disabilities (NIH) faced in 1987 when they met in Washington, D.C., to update the 1967 definition. Although the revised definition has certain shortcomings, such as not specifically including impaired social skills and attention deficit disorders, the committee believed that the definition reflects the conceptual advances that have emerged from research in the past two decades:[11]

> Learning disabilities is a generic term that refers to a heterogeneous group of disorders manifested by significant difficulties in the acquisition and use of listening, speaking, reading, writing, reasoning, or mathematical abilities. These disorders are intrinsic to the individual and presumed to be due to central nervous dysfunction. Even though a learning disability may occur concomitantly with other handicapping conditions (e.g., sensory impairment, mental retardation, social and emotional disturbance) or environmental influences (e.g., cultural differences, insufficient or inappropriate instruction, psychogenic factors), it is not the direct result of those conditions or influences.

The scope of this "definition" is indeed all inclusive; however, as a theoretical model it is ambiguous and not testable. It would be very difficult to establish the criteria for either meaningful deficits or gains in the skills enumerated. When one combines the "handicapping conditions," "environmental influences," and central nervous system dysfunctions with the learning disabilities enumerated, it is hard to imagine arriving at a common denominator for this group of diverse disorders. Further, many different professional specialties are involved in the diagnosis and treatment of learning disabilities and the factors that influence learning disabilities, and each has its own theoretical perspective. It is unlikely that an educational specialist, an audiologist, a developmental linguist, a neurologist, a neuropsychologist, and an optometrist would share a totally common view of what constitutes learning disabilities. This definition, which has been promulgated by the Interagency Committee on Learning Disabilities (NIH), may be useful for the purpose of identification and classification of learning disabilities in the classroom when the need arises but will be of little help in enhancing our understanding of learning disabilities and facilitating the discovery of fundamental factors that cause them.[12]

PREVALENCE AND INCIDENCE OF LEARNING DISABILITIES

Because the definitions of dyslexia and learning disabilities are not statements of the amount of deficit that constitutes a disability, it has been virtually impossible to establish the number of affected persons in a particular population at a particular time. That is, prevalence varies when different case definitions of the conditions are used, different populations are studied, or studies are done at different ages. The Interagency Committee therefore found that "the studies conducted to date to be totally inadequate to provide anything more than a wide-ranging estimate of this number (10-15% in the elementary school), and concluded that further study is necessary to provide an accurate estimate of the prevalence of learning disabilities in this country. Furthermore, such an endeavor should not be undertaken until there is a national consensus on a definition of learning disabilities, and inclusionary and exclusionary criteria have been agreed upon and standardized."[11]

ETIOLOGICAL CONSIDERATIONS AND TREATMENT APPROACHES

A number of etiological factors have been associated with reading and learning disabilities. These include genetics, nutrition, low birth weight, psychological status, impulsivity, hyperactivity, distractibility, attention deficit disorder, maturation of the nervous system, and dyslexia. Along with this discussion of etiology I will outline some therapy approaches that have been proposed in an attempt to address these underlying conditions.

Genetics

> What is inherited is not this or that phenotypic trait or character but a genotypic potentiality for an organism's developmental response to its environment. Given a certain genotype and a certain sequence of environmental situations, the development follows a certain path. . . . The observed phenotypic variance has both a genetic and an environmental component.[13]

The genetic aspects of reading and learning disabilities represent a complex and challenging topic, since these disabilities compose a *group* of disorders with both significant genetic and environmental determinants. The accumulation of correlational data between genetic and clinical findings will ultimately yield more precise delineation of specific reading and learning disabilities. At the very least, increased understanding of these disorders through genetic analysis should enable the clinician to intervene earlier with more effective preventive and corrective procedures.[14] It is hoped that genetic research will further refine the definition of the phenotype to get closer to the actual gene effects. Since the current definition encompasses many heterogeneous entities that include the central nervous system, phenotype definition is one of the principal issues facing the genetic studies of learning disabilities at this time. Smith concludes that such inability to determine the phenotype makes any effort to elucidate underlying genotypes futile.[15]

Family studies to explain the genetics of a disorder are further complicated by reduced penetrance (not everyone with the genotype exhibits the phenotype), age of onset of disorder, and developmental changes in the manifestations of the disorder. The ideal phenotype (marker phenotype) for family studies is one that is fully penetrant, manifests early in development, and persists in similar form throughout development. Learning disabilities, dyslexia, and hyperactivity frequently show remission. Family history, on the other hand, is very significant in predicting whether a child will become reading or learning disabled. When combined with other risk factors normally included in a comprehensive case history, such as complications of pregnancy and early developmental milestones, family history of reading and learning disabilities can be especially helpful in the early identification of individuals at risk. Early identification with effective preventive intervention is likely to enhance the prospects of academic success in this population of "at-risk" children.[16]

It should be stressed that familial disorders may be caused by heredity or environment. Although the definition of learning disabilities tends to rule out environmental and emotional determinants, there remains the potential for very early psychosocial and biological environmental factors to interact with genetic factors. Oliver, Cole, and Hollingsworth reported in a study, involving 101 learning-disabled children and 171 controls, that a family history of learning problems may be interpreted as consistent with, though not unequivocally supportive of, genetic factors as determinants.[17] In an earlier study, Lewitter, DeFries, and Elston analyzed the data of 133 reading-disabled children and their nuclear families. Their findings supported the hypothesis that reading disability is a genetically heterogeneous disorder (two or more fundamentally distinct genetic antecedents with essentially one phenotype). Analyzing the children's data separately, however, indicated that they are consistent with both genetic and environmental determination.[18] Recent investigations by Pennington and his colleagues strongly support the concept of genetic heterogeneity.[19,20]

Unlike family studies, twin studies can provide more accurate estimates of environmental and genetic contributions to the phenotype, since it is based on the fact that monozygotic (MZ) twins are identical twins and share the same exact genotypes. Same-sex dizygotic (DZ) twins are fraternal twins and share on the average only 50% of their genes. Therefore, if MZ and DZ twins show the same degree of similarity for a trait such as reading disability, we may conclude that the greater degree of genetic similarity of the MZ twins has *not* played an important etiological role in the development of this disorder. On the other hand, if the degree of similarity (concordance) between the MZ twins is significantly greater than that for the DZ twins, genetic factors are playing an important role in the cause. Of course, we must assume equal environmental similarity for the two types of twins.[21]

In an interesting longitudinal study, Matheny, Dolan, and Wilson confirmed that the probability of both twins in a pair being reported to have academic problems was greatly increased if the twins were identical ($p <$ 0.001) or same-sex fraternal ($p <$ 0.01). Furthermore, the identical twins were more concordant than same-sex fraternal twins for all the preschool behaviors such as activity level, distractibility, and feeding and sleeping problems. Although 76% of the MZ pairs were concordant for academic performance, the DZ twins showed a pairwise concordance rate of just 20%. None of the opposite-sex dizygotic twin pairs were concordant.[22] It should be recalled that there are other environmental factors operating in conjunction with the genetic predisposition of the children. For example, compared to singletons, twins are more liable to biological insults in the prenatal and intranatal periods.[23]

During the past 10 years, reports of identification of an inherited form of dyslexia through linkage analysis have appeared. (Linkage analysis tests whether the trait in question is transmitted in nonrandom fashion with another trait that is known to be genetic. The linkage results when two genes are located close to each other on the same chromosome.) Linkage analysis in nine families (84 persons) with apparent autosomal dominant reading disability was reported in 1983. The results strongly supported that a gene on chromosome 15 plays a major etiological role in one form of reading disability.[24] This investigation is continuing, and Pennington has reported that linkage data on 245 individuals in 21 extended families have been completed. The results continue to support genetic heterogeneity. Researchers are also currently testing for a second possible locus on chromosome 6. Apparently, there is evidence for both linkage and genetic heterogeneity.[25]

The genetic transmission of visual and perceptual deficits that have been associated with learning disabilities and dyslexia also need to be investigated with twin research designs. The hereditary component of intelligence, the high correlation between intelligence and reading, and the probability that visual efficiency, visual perceptual, and attentional disorders may have their own genetic models all tend to contribute to the outcome of genetic studies. Equally important, the results could be helpful in refining the definition of the phenotype. A pedigree analysis by Omenn and Weber revealed a pattern of inheritance compatible with an *autosome-dominant* mode of transmission. It is interesting that visual-predominant dyslexia clustered in families of dyslexia with that subtype. This finding indicates that there may be genetically distinct subgroups among dyslexics.[26]

Although twin studies provide us with a "natural experiment" in which the environmental similarity is equal and the degree of genetic similarity is known, not all co-twins of learning disabled MZ twin children are affected. To some extent, we are always dealing with a heterogeneous disability whose phenotype remains to be defined. Furthermore, environmental influences that are difficult to control may impair the ability of the child to respond to academic teaching. For example, although the potential for stature and intellect may be strongly influenced by the genes we inherit, each may be substantially modified by a child's nutritional environment.

Nutrition

Since many children who are identified as reading and learning disabled are also socially and economically disadvantaged, it is imperative for the optometrist to be aware of some of the ways in which food nurtures brain growth. Children who are poorly fed may survive preschool years, but their subsequent failure in school is almost foreordained. *For maturation and growth to be maintained, nutrition must be adequate.* Nutrition is a prime factor in the actualization of the biological and psychological potentialities. Although the former includes a sound physical and neurological base, the latter embraces psychomotor, perceptual, cognitive, and affective maturation. The effects of inadequate nutrition on growth and mental development depend to a large extent on the point in the continuum at which the deprivation occurs, the severity and duration of the deprivation, and the nutrient of which the organism is deprived.[27]

Effects of malnutrition. Two principal strategies have been used to study the consequences of poor nutrition. One approach is to infer a history of malnutrition from deviations of height for age. Short (stunted) children have been assumed to be at greater risk nutritionally than taller ones in communities where malnutrition is endemic. An alternative method is the use of follow-up studies several years after infants have been hospitalized for malnutrition. The identified children are compared to siblings close in age, classmates, or neighbors who do not have a similar history of malnutrition but who reside in communities where the nonnutritional social and economic variables are equally hostile.[28]

Hertzig and associates,[29] using this experimental design, concluded that children who have experienced severe malnutrition in the first 2 years of life have statistically lower intelligence scores at school age than their siblings and classmates have. No association between intellectual level and the ages at which the children were hospitalized for the treatment was revealed by the study. Brain vulnerability therefore is not limited to the first year of life.

Croviato and DeLicardie[30] reported significant differences in intersensory development between malnourished and matched controls.[31] They also reported that tall children (upper quartile of height) performed at a higher level of competence on tests of intersensory integration than stunted children (lower quartile) did. Of particular interest to the optometrists is the implication that functional lags could result from mild to moderate degrees of protein-calorie malnutrition and may not be limited to the extremely severe cases. Serial studies of sensorimotor development have also shown that as recovery from malnutrition takes place developmental quotients, which are much lower than those obtained in nonmalnourished children of similar age and social class, increase in most subjects.

In a more recent study,[32] the motor, perceptual, and cognitive abilities of 99 Filipino children, 4 to 6 years of age, with a documented history of malnutrition were measured using the Revised Manila Motor-Perceptual Screening Test. The children were classified into four groups: normal, acutely malnourished, stunted but not malnourished, and chronically malnourished. Thirty-one normal children of comparable ages and background were similarly tested and served as the control group. Motor and perceptual skill scores were statistically lower in the malnourished than in their normal counterparts, especially in the chronically malnourished group. This research demonstrates the influence of malnutrition on children's development, especially functional skills. Interestingly, cognitive abilities were not affected to the same degree by the malnutrition. A similar study involving somewhat older children, 6 to 8 years of age ($n = 1336$), yielded cognitive performance levels that were quite different.[33] Mean fullscale, verbal, and performance IQs as well as the scores for various subtests decreased with the severity of malnutrition. The authors further observed that even a moderate degree of malnutrition (undernutrition) influences IQ scores. Its effect, however, is of a higher magnitude on immediate memory, visual perception, and visual-motor integration than on verbal reasoning and comprehension. These same children were required to complete seven piagetian tasks covering the mental processes of the concrete operational period.[34] The percentage of malnourished children who remained in the lower preoperational stage of development was significantly higher than that of well-nourished children. A higher percentage of the latter group had advanced to the concrete operational stage. The effect of nutrition on the conservation tasks revealed poor visual and verbal reasoning and conceptualization in malnourished children. Overall, one develops the impression that poor nutrition appears to have a significantly greater influence on mental development in poor social conditions than in good social conditions.[35]

Effects of vitamin and mineral supplements. Studying the effects of vitamin and mineral supplementation on intelligence of school children has yielded some interesting results. Benton and Roberts[36] administered either a vitamin-mineral supplement or a placebo to 90, 12- and 13-year-old adolescents. Although the effect on the verbal IQ was not statistically significant after 8 months, the nonverbal intelligence increased significantly. It is of particular interest that the original diet of this sample of children was typical of British society. The authors do not, however, speculate which specific element was most effective. In commenting on this article, Conners[37] observed: "Unlike verbal IQ, non-verbal IQ depends much less upon the child's exposure to information, language, and unique cultural environment, and it is therefore considered a more 'culture free' and fluid form of intelligence; unlike verbal IQ, which develops rapidly very early in life, non-verbal IQ appears to continue developing through adolescence."

Is it important for a child to eat breakfast before going to school? The effect of omitting breakfast on cognitive functions of three groups of children—stunted, nonstunted, and previously severely malnourished—was examined by Simeon and Grantham-McGregor.[38] The results indicated that cognitive functions are more vulnerable to missing breakfast in poorly nourished children. According to Conners, normal children can miss breakfast without seriously impairing mental functions as measured on a continuous performance test or an arithmetic test. But they do so at the cost of diminishing the probability of functioning optimally. Children whose attention is already impaired and have learning and impulse-control problems are even more likely to suffer from missing breakfast than normals. Compared to normals, hyperactive children are especially vulnerable to impairment in attention after a pure carbohydrate meal. Studies show that protein in breakfast is important, and swamping a child with too much carbohydrate should be avoided.

Effects of dietary modifications. The role of nutrition in ameliorating hyperactivity has been a topic of investigation for almost two decades. Feingold,[39] an allergist, reported a preliminary study in 1974 that suggested a relationship between salicylates, food colors, and additives, and hyperactivity in children. Subsequently, Feingold carried out at least five studies,[40] which, at the very least, support his hypothesis, though they lacked scientific rigor (such as "Four children responded dramatically and 12 had a favorable response"). The structure of the studies was too subjective and global. Parents and teachers were aware of the diet, and therefore certain expectations were present. Feingold was ambiguous on several points: Was he dealing with an allergic or a toxic reaction? How did he define the hyperkinetic syndrome and learning disabilities? What was the role of salicylates?[41] Finally, Feingold's experiments were not controlled for the *placebo effect,* which may run as high as 35%. Several additional studies were completed, but the results were not consistent. A group headed by Conners[42] tested Feingold's hypothesis using a double-blind experimental design. Both parents and teachers reported fewer hyperkinetic symptoms on the Feingold diet as compared to the pretreatment base-line values. The teachers noted a highly significant reduction of symptoms as compared to the control diet. However, the investigators reported some reservations about the experimental design. A subsequent study by Harley et al.[43] obtained teacher ratings, objective classroom and laboratory observational findings, and other psychological measures on 36 school-aged hyperactive boys under experimental control and diet conditions. Although the laboratory observations showed no diet effect, the parents' behavioral ratings indicated a positive response to the experimental diet. Ten of 10 mothers and 4 of 7 fathers of the preschool sample rated their children's behavior as improved on the experimental diet. Mattes and Gittleman[44] sought to maximize the likelihood of demonstrating behavioral effects of artificial food colorings (1) by studying only children who were already on the diet and were reported to respond greatly to artificial food colorings, (2) by attempting to exclude placebo responders and (3) by administering high dosages of colorings. Eleven children participated in this double-blind crossover experiment. Evaluations by parents, teachers, and psychiatrists and psychological testing yielded no evidence of a food-coloring effect. Conners (see ref. 38) performed a second study from which he concluded that his and most other studies find that a small number of hyperactive children among those who showed improvement on Feingold's diet also react adversely when given a challenge of the coloring in a double-blind study. These children do have some specific sensitivity to artificial colors. In their review of the subject, Lipton and Mayo[45] recommended:

> Since the food additive free diet has no apparent harmful effects and since the non-specific placebo effects of this dietary treatment are frequently very beneficial to families, there is no reason to discourage families that wish to pursue this type of treatment as long as they continue to follow other therapy that is helpful.

Effect of orthomolecular therapy. The efficacy of orthomolecular medicine (megavitamin therapy) in helping the learning-disabled child is another area where the treatment outcome has often been supported by either anecdotal evidence or experimental results that are less than rigorous. Dr. Allan Cott,[46] a leading proponent of orthomolecular medicine describes the therapy as ". . . the treatment of disease or disability by intensifying the concentration of substances normally present in the human body and required for good health and optimum mental functioning". He postulates that the orthomolecular approach basically corrects an imbalance of brain chemistry that does not exist among other children. Although he has a specific list of substances, primarily vitamins and minerals that are sugar- and starch-free without artificial colors or flavors, he approaches each child's medical problem on an individual basis and prescribes the items in appropriate dosages to fit each child's needs. He stresses that none of the substances he recommends is a drug or a medication. He considers them to be food items, not pharmacological compounds.

Unfortunately, Dr. Cott's published reports are anecdotal,[47] and it has been difficult to replicate his hypothesis with the usual experimental methods. Brenner's study[48] was not double blind, and therefore the 25% who showed a "dramatic response" were well within the placebo range (30%

to 35%). After following some of his patients for as long as 4 years, he concluded that the hyperkinetic syndrome comprises a greatly heterogeneous group, some of whom will benefit from a program of B-complex vitamins. In a double-blind crossover experiment that was carried out by Haslam and his associates,[49] the results revealed no beneficial effect for children with attention deficit disorder (ADD).

Since there have been some children who have shown significant improvement from megavitamin therapy, as was the case with the Feingold diet, further research is warranted. Conners[38] raises an important ethical issue relating to some of the negative conclusions: "There are no clear cut results, yet the scientific papers, in their abstracts and summaries, talk as though there were." It is important to make a distinction between rigorous statistical reports and anecdotal reports, but optometrists should not, *a priori*, dismiss all anecdotal reports as meaningless, especially when they are reported by experienced clinical observers. Susser observed that the causal relations of nutrition and mental development have been a matter of concern and dispute for the past two decades. In the world at large, however, nutritional and social deprivation go hand in hand.[50] It is apparent that children who survive a severe episode of malnutrition early in life are handicapped in developing skills in reading and writing and are less able to profit from the cumulative knowledge available to the human species in general and to their socioeconomic group in particular.[51]

Low birth weight

Defined as a birth weight less than 2500 grams, low birth weight (LBW) appears as a ubiquitous risk factor when evaluating children who are identified as learning disabled. Although it has more frequently been associated with lower socioeconomic groups, vulnerability includes a broad range of social classes. Low birth weight is most often associated with pre-term birth, equal to or less than 37 weeks. It is not a one-dimensional variable. Within this group, the infant's weight may be appropriate for gestational age (AGA) or small for gestational age (SGA), the latter having a different cluster of antecedents and problems. In every study reviewed, the mean IQs of the LBW children were lower than those of the controls. A double gradient appears to be present: For a given social class, the lower the birth weight (< 2000 g), the lower the IQ is; for a given birth weight, the lower the social class, the lower the IQ. For example, the IQ data of Drillien and associates[52] provide clear birth weight differences between social classes *and* social-class differences within each birth-weight group. LBW children scored worse than the control children of the same social class, but even larger IQ differences were found between social-level groups than between birth-weight groups. The evidence is overwhelming that LBW children who come from disadvantaged socioeconomic groups are more adversely affected than LBW children who come from middle-class homes.[53]

Of special interest to the developmental optometrist is the relationship of perceptual and visual motor skills to low birth weight. Taub, Goldstein, and Caputo[54] reported that, for children with a history of prematurity, verbal IQ scores were not significantly different from those born at term, but performance IQ scores that require visual spatial skills were significantly lower. Poor visually mediated functioning and perceptual organization were also noted on the Visual Motor Gestalt Test. The impairment of visual experience in low birth weight infants, or any infants, has many implications. Therefore it is not unreasonable to speculate that the lag in the maturation of visual function in low-birth-weight infants would contribute to the lower-performance IQ scores, an implication that warrants further research.

Despite warnings by the surgeon general of the USA,[55] cigarette smoking during pregnancy continues to be a problem. It is known to contribute to prematurity, low birth weight, learning disabilities, and certain congenital anomalies.[56] Further, cigarette smoking during pregnancy has been associated with specific decrements in reading and arithmetic, reduced IQ, hyperactivity, impulsivity, and neurological soft signs during childhood.[57] Still, smoking is perceived to pose a lesser risk to pregnancy than alcohol, particularly by women with less education.[58]

Numerous studies are in agreement that low and moderate maternal alcohol use during pregnancy, after adjustment for smoking, produces numerous effects on infant health and development. The following are some of the alcohol-related findings: smaller infant size (birth weight, length, and head circumference), lower Apgar scores, decreased sucking pressure, and increased tremors.[59] By 4 years of age, developmental lags in gross-motor (balance) and fine-motor (motor steadiness) development are evident in children of mothers whose drinking habits can best be described as social drinking.[60] In 7-year-old children, a history of maternal consumption of 2 drinks per day or more on the average was related to a 7-point decrement in IQ even after statistical adjustment for appropriate covariates. In this study, the investigators traced the roots of one important cause of learning problems in young children to their prenatal alcohol exposure.[61] It is of further interest that an additional effect of prenatal alcohol exposure on 7-year-old children is poorer reaction-time and attention scores as measured on a computerized continuous-performance test.[62] Statistically significant effects of prenatal alcohol exposure on subtle measures of attention, visual and verbal memory, and cognitive processing in school-aged children also have been demonstrated.[63] All these developmental factors have serious implications for classroom learning. As is the case for maternal smoking during pregnancy, there is abundant evidence that implicates maternal drinking and supports the surgeon general's recommendation that women should not drink during pregnancy.[64]

Psychological status

Have you ever been in a situation where so much of what you did or said "came out" wrong, no matter how hard you tried? Such is the daily life of the learning-disabled child. In addition to not being able to perform up to expectations in his primary responsibility, the classroom, the LD child has many other burdens troubling an emotional system that becomes more and more fragile. Ultimately, the weight of this developmental ordeal manifests itself in various secondary psychogenic manifestations. Other behaviors that have been associated with learning and emotional disorders are lags in gross and fine motor development and motor planning, impulsive and unpredictable behavior that lacks prior consideration of the consequences of the behavior, and poorly developed social skills and interpersonal relations in school and at home. It is no wonder that Silver described the handicaps of the LD child as "not just school disabilities; they are *life disabilities*."[65]

Although the primary role of the optometrist is to diagnose and treat visual efficiency and visual information processing problems that contribute to the LD child's dysfunctions, it is important to be aware that children with learning problems may have primary or secondary emotional difficulties. Before an optometrist makes a decision about treatment of a vision disorder, he should try to determine if emotional or psychological problems are present.

The school psychologist is another important resource for this information. The optometrist may be concerned about whether the behavior is secondary to the learning problem because the child is failing and frustrated, or that there is a primary emotional disorder. In either case, it should be suggested that the child be seen by a psychologist or psychiatrist for a complete evaluation (Chapter 12). It is important for the optometrist to maintain a collaborative tone during these discussions. The urgency depends on the other parameters involved such as age, degree of hyperactivity and impulsivity, the child's grades and the extent of language deprivation if reading disability is present, and developmental, social, and family history. The inclusion of the mental-health specialist is necessary for the diagnosis and for future treatment. If medication is indicated (discussed later in this chapter), the psychiatrist can make appropriate recommendations.

Gardner[66] recommends that the treatment of children with psychological problems involves a hierarchy of four sequential steps: (1) medication, (2) education, (3) parental guidance, and (4) psychotherapy. The critical question, according to Silver,[67] is whether emotional, social, or family problems are *causing* the academic difficulties or are the *consequences* of the frustrations and failures brought on by the learning disorder. If the emotional, social, or family problems persist after issues 1, 2, and 3 above are treated, some form of psychotherapy may be needed. Wender[23] also subscribes to these procedures but emphasizes the limitations of psycho-therapy. He stresses explaining the child's problem to the child, explaining the drug treatment, and giving therapy to enhance interpersonal relations and ego development to offset the usual history of academic and social trials. He has strong feelings opposing "release therapy," which diminishes the weak controls in these children. In addition, he advocates that the parents follow a firm consistent program to improve the organization at home:

1. Establish a hierarchy of importance, distinguishing between misdemeanors and felonies. Parents must decide what is trivial, what is important, what is essential. Such distinctions allow the child some breathing room.
2. Decide in advance upon a plan for rewards and punishment. The rewards and punishment must be commensurate with the behavior. Also, it should be remembered that either provides attention; thus punishment is more rewarding than ignoring.
3. The one-time principle: By proscribing and prescribing behavior only once before rewarding or punishing, the child is provided with a predictable environment thereby decreasing limit testing.
4. Both parents must predecide to abide by the prescribed course of action.

When minimal problems appear in a child, the optometrist can provide parents with a copy of Wender's four simple rules. Additionally, the optometrist should be familiar with a few of the adaptive behaviors that are characteristic of children with learning disabilities.

Withdrawal reaction. By not participating in classroom and life experiences that could lead to failure or frustration, the child learns to avoid situations (such as reading and math) that are stressful. Sometimes the child reverts to inner fantasy that is perceived as daydreaming by the teacher. In either case the withdrawn child is not available to acquire academic skills that he or she is capable of learning.

Clowning reaction. When a mother describes symptoms that indicate that a child is clowning in school, the optometrist is probably dealing with a serious problem. Here, the child can rationalize that he is not learning because he has *chosen* not to learn. Peer reinforcement is always available, since the lesson is disrupted. Teacher reinforcement may also be present if the child is asked to leave the room, especially if he or she will miss a turn to read.

Regression reaction. The child tries to avoid the potential embarrassment of not being able to perform at an acceptable level by regressing to a less mature level of social and emotional development. Behaviors such as enuresis, baby talk, and silliness reappear, and age-appropriate skills such as dressing and doing chores disappear. This adaptation helps to rationalize a decreased level of class performance and should not be encouraged.

The LD child is at risk on a daily basis. Lowered expectations from peer groups, teachers, and family remind the child that he or she is not taken seriously socially or academically. This self-reinforcing loop ultimately obliterates competencies as well. The optometrist can be therapeutically helpful by planning visual and perceptual programs so that they are success oriented. The child should continually be made aware of progress and taught to recognize increasing mastery of a skill that is being acquired, not only in the vision therapy session, but also in school and at home. This secondary reinforcement ultimately leads to intrinsic motivation. On the other hand, it is necessary to distinguish between "good try" and "good job." Compliments not based on accomplishments that the LD child can recognize are ego-debasing. Visual and perceptual therapy programs, therefore, can play an important role in enhancing the psychological development of the LD child.

Impulsivity, hyperactivity, distractibility, and attention deficit hyperactivity disorder (ADHD)

Most clinicians would agree that the degree to which inattention, impulsiveness, and hyperactivity are implicated in a particular individual varies considerably. Although recollections of the excessively hyperactive children who have been treated are always the most vivid, distractibility and impulsivity are present in a greater share of the learning-disabled children. They are more manageable than the hyperactive children in that their behaviors are more readily modified by the various treatment alternatives that are available. It is also possible that the structured environment in an optometric office where individual (one-to-one) attention is the rule also tends to minimize aberrant behavior.

The definition of impulsivity is situation specific. For example, Wender[23] defines the child's ability to inhibit the performance of an act long enough to become concerned about the consequences of his behavior as *social impulsivity*. Kagan,[68] on the other hand, in discussing cognitive style *(academic impulsivity)* observes that impulsive children "select and report solution hypotheses quickly with minimal consideration for their probable accuracy. Other children, of equal intelligence, take more time to decide about the validity of solutions. The former has been called impulsive, the latter reflective." The premature closure that the optometrist observes signals a failure of the child to process incoming information fully. This lack of assimilation serves to interfere with the ability to generalize. Fortunately, the impulsivity-reflectivity balance most often improves with age in normally achieving children. LD children, however, often find it very difficult to learn to delay their response; they don't "stop and think." As we shall see, this is teachable.

Strauss and Kephart[69] likened the nervous system to a servomechanism that is used in electronic guidance. He postulated that a similar closed-loop system involving feedback control is operative in the perceptual process. Information from the output end of the system is fed back to the input:

> The central nervous system no longer appears as a self-contained organ, receiving inputs from the senses and discharging into the muscles. On the contrary, some of its most characteristic activities are explicable only as circular processes, emerging from the nervous system into the muscles, and re-entering the nervous system through the sense organs, whether they be proprioceptors or organs of the special senses.

That the amount of feedback is variable is particularly significant. At the extremes, there are two distinct possibilities: (1) That all or almost all of the output is fed back to the input, and no motor response takes place (motor regulation). In this case, the child's behavior is *reflective*, since the perceptual process is permitted to continue until a suitable perceptual-motor match has been made. (2) That none of the output is fed back to the input, and the child's motor system responds *impulsively* (Figure 4.1). Since perceptual feedback provides the "next" stimulus in the completion of a task, it is an elemental component of the perceptual-motor match.

The issue of impulsivity, hyperactivity, and distractibility has become a major focus in recent years for clinicians dealing with learning-disabled children. A common term being used today to describe children with learning difficulties is "attention deficit hyperactivity disorder" (ADHD). According to the current definition of ADHD, for a child to be diagnosed as having ADHD he must display a problem for at least 6 months in at least eight of the following characteristics starting before 7 years of age.

1. Often fidgets with hands or feet or squirms in seat (in adolescents this may be limited to subjective feelings of restlessness).
2. Has difficulty remaining seated when required to do so.
3. Is easily distracted by extraneous stimuli.
4. Has difficulty awaiting turn in games or group situations.
5. Often blurts out answers to questions before they have been completed.
6. Has difficulty following through on instructions from others, such as failing to finish chores.

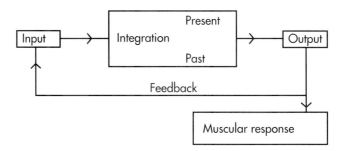

FIGURE 4.1 Diagram of feedback mechanisms in preception.

From Kephart NC: *The slow learner in the classroom,* Columbus, Ohio, 1971, Charles E. Merrill Books.

7. Has difficulty sustaining attention in tasks or play activities.
8. Often shifts from one uncompleted activity to another.
9. Has difficulty playing quietly.
10. Often talks excessively.
11. Often interrupts or intrudes on others, such as butting into other children's games.
12. Often does not seem to listen to what is being said to him or her.
13. Often loses things necessary for tasks or activities at school or at home (toys, pencils, books).
14. Often engages in physically dangerous activities without considering possible consequences, such as running into the street without looking.

A second category is referred to as ADD, or attention deficit disorder without hyperactivity. In these children the primary characteristic is inattentiveness without signs of hyperactivity. It is sometimes referred to as "undifferentiated attention deficit disorder."

ADHD can have a very significant effect on school performance. In the school setting children are asked to sit still, to attend, to concentrate, to comply, to keep quiet, and generally to contain themselves in an effort to learn. A teacher's expectations frequently conflicts with the ADHD child's natural momentum of restless activity or extreme inattentiveness. Teachers often report that these children do not finish their assignments, have trouble following directions, constantly fidget in their seats, carelessly drop materials on the floor, are very curious and distracted by activities around them, and most noticeably talk excessively in the classroom. Sometimes, ADHD children show fine-motor difficulty that can result in poor handwriting and an aversion to written assignments. They also tend to lose their place a great deal more often when reading.

These last two problems relate well to the optometric findings that are commonly found in a child with ADHD. Clinical experience confirms that children with ADHD problems tend to have poor ocular motility and visual perceptual disorders.

In the past, learning-disabled children have been labeled as suffering from minimal brain dysfunction, dyslexia, or neurological impairment. As is the case with dyslexia, the terms ADHD and ADD are sometimes overused. Today, too many professionals use these terms as a synonym for learning problems, regardless of the true nature of the learning problem. It is important for the optometrist to determine whether or not a psychologist or other professional actually reached the diagnosis of ADHD or ADD.

Treatment of impulsivity and ADHD. The treatment program for ADHD is multidimensional and interdisciplinary and may include multiple factors including educational intervention, psychological counseling, behavior modification, optometric intervention, and medication.

There are no simple rules for treating the child who has been identified as impulsive. The concept of a simple dichotomy such as fast/inaccurate and slow/accurate is an oversimplification of decision time that does not take into account either the specific context of the problem or the child's analytic style.[70] For example, Kagan noted that if a child's anxiety over a possible error is much stronger than a desire for quick success he or she will be reflective. If the anxiety over committing an error is weak in relation to the desire for quick success, he or she will be impulsive. The exception is the child who has had a long history of failure and therefore *expects* failure.

Kagan et al.[71] reported that the consequences of trying to modify impulsive behavior with training have been mixed. It may seem like a good place to begin, but delaying response alone is not necessarily a potential "cure" for impulsiveness. Although the training produces response latencies that match those of reflectives, the effect on quality of performance is minimum, since the scores are not significantly affected by the training. (The child may make an instantaneous decision but postpone the response for 15 seconds.) In the second procedure, the examiner tries to serve as a model by persuading the child that the two have common interests, likes, and dislikes. The dialog is accompanied by the examiner displaying reflective behavior throughout the training sessions that include haptic-visual matching, design matching, and inductive reasoning tasks. The effect of modeling in this study is of borderline significance. Egeland[72] trained impulsive children by developing more efficient scanning techniques. His procedures are, in many ways, applicable to optometric vision therapy. Numerous primary-grade children seen by optometrists present with difficulties in taking standardized tests that involve multiple choice responses. They fail to consider carefully all alternatives before making a selection. The children in his study who learned better scanning techniques made significant improvements on standardized reading and vocabulary tests and continued to maintain the improvement 2 months after training.

Cognitive therapy for the management of impulsivity. The efficacy of cognitive self-instructional training procedures in altering impulsive behavior, as developed by Meichenbaum,[73,74] has been especially effective. They provide the child with a mechanism to progress from external to internal control of behavior. The developmental hierarchy starts with overt verbalizations by the therapist, followed by the child's self-verbalization, to covert self-verbalization that results in the child's own verbal control of his nonverbal behavior. In the first of the five steps for completing a block design with design cubes, the therapist talks about what he is doing as he performs the task. Then the child constructs a design as the examiner explains the task. Next, the child describes the task as he performs it. Then the child whispers while performing instead of talking. Finally, the child talks to himself without lip movements as the task is performed. This sequence is sometimes called "fading." The effect is a hierarchical shift in the processing of information that proceeds from external organization to internalization as the child learns to generalize these skills beyond the therapy room. Usually, optometric visual and perceptual therapy extends over a period sufficiently long to bring the various skills under the child's own verbal or discriminative control. Furthermore, the increased success experienced by the child in school, as therapy continues, provides significant behavioral reinforcement. Since the training primarily involves developing learning methods rather substantive abilities, they are known as metacognitive skills.

In treating the problems that result from an impulsive cognitive style in children, optometrists are in the unique position of being able to add another dimension to their therapeutic regimens. Optometrists should consider the potential value of training reflectivity in conjunction with the visual skills being developed with a view toward making a significant difference in the child's academic performance.

Effects of psychostimulants on impulsivity, hyperactivity, and distractibility

Although most people prefer alternatives to the use of medication, the cautious use of certain medications for impulsivity, hyperactivity, and ADHD has been shown to be of benefit at times. More than five decades have past since Bradley[75] observed that amphetamine sulfate (Benzedrine) appeared to have a salutary effect on academic achievement. During the past 20 years, however, research techniques have become much more sophisticated, and the benefits derived from the treatment are more differentiated. Since an estimated 500,000 children who have been identified as learning disabled *and* attention deficit disordered (ADD), with and without hyperactivity, receive psychostimulants,[76] it is important for the optometrist to become familiar with their clinical and behavioral effects. Although psychostimulants are primarily prescribed for hyperactive children who are having academic problems, this therapy is frequently used for children who are distractible or impulsive, or both. It is not usually prescribed for academic underachievement alone.

The psychostimulants that are prescribed most often are methylphenidate (Ritalin), dextroamphetamine (Dexedrine), and pemoline (Cylert). The first two are available in sustained release form, Ritalin SR and Dexedrine spansules. The optimum dosage should be carefully determined by the prescribing physician with help of the parent's and teacher's observations of the child. Since the child's behavior influences all aspects of his or her life, the medication should not necessarily be limited to the school day. Silver[66] points out that hyperactivity and distractibility are not just school disabilities they are life disabilities that interfere with every aspect of family and social life. The problems associated with children who have been so identified are evident at home, with groups of friends, in food markets, and in restaurants. Optometrists who treat children receiving psychostimulant medication should emphasize to the parents the importance of compliance and continuous monitoring of the drug's effectiveness. The action of psychostimulants in modifying a child's behavior has been described as paradoxical, since one would not anticipate that a stimulant could have a salutary effect on hyperactivity, distractibility, and impulsivity. In addition, the child exhibits increased goal-directed activity that results in an increase in completed tasks. The child is more sociable and responsive to both reward and punishment. But most important, as Silver[64] points out, the child is more available to learn. On the other hand, in some children temporary appetite reduction has been reported. Occasionally, sleep disturbances, nail biting, and other tension behaviors are observed initially. Overall, the positive effects significantly outweigh the possible negative effects in most children.

There appear to be two separate issues that have been addressed in the research. The first relates to behavioral changes that have been observed as the result of psychostimulant medication. The second question is concerned with whether the improvement in reading and academic skills is statistically significant. For example, Dykman and Ackerman[77] showed that methylphenidate benefited children who were identified as ADD with and without reading disability. The medication ameliorated hyperactive and aggressive behavior, as well as attentional difficulties. Kavale's[78] review of 135 studies using metanalysis demonstrated "beneficial effects for hyperactive children treated with stimulant drugs." Significant improvements were obtained in perception including visual and auditory memory, motor behavior, and long- and short-term memory with the average drug-treated subject showing a 67% gain. Large positive gains were also found for the Bender Visual Motor Gestalt Test and Frostig Developmental Test of Visual Perception. The notion that methylphenidate improves auditory processing in children with hyperactivity received further support in a comprehensive study of 20 elementary grade children.[79] The effects of methylphenidate in combination with reading remediation on children who do *not* have behavioral disorders were addressed by Gittelman, Klein, and Feingold.[80] The pretreatment and posttreatment increments for the medication group were not significantly different from the placebo group for reading comprehension, auditory discrimination, or oral reading, but in arithmetic the medication group obtained significantly higher scores. It is of special interest to the optometrist that although there was no significant difference between the two groups on the Verbal IQ of the WISC-R, methylphenidate led to improved scores on the Performance IQ where the subtests predominantly require visual spatial processing. The medication may have improved attention, but the acquisition of reading skills was not enhanced in this sample of children with pure reading disorders, and the improvements in mathematics were no longer evident at the 2-month follow-up testing. Brown et al.[81] reported a similar rapid dissipation of measurable effects of stimulant medication upon the discontinuation of pharmacotherapy.

The next logical step would be to show that using methylphenidate to treat hyperactive children who have reading disorders would result in long-term improvement in reading and academic achievement. Richardson et al.[82] concluded that successful methylphenidate treatment of the behavioral symptoms of ADD with hyperactivity in elementary school children is associated with improved academic learning. Measurement of reading achievement, however, was limited to improvement in reading vocabulary. Gadow[83] concludes that although stimulants may increase academic productivity and improve certain behaviors the effect on standardized achievement test scores is not particularly robust. This same point of view is expressed by Swanson et al.[84]:

> Even though it has been established that stimulants do improve *productivity*, it is still unclear whether stimulants alone improve long term academic *achievement*. It remains to be determined whether drug induced enhanced attention during drill and practice operates to produce improvements in basic learning skills, and whether large drug induced increases in short term academic productivity translate into long term increases in academic achievement.

Although there appears to be little controversy as to whether stimulant medication is capable of positively modifying behavior in children who have been identified as hyperactive, the potential for the medication to result in improved academic performance, especially reading, remains unclear. Teaching a child to read who has previously failed is an extremely difficult task, one that includes many complex variables. Even though certain perceptual and cognitive subskills that easily fit into the standardized design of experimental psychologists may reveal positive associations, unless individual supplementary instruction in reading *that meets the individual needs of each subject* is provided in the study, the outcome is foreordained to failure. Unfortunately, most research studies do not lend themselves to matching intervention methods to the cognitive and behavioral strengths and weaknesses of individual children. The need for consistent treatment often is not compatible with optimal remediation.

In 1978, Denckla[85] proposed that stimulants are less than one fourth of the treatment program and until the other three fourths are in progress in home and school it will not even be possible to perceive or report the benefits of that one fourth treatment. Such a perspective on stimulants is a middle-of-the-road position: stimulants are useful adjuncts but not decisive or exclusive cures. Denckla's position is supported by the American Academy of Pediatrics Committee on Children with Disabilities,[86] which recommended that medication for children with attention deficit disorders should never be used as an isolated treatment. As a member of the interdisciplinary team treating the LD child, the optometrist is responsible to recognize when a child can be helped by psychostimulants and, equally important, communicate with the prescribing physician when the dosage appears to require monitoring, perhaps as the result of perceptual therapy.

Maturation of the nervous system

Earlier, in defining learning disabilities, I referred to Piaget's premise that learning is a function of an individual's biological maturation, especially neurological maturation and the development of mental functions. Piaget called this process *embryogenesis.*[5] If Piaget was correct that development is a process that affects the totality of the structure of knowledge, any biological insult that jeopardizes the integrity of the nervous system is of concern to us. In this respect, the vulnerability of the developing fetus and neonate has been particularly evident. In a controlled retrospective study that compared the hospital records of 205 poor readers with those of 205 good readers, Kawi and Pasamanick[87] reported significant differences between the two groups. Mothers of 16.5% of the children who were poor readers had experienced complications during pregnancy or delivery, usually related to a reduction of oxygen supply to the fetus or neonate, compared to only 1.5% of the good readers. And, conversely, not all children who are the product of difficult pregnancies are reading and learning disabled. Why some children are affected by the increased risk whereas others escape remains to be explained. It is possible that the affected children have a greater genetic predisposition for learning problems, and the combined risk is too much to overcome. Neurological development is further compromised by an assortment of medical episodes such as convulsions, concussions, high fevers, and chronic ear infections. The effects of low birth weight have been discussed earlier. The appalling rate of infant deaths in the United States is also a matter of concern, since the high level of infant mortality in any population is suggestive of an increased risk of central nervous system damage to the survivors. The persistently higher infant mortalities for nonwhites whose per capita income levels are lower lend support to the notion that learning disabilities are related to socioeconomic status.[88]

Another area that deserves attention is the so-called soft neurological signs that Strauss[3] identified as exogenous disorders a half a century ago. Such signs are observed by optometrists regularly during developmental evaluations. They include lags in balance and coordination, poor left-right directionality, excessive motor overflow, and a history of delayed early motor and speech and language development.[89] Bender[90] applied the concept of *plasticity* to neuromaturational lag in a way that embryologists use the term: ". . . being as yet unformed, but capable of being formed . . . and carrying within itself the potentialities of patterns which have not yet become fixed." It is as though we were examining a younger child. Our patient shows a broad spectrum of *dysfunctions* but lacks the necessary evidence of *damage* to the central nervous system. Nowhere is the concept of developmental soft signs demonstrated more vividly than among children whose testing reveals a slower than expected differentiation of their perceptual patterns.

Dyslexia

Learning to read is a special and complex kind of learning. Although the stimulus requires visual processing, the final product of reading is dependent on language processing. *Pure dyslexia* may be defined as a severe language-based reading disability usually in the absence of any other specific learning problem. On the other hand, reading disability (RD) will be thought of as a prominent and ubiquitous disorder that is a subset of learning disabilities and may be accompanied by other academic disorders in varying degrees. Clinicians who treat dyslexics generally agree that there exists a population of children who fail to learn to read despite average or better-than-average intelligence, adequate or even abundant educational opportunities, normal sensory development (auditory and visual), normal culturation, no frank brain damage, and no primary emotional disturbance.[91] Although RD may occur concomitantly with other handicapping conditions, mental retardation, emotional disturbance, educational deprivation, hearing impairment, and visual handicaps are eliminated as *primary* determinants in most persons. Reading disability as the diagnosis is dependent on fundamental cognitive disabilities that are frequently of constitutional origins.[92] These constraints may, at first, appear to be substantial; however, they should not suggest to the reader that reading disorders form a homogeneous group of individuals. It is the heterogeneity of the disorder that causes children with different types of reading disability to respond differently to a given assignment. Depending on the definition, it has been estimated that between 2% and 16% of all school-aged children require special educational assistance in reading. (The higher figure is more realistic.) Most contemporary researchers would probably agree that *pure dyslexia* is a relatively rare disorder that affects 3% to 6% of school-aged children and may be related to neurodevelopmental deficits.[93]

In his explorations into the pathogenesis of dyslexia, Galaburda[94] concluded that dyslexics exhibit aberrations in the development of cerebral dominance. The expected anatomical asymmetry in the brain, especially the area in the temporal lobe that accounts for the predominant localization of speech and language, the *planum temporale,* failed to develop appropriately. In a normal right-handed nondyslexic infant, the *planum temporale* located in the left fissure of Sylvius is larger than the homologous area in the right hemisphere. Ordinarily, the left hemisphere develops more slowly than the right, has a greater number of neurons, and is therefore larger. In the dyslexic brain, the right planum is equal in size to the left, making the two symmetrical. Galaburda postulated that this anomalous developmental process may have a genetic origin. The symmetry is caused by disordered prenatal neuronal migration in the left temporal region that resulted in abnormally placed neurons (ectopias) and distorted cortical architecture (dysplasias). This microdysgenesis in those persons destined to become dyslexic is rarely seen in normal brains. It encourages the development of the right hemisphere and may even increase the potential for such a person to become gifted in skills normally attributed to the *right* hemisphere such as mathematics, music, and painting. Symmetry displaces asymmetry. Geschwind and Galaburda speak of this as the "pathology of superiority."[95]

In addition to the individuals just discussed, those who are deficient in verbal and language skills, there exists a second group of dyslexics who have been shown to have weaknesses in visual perceptual,[96] spatial, and oculomotor functions.[97] Pirozzolo has referred to the two subtypes as auditory-linguistic and visual-spatial dyslexics.[98] In the former, the dyslexics show an eye-movement pattern characteristic of young children who are just learning to read: increased number of fixations and regressions and longer durations of fixations. The inefficient eye-movements in these individuals are believed, by some investigators, to be the result of the dyslexia. (A quick test is to remeasure using a lower grade level selection and note the improvement in eye movements.) In visual-spatial dyslexics, on the other hand, one observes increased numbers of regressions and poorly formed return sweeps (reversed staircase) from the end of one line to the beginning of the next line.[91] These findings are in agreement with other spatial findings in the individual and are suggestive of directional disorientations. It should be noted that observations of visual-spatial disorders in dyslexics, especially in the elementary school grades, are not limited to eye movements.[99,100]

Pavlidis[101] postulated that faulty eye movements in dyslexics are the results of a generalized problem involving sequential processing, naming, phoneme identification, and reading. That is, motor sequencing is part of an overall sequencing deficit. If this is true, dyslexics should make significantly more regressions in a nonreading task than normal and retarded readers do. Using five sequentially illuminated lights equidistantly placed in a horizontal array, Pavlidis's 14 dyslexics (mean age, 11 years; mean full-scale IQ, 102) made significantly more eye movements than matched normal readers, but the most prominent difference was the increased number of regressions. Pavlidis concluded that the eye-movement patterns found in dyslexics are not solely caused by problems with reading, but are also relatively independent of the reading material. He proposed that eye-movement patterns and characteristics in the nonreading "lights" test can differentiate dyslexics from normal and other subtypes of retarded readers, possibly even before learning to read.

Failure to learn to read is the most predominant and important subtype of specific learning disability. Even after a century of concern, this enigmatic educational problem has eluded solution. This discussion has addressed the antecedents and characteristics of two of the major subtypes of reading-disabled individuals, auditory-linguistic and visual-spatial. Refractive and binocular dysfunctions are discussed in subsequent chapters.

Irlen filters (tinted lenses) and reading

During the past few years, the use of tinted glasses or plastic overlays has become a "fashionable" treatment approach for children with reading disorders. The term "scotopic sensitivity syndrome" was introduced by Irlen[102] and described as a perceptual dysfunction related to subjective difficulties with light source, luminance, intensity, wavelength, and color contrast. According to Irlen, individuals with this condition are inefficient readers who see the printed page differently from the way the normal reader does and therefore must use more effort and energy when reading. The difficulties they experience may lead to fatigue, discomfort, and inability to sustain attention for extended periods of time.

In addition to their reading difficulties, individuals with scotopic sensitivity syndrome complain of symtoms such as sensitivity to light, eyestrain, difficulty focusing, unstable appearance of the print, words moving on the page, and words appearing as washed out.

In her paper, Irlen[102] claimed that approximately 50% of the reading-disabled and dyslexic populations have this syndrome and that this key factor interferes with the reading process. Irlen has suggested that most individuals with this disorder can be successfully treated using appropriately tinted lenses selected from a range of 150 color possibilities. The lenses that are used to treat patients with scotopic sensitivity syndrome are referred to as "Irlen Filters/Lenses." The objective of this treatment procedure is to eliminate the visual discomfort associated with reading and to improve reading performance.

Although Irlen Filters/Lenses have been publicized in the press, radio, and television as a sucessful treatment for reading disorders, there is a dearth of scientific research available to validate either the syndrome or the treatment approach. A literature review by Evans and Drasdo[103] concluded that because of the poor quality of much of the supporting research, the claims for the efficacy of these procedures cannot be proved or disproved. Recently, a carefully controlled study by Manacker et al.[104] was unable to substantiate the effectiveness of tinted-lens therapy in a well-defined group of children with dyslexia.

Optometrists have raised the issue that subjects diagnosed as having scotopic sensitivity syndrome may simply have a refractive, accommodative, binocular vision, or ocular motility disorder that has not been properly diagnosed.[105] The reason for this concern is the pronounced similarity between the symptoms of Irlen's scotopic sensitivity syndrome and the symptoms associated with accommodative, binocular vision, and ocular motility disorders. Specifically, the following symptoms have been reported to be associated with both scotopic sensitivity syndrome and these vision problems: headaches, eyestrain, excessive blinking, excessive rubbing of the eyes, squinting, intermittent blur, occasional double vision, movement of words on a page, frequent loss of place, skipping lines, inability to sustain effort and concentrate, and re-reading the same words or lines unintentionally.

A recent study by Scheiman et al.[105] demonstrated that 95% of subjects identified as candidates for Irlen filters had significant and readily identifiable vision anomalies ($n = 39$). It is important to stress that Irlen advocates specifically claim that scotopic sensitivity syndrome is an entity separate from vision problems that could be identified in an optometric evaluation. The Irlen brochure implies that each client first receives a complete vision examination and that vision problems are treated before Irlen diagnostic testing. The study by Scheiman et al. addresses this issue. They found that 57% of their subjects either had periodic vision care or at least one eye examination within a year of the study. Of these subjects, 90% had significant uncorrected vision problems. Simply recommending an eye examination is insufficient to rule out an accommodative, binocular vision, or ocular motility disorder. It is also necessary that the appropriate testing be performed to detect the underlying vision disorders.

Our current understanding of Irlen Filters leads to the following conclusions:

- In most cases, persons who believe that they would benefit from Irlen filters probably have accommodative, binocular, ocular motility, or refractive conditions that require traditional optometric care.
- There is not sufficient research evidence to demonstrate that the use of Irlen filters leads to improved reading performance.
- The use of Irlen filters does appear to lead to improved visual comfort in a significant number of patients. The basis for this improvement is unclear.

Clinicians and researchers are currently studying the reason why some subjects feel more comfortable with Irlen filters. The most prominant theory at present us that a transient system processing deficit exists in many reading-disabled individuals and the use of colored filters may have a salutary effect on this disorder.[106]

Transient and sustained processing: a duel subsystem theory of reading disability

The transient and sustained processing systems are two interactive parallel, albeit segregated, visual pathways that operate from the retina via the lateral geniculate nucleus to the visual cortex, extrastriate area, and perhaps the higher visual centers.[107] Retinal images are sampled at least twice by the visual system but not in a redundant manner. The transient subsystem is characterized as motion sensitive, and the sustained subsystem is described as pattern or form sensitive. At first the information is sampled globally by the transient, and then the retinal images are sampled for fine detail by the sustained channel. Any alteration of the normal or-

Characteristics of Transient and Sustained Subsystems

Transient

Short latency and short response persistence.
Sensitivity to low spatial frequencies and high temporal frequencies.
Response to quickly moving targets.
Rate of processing increases as wavelength of light decreases.
Preparation of visual system for input of slower detailed information that follows.

Sustained

Pattern-detection system.
Sensitivity to stationary or slow-moving stimuli.
Response subsequent to transient output and dependence on transient output.
Central (foveal) vision dominant, with detailed visual information and color vision being important functions.
Response during and after stimulus presentation; long response persistence.

der and timing or processing speed of the two pathways can result in a visual processing defect.

Lovegrove et al.[108] has identified a transient deficit in subjects with specific reading disability (SRD). A transient system deficit occurs early in the information processing sequence and is considered to be preattentive. This implies that the input is processed before allocations of significant attentional processes or higher cognitive analysis. The transient system has a major function in all reading tasks that require eye movements. The slower sustained-response system is generated during fixations and extracts the details of the text. Reading requires integration of information across saccades. Transient channels, which are very sensitive to stimulus movements across the retina, diminish the visual persistence effect of sustained channels by erasing the pattern information that persists from the previous fixation. Therefore information extracted during each fixation is separate and processed in proper sequence, thus maintaining clear vision in each fixation. In the presence of a transient-system deficit, the preceding pattern is not erased and the two successive patterns overlap (mask). Significant masking makes the reading process confusing and inefficient.

Researchers have reported that reducing the contrast of text materials with frosted acetate or using short wave (blue)–colored overlays in books and computers normalizes the timing between the transient and sustained systems and leads to improvement in reading performance.[109,110] The former (image blurring) delays the sustained process, whereas the latter increases the rate of processing in the transient-on-sustained system to create the temporal separation between the two subsystems necessary to compensate for the transient processing deficit. The transient processing deficit has been reported to be present in 70% of the population with specific reading disability. Current preliminary research reports that, unlike the

Irlen filters, only blue filters affect the transient system and gray filters or frosted acetate has a beneficial effect on the sustained system.[106] The need for additional research provides a special challenge to optometry.

LEGISLATION AND RIGHTS OF CHILDREN WITH LEARNING DISORDERS

Federal and state laws mandate that each exceptional child has the right to a free and appropriate education to meet the child's unique learning needs from birth to 21 years of age. Many of these rights are defined in U.S. Public Law 94-142 and subsequent legislation (Individuals with Disability Education Act, 1993).[111] The provisions include eligibility, assessment, specially designed classroom instruction, and the related services necessary for the child to benefit from the classroom program in the least restricted educational environment. Exceptional children and their parents are also entitled special protections known as "due process" to assure that their opinions are considered by school officials.

Purpose of the evaluation

In order for a child to be classified under the law, a minimum assessment of the child's cognitive abilities and performance levels in reading, mathematics, and written language must be completed by an interdisciplinary child study team. The classroom teacher or the school psychologist may recommend to the Child Study Team that a child be assessed. It is important that the child and the parent understand the reason for the testing. To thoroughly appraise the child's strengths and weaknesses, many school districts administer much more in-depth evaluations before recommending a child for special education. From the results of the evaluation, the team determines whether the child is exceptional and, if so, the nature of the disability, or whether the child is gifted. An evaluation should also provide information concerning the child's learning style, the type of instruction that would be successful, and a history of previous intervention.

Usually, the child is evaluated under the supervision of a certified school psychologist. Other evaluations may also be needed. For example, a child with a hearing impairment will require the services of an audiologist or otologist or both, and a child with a health or physical impairment may need an examination from a physician. Optometrists may perform perceptual evaluations or may participate under related services (see below).

Parents can request this evaluation by writing a letter to the school that states that they are not satisfied with their child's progress. The school district is responsible to provide the evaluation in a timely manner.

The individualized educational program (IEP)

After the child qualifies for special education, the interdisciplinary child study team in consultation with the parents formulate the individualized education program (IEP). The IEP is a written plan that carefully describes the educational program and services the child will receive. Each year the

IEP is reviewed and, when needed, is revised by the IEP team. The IEP lists the long-term goals, short-term objectives, services to be provided, and evaluative criteria *in detail* that are necessary to meet the child's individual needs as determined during the evaluation. The school officials are responsible to monitor the program carefully. If a child moves from one school district to another, the IEP "moves" with the child, unless the parent and district mutually agree to some other arrangement.

Related services

Related services are usually support services that are necessary to help the student benefit from the education program. They can include transportation to and from school or around the building; physical, occupational, and speech therapy; counseling or psychological services; and school health services. Families may not be charged for related services whether the school district provides them directly or through a private source. If the child has needs that are so complex that the child's home district cannot provide them, the district must assign the child to a program run by a neighboring district, an intermediate unit, or a private school. Vision care by an optometrist, mandated only in California and Massachusetts, is sometimes "contracted out" by the school district to diagnose and treat refractive problems and binocular and perceptual dysfunctions.

Due process

Sometimes school districts do not respond to a child's educational needs in a timely manner. In other cases, the appropriate placement recommended by the child study team is delayed or the implementation of the program is incomplete. The parent can request a hearing. The district is responsible for responding to a written request in 30 days during which time the child continues to attend school in his previous setting. The parents must be notified of the hearing officer's decision within 10 days.

SUMMARY

This chapter concludes the section on *background information*. How the optometrist treats the child who has been identified as learning disabled depends, to a large extent, upon how he or she conceptualizes the problem. Before one can understand aberrant behavior, one must have an understanding of normal behavior. In addition, the effective management of the LD child requires that optometrists must be aware of the contributions of other disciplines, each with its own professional bias. Of special concern is the rendering of appropriate professional care to the economically impoverished and socially disadvantaged children. As long as society continues to deny the poverty that is so pervasive, the role of the optometrist and other professionals in treating children will be limited by nutritional and social constraints. It would be far more economical to treat the causes of many of our educational problems than the product.

Optometrists in practice and in research are cautioned against conceptualizing and treating reading and learning problems in terms of a single factor theory. Research and clinical experience tells us that unidimensional conceptions of learning disabilities are not valid. Problems involving reading disabilities especially, characteristic of many LD children, are often so complex that no theory positing a unitary deficit hypothesis is acceptable. If we are to provide LD children with optimal care, we must facilitate the complete mobilization of our *combined* professional skills so that the benefits of a multidisciplinary approach will accrue to each learning-disabled child.

CHAPTER REVIEW

1. Although optometrists do not prescribe medications such as methylphenidate (Ritalin) to ameliorate impulse disorders and hyperactivity in prepubertal children, those who examine and treat children are often asked for information.
   a. What is meant by the paradoxical effect of stimulant drugs?
   b. Briefly discuss a few positive and negative side effects of stimulant drugs on children with these syndromes.
   c. Under what circumstances would you (or would you not) refer a child under your care to a pediatric psychiatrist or neurologist for the purpose of possibly prescribing Ritalin?
2. Since many children who are identified as reading and learning disabled are also socially and economically disadvantaged, it is imperative for the optometrist to be aware of some of the ways in which food nurtures brain growth. How do you envision the role of optometry and the optometrist in minimizing the effects of inadequate nutrition on growth and visual and mental development?
3. What can the practicing optometrist who treats learning disabled and other children who require special educational services do to assure that their rights are protected with respect to eligibility, assessment, special classroom and supplementary instruction, and related services?
4. The prevalence of reading disorders among children who have been identified as learning disordered is very high. How may the optometrist contribute to the diagnosis and treatment of children who present with a history of reading problems?
5. Many children seen by optometrists for visual and perceptual therapy exhibit social and academic impulsivity, hyperactivity, distractibility, and attentional deficits. All these characteristics can interfere with a student's ability to process information and respond to classroom instruction. In addition, they are also socially disruptive in school and at home. Explain how optometric vision therapy can make a significant difference in these children's academic performance and behavior.

ACKNOWLEDGMENT

The author expresses his gratitude to the staff of the Harold Kohn Vision Science Library at the State College of Optometry State University of New York, for their valued assistance in obtaining many of the references cited in this chapter.

REFERENCES

1. Sequin E: *Idiocy and its treatment by the physiological method,* 1864. Reprinted in 1907 by Teachers College, Columbia University, New York.
2. Binet A, Simon TH: *Mentally defective children.* (Translated by WB Drummond.) London, 1973, Edward Arnold.
3. Strauss AA, Lehtinen LE: *Psychology of the brain-injured child*, vol 1, New York, 1947, Grune & Stratton.
4. Werner H: *Comparative psychology of mental development*, New York, 1948, Science Edition.
5. Piaget J: Development and learning. In Ripple R, Rockcastle V, editors: *Piaget rediscovered*, New York, 1964, Cornell University Press.
6. Jensen AR: Understanding readiness. In Solan HA, editor: *The psychology of learning and reading difficulties*, New York, 1973, Simon & Schuster.
7. Birch HG: Dyslexia and the maturation of visual function. In Money J, editor: *Reading disabilities*, Baltimore, 1962, Johns-Hopkins University Press.
8. Sherrington C: *Man on his nature,* ed 2, Cambridge, 1963, Cambridge University Press, p 175.
9. Birch HG, Belmont L: Auditory visual integration, intelligence and reading ability in school children, *Percept Mot Skills* 20:295-305, 1965.
10. Solan HA, Mozlin R, Rumpf D, et al: The auditory-visual integration test: intersensory or temporal spatial? *J Am Optom Assoc* 54:607, 1983.
11. Learning disabilities: a report to the U.S. Congress, prepared by the Interagency Committee on Learning Disabilities, National Institutes of Health, 1987, p 221.
12. Duffy FH, McAnulty G: Neuropsy-chological heterogeneity and the definition of dyslexia: preliminary evidence for plasticity, *Neuropsychologia* 28(6):555-571, 1990.
13. Dobzhansky T: On genetics, sociology, and politics. In Solan HA, editor: The psychology of learning and reading difficulties, New York, 1973, Simon & Schuster.
14. Moser HW: Genetic aspects of learning disabilities. In Lewis M, editor: Learning disabilities and prenatal risk, Urbana, Ill, 1986, University of Illinois Press.
15. Smith SD: Genetics and learning disabilities, San Diego, Calif, 1986, College-Hill Press, Chap. 1 and 9.
16. Volger GP, DeFries JC, Decker SN: Family history as an indicator of risk for reading disability, *J Learning Disabilities,* 17(10):616-618, 1984.
17. Oliver JM, Cole NH, Hollingsworth H: Learning disabilities as functions of familial learning problems and developmental problems, *Except Child* 57(5):427-440, 1991.
18. Lewitter, FI, DeFries JC, Elston RC: Genetic models of reading disability, *Behav Genet* 10(l):9-30, 1980.
19. Pennington BF, Smith SD: Genetic influences on learning disabilities: an update, *J Consult Clin Psychol* 56(6):817-823, 1988.
20. Pennington BF, Gilger JW, Pauls D, et al: Evidence of major gene transmission of developmental dyslexia, *JAMA* 266(11):1527-1534, 1991.
21. Decker SN, Bender BG: Converging evidence for multiple genetic forms of reading disability, *Brain Lang* 33(2):197-215, 1988.
22. Matheny AP Jr, Dolan AB, Wilson RS: Twins with academic learning problems: antecedent characteristics, *Am J Orthopsychiatry* 46:464, 1976.
23. Wender PH: *Minimal brain dys-*

function in children, New York, 1971, Wiley-Interscience.

24. Smith SD, Kimberling WJ, Pennington BF, Lubs HA: Specific reading disability: identification of an inherited form through linkage analysis, *Science* 219(4590):1345-1347, March 18 1983.

25. Pennington BF: Annotation: the genetics of dyslexia, *J Child Psychol Psychiatry* 31(2):193-201, 1990.

26. Omenn GS, Weber BA: Dyslexia: search for phenotypic and genotypic heterogeneity, *Am J Med Genet* 1:333-342, 1978.

27. Raman SP: Role of nutrition in the actualization of the potentialities of the child, *Young Children* 31(1):24-32, Nov 1975.

28. Solan HA: Learning disabilities. In Rosenbloom AA, Morgan MW, editors: *Principles and practice of pediatric optometry,* Philadelphia, 1989, J.B. Lippincott.

29. Hertzig ME, Birch HG, Richardson SA, et al: Intellectual levels of school age children severely malnourished during the first two years of life, *Pediatrics* 49:814, 1972.

30. Cravioto J, De Licardie ER: Nutrition, mental development and learning. In Falkner F, Tannen J, editors, *Human growth,* vol 3: *Neurobiology and nutrition,* New York, 1979, Plenum Press.

31. Cravioto J, Gaono-Espinosa C, Birch HG: Early malnutrition and auditory-visual integration in school age children, *J Special Educ* 2:75, 1967.

32. Reyes MR, Valdacanas CM, Reyes OL, Reyes TM: The effects of malnutrition on the motor, perceptual, and cognitive functions of Filipino children, *Int Disabil Stud* 12(4):131-136, 1990.

33. Upadhyay SK, Agarwal DK, Agarwal KN: Influence of malnutrition on intellectual development, *Ind J Med Res* 90:430-441, 1989.

34. Agarwal DK, Upadhyay SK, Agarwal KN: Influence of malnutrition on cognitive development assessed by Piagetian tasks, *Acta Paediatr Scand* 78(l):115-122, 1989.

35. Carson DK, Greeley S: Not by bread alone: reversing the effects of childhood malnutrition, *Early Child Dev Care* 30:117-131, 1988.

36. Benton D, Roberts G: Effect of vitamin and mineral supplementation on intelligence of a sample of school children, *Lancet* 1(8578):140-143, Jan. 23, 1988.

37. Conners CK: *Feeding the brain: how foods affect children,* New York, 1989, Plenum Press.

38. Simeon DT, Grantham-McGregor S: Effects of missing breakfast on the cognitive functions of school children of differing nutritional status, *Am J Clin Nutr* 49(4):646-653, 1989.

39. Feingold BF: Hyperkinesis and learning difficulties (H-LD) linked to the ingestion of artificial colors and flavors, Paper presented at the annual meetings of the American Medical Association, section on allergy, Chicago, June 24, 1974.

40. Conners CK: Food additives and hyperactive children, New York, 1980, Plenum Press.

41. Wender EH: Food additives and hyperkinesis, *Am J Disabled Children* 131:1204-1208, 1977.

42. Conners CK, Goyette CH, Southwick DA, et al: Food additives and hyperkinesis: a controlled double blind experiment, *Pediatrics* 58(2):154-166, 1976.

43. Harley JP, Ray RS, Tomasi L, et al: Hyperkinesis and food additives: testing the Feingold hypothesis, *Pediatrics* 61(6):818-827, 1968.

44. Mattes JA, Gittleman R. Effects of artificial food colorings in children with hyperactive symptoms, *Arch Gen Psychiatry* 38:714-718, 1981.

45. Lipton MA, Mayo JP: Diet and hyperkinesis—an update, *J Am Diet Assoc* 83(2):132-134, 1983.

46. Cott A: Dr. Cott's help for your learning disabled child: the orthomolecular treatment, New York, 1985, Time Books.

47. Cott A: Megavitamins: the orthomolecular approach to behavioral disorders and learning disabilities, *Acad Therapy* 7:245-258, 1972.

48. Brenner A: The effect of megadoses

of B-complex vitamins on children with hyperkinesis: controlled studies with long term follow-up, *J Learning Disabilities* 15:258-264, 1982.

49. Haslam RHA, Dalby JT, Rademaker AW: Effects of megavitamin therapy on children with attentional deficit disorders, *Pediatrics* 74:103-111, 1984.

50. Susser M: The challenge of causality: human nutrition, brain development and mental performance, *Bull NY Acad Med* 65(10):1032-1049, 1989.

51. Cravioto J, De Licardie ER: Mental performance in school age children, *Am J Disabled Children* 120:404-410, 1970.

52. Drillien CM, Thomson AJM, Burgoyne K: Low birth weight children at early school age, *Dev Med Child Neurol* 22:26-47, 1980.

53. Cohen SE: The low birth weight infant and learning disabilities: a longitudinal study. In Lewis M, editor: *Learning disabilities and prenatal risk,* Urbana, Ill, 1986, University of Illinois Press.

54. Taub HB, Goldstein KM, Caputo DV: Indices of prematurity as discriminators of development in middle childhood, *Child Dev* 48:797-805, 1977.

55. Surgeon General's advisory on the health consequences of smoking for women, 1980, U.S. Department of Health and Human Services.

56. Johnston C: Cigarette smoking and the outcome of human pregnancy: a status report on the consequences, *Clin Toxicol* 18:189-209, 1981.

57. Butler NR, Goldstein H: Smoking in pregnancy and subsequent child development, *Br Med J* 4:573-575, 1973.

58. Fox SH, Brown C, Koontz AM, Kessel SS: Perceptions of risks of smoking and heavy drinking during pregnancy: 1985 NHIS findings, *Public Health Reports,* Hyattsville 102(l):73-79, 1987.

59. Streissguth AP, Martin DC, Martin JC, Barr HM: The Seattle longitudinal prospective study on alcohol and pregnancy, *Neurobehav Toxicol Teratol* 3:223-233, 1981.

60. Barr HM, Streissguth AP, Darby DL, Sampson PD: Prenatal exposure to alcohol, caffeine, tobacco, and aspirin: effects on fine and gross motor performance in 4-year-old children, *Dev Psychol* 26(3):339-348, 1990.

61. Streissguth AP, Barr HM, Sampson PD: Moderate prenatal alcohol exposure: effects on child IQ and learning problems at age 7½ years, *Alcohol Clin Exp Res* 14(5):662-669.

62. Streissguth AP, Barr HM, Sampson PD, et al: Attention, distraction and reaction time at age 7 years and prenatal alcohol exposure, *Neurobehav Toxicol Teratol* 8:717-725, 1986.

63. Streissguth AP, Bookstein FL, Sampson PD, Barr HM: Neurobehavioral effects of prenatal alcohol: Part III.PLS Analyses of neuropsychologic tests, *Neurotoxicol Teratology* 11:493-507, 1989.

64. Surgeon General's advisory on alcohol and pregnancy: *FDA Drug Bull* 2, 1981.

65. Silver LB: The child psychiatrist's role. In Solan HA, editor: *The treatment and management of children with learning disabilities,* Springfield, Ill, 1982, Charles C Thomas.

66. Gardner RA: MBD: the family book about minimal brain dysfunction, New York, 1973, Jason Aronson.

67. Silver LB: The misunderstood child: a guide for parents of learning disabled children, New York, 1984, McGraw-Hill.

68. Kagan J: Reflection-impulsivity: the generality and dynamics of perceptual tempo, *J Abnorm Psychol* 71(1):17-24, 1966.

69. Strauss AA, Kephart NC: Psychopathology and education of the brain-injured child, vol 2, New York, 1955, Grune & Stratton.

70. Messer SB: Reflection-impulsivity: a review, *Psycholog Bull* 83(6):1026-1052, 1976.

71. Kagan J, Pearson L, Welch L: Modifiability of an impulsive tempo, *J Educ Psychol* 57(6):359-365, 1966.

72. Egeland B: Training impulsive children in the use of more efficient scanning techniques, *Child Dev* 45:165-171, 1974.

73. Meichenbaum DH, Goodman J: Training impulsive children to talk to themselves: a means of developing self-control, *J Abnorm Psychol* 77(2):115-126, 1971.

74. Meichenbaum D: Cognitive-behavior modification: an integrated approach, New York, 1979, Plenum Press.

75. Bradley C: The behavior of children receiving Benzedrine, *Am J Psychiatry* 94:577-585, 1937.

76. Sprague RL, Gadow KD: The role of the teacher in drug treatment, *School Rev* 85:109-140, 1976.

77. Dykman RA, Ackerman PT: Attention deficit disorder and specific reading disability: separate but often overlapping disorders, *J Learning Disabilities* 24(2):96-103, 1991.

78. Kavale K: The efficacy of stimulant drug treatment for hyperactivity: a metaanalysis, *J Learning Disabilities* 15(5):280-289, 1982.

79. Keith RW, Engineer P: Effects of methylphenidate on the auditory processing abilities of children with attention deficit hyperactivity disorder, *J Learning Disabilities* 24(10):630-636, 1991.

80. Gittelman R, Klein DF, Feingold I: Children with reading disorders: II. Effects of methylphenidate in combination with reading remediation, *J Child Psych Psychiatry* 24(2):193-212, 1983.

81. Brown RT, Borden KA, Wynne ME, et al: Methylphenidate and cognitive therapy with ADD children: a methodological reconsideration, *J Abnorm Psychol* 14(4):481-497, 1986.

82. Richardson E, Kupietz SS, Winsberg GG, et al: Effects of methylphenidate dosage in hyperactive reading disabled children: II. Reading achievement, *J Am Acad Child Adolesc Psychiatry* 27:78-87, 1988.

83. Gadow KD: Effects of stimulant drugs on academic performance in hyperactive and learning disabled children, *J Learning Disabilities* 16(5):290-299, 1983.

84. Swanson JM, Cantwell D, Lerner M, et al: Effects of stimulant medication on learning in children with ADHD, *J Learning Disabilities* 24(4):219-230, 1991.

85. Denckla MB: Minimal brain dysfunction. In Chall JS, Hirsky AF, editors: *Education and the brain:* the 77th yearbook of the National Society for the Study of Education, part II, Chicago, 1978, University of Chicago Press.

86. Committee on Children with Disabilities, Committee on Drugs, American Academy of Pediatrics: Medication for children with attention deficit disorder, *Pediatrics* 80(5):758-760, 1987.

87. Kawi AA, Pasamanick B: Association of factors of pregnancy with reading disorders in childhood, *JAMA* 166(12):1420-1423, 1958.

88. Birch HG, Gussow JD: *Disadvantaged children: Health, nutrition, and school failure*, New York, 1970, Grune & Stratton.

89. Gardner RA: *The objective diagnosis of minimal brain dysfunction*, Cresskill, NJ, 1979, Creative Therapeutics.

90. Bender L: Specific reading disability as a maturational lag. In Hoch PH, Zubin J, editors: *Psychopathology of education*, New York, 1958, Grune & Stratton, Chap 11.

91. Stark LW, Giveen SC, Terdiman JF: Specific dyslexia and eye movements. In Stein JF, editor: Vision and visual dysfunction: vision and visual dyslexia, vol 13, Boca Raton, Fa, 1991, CRC Press.

92. Critchley M: *The dyslexic child*. London, 1970, William Heinemann Medical Books.

93. Hynd GW, Cohen M: *Dyslexia: neuropsychological theory, research, and clinical differentiation*, Orlando, Fla, 1983, Grune & Stratton.

94. Galaburda AM: The pathogenesis of childhood dyslexia. In Plum F, editor: *Language, communications, and the brain*, New York, 1988, Raven Press.

95. Geschwind N, Galaburda AM: *Cerebral lateralization: biological mechanisms, associations, and pathology,* Boston, 1987, MIT Press.

96. Mattis S, French J, Rapin E. Dyslexia in children and young adults: three independent neuropsychological syndromes, *Dev Med Child Neurol* 17:150-163, 1975.

97. Pirozzolo FJ, Rayner K: The neural control of eye movements in acquired and developmental reading disorders. In Whitaker HA, Whitaker H, editors: Studies in neurolinguistics, vol 4, New York: Academic Press, 1979.

98. Pirozzolo FJ: Visual spatial and oculomotor deficits in developmental dyslexia: evidence for two neurobehavioral syndromes of reading disability, Ann Arbor, Mich, 1980, University Microfilms International.

99. Satz P, Rardin D, Ross J: An evaluation of a theory of specific developmental dyslexia, *Child Dev* 42: 2009-2021, 1971.

100. Mattis S, French JN, Rapin I: Dyslexia in children and young adults: three independent neuropsychological syndromes, *Dev Med Child Neurol* 17:150-163, 1975.

101. Pavlidis GTh: The role of eye-movements in the diagnosis of dyslexia. In Pavlidis GTh, Fisher DF, editors: *Dyslexia: its neuropsychology and treatment,* New York, 1986, John Wiley & Sons.

102. Irlen H: *Successful treatment of learning disabilities,* Unpublished manuscript presented at the ninety-first annual convention of the American Psychological Association, 1983.

103. Evans BJW, Drasdo N: Tinted lenses and related therapies for learning disabilities—a review, *Ophthalmic Physiol Opt* 11:206-217, 1991.

104. Menacker SJ, Breton ME, Breton ML, et al: Do tinted lenses improve the performance of dyslexic children? *Arch Ophthalmol* 111:213-218, 1993.

105. Scheiman M, Blaskey P, et al: Vision characteristics of individuals identified as Irlen Filter candidates, *J Am Optom Assoc* 61:600-604, 1990.

106. Williams MC, Lecluyse K, Rock-Faucheux A: Effective interventions for reading disability, *J Am Optom Assoc* 63:411-417, 1992.

107. Breitmeyer B, Ganz L: Implications of sustained and transient channels for theories of visual pattern masking, *Psychol Rev* 83:1-36, 1986.

108. Lovegrove W, Martin F, Slaghius W: A theoretical and experimental case for a visual deficit in specific reading disability, *Cogn Neuropsychol* 3:225-267, 1986.

109. Williams MC, Brennan J, Lartigue E: Visual search in good and poor readers, *Clin Vis Sci* 1(4):367-371, 1987.

110. Williams MC, Lecluyse K: Perceptual consequences of a temporal processing deficit in reading disabled children, *J Am Optom Assoc* 61:111-121, 1990.

111. Lemer PS: Education for All Handicapped Children Act, *J Behav Optom* 1:150-153, 1990.

PART TWO

RELATIONSHIP BETWEEN VISION AND LEARNING

CHAPTER **5**

General Issues

NATHAN FLAX

KEY TERMS

vision and learning	**accommodation**
learning problems	**fusion**
visual perception	**handwriting**
attention	**spelling**
dyslexia	**mathematics**
ocular motility	**sensorimotor**

Much of the confusion surrounding the relationship between vision and learning stems from simplistic analysis of both vision and learning. Each is an exceedingly complex function, difficult to define and specify and even more difficult to measure appropriately. As a consequence it is not unusual for researchers to select a few subfactors within the vision complex and assume that these represent the overall entity. Similarly, a single component of the learning process is often utilized to represent learning in its broadest sense. It is no wonder that confusion abounds. It is illogical to assume that all aspects of visual function would relate to all aspects of the learning complex. Too often, the determination of what visual factor or what learning factor to consider is predicated upon the ease of testing or the availability of a particular test instrument rather than careful analysis of why that particular visual function logically relates to the learning task at hand. This chapter will attempt to explore some of the relationships between vision and learning and will emphasize the importance of using a task analysis approach. Each visual function will be analyzed in terms of its potential contribution to the specific learning task addressed.

This chapter is written from the vantage point of an optometric clinician who views the educational process with an orientation that has been shaped by an understanding of vision. The categories utilized may or may not coincide with the way that an educator assesses the problems but nonetheless have proved exceedingly useful in both understanding patient complaints and, even more importantly, being able to explain patient behaviors and predict the outcome of optometric interventions. These are really the major objectives of the clinician: to analyze the nature of the learning task that is deficient, to determine if there is a visual component to the learning dysfunction, and, if such exists, to offer appropriate treatment or management of the problem. This is difficult if not impossible to do if there is failure to establish the fundamental problem itself.

Patients present with complaints such as "doing poorly in school," "failing," "not working up to potential," "has been diagnosed as learning disabled," "hates school work," "has a school problem," or other similar generalized statements. The first objective in this task analysis approach is to gain specific understanding of just what the school problem is.

DEFINING THE NATURE OF THE LEARNING PROBLEM

Learning problems come in a wide variety of styles, and it is necessary to conduct a probing case history to ascertain just what is wrong. For instance, a youngster might present with a "reading problem." What is the nature of this reading problem? Is it failure to learn to read, or an inability to read lengthy assignments at a more sophisticated level? Is it a failure to recall previously encountered words or is it an inability to utilize phonetic analysis to decode an unfamiliar word? Is the youngster able to pronounce all words but not understand what is being read? Are words omitted or other words inserted? Does the length of the reading passage make a difference? Does the size of the type make a difference? These and similar questions must be asked so that one can understand the nature of the reading difficulty.

At the most basic level it is important to determine if visual considerations are likely to be contributory at all. For instance, a patient presents with the complaint of "reading problem with poor comprehension." During the history it is established that there is no difficulty with pronouncing each word correctly regardless of the grade level or difficulty of the word. There are no indications of fatigue, the child works for hours quite diligently but does not seem to understand what is being read. He can pronounce words but not define them. He does no better when the reading passage is read aloud to him. When attempting to explain what has just been read, he repeats the very same words that were in the text but does not offer synonyms, alternative phrases, or anything suggesting insight despite the fact that the mechanics of reading seem to be intact. Given this history, are visual factors likely to be major contributors to this youngster's reading problem? Probably not.

Contrast this with a second youngster who also has a "reading problem" that the teacher has identified as being "poor comprehension." This child can also identify single words in isolation quite effectively. This child can decode unfamiliar words. But this child shows a decline in efficiency on longer assignments and reading comprehension becomes even worse on smaller type. This child frequently omits words, rereads the same line, and skips lines. This youngster loves being read to and can discuss and recall effectively when material is read aloud to him. This child can define words, give synonyms, and has good understanding of anything that he hears. His problem occurs when he has to read several pages of text. It is at this point that reading comprehension suffers. This child's problem cries for optometric intervention.

Both of these youngsters entered your office identified as having reading comprehension problems. Both would score satisfactorily at those reading tests that probe the ability to correctly identify words in isolation. Both would score poorly on those reading tests that measure comprehension. The first is not likely to show a visual problem as the cause of the comprehension difficulty, whereas the second child almost certainly has a contributory vision problem.

Language factors or even low intelligence are more likely to be the cause of the first child's problem. His ability to repeat almost verbatim indicates that there is no problem with visual intake of the reading material. There are no signs suggestive of visual fatigue, nor does anything point to high probability of visual factors playing a major role here. The second youngster, on the other hand, shows many signs of potential visual interference. This child shows good language ability, and, importantly, when the material is heard rather than seen, there is no comprehension problem. This is a very rudimentary distinction that is often overlooked by both teachers and parents. It certainly should not be overlooked by optometrists. The history of the second child indicates the possibility of difficulty with ocular motility, fusion, or accommodation. There may even be contribution because of uncorrected refractive conditions. There does not seem to be any lack of the fundamental language and integrative skills necessary for reading comprehension but rather an input problem. This youngster cannot acquire the reading material accurately for long enough periods of time to facilitate reading comprehension. Is this second child apt to have usual asthenopic symptoms? Maybe yes and maybe no. This would depend on other factors.

If the second child just stops reading each time that the task becomes difficult, there will not be any report of overt symptoms such as discomfort or blur. On the other hand, if the second child has high drive, or is forced to persist at reading by either parents or teacher, there is a greater likelihood of asthenopic symptoms. Keep in mind that asthenopic symptoms do not derive directly from aberrant visual measures but rather reflect the effort or frustration of attempting to overcome a visual dysfunction. You do not get a headache just because accommodation is low unless you attempt to accommodate. You do not get a headache from a fusion problem if you manage to suppress successfully. It takes effort to become uncomfortable, and many youngsters avoid discomfort by withdrawal from the task that might produce it. Others adapt within the visual process itself. Suppression and myopia (or pseudomyopia) attributable to accommodative spasm are examples of adaptations that reduce symptoms.[1] Although the pattern of measurements can usually disclose if there has been effort to overcome the problem either by adaptation or by withdrawal from the task to avoid symptoms, this information can also be gleaned during the case history.

Learning to read versus reading to learn

The two previous examples were cited to demonstrate how the case history can sort those with visually based learning problems from those whose learning problems are caused by other factors. Utilization of a task analysis approach can also give insight into the specific nature of a visually related learning problem. I find it helpful to make a distinction between learning to read and utilization of reading as a tool for learning, since these two aspects of reading present very different visual task requirements.

The early phases of learning to read place great demands on visual perception factors (see box). The beginning curriculum is heavily loaded with tasks requiring recognition, matching, and recall of shapes. The ability to deal with directional orientation of visual stimuli is an important factor. These skills are fundamental to acquisition of basic reading ability. Their

---

Learning to Read

Task requirements:

Major emphasis on word recognition and recall.
Large type with few words on each page.
"Look-and-say" methods of teaching place premium on visual memory.
Phonic methods require careful scrutiny of internal details of individual words.
Activity usually does not extend over long periods.
Writing may be utilized to reinforce reading.

Important visual factors:

Accurate oculomotor control.
Visual form perception and visual discrimination, including the ability to deal with directional orientation.
Visual-memory.
Accommodation and binocular vision are usually not critical factors unless there is heavy utilization of ditto sheets or similar teaching aids.
Ability to integrate auditory and visual stimuli.
Eye-hand coordination becomes important when writing is used as a reinforcer for reading.

contribution lessens as the primary emphasis in reading shifts from word analysis to sustained reading for comprehension. The degree of loading on visual perceptual skills is also influenced by the particular teaching method being utilized. A "look-and-say" method of teaching reading places a high premium on the ability to recall word shapes. This is somewhat less if the early reading strategy involves a phonetic approach. Similarly, words presented in isolation do not permit utilization of context cues to assist the beginning reader in word recognition. This tends to place a very high demand on visual recall particularly when phonetically irregular words are presented. Unfortunately, many of the more commonly utilized words in English cannot be analyzed using phonics and must be recalled based upon the *Gestalt* ('shape') of the word.

Some reading programs are based upon linguistic and semantic approaches that also offer cues to assist in deciphering the unknown word. Those approaches that offer such help tend to reduce dependence on visual configuration as the sole clue to word recognition. As a consequence, a kindergarten or first grade child being exposed to a "look-and-say" method of reading instruction who shows inadequate or delayed visual perception ability can be severely handicapped. The same child might be less handicapped if the instructional approach is based upon a "whole-language" method or offers opportunity for utilization of other cues to assist in visual recognition. This is not meant to advocate one particular method of teaching reading over another. There are many different approaches to teaching early reading, each of which has some advantages as well as disadvantages. From an optometric point of view, however, it is useful to know the particular system being encountered by the patient because this permits more insightful analysis of how specific visual dysfunctions might play a role. There are children who fail to learn to read because the teaching program assumes a level of competence in visual recognition and recall that they may not possess. In such instances, alternative teaching strategies as well as appropriate remediation of the deficient visual function can be exceedingly helpful. Although the degree to which the curriculum calls upon visual perception skills is dependent on the instructional method used, visual form perception plays a major role in acquiring rudimentary word recognition facility.[2]

Those aspects of vision that relate to the ability to maintain prolonged attention are not usually of primary importance in the lower grades. Most teachers do not expect prolonged, sustained attention from their students and change activities frequently. The text material utilized has very large type. As a consequence, accommodation and binocular vision are not taxed greatly. This changes when the teaching program is centered around desk work or individual workbooks, which do require prolonged attention. Poorly printed ditto sheets with very low contrast are difficult to see clearly. Eye-hand control can also become important when writing is utilized as a reinforcer for reading, as when a new word is written five times. A child with very poor graphomotor control can become easily frustrated during this activity.

As reading proficiency increases and more strategies can be brought to bear on word analysis, the relative contribution of visual perception tends to become reduced (see box). Other visual factors increase in importance. As a general rule, binocular vision and accommodative dysfunctions increase in their potential contribution to reading disorders as the demands of the reading task shift from emphasis on word recognition and word analysis to sustained reading for longer periods of time. It is quite possible for a youngster to enter school with binocular or accommodative problems and for the visual dysfunction to play a minimal role. It is only when this child acquires word recognition ability and attempts to sustain reading for longer periods of time on smaller type that the fusion or accommodative problem becomes critical. I have seen many children who learn to read but begin to fall apart at about third- or fourth-grade level. It is at this point that the size of the type is reduced along with increased length of reading assignments. Now the ability to sustain comfortably becomes the dominant consideration, and the deficient visual skills interfere. In the early grades there is generally less need for sustained attention.

Recent changes in the field of education are modifying the role of vision. Kindergarten as a transitional readiness program is giving way to formal reading and writing instruction, sometimes even at the prekindergarten level. Additionally, the traditional teacher in front of the classroom presenting material at the chalkboard is being replaced by more individualized workbook activities. The manifestation of visual problems that produce fatigue has been moved forward in the school experience so that binocular vision and accommodative problems sometimes interfere well before fourth grade. It is very important to know the educational program

---

Reading to Learn

Task requirements:

Longer reading assignments.
Smaller type.
Context cues become increasingly important to word recognition.
Phonic and linguistic cues are more readily available.
Word analysis becomes more automatic with less need to depend primarily on
  form perception.
Emphasis shifts to comprehension and speed.

Important visual factors:

Accommodation and binocular vision become more important.
Oculomotor control is important to keep place and preserve continuity of input.
Form perception plays a decreasing role.

as well as the reading level of the patient for proper assessment of the contribution of binocular vision and accommodative problems to reading difficulty.

Dyslexia

There are some people who have an inordinate difficulty learning to read. They are intelligent enough, have been exposed to sound education, and show no obvious problems in seeing, hearing, or maintaining emotional control. This group of people has attracted considerable attention and has been the subject of speculation and investigation by many professional disciplines. At best, this is a confused area with disagreement among professionals. The problem begins with definition. Most workers in the field utilize an exclusionary definition, ruling out other causes for the problem and labeling those who show no other cause for their severe reading problem as suffering from dyslexia. Genetic factors are often believed to be present. Although all agree that such a population exists, there is much less agreement as to the prevalence of the condition, appropriate methods of identifying them, and even if they are actually a single group, since there is no fully agreed upon classification system. The confusion associated with dyslexia is compounded by frequent utilization of the label to describe anyone with reading difficulty, without even applying the exclusionary definition.

Traditionally, the term had been reserved for those showing massive delay in acquiring rudimentary word recognition ability. There is a welter of confusion and disagreement in the literature because investigators have come to the problem from many different disciplines and from varied experiential backgrounds within disciplines. Some believe dyslexia to be a language-based congenital disorder, often associated with delayed language development. They completely discount the possibility of any visual component to the problem and may screen out of their dyslexic research population those who show performance IQ lower than verbal IQ. This effectively precludes visual perception deficiency as a causative factor. There is nothing wrong with this, except that they then generalize and assume that all who fail to read have this type of dyslexia.

Others recognize different types of dyslexia, with the two major types being dysphonetic and dyseidetic. The *dysphonetic* show language deficits and generally do not have visual factors as the primary cause of their failure to read. This does not mean that visual conditions do not play a contributory role in their overall reading difficulty. There are often associated problems with oculomotor control, accommodation, and binocular vision that interfere even if they are not primary. *Dyseidetic* dyslexics are a different group. They may show significant visual perception and visual memory deficits. Those with delayed visual perceptual development frequently demonstrate associated problems in oculomotor control that reduces their attentional capability. Both types of dyslexics show poor ability to integrate visual and auditory stimuli. They may have subtle or more overt neurological problems and have not established proper cross-modal linkages. This should be investigated if dyslexia is suspected. Major difficulty with spelling as well as reading should alert the examiner to the possibility of dyslexia.

It is important to sort the symptoms and behaviors of the patient to be sure that there are no significant visual complicating conditions for a patient presenting with a diagnosis of either dysphonetic or dyseidetic dyslexia. Many dyslexics can be helped with optometric training to improve visual perception and visual-auditory integration as well as oculomotor control so that they can then become more responsive to appropriate pedagogical help. Accommodative and binocular deficiencies that are contributory should also be treated, since this will make it easier for the patient to sustain accurate attention.

RELATING VISUAL FACTORS TO READING
Oculomotor control

Accurate oculomotor control is important for beginning reading. The neophyte needs to scrutinize internal details of words and even letters, which the more advanced reader does not have to attend to.[3] Sophisticated readers make use of a variety of different cues to assist in word recognition. Familiarity with the linguistic code of the language permits experienced readers to utilize perceptual filling. Words and phrases can be read despite blurred or obliterated letters, such as those often encountered on poorly reproduced ditto sheets. Good readers are hardly handicapped if the lower half of a line of print is blocked off. Practice in reading English leads one to anticipate that the letter following *q* will be *u*. There are a host of probabilities that are unconsciously mastered as one develops reading proficiency. Certain combinations are far more likely to appear than others. The beginner does not as readily appreciate these relationships and may have to scrutinize each letter in unfamiliar words.

Successful readers automatically utilize context and semantic cues. They may respond to the overall configuration of a word or phrase because they anticipate what is written. These abilities develop with experience and growth of vocabulary, largely as a function of reading itself. As a consequence, the beginning reader is more closely limited by the sharply peaked resolving capability of the human eye, necessitating accurate oculomotor control to ensure foveal fixation of the word being decoded. The ability to read utilizing poorly resolved peripheral cues requires experience. This does not mean that the beginner is incapable of responding to the overall word configuration without attending to internal details. Some teaching strategies emphasize this method of word recognition, but the beginner cannot be as good as the experienced reader. *Many* and *Mary* have the same general shape. Context will lead the more advanced reader to the correct choice, whereas the beginner may have to actually inspect each letter to be sure of the word.

Precise oculomotor control is needed to accomplish accurate decoding when learning to read. Phonic analysis requires careful viewing to properly match grapheme to phoneme. The eyes must be aimed with precision in order to allow the sequential foveal inspection needed to accomplish this task. Although this will be referred to as "oculomotor control," it should be realized that the activity is not simply limited to the extraocular muscles, but rather involves all the motor systems utilized when a person looks at a particular object or shifts attention between two objects. Head and body movement systems are involved as well. It is possible for the pursuit, saccadic, and vergence motor systems each to be physiologically intact and still the patient may have difficulty coordinating extraocular motor movements with head and body movements with sufficient accuracy to permit effective reading. This is particularly so when the student is dependent on inspection of each internal detail of the printed word. As words become more familiar, the store of "sight" words increases, reducing dependence on letter-by-letter analysis.

A second aspect of oculomotor control that is important to beginning reading is its relationship to attention.[4] A dominant characteristic of children who fail to learn to read in the early grades is inability to sustain attention. This is particularly true of those youngsters who are immature or who show developmental disturbances. Often the major complaint reported by the classroom teacher is distractibility when faced with visually demanding tasks. The child is unable to sustain attention on the work at hand long enough or consistently enough to respond to instruction.

When analyzed in terms of the development of oculomotor control, this inattentiveness often can be better understood as "inappropriately attentive." There are reflex oculomotor behaviors at birth that serve to force multisensory attention. Vestibular reflexes permit maintenance of fixation despite body movement. Oculo-auditory reflexes center both visual and auditory space at the same point of interest. The infant's attraction to novelty, complexity, and movement are all responses that, in a normal child, force multisensory exploration of the external environment. Indeed, without a preprogrammed system to force simultaneous exploration by vision, hearing, touch, and even smell and taste, the newborn would be adrift in a world of conflicting stimuli and would never be able to associate, for example, the visual and auditory schemas that later become the basis for sophisticated matching of print and auditory language, which is the core of reading.

The early multisensory explorations, however, are determined by reflexes and driven by the strength of the external stimuli as measured in physical terms. It is the loudness of the noise, the unusualness of the stimulus, the motion of the stimulus, the brightness of the stimulus, and other such factors that capture attention and trigger a fixation reflex. This reflex behavior is never fully lost but rather must be overridden in favor of socially acceptable attention. The classroom teacher may point to the word on the blackboard and tell the youngster that it is important, but the biological system is programmed to attend to the bright light coming through the window or the noise of passing children in the hallway. The word that the first grader is asked to look at does not have physical characteristics that distinguish it from its surround but is rather made important by the teacher calling attention to it.

Under usual circumstances, children develop the facility to inhibit the more reflex oculomotor stimuli in favor of attending to the task at hand. Not all children make this transition from preprogrammed multisensory attention to the ability to attend utilizing vision selectively. These are the ones who are labeled as having attention deficits when, in fact, they are behaving quite appropriately at what is actually an earlier stage in development. Our educational establishment pays lip service to individual differences, but our schools have precious little tolerance for those who do not show appropriate readiness at the time they become chronologically (not developmentally) old enough for formal instruction. There is even little or no allowance made within a grade level for those whose birthday may be almost a year later than their classmates. One of the hallmark characteristics of developmentally delayed children is inadequate oculomotor control. They cannot function adequately in a classroom that places a premium on sustained visual attention while at the same time inhibits movement, touch, and auditory support for the object of interest. This problem has become exacerbated in recent years with introduction of formal learning ever earlier in the curriculum.

We measure deficient pursuit or saccadic fixation ability in these children, but this does not necessarily mean that there is a fundamental defect in the oculomotor system. In my experience, the deficiency is generally not an ocular motor problem per se, but rather an inability to utilize the eye-motor system to aim the eyes effectively and appropriately for classroom demands. The problem is most often an inability to utilize a neurologically intact system to make the needed eye movements for successful reading. Fortunately, this is highly trainable. The most dramatic change brought about by oculomotor training with beginning readers is improvement in the accuracy and span of attention of the child.

The contribution of oculomotor control to reading disorder does not end once a youngster has mastered basic word recognition facility (see box). Eye-aiming problems still play a role, but their influence on the reading process changes. Once word analysis is mastered, inaccurate oculomotor control continues to contribute to loss of place. Many reading errors are directly related to this, with words being omitted and lines reread or skipped (along with errors at copying from a book or from the blackboard). Different patients may react differently. Some persist at finger pointing, whereas others who are chastised for doing so become "closet"

Relating Oculomotor Control to Learning

Beginning reading:

Beginner needs to attend to internal details of words, requiring precise oculomotor control.

Accurate sequential inspection of words is necessary for utilization of phonic analysis.

Oculomotor control is related to the ability to maintain attention.

Sophisticated reading:

Less dependence on precision eye aiming to attend to internal details of words, since more methods can be utilized to identify words.

Oculomotor control becomes important for keeping place.

Omissions, substitutions, and "careless" errors may be attributable to inaccurate oculomotor control.

Reading comprehension can be adversely effected by poor oculomotor control.

One compensation for erratic oculomotor control is to slow the reading rate to avoid errors.

Arithmetic:

"Careless" errors such as miscopying, shifting over one integer when adding columns, or misplacing answers on Scantron marked tests may be attributable to oculomotor difficulty.

---

finger pointers by surreptitiously running a thumb across the page well below the line of print. Still others abandon the use of pointing and persist in "careless" errors. The reading problems that ensue are directly related to the interference in the flow of material from the page.

Comprehension suffers in all but very bright children. Erratic oculomotor control interferes with appropriate sequential acquisition of the reading material. Just how much this influences reading is dependent on nonvisual parameters such as intelligence, language facility, and personality style of the child. Bright children, with good language facility, who can delay making closure can often mask the interference of erratic oculomotor control. They can retain jumbled inputs in short-term memory long enough to make sense of them by utilizing context or linguistic analysis. Although their reading may not be maximally efficient, it may be good enough so that they escape detection unless an observant teacher notices a discrepancy between their potential and actual reading score, or error patterns such as "logical substitutions" indicating that they may have deficiencies in visual input.

On the other hand, a youngster who is less bright, not as adept with language, or whose personality style demands immediate rather than delayed closure, can become a frustrated and dismal failure at reading because of the same degree of oculomotor dysfunction that merely reduces efficiency of his classmate. Tests for oculomotor efficiency may give identical results in two children but have a greatly different influence on reading ability. Although this difference may plague the researcher, it is a fact of life for the clinician. It is necessary to understand the dynamics of a particular patient in order to assess appropriately the role of oculomotor difficulty. Some youngsters compensate for this type of problem by an abnormal slowing of all reading to a word-by-word rate so as to avoid losing place. They score well at what they read but cannot complete assignments. Others will gallop through material with major disruption of comprehension simply because they are not sampling all of the text or are sampling in incorrect sequence.

Oculomotor disorders can be found at all ages, even among reasonably successful adults. Frequent "careless" errors, persistent need for finger pointing or a line guide, abnormally slow reading to maintain comprehension are tell-tale markers. Those who adapt by head turning are usually somewhat more successful than those who do not. Those who are fairly successful academically despite inaccurate fixation tend to read more in a skimming mode than with careful attention to all details. Although they mask their problem, they are not nearly so efficient as they might be.

Accommodation

Accommodative dysfunctions are quite prevalent among school-aged children and are related to discomfort symptoms.[5] They tend not to be so debilitating in kindergarten and first grade as they will be later on. Standard text material at the primer level is quite large with a good deal of leading between lines or space around individual words and letters. With progression through the grades, the typeface is made smaller, words and letters are closer together, and the length of the reading passage increases. It is at approximately third or fourth grade that accommodative dysfunctions begin to show a great influence, though this can occur earlier with the downward transfer of formal education into lower and lower grades. Then the problem becomes one of maintaining high-level attention. Very rapid fatigue is encountered, sometimes measurable in minutes. Careful questioning of parents often discloses that the youngster's behavior changes at homework assignments after the first 6 or 7 minutes of the activity. It is then that fidgetiness and distractibility enter the picture. Distractibility brought on by visual fatigue should be differentiated from that attributable to more central causes (see box).

Accommodative disorders typically show strong relationship to time at task. One question that is useful to ask is whether reading efficiency declines as a function of time at the activity independent of level of difficulty of the material. Children who read well for the first two or three pages and then show collapse of all reading skills are strongly suspect of an accommodative dysfunction. Children who have no difficulty learning to read but who begin to fall back at about third or fourth grade should be checked carefully for accommodative or binocular deficiency.

The presence of an accommodative dysfunction does not necessarily

---

Relating Accommodation to Learning

Beginning reading:

Large type utilized.

Blur rarely reported even if accommodation is deficient.

Most lessons are of short duration minimizing the effects of fatigue from accommodative problems.

Extensive use of ditto sheets may change this and cause accommodative disorders to interfere.

Short attention span more likely than blur or asthenopia.

Sophisticated reading:

The emphasis in reading shifts from decoding to speed and comprehension.

Smaller type and longer time at reading make accommodation very important.

Fatigue often manifest as the primary symptom.

Abrupt decline in reading efficiency as a function of time at task.

Intermittent blur may be reported.

Asthenopia present when patient persists at reading despite accommodative inefficiency.

Mild brow headaches are common.

Symptoms can be avoided by just not reading.

Accommodative spasm may develop as adaptation among those who persist at reading despite asthenopia.

---

mean that there will be asthenopic symptoms. Blur is not frequently reported by very young children though sometimes it can be elicited by careful questioning. I have encountered youngsters who have suffered chronically from transient near-vision blur but who accepted this as a normal part of the reading process. Needless to say there have been some very surprised parents when this information is disclosed during the case history. Having no basis of comparison, these children associate blur and discomfort with the reading process and think that everybody sees that way.

The major reason that young children do not report blur or asthenopia is simply that they do not experience them. At the first sign of difficulty, withdrawal from the task is the simplest and most convenient response. They stop doing the thing that bothers them and as a consequence symptoms and adaptive changes within the visual system are minimal. These youngsters show what look like very normal measurements unless the examination probes deeply. Accommodative facility is more likely to be deficient than amplitude is. They may even give satisfactory accommodative responses to an initial or even second trial but then show rapid depletion in accommodative ability. The time to clear minus lenses on flipper-lens testing may increase with each successive flip.

Accommodative dysfunctions in older and more motivated children are more likely to produce discomfort. Headache complaints are frequent. Usually the pain is localized above the eyes and is not severe. Over-the-counter medications such as aspirin or Tylenol will relieve them, as will resting for a few minutes. Patients who are highly motivated will often work right through the brow headache caused by an accommodative problem. Those who are extremely motivated and diligent can often maladapt in a manner so that discomfort symptoms eventually disappear. Myopia can be a useful and reasonably successful adaptation to accommodative infacility. I routinely question beginning myopes about the possibility of unanswered headache and ocular fatigue 6 months to a year before the first awareness of distance blur. It is not unusual to find that this is indeed the case. There was a period of discomfort, generally characterized by mild brow headache, that seemed to resolve spontaneously. Unfortunately the resolution brought its own problem of distance blur. The time delay between headache and distance vision blur makes these two events seem unrelated to the patient or parent.

Other youngsters do not adapt and persist with more typical discomfort symptoms. These are, in my estimation, the more fortunate ones provided that the examiner is sensitive to the possibility of accommodative dysfunction and treats it appropriately. Far too frequently this is not the case, and symptoms persist unanswered. The sadness is that simple accommodative dysfunctions are relatively easy to treat with vision therapy and lenses.

Untreated accommodative dysfunctions can sometimes continue for many years while the youngster goes through the school system by learning aurally instead of visually. There is a substantial population of "good nonreaders." These are people who have mastered basic reading and decoding skills and who should be proficient readers but who tend to do as little as possible simply because they experience discomfort. If they are bright enough they do well at school though not nearly to their potential. These are youngsters who count the pages before beginning a reading assignment and read the bare minimum necessary to get by. Children with long-standing accommodative problems often break down as they enter young adulthood, particularly when they enter a demanding college program that does not permit them to get by merely by listening. Adult-onset myopia (AOM) is now an accepted phenomenon. Most myopia that begins in the late teens or early twenties is probably preventable with appropriate management of accommodative disorder.

Binocular vision

Binocular dysfunction plays a somewhat similar role in the reading process just as accommodative deficiency does. The greatest influence is on the more advanced reader though it can and does play a role in the very beginning reader when severe enough to disrupt attention processes. Young children usually do not report typical asthenopic symptoms. They are more likely to show a very short attention span at desk work. Some children will become disruptive and talk or wander about the room rather than completing their work. More often, binocular problems are noticed as the individual moves from the learning-to-read stage to the reading-to-learn stage and where sustaining ability and maintaining comprehension over time becomes important. They can be present previously and not interfere, or they can develop as part of a syndrome brought about by the stress of heavy near work demands (see box)

Binocular problems can produce asthenopia, diplopia on occasion, and seriously degrade reading efficiency. Loss of place despite reasonably good oculomotor control may occur, particularly with high exophoria. Individuals with convergence insufficiency may present with a very interesting reading pattern. Most people can alter reading speed depending on the specific needs of the reading task. Facile readers operate at more than one speed and adjust that speed to the needs of the moment. Patients with convergence difficulty often cannot do this. They can comprehend only when they read very slowly. Instead of a gradual tradeoff of comprehension for speed, they experience a precipitous comprehension drop with any attempt to accelerate. They can read the lead article in *The New York Times* and not be sure of whether it was a foreign policy article or had something to do with domestic taxes. They must read very slowly or read everything twice. Flexibility in their reading pattern is what is most influ-

---

Relating Binocular Vision to Learning

Beginning reading:

Emphasis is on decoding and not sustaining.
Binocular vision problems may not always be a major factor even when present.
Binocular fusion problems can interfere when there is great emphasis on workbooks or ditto sheets with lengthy assignments.
Asthenopic symptoms are rare.
Avoidance, short attention span, or disruptive behavior are more common.

Sophisticated reading:

Reading emphasis is on speed and comprehension.
Sustaining ability becomes important.
Binocular dysfunctions become increasingly important as the work load increases.
Comprehension is adversely affected, and there may be need for excessive rereading.
Reading in a moving vehicle can produce nausea.
Headaches can be more severe than with accommodative problems and may be occipital as well as frontal or temporal.
Loss of place may occur, particularly if there is a high phoria.
Suppression is an adaptive response that can permit reading despite a binocular deficiency.
There may be an inverse relationship between the degree of binocular vision problem and the influence on reading.
Smaller and less obvious deficiencies in binocular vision can seriously reduce reading efficiency.

enced by the convergence problem. Some do well even at college level reading provided that they are willing to plug and work long enough hours. Their performance on standardized tests is typically adversely effected because they cannot function under time constraints and are penalized by slow reading.

Many patients with fusion difficulty are symptomatic in terms of usual asthenopic or discomfort indices. They may show mild brow headache similar to those with accommodative disorder, but occipital and temporal headaches are also reported. These tend to be more severe and lasting than the very mild pain over the eyes associated with accommodative problems. They may persist for some time after reading is completed. Other patients with fusion problems do not report pain but just manifest lower reading efficiency, which they tend to attribute to anything but vision.

Just as some people adapt to accommodative disorders by developing myopia, so too is adaptation possible for binocular problems. This often confounds research efforts. Lesser degrees of binocular instability may have a far greater influence on reading efficiency than more obvious disorders. Constant strabismics, as a group, do not have any particular problem with reading because of their binocular deficiency.[6] This poses an enormous problem in the research domain and is one of the leading causes of confusion in the literature. Typically research, to investigate the relationship between vision and reading, scores the visual factors on a scale based upon departure from clinically normal. Under these circumstances the individual with a minor binocular problem falls in between those with no binocular deficiency and the more obvious extreme binocular problem characterized by strabismus. From a task analysis point of view, however, this ordering of the data is not appropriate. Reading could be accomplished quite nicely with a single eye. The problem occurs when there are inconsistencies in binocular input that serve to degrade the information flow from the paper. This is exactly what happens when one deals with fusion deficiency to which the patient has not successfully adapted. Small degrees of imbalance in binocular coordination and, more particularly, small deficiencies in the interplay between accommodation and convergence can sometimes have a disproportionately large adverse effect on reading efficiency.

The influence of binocular dysfunctions on reading performance is similar to that of accommodation, but the manifestations may take a bit longer to become apparent. Fatigue comes on somewhat more slowly than fatigue from accommodative dysfunction does. Among older students and adults, binocular problems may make it impossible to read in a moving vehicle, sometimes producing symptoms of nausea, or general malaise after reading. Head turning, covering one eye, or even closing an eye while reading are frequent unconscious attempts to deal with the fusion difficulty. Adaptations within the visual complex itself are observed for those who persist at reading and manage to work through initial discomfort.

Suppression and general degradation of binocular function, including changes in vergence findings, sometimes occur as reading proficiency increases. This should not be surprising since adaptive changes typically are brought about to resolve an immediate dilemma. Unfortunately, many of these adaptations are self-limiting and ultimately create their own problems.

Visual Perception

The role of visual perception deficiencies in reading disorders is strongly dependent on the child's current reading level. Visual perception deficiencies relate most closely to early acquisition of fundamental reading skill. Their influence tends to diminish with maturation and sophistication in reading (see box). This leads to confusion as to the appropriate role of visual-perceptual-motor treatment. Going back to our task analysis approach, it should be kept in mind that normal 6-year-olds possess sufficient perceptual motor competency to learn to read. They may not as yet have reached full maturation in visual perception, but they do possess the minimum competency necessary to learn word recognition. The key here is "minimum competency." This may be lost sight of when seriously retarded readers are examined at an older age.

It is not unusual to find that very severely impaired readers show significant developmental delays in visual-form perception. An 11-year-old, for example, may score at an 8-year-old's level on a standardized test, displaying a major visual perception problem. One could infer, probably quite correctly, that when this youngster was in first grade the perceptual abilities were inadequate to permit response to standard pedagogical approaches and that the visual perception problem may have played a significant role in the cause of this child's learning disorder. Although this is exceedingly helpful in understanding the cause of the learning disorder, the optimum intervention may not be quite as obvious.

This 11-year-old can be viewed in two different ways. He can be looked at as having a substantial lag in visual-motor development, which must be remediated before the child can learn to read. On the other hand, this same child can be viewed as now possessing sufficient minimum competency in visual perception so as to be able to learn to read at an elementary level. The visual perception problem may have been fundamental to the learning disorder, but by maturation this child has acquired sufficient visual perception capability to function at the lowest levels of learning word recognition. Basic remedial reading assistance directed toward teaching the initial word-recognition methods that this child could not master when they were initially presented might now be effective, provided that there are no other visual deficiencies present.

If this youngster was placed into a program to remediate the developmental lag in visual perception, the treatment might successfully accomplish its objective but not lead to improvement in reading because the

Relating Visual Perception to Learning

Beginning reading

Word recognition is a major task.

Although there are many different cues to recognizing and recalling a word, visual perception factors are often primary.

Recalling and matching shapes is important.

Ability to deal with directional orientation is necessary.

The teaching method employed influences the degree to which visual perception is important.

Regardless of teaching strategy, many commonly used words must be learned by memorization of their shape because they are phonetically irregular.

Most children have sufficient visual perception capability to read by about 6 years of age.

Treatment of visual perception deficiencies has greatest carryover when done in the early grades.

Sophisticated reading

Emphasis shifts from decoding as the primary demand to speed and comprehension.

Visual perception factors decrease in importance as reading level increases.

Very bright children may progress to sophisticated reading by utilizing alternative strategies to work around a visual perception deficit.

Mathematics

Visual spatial ability is important to development of the appreciation of numbers as quantities.

Visualization is important to understanding spatial relationships in trigonometry and geometry but is not the only way that these subjects can be learned.

Spelling

Some people spell by visualizing the word, others by sequential memorization of the letters.

Spelling errors that are based on the sound of the word are strongly suggestive of visual perception deficiency.

People with severe perceptual problems may ultimately learn to read but poor spelling often persists.

Writing

Some children score poorly on perceptuomotor tests simply because of faulty fine-motor control.

Early optometric treatment can be very effective for children who show developmental delays.

Defective visual perception should be differentiated from delayed development, since the prognosis is not the same.

pedagogical gaps caused by the initial impairment in vision perception remain. The optometrist should be alert to the many situations where optometric intervention, by itself, cannot be expected to produce reading improvement. Optometric treatment is directed toward improvement in visual function. The task-analysis approach includes realistic assessment of what changes might be brought about if treatment were optimally successful. Optometric training will not ensure reading for someone who may have been sitting in the classroom but was unable to respond to the instruction offered. The cause of the inability to respond might very well have been inadequate visual perception abilities. Several years later, however, improving those visual perception abilities will not provide the reading skills that were not learned when initially presented to the child. Appropriate educational help will have to be supplied along with optometric treatment.

Although the visual perception problem may have been fundamental to the learning disorder, the most effective treatment strategy may not be treatment based primarily on developing visual perception capability. The minimum competency concept comes into play. Presented with an 11-year-old who has visual perception capabilities commensurate with that needed to learn to read (albeit very much delayed in development), the most effective optometric intervention may be to focus on the associated visual problems that intrude on maintaining attention. I have found that improving the erratic oculomotor control, inefficient accommodation, and sometimes fusional instabilities, which often accompany the massive delay in visual perception, provides higher leverage when remediated than perceptual training does. The initial therapeutic strategy will be directed primarily toward improvement in "visual skills," since this will permit the youngster to respond to appropriate instruction. Visual perception factors will be treated, but these are of secondary importance. Initial emphasis in treatment is on those visual abilities necessary to attend effectively so as to be able to use the minimum competency in visual perception that is already present. More can be accomplished faster by relieving the information-collecting aspects of the visual problem first.

This is not necessarily the optimum strategy for a youngster who is developmentally delayed in kindergarten, first grade, or second grade. At this stage in the youngster's education, normalization of visual perception capabilities can have enormous carryover into improved academic performance, since the curriculum is still emphasizing word recognition and decoding.

Improvement in visual-form perception and associated skills at this stage generally has direct carryover because the classroom activities are dependent on and utilize the skills that the vision therapy improves. The timing of optometric treatment is an important consideration. In general, perceptual motor training has its greatest direct carryover effect when done early in the school career with decreasing effect, insofar as reading is concerned, later in the school career. Perceptual training for older children may have a positive influence on other aspects of the curriculum even up into adulthood. When dealing with severely impaired readers, where the educational objective is to develop fundamental elementary word recognition ability, the minimum competency concept may allow prediction of more immediate benefit from improvement in fixation, accommodation, and fusion than that from perceptual training.

There is a group of children who may show lags in perceptuomotor development and yet not demonstrate problems in learning to read. I have encountered highly verbal youngsters who score very poorly on copying tests of visual perception and show a major discrepancy between verbal and performance IQ scores and yet become early readers, sometimes self-taught. The key characteristic seems to be verbal IQ of 125 or greater. Apparently, these children are so bright and have such advanced language facility that they read despite their perceptual deficiency. They do not, however, succeed at writing.

RELATING VISUAL FACTORS TO MATHEMATICS

Vision relates to mathematics in several ways. The spatial aspects of vision are important for the appreciation of numbers as representative of quantities rather than abstractions. Memorization that 2 plus 2 equals 4 has little utility unless the 2 and 4 stand for magnitudes and can be appreciated as such. Early teaching of arithmetic generally incorporates procedures to permit utilization of visual cues to magnitude. Children unable to visualize spatially may have difficulty acquiring fundamental understanding of the relationship between numbers and quantity. Remedial mathematics programs incorporate concrete objects such as blocks or sticks of different lengths to develop spatial appreciation of the number values. Although not necessarily identified as such, these procedures would serve to improve deficient visual function and are similar to some activities that are utilized in an optometric treatment program for children with visual development lags.

Apart from arithmetic, there are other aspects of mathematics that are best accomplished utilizing spatial thinking. Trigonometry and geometry are examples. The ability to visualize and mentally manipulate shapes is important to full understanding. Although best managed by spatial thinking, this is not the only way to solve problems. There are bright people, adept at sequential-logical thinking, who score very well at geometry despite the fact that they cannot intuitively understand the spatial relationships involved. Most geometry problems can be solved when a sequence of logical steps is followed and the correct answer is reached even with perceptual deficiency. If we keep in mind our task-analysis approach, it is possible to score well on geometry tests even with visual perception weakness. There are students who achieve excellent grades in this subject with little deep understanding. They can benefit from optometric treatment but not show the dramatic gains registered by their less intelligent classmates with comparable visual perception weakness who may go from failure to success after optometric therapy.

Oculomotor difficulty can intrude by the introduction of "careless" errors such as omission of a number, or inadvertent shifting over of one integer when adding or subtracting is performed. This difficulty is most likely to occur when the numbers are far apart, as at long division. Problems may be copied incorrectly from the blackboard or book. Just as in the case of reading difficulty, it is vital to probe to find the specific nature of the academic problem in math. An inability to memorize multiplication tables even with considerable oral rote practice is not likely to be caused by a primary visual problem. Good performance at oral arithmetic with poor performance at written arithmetic is highly suspect for visual interference. Careless errors, fatigue, or low scores on Scantron marked tests are suggestive of the possibility of visual inefficiency.

As in the case of reading disorder, it is vital that the optometrist fully understands the nature of the patient's math difficulty in order to relate the results of the vision evaluation to the learning problem. Generalized statements that the child is poor at arithmetic do not automatically mean that there is a vision problem, or if there is a vision problem that it is the basis for the math problem. Fusion difficulty does not explain an inability to learn the basic number facts such as $2 + 3 = 5$. It can explain low scores on standardized achievement tests that may require more than an hour of sustained attention. Inaccurate eye aiming can account for low scores on a standardized test where the answers are filled in on a page of dotted lines and the child's teacher believes that the material is well within the child's demonstrated capacity in the classroom. The child may be failing the test format rather than the subject material. Perceptual problems can and do interfere with math, but be sure that the low math score isn't just another manifestation of a reading problem. Find out if math problems can be solved if the questions are read to the child.

RELATING VISION TO SPELLING

Spelling can be accomplished in several different ways. Some people memorize the sequence of letters and use aural reinforcement; others use visualization. When asked to spell a word, there are those who spell the word aloud as is done on a spelling bee. Others reach for a pencil to write the word so as to see if it is spelled correctly. Ideally, it might be best to be able to utilize either method, but not all can do so. When the ability is functioning properly, visualization is most efficient, particularly for phonetically irregular words. Patients who cannot spell may suffer from deficient visualization ability or may be dyseidetic. One sign of a visual memory problem is spelling that is completely based on the sound of the word, with errors that still permit the word to be identified by reading it aloud. If so, optometric treatment can be efficacious in helping to improve spelling, provided that there is sufficient familiarity with written language. Although the primary objective of vision therapy is to improve visual memory and visualization, there are instances where spelling improvement occurs after improvement of these abilities. Naturally, improvement in visualization cannot replace the need for exposure to written material.

A word cannot be visually recalled if not experienced. A major nonvisual basis for spelling difficulty is lack of reading.

The same visual perception factors that interfere with learning to read can continue to intrude in spelling even after basic reading has been mastered. Many seriously retarded readers who show dyslexic traits have been taught by teaching approaches that stress phonic analysis and rote learning of words. They learn to read but may spell atrociously. Cursive writing, rather than printing, can help spelling, since the word is learned as a single entity using kinesthetic cues. Dyseidetic dyslexics are often taught to work around their problem by utilization of spelling rules (such as "*i* before *e* except after *c*") or kinesthetic reinforcement. This is an example of a pragmatic educational approach to teach around an often undiagnosed visual deficiency. Visual perception deficiencies can be part of the dyseidetic syndrome.

I have learned to be cautious about predicting spelling improvement with optometric training even after establishing that deficient visual memory and poor visualization is present. Some patients show dramatic improvement in spelling after treatment, whereas others show improvement in visual abilities with little transfer. My suspicion is that there are style factors present that may be based upon an innate predilection to be a visual, auditory, or kinesthetic learner. There may be some whose style is inborn and not just a consequence of visual dysfunction. The dramatic improvement may occur among those who have the propensity to be visual but who had visual difficulty. The failure to transfer may indicate the innate propensity to be auditory, in which case the newly acquired visualization ability is not readily utilized. Those who cannot utilize visualization are truly dyseidetic dyslexics.

RELATING VISION TO HANDWRITING SKILLS

Handwriting is greatly influenced by perceptual-motor development. Most children achieve sufficient facility to learn to write by first grade, but some do not. Optometric vision therapy can be quite effective for those who show developmental lags in eye-hand coordination. Perceptual training can lead to handwriting improvement when done in kindergarten or first, second, or even third grade. When treatment begins later, transfer to better handwriting is problematical. The reason is that the nature of the task changes. Improvement in visual perception and eye-hand facility when the child is still actively and consciously controlling hand movements leads to immediate improvement in writing skill. Later, however, writing becomes increasingly dependent on motor memory and is no longer directly controlled utilizing visual steering when forming letters. This is the reason why adults generally do not show handwriting improvement, unless they make a systematic effort to relearn writing. Most children will not make this effort, particularly if the activity is difficult to begin with.

It is possible to overcome a developmental lag by dint of sheer repetitive effort. A death grip on the pencil, immobilization of the wrist of the writing hand, and writing solely with finger movements is suggestive of this adaptive response. Ideally, handwriting should represent the culmination of a gradual shift from gross to fine motor activity. This would be consistent with normal development and lead to writing accomplished with minimal effort. Children not yet physiologically ready to write, but who are forced to perform by parental or teacher pressure, can sometimes master writing by exerting unusual effort. Others cannot mount the necessary effort and retreat from the task, do as little writing as is possible, and go through life with illegible writing. They are often accused of being lazy, and yet their illegible scribbles require more effort than they are ever given credit for. Sadly, the graphomotor disability limits development of the literary side of writing. These children will not edit or rework a piece simply because of the tediousness of getting their ideas on paper. They use the shortest answers available to them—those requiring the fewest number of written words. Asking such a child to rewrite a paper to make it neat is almost a form of child abuse.

Establishing the diagnosis for a young child who shows poor handwriting is not always easy. It is necessary to differentiate between the perceptual and motor components of the perceptual-motor complex. If the problem is attributable to delayed perceptual development, optometric treatment may produce improvement in handwriting as perceptual abilities improve. In some instances, however, the problem is more in the motor capability itself rather than perceptual deficiency. Careful observation is needed in addition to the scored results of standardized tests of visuomotor integration. I prefer to do such testing personally rather than delegating it to an assistant in order to gain insight into the nature of the problem. There are some children who actually give themselves verbal instructions as they copy geometric forms and who are immediately aware of their errors as they make them. Tests of hand motor facility itself will also help to differentiate the perceptual from the motor. If the problem is primarily motor, the degree of impairment as well as general motor facility will determine the maximum improvement possible with therapy. Genetic factors may also play a role. A family history of motor deficiency should make for cautious prediction of the degree of improvement expected.

Attention must also be paid to differentiating between delayed and abnormal sensorimotor performance. They are not the same. Children with an organic brain syndrome (minimal brain dysfunction) show characteristic response patterns at copying tests of visual perception that differentiate them from those merely lagging in development. Severe problems with angulation, characteristic "ears" on diamonds that are repeated in a perseverating manner, and dissociation of the elements of more complex figures are qualitatively different in those with minimal brain dysfunction than in those with simple developmental delays. Although both groups can be helped with vision therapy, the final outcomes will not be the same.

Those with underlying neurological dysfunction will improve greatly, but remnants of the fundamental problem will persist even after successful treatment.

The task-analysis approach can be helpful in predicting the outcome of treatment. If the child is still at the stage of active visual guiding of the motor movements of writing when forming letters, carryover in the form of more legible handwriting may be possible. If the child is no longer consciously planning letter formation but rather has moved to the stage where the hand and finger movements are largely automatic, easier, more regular writing can be anticipated but not necessarily better letter formation. The grade level, emphasis (or lack of emphasis) on writing at school, and personal style of the patient will all influence the way in which optometric treatment will affect on writing.

Some schools or individual teachers make an absolute fetish of neat, legible writing. Others are so unconcerned about the mechanics of writing that they do not even care if the letters are formed in any standard way. Some spend considerable time on writing drills, whereas others are interested solely in the creative side of writing—the message and literary content of the piece. It is vital that the optometrist be aware of the true demands being place on the patient. In the case of a bright child with slight lag in fine motor development, just apprising a sympathetic teacher of the problem and allowing for maturity may be all that is needed. Deemphasis of demands for neatness, allowance for crossing out without the need to recopy an entire page, and other similar minor modifications can unburden a child so that the normal maturational process can continue. There are times when this can be more effective than active treatment undertaken in an attempt to make it possible for the child to meet unrealistic immediate goals.

SUMMARY

Visual factors impinge on the learning process in a variety of ways. This chapter is an attempt to indicate some of the complex relationships that the clinician should be aware of when evaluating a patient who presents with academic or learning problems. The evaluation must include clear delineation of the specifics of the learning problem to guide the testing to be done and also to make sense of the data collected. It is not sufficient to assume automatically that any particular visual deficiency relates to any and all learning problems. Different visual skills are required for proficiency in various academic tasks. There is no overall single index of vision that correlates with the multiple demands of the classroom. Learning to read is a very different visual task from reading as done by a successful college student. Mathematics, spelling, and writing depend on utilization of different visual skills in different ways. Insightful analysis of the specific learning problem encountered is requisite for appropriate examination and still more important for analyzing the results of the visual examination.

Four major aspects of vision have been discussed in terms of their relationships to the learning process. It is assumed that ocular health and refraction will always be checked as part of any primary care evaluation and that refraction will be attended to as needed. This discussion has intentionally not discussed refractive error as a separate category, though there is the obvious relationship between refraction and accommodative or binocular problems. The focus of this chapter has been on the ways in which oculomotor, accommodative, binocular vision, and perceptual problems relate to different demands of the school curriculum. A task-analysis approach has been utilized to offer specific relationships based on the visual demands of different academic subjects. Even within subject areas, the interplay between visual and learning problems is influenced by grade level, since specific curricular demands change as a student progresses. A further complication has to do with the specific teaching methods and materials being used. It is important to be aware of each of these considerations when faced with the clinical task of evaluating the influence of a visual dysfunction on the learning problem of a patient.

Finally, there are individual differences among patients that also determine the way in which visual dysfunctions impinge on learning. Intelligence, language facility, and personality style all contribute. The same visual profile can affect two patients in very different ways, depending on their particular personalities and nonvisual capabilities.

Fortunately, an optometric evaluation provides an excellent opportunity to gauge the style of the patient at the same time as one is collecting standard data. Speed of response, accuracy rate, willingness to guess as thresholds are reached, choice of language, impulsivity tendencies, reflective tendencies, and other similar behavior patterns are evident throughout the examination sequence. It is necessary to pay attention to the qualitative aspects of the patient's responses in addition to the recorded quantity. Careful observation during the examination sequence can disclose a good deal about intelligence, language facility, and characteristic response style. In addition to these insights from the optometric testing, additional input should be sought from school records or other professionals. This information is usually available from school or other psychoeducational evaluations. Understanding the patient makes it possible to relate specific visual dysfunctions more accurately to specific learning difficulties.

Subsequent chapters will deal with the role of individual visual factors in greater detail. At all times, analysis must be based on the specific visual task demands, the teaching strategies and environment, and the personality and nonvisual strengths and weaknesses of the specific patient being evaluated. Only in this manner can visual considerations be properly assessed for their influence on learning. This approach leads to insightful diagnosis and effective intervention that can minimize the influence of visual problems on learning.

CHAPTER REVIEW

1. How can the case history assist in determining the influence of visual conditions on a child's learning disability?
2. How do language facility, IQ, and teaching method influence the role played by vision in a learning disability?
3. How does the importance of visual perception deficits change during a person's school career? Why?
4. Why do binocular difficulties sometimes interfere with scholastic performance and at other times have little influence?
5. Discuss the role of ocular motility in learning disability.

REFERENCES

1. Birnbaum MH: Nearpoint visual stress: clinical implications, *J Am Optom Assoc* 56:480-490, 1985.
2. Spache GD: *Diagnosing and correcting reading disabilities*, Boston, 1976, Allyn & Bacon, p 208.
3. Flax N: Problems in relating visual function to reading disorder, *Am J Optom* 47:366-372, 1970.
4. Richman JE: Use of a sustained visual attention task to determine children at risk for learning problems, *J Am Optom Assoc* 57:20-26, 1986.
5. Hennessey D, Iosue RA, Rouse, MW: Relation of symptoms to accommodative infacility of school-aged children, *Am J Optom* 61:177-183, 1984.
6. Simons HD, Grisham JD: Binocular anomalies and reading problems, *J Am Optom Assoc* 58:578-587, 1987.

CHAPTER **6**

The Relationship Between Visual Efficiency Problems and Learning

RALPH GARZIA

KEY TERMS

reading disability
visual efficiency problems
oculomotor disorders
accommodative dysfunctions
vergence dysfunctions

Matthew effect
vision therapy
saccadic eye movements
case controls studies
correlational studies

Learning disability is the most common childhood disorder requiring special education services. Learning problems encompass a diversity of disorders, including mathematics, written or oral language difficulties, reading disability, perceptual problems, and disorders of attention. Estimates of the prevalence of learning difficulties varies widely depending on identification procedures and qualifying criteria. Information from the United States Department of Education indicates that approximately 5% of total school enrollment is learning disabled. In a study of over 3000 second-grade children in 110 classrooms across eight states, Meier[1] identified 15% with learning disabilities.

Reading disability is the most frequently encountered learning disability and is the focus of this chapter. In a recent attempt to differentiate sex-dependent prevalence rates based on a discrepancy between IQ and reading achievement, reading disability was found in approximately 7.5% of a sample of second- and third-grade children.[2]

Optometrists and educators have been interested in the relationship between visual efficiency and the acquisition of reading skill for nearly a century. This relationship is axiomatic. Visual processing must be considered a fundamental part of the reading act. There can be little question that

153

the initial phases in reading, before phonological encoding, are visual, involving visual sensory processes. Vision is not obligatory for all types of reading-like activity as evidenced by braille reading, but in the more typical situation, visual processes must operate automatically and effortlessly for facile reading.

As is the nature of most cause-and-effect relationships in medicine and optometry, vision problems are neither a necessary nor a sufficient cause of reading disability. Reading disability can occur in the absence of significant vision problems, and not all persons with vision problems develop reading disability. Rather, vision problems as a cause of reading disability are primarily contributory. The presence of anomalies of visual efficiency, perhaps at some critical period of reading development enhances the probability for occurrence of reading disability.

Knowledge about visual skills and reading is important for an optometrist because they are frequently the first collateral professional to evaluate a child with difficulties in reading. Informed teachers and parents request an examination if a child is not making appropriate progress in reading skill acquisition or subsequent to a formal educational diagnosis of reading disability. With increasing frequency, a vision evaluation is included in a comprehensive multidisciplinary assessment of the child. The goal is to establish the degree of involvement of visual abnormalities or visual efficiency problems in failure of anticipated reading achievement.

DEFINING VISUAL EFFICIENCY PROBLEMS

The assessments of visual acuity, refractive error, ocular motility, accommodation, and binocular vision are standard features of a functional vision examination. Together these visual components are important contributors to visual efficiency. Abnormalities or dysfunctions in one or more of these functions forms the core of learning-related vision problems; that is, they are capable of disturbing the visual environment in which reading development, instruction, or activity takes place.

Accommodative and vergence dysfunctions

Accommodative and vergence dysfunctions can be either primary or secondary. Primary dysfunctions occur in the absence of influential uncorrected refractive error. Vergence dysfunctions can also be secondary to the disrupting effects of uncorrected refractive error. For example, uncorrected hyperopia increases the amount of accommodation for near-point tasks and creates an esophoric tendency. The increased demands on accommodation and negative disparity vergence can disrupt normal self-regulatory behavior, creating the clinical portrait of an accommodative or vergence disorder.

The taxonomy of accommodative and vergence anomalies are presented in the following box. Accommodative disorders are classified into patterns of inadequate response to stimulation, relaxation, or both. Ver-

Accommodation syndromes

Accommodative insufficiency
Accommodative excess
Accommodative infacility

Vergence syndromes

Convergence insufficiency
Convergence excess
Divergence insufficiency
Divergence excess
Basic esophoria
Basic exophoria
Fusional vergence dysfunction

Oculomotility disorders

Fixational instability
Saccadic dysfunction
Pursuit dysfunction

gence disorders are classified according to the magnitude and direction of the distance and near-point heterophorias.

Oculomotor disorders

Oculomotor skills are typically tested by chairside assessment of fixation stability, smooth pursuit, and saccadic eye movements (see box). Although saccades are required for conventional reading, testing of smooth pursuit is important in reading-disabled children. Smooth-pursuit ability mirrors attentional capability. Tracking an object across a stationary, textured background (often the examiner) requires a conscious effort. These voluntary eye movements require attentional processing.

It has been proposed that the control of smooth pursuit is a magnocellular pathway function, from retinal ganglion cells, to the magnocellular portion of the lateral geniculate nucleus, to the middle temporal cortex, to the posterior parietal lobe, frontal eye fields, and dorsolateral pontine nuclei.[3] This has important implications because this magnicellular pathway (transient system) has been shown to be deficient in the reading disabled.[4]

The Southern California College of Optometry (SCCO) system is a quick and convenient testing and rating method for pursuits on a 4+ scale.[5] For a more detailed analysis, the Maples's Northeastern State University College of Optometry (NSUCO) system is recommended.[6] Both of these involve tracking a circularly moving target. Evaluation of performance is by gain (eye velocity in relation to target velocity) and number of disruptions in tracking by catch-up saccades. Errors of initiation occur in some children. As a result, they have great difficulty with the initial phases of target movement. Because of the uniformity of target movement, prediction of its movement becomes possible. Prediction is an extrapolation of target movement based on the current stimulus to the smooth pursuit system. A brief continuation of pursuit eye movement after sudden stopping of the target, as occurs in the reversing of movement direction after one revolution, is suggestive of an ability to use a predictive method and further indicates smooth pursuit competency.

Saccadic eye movements have a more direct application to reading. Clinical testing usually involves predictive saccades between two targets. The SCCO and NSUCO systems are also available for analysis of saccadic performance. Evaluation of performance is by saccadic accuracy. Hypometric saccades are commonly found in individuals with poor saccadic eye movement control.

To simulate reading, rapid number-naming tasks have been adapted to assess oculomotor function.[7] These tests place a higher demand on saccadic accuracy because of the quasi-unpredictability of the target. The relationship between these tests and chairside tests of saccadic eye movements remains to be elucidated.

ASSOCIATED SIGNS AND SYMPTOMS

Uncorrected refractive error, particularly hyperopia and anisometropia, accommodative and vergence anomalies, and oculomotor dysfunction can produce a coterie of clinical signs and symptoms.

Clinical signs

Parents and teachers will frequently observe and report manifestations of visual inefficiency in children at home or in the classroom. Squinting, frowning, excessive blinking or eye rubbing, covering an eye, or tilting the head are examples. The clinician should be attentive to these signs during an examination because they are indicative of poor quality of response, despite apparently normal quantitative test results.

A very common observation is an excessively close (rarely farther away in children) working distance when reading. Although there are several alternative explanations for this behavior, the clinician should be very suspicious of a visual dysfunction.

Ocular symptoms

It is imperative that the clinician consider the difficult chore children have in understanding or describing the nature of their symptoms. This is compounded in children with a history of reading disability because of the potential for limited expressive vocabulary development and episodic memory. The caveat becomes, "Limit reliance on symptoms as the dominant indicator of visual function and in the determination of the clinical testing regimen."

The most common ocular symptoms of visual efficiency problems are blur and diplopia, particularly at near point. These occur with reading, or more likely after a period of protracted reading. Asthenopia, or localized eye discomfort, can accompany the blur or diplopia or be an unrelated occurrence. Headaches are also frequently reported. They are typically frontal and are initiated or exacerbated by reading.

Perceptual symptoms

Unusual disturbances of visual perception reported during reading are not unusual. These perceptual anomalies range from illusory movements of the text to spatial distortions of letters or words. Text movement may be in the form of oscillations or even words seen "jumping" from one point to another. Individual letters may be seen as misshapen, deformed, or ill proportioned to the point of hindering their identification. Words are perceived as overlapping or not occupying their proper location or relative position in a line of text.

Behavioral signs

Behavioral signs are another important indication of possible problems with visual efficiency. For example, if sustained near work creates asthenopia, some children will quickly learn to limit such activity to reduce susceptibility to discomfort. This will gradually become a habitual pattern of avoidance. This behavior may be construed in the classroom as a disorder of attention. Children with visual efficiency problems have more difficulty in coming to attention and sustaining attention than children with normal visual efficiency.[8] Easily distractible children or those labeled with an attention deficit may be literally unable to stay focused on the task because of limitations fashioned by visual efficiency problems. These children should be carefully examined and treated promptly. The effectiveness of treatment on attention should be assiduously monitored.

Oculomotor symptoms

Although oculomotor disturbances can create similar signs and symptoms as those described above, there are distinctive features. There is a proclivity, during reading, to omit small words or to transpose word order or letter sequences. This contributes to an overall pattern of reversals.

Losing place, particularly with the return sweep, is common. This results in omission of whole lines of text or rereading of the same line. A frequently encountered adaptation for poor oculomotor control is the use of finger guidance to maintain place.

One explanation for this difficulty in the return sweep phase of reading may be the particular nature of binocular saccadic eye movements. During the return sweep, binocular saccades show an abduction-adduction asymmetry.[9] This represents a dynamic violation of Hering's law.[10] During abduction, saccades are slightly larger, with a higher peak velocity and shorter duration. As a result, the eyes diverge transiently during saccades, creating exophoria. A transient loss of vergence signal during saccades has been suggested as an explanation for this phenomenon. Readers making frequent return-sweep errors may have difficulty reestablishing binocular alignment because of less efficient vergence responses.[11] High exophores have a greater magnitude of these return sweep anomalies,[12] and, more significantly, symptomatic high exophores have even greater difficulty.[13]

There have been few studies of the frequency of signs and symptoms of visual inefficiency in reading-disabled children. In one report, Meier surveyed classroom teachers for the observed behaviors of 284 learning-disabled children.[1] Those questions with a strong visual component are listed in Table 6-1. As can be seen, some of the behaviors listed occurred quite frequently.

GENERAL INFLUENCE OF VISUAL EFFICIENCY PROBLEMS ON LEARNING

Uncorrected refractive error, particularly hyperopia and anisometropia, accommodative and vergence anomalies, and oculomotor dysfunction can have an effect on the reading process either in isolation or, more commonly, in combination. Their specific influence on reading is dependent on the nature of the visual problems, their severity, and the particular stage of reading development at which they occur. Visual inefficiency can be either a dominant factor in the genesis of a reading disability, a contributory factor of variable degree, or an insignificant factor. There are several hypothetical modes of influence.

Matthew effect

Ocular discomfort when reading may reduce the amount of time in reading activity. This most certainly contributes significantly to Matthew effects in reading.[14] This refers to a biblical passage about the parable of the talents from the gospel of Matthew (25:29, "For to everyone who has, more will be given and he will grow rich; but from the one who has not,

TABLE 6.1   Prevalence of classroom behaviors of learning-disabled children

1. Reverses or rotates letters, numbers, and words (writes *p* for *q*, *saw* for *was* far more frequently than peers)	52%
2. Points at words while reading silently or aloud	49%
3. Avoids work requiring concentrated visual attention	39%
4. Loses place more than once while reading aloud for 1 minute	38%
5. Omits words while reading grade-level material aloud	38%
6. Facial contortions with visual tasks (including squint)	28%
7. Moves head or trunk excessively during visual tasks (instead of moving eyes)	19%
8. Head forward or tilted to one side when reading	18%
9. Holds book too close (6 inches or less)	17%
10. Rubs eyes often when reading	14%
11. Can read better when print is turned upside down	8%

even what he has will be taken away."). This describes the effect of reading volume on vocabulary growth and reading skill, and vice versa. Better readers with good vocabularies will read more, expand their vocabulary and reading skill, read even better, and enjoy it, leading to even more reading. The visually symptomatic child who reads less will have diminished opportunity to develop reading skill. From a behavioral perspective, a child may begin to associate reading with discomfort, further contributing to a dislike or frustration with reading.

Attention allocation

Seeing text as blurred or diplopic or having discomfort associated with visual inefficiency may interfere with automatic information processing required for successful reading.[15] This concept supposes the availability of a limited-capacity attentional pool. With efficient visual function, the allocation of attention can remain at the semantic level to maximize reading comprehension. It need not be depleted by peripheral visual system dysfunctions to correct or adjust binocular or oculomotor function.

Children with preexisting attentional deficits may be particularly at risk for the "distracting" effects of visual inefficiency.

Word-Recognition speed

It has been convincingly demonstrated that optically degraded text has an adverse effect on speed of word recognition.[16] Reduced speed of word recognition of course slows the entire reading process. If attention has to be directed to the word recognition process, ongoing reading comprehension will be hampered. Correcting significant hyperopia (>2.00), a condition with a real potential for evoking near-point blur has been found to enhance speed of word recognition measured tachistoscopically.[17]

Shifting to more top-down processes

Competent reading requires interaction between bottom-up (visual) and top-down (cognitive) processes.[18] It requires simultaneous visual pattern analysis, that is, translating visual symbols into phonological codes, with higher order knowledge of the lexicon, syntax, semantics, and the ongoing contextual flow. Blurred, diplopic, or otherwise distorted text may reduce visual processing, with greater demand placed on contextual facilitation for comprehension. The slower the word-decoding process, the more the reader must draw on contextual information as compensation. This may be particularly troublesome in weakly constraining text. This is analogous to reading poorly produced, low-contrast mimeographic work sheets.

Oculomotor inaccuracy

Eye-movement control during reading involves the selection of the next word to fixate and the most appropriate landing location within that word for maximum efficiency of word recognition.[19] The optimal landing site is near the center of the word for words up to eight letters in length. Any error, even a letter or two from this optimal site will increase the likelihood of refixating that word, delaying word recognition, and slowing comprehension.

SPECIFIC RELATIONSHIPS BETWEEN VISUAL EFFICIENCY AND LEARNING

Limitations of previous research

Over the years there has been a considerable literature devoted to answering the epistemological question on the role of vision abnormalities or dysfunctions in the genesis of reading disability. However, these research endeavors are honeycombed with confusion and misunderstanding. Experimental design flaws, the complexity of reading processes and a general nescience of clinical visual physiology have all contributed to the muddle. Unfortunately this confusion has been malinterpreted to mean that vision and more specifically visual function has a minor role or no role at all in reading achievement. This has been extended to the clinical domain by the general inattention directed to the visual efficiency of children experiencing difficulty learning to read.

There have been primarily two research approaches to explore the relationship between vision and reading, the case-control study and the correlational study. In the majority of case-control studies, reading level was the independent variable. The prevalence rate of certain visual functions or abnormalities (or arbitrarily defined levels of performance) was then compared between a poor reading and a control group of normal readers. Presumably, a greater prevalence of visual dysfunctions or abnormalities among poor readers would indicate the capacity for vision to influence reading ability. The second prominent research design has been the correlational study.

In correlational studies, quantitative measures of a visual function are related to reading level in a designated sample. The correlation coefficient denoted by the Pearson *r* is the descriptive measure of association in correlational studies. An anticipated correlation assumes that the more profound the reading disability, the greater the degree of visual abnormality. From a clinical perspective, this is an untenable hypothesis. For instance, most clinicians would agree that the variance between two and four prism diopters of near-point exophoria in most respects is not significantly differential in creating a visual dysfunction. In actuality, for this example, 2 prism diopters (pd) exophoria is more deviant from the expected level of near phoria. Significant deficits in accommodative or vergence function may not even be reflected in the heterophoria. Yet, a correlational statistic would demand that the higher exophoria be associated with poorer reading.

Likewise, there is no logic in the proposition that higher levels of anything would necessarily be more strongly correlated to lower levels of reading achievement. The correlational approach to understanding the relationship between vision and reading is categorically the wrong approach.[20] Clinical experience has taught that the magnitude of an individual test result is not necessarily the singular determinant of visual efficiency. Visual inefficiency is not based on minor differences from the norm but when some threshold level of dysfunction is reached.

By way of a specific example, Robinson[21] correlated reading scores and visual skills for 100 pupils each from elementary grades one through eight. Visual acuity, refractive error, stereopsis, vertical and lateral heterophoria, and vergence ranges were determined. Correlation coefficients were small and in the range from $+0.25$ to -0.25. These results are consistent with the majority of correlational studies. However, when a subsample of the best readers (2 grades above expected) and the poorest readers (greater than 1.6 grades below) were compared, significant differences between the groups materialized. The poorer readers were more hyperopic, had lower vergence ranges, and had phorias that deviated significantly from the normal range than the better readers.

Another influence is that of the variability of visual functions under investigation. For example, low hyperopia is the norm for the majority of school-aged children. The range and variability of refractive status is necessarily limited in this age group. The low variability in refractive error relative to the variability of other factors that determine reading ability (such as language ability) means that refractive error will not be as strongly related to individual differences in reading ability, despite its importance as an underlying factor in every child's reading performance. The same is probably true of other visual functions. If the variability of one factor is restricted, other factors will necessarily be more strongly related to differences in reading achievement.

Other difficulties encountered in studies relating vision and reading is the use of arbitrary or nonuniform criteria for designating normal and abnormal visual function. The most recent example, and one that has been widely cited, is a publication of Helveston, Weber, Miller, et al.[22] In an evaluation of 1910 first-, second-, and third-grade children, they found that visual function and reading performance were not positively related. Concerns about their conclusions are raised by the tests selected to evaluate visual function and their arbitrary selection of normal versus abnormal criteria. For example, Titmus stereoacuity of 140 seconds, near point of convergence of 10 cm, and amplitude of accommodation of 11 diopters (independent of age) were all considered normal findings. Most optometrists would unequivocally reject this classification system in this age group. Moreover, the one visual function, namely, refractive status, that through the years has shown the most meaningful relationship with reading achievement (see below) is not even reported in the paper, even though noncycloplegic refractive error was determined.

Few studies have used comprehensive clinical testing or complete diagnostic classification. There has been an overreliance on inadequate tests of visual function, for example, information obtained on vision screenings. The use of screening instruments whose reliability has been challenged makes these results questionable.[16] The effects of stress or fatigue or the capacity of vision to function efficiently under sustained reading conditions have been largely ignored. This has created the tendency to view each visual function separately and as being presumably neither interrelated nor interdependent. Nor are functions typically grouped together as a syndrome or cluster of skills, as is commonly done clinically.

Previous research efforts have also been hampered by definitional complications surrounding reading disability. There is a myriad of causes of reading disability.[23] These include physical factors, cognitive and language factors, and emotional, environmental, and educational factors. There are almost certainly complex interactional effects that contribute differentially to an individual child's reading difficulties.

Similarly all reading disabilities cannot be equated. The difficulties encountered in reading are expressed in diverse forms. A circumscribed classification scheme includes faulty word identification and recognition (sight vocabulary, phonics), deficient basic comprehension abilities, deficient study skills, deficient rate of reading with comprehension, differences in silent versus oral reading, and deficient adaptation to the reading needs of content fields. Visual inefficiency may be differentially related to each of these expressions of reading disability. Actually, two children can score similarly on reading achievement tests but perform differently in the classroom environment.

There is no distinct delineation to distinguish children with reading disability from normal readers. The condition is not an all-or-none phenomenon, but reading ability must be considered as occurring along a continuum. This is the reason why the criteria and methods used for sample selection differentiating poor readers from normal readers is crucial to interpreting research results. Children at the lower extreme of the distribution of reading ability and having the most profound disability are certainly not typical, and it would not be expected that visual dysfunction would have a significant etiological role. Norn, Rindziunski, and Skydsgaard,[24] for example, found no differences in refractive error, heterophoria, and vergence amplitude between 117 children diagnosed with, in their terms, specific dyslexia or congenital word blindness and 117 controls from an affluent suburb of Copenhagen. The reading-disabled children were enrolled in a specific remedial reading class and their mean school grade was 5.4. The mean reading grade level of the experimental group was 2.5. But, using Bond and Tinker's[23] reading expectancy grade level, which is based on the years in school and IQ, the mean discrepant reading level for the reading disabled was 4.5 grades. That is, the experimental group of fifth grade children, was reading at a first grade level. This then represents a group of profoundly disabled readers. In fact, a familial pattern was present in one or more relatives of about 73% of the children. The negative results should not be generalized to the more typical "garden-variety" reading disabled.

In addition to these methodological handicaps in defining a reading-disabled sample for study, other uncontrolled confounding variables that affect reading achievement are present, for example, the child's intrinsic motivation, the effectiveness of compensatory cognitive and educational strategies, and the often-ignored effects of pedagogy (such as teaching styles and auditory versus visual classroom orientation).

A review of the literature in this field will also find appalling examples of egregious experimenter bias. In an oft-quoted study supporting a lack of association between visual function and reading achievement, Blika[25] examined 200 primary-grade good readers and 41 nominal* poor readers. He found no significant differences in visual acuity, refractive status, heterophoria, and vergence ranges between the two reader groups. However, he stated quite clearly the purpose of the investigation:

> . . . an increasing amount of parents pay huge sums of money to non-medical persons who claim to be able to cure reading disabilities by eye muscle exercise and glasses. In our country [Norway] this sort of "therapy" is carried out by a small number of opticians, assisted by some teachers and psychologists. The increasing amount of useless glasses being given was the reason why this investigation was undertaken.

When the appropriateness of spectacle correction was evaluated, Blika[25] concluded that "44% of the spectacles in the good reader group and as many as 71% of the spectacles in the poor reader group were unnecessary . . . 86% of the unnecessary spectacles had with certainty been prescribed by opticians, 6% by ophthalmologists."

There are even unmistakable examples of ignoring positive results. Norn, Rindziunski, and Skydsgaard[24] concluded that visual deficits were not more frequently encountered in a reading-disabled sample. However, a review of their data indicates that the reading-disabled sample did have a higher prevalence of significant heterophorias ($\chi^2 = 7.28$, $p = 0.007$). In addition, there were greater subjective complaints during reading, approaching significance ($p = 0.06$).

Nevertheless, despite these difficulties noted in research efforts, a credible pattern of association between visual skills and reading ability emerges. In an extensive study-by-study narrative review of the literature, Grisham and Simons[5,26] concluded that there is a relationship between refractive status and binocular vision and reading. This was further supported by a metanalysis of the same literature.[27] For the discussion in this

---

* The word "nominal" will be used to describe those subjects identified as reading disabled but in which the author does not adequately describe selection criteria, or if no specific reading achievement test was stated or utilized in the study.

chapter, those studies that included professional testing in a nonscreening environment will be primarily considered.

OVERALL INDICES OF VISUAL FUNCTION

Park and Burri[28] randomly selected 250 primary school-aged children from Chicago public schools. Visual acuity, cycloplegic refraction, heterophoria (cover test, Maddox rod), and vergence ranges were assessed. Each deviation from normal was considered an eye defect. Any heterophoria was considered a defect. Passable vergence levels were at distance, base out, 24/16 break/recovery; base in, 8/5. Overall, 14 skills were evaluated. Reading tests were administered by school personnel. The students were ranked into 8 reading categories, and the percentage of students with eye scores lower than the mean for each group (6) was determined. In children with greater reading abilities, there were fewer with eye scores lower than the average and that the lower the reading scores, the more likely it was that the child had a peripheral ocular defect ($\chi^2 = 46.45$, $p < 0.001$). Using a similar paradigm of assembling a composite visual profile of 225 children, Park and Burri[21] found a significant correlation coefficient between reading expectancy level and total eye score ($r = 0.47$).

In arguably the most compelling research effort to explore the relationship between vision and educational performance, O'Grady[29] reported the results of a joint study conducted by the Education Department of Tasmania with local optometrists. A random sample of 227 second-grade children were selected from 74 schools. The students were given a series of educational tests and a comprehensive office-based visual examination, including accommodative facility and fixation disparity but not vergence ranges. Each visual examination was provided by one of 26 optometrists. The vision tests were selected and standardized by the participating optometrists. The visual status of each child was categorized as normal, borderline, or suspect with a full examination recommended. After the examination, 16.2% of the sample were judged as requiring additional vision care. Although four individual vision variables discriminated educational performance, the most interesting conclusion was that optometric recommendations based on overall assessment of vision status was related to reading and mathematics performance ($p = 0.05$). The suspect category of children were found to perform significantly poorer on the educational tests than the other children.

In a study with a negative result, Wilson and Wold[30] performed a modified clinical screening with 160 third, fourth, and fifth graders. The children were divided into the highest and lowest quartile according to the Stanford Reading Achievement Test. With the Orinda Study–formulated criteria being used, no significant differences in failure rate were noted between the two groups. However, as discussed above, there are limitations imposed by the use of vision screening data in defining visual function.

VISUAL ACUITY

There is negligible reason to suspect that distance visual acuity would influence reading performance, except as it mirrors dysfunction in accommodation and vergence control. Most of the published research corroborates this.[31] Paradoxically, there has been little attention directed to near point visual acuity and reading. In a substantive, well-controlled report, which deserves mention, Fendrick[32] used a modified Jaeger chart to measure near-point visual acuity (among other tests) in 64 disabled readers and an equal number in a control group matched for age, sex, school attendance, years in school, and IQ. The Paragraph Reading subtest of the Gates Primary Reading Test battery was administered to all the children. He found a higher prevalence of reduced near acuity among the disabled readers ($p < 0.05$ for binocular acuity). Diminishing the strength of this study, these data were collected in a nonprofessional screening.

In a more recent well-conducted case control study of 172 Swedish second-grade school children (mean age 9.4 years), disabled readers were found to have a lower prevalence of best corrected visual acuity at the 20/20 level than controls. The effects were noted for distance and near fixation and monocularly and binocularly. At near point, nearly all the control subjects could obtain at least a 20/20 level of visual acuity. However, there were a significant number of reading disabled (approximately 10%) who could not.[33]

It has been known for some time that reading disabled children have reduced contrast sensitivity for low spatial frequency gratings.[4] These studies have been conducted under laboratory conditions with briefly displayed stimuli. Of note from the Swedish study, Ygge et al. have demonstrated these contrast deficiencies under more typical clinical condition.[33] Using the near-point Vistech test with best corrected visual acuity, reading disabled subjects had reduced contrast sensitivity for the 1.5 and 3.0 cycles/degree gratings. Contrast-sensitivity reductions were also found for the highest spatial frequency grating tested (18 c/deg). Although this latter result is somewhat surprising and atypical, it probably reflects the reduced near-point visual acuity in this particular sample of reading disabled. One may account for these results by postulating an accommodative insufficiency in these subjects. Overall, these results indicate that testing of contrast sensitivity should be given greater emphasis in the visual examination of those individuals with reading disability.

REFRACTIVE ERROR

Among those studies finding a relationship between refractive error and reading, none have reported an association of hyperopia with good reading and myopia with poor reading. Myopia appears to be associated almost completely with normal or above-normal reading achievement.

Thomas H. Eames, optometrist, physician, and educator has contributed considerably to the understanding of the relationship between vision and reading. In his first report (1932), Eames[34] compared the refractive distribution of 114 nominal reading-disabled children selected from a private practice and a university clinic with 143 controls. He found a significant difference ($p = 0.001$) in the prevalence of hyperopia between the reading disabled and the control group (43% versus 27%). A subsequent report (1935) largely duplicated these results.[35]

These results have been criticized because of the lack of information concerning the selection of the samples, their reading levels, and their control of IQ. In a later report (1955), Eames[36] compared a remarkable number of nominal reading-disabled children (1000) with 150 controls. The nominal poor readers had a median age of 9.67 years as compared to the controls who were 1 year older. The same professional (probably Eames himself) performed all the visual examinations, including retinoscopy and a subjective refraction. The results nearly match the previous findings. The prevalence of hyperopia was much greater among disabled readers (43%) than the control group (13%). In this study, the median IQ was somewhat higher in the control group (109 versus 102).

This phenomenon of slightly lower IQ scores among reading disabled is a common phenomenon in educational research. Therefore, most research efforts, even those that have attempted to match IQ, have been conducted comparing a reading disabled sample with slightly lower IQ scores to a normal control group. Other than refractive error, there has been no suggestion that other visual functions are related significantly to IQ.

There has been much interest in the relationship between intelligence and refractive error.[37] Nadell and Hirsch[38] reported a correlation coefficient of -0.082 between California Test for Mental Maturity scores and refractive error in high school students (the negative correlation can be interpreted to mean that myopia was associated with higher IQ scores). Using the California Test and the Stanford-Binet on a sample of 554 school children (6 to 17 years of age), Hirsch[39] found a correlation of -0.19. One interesting result was that in the 14- to 17-year-old group: those with more than 2.00 D of hyperopia had an average IQ score 17 points lower than those with 2.00 D of myopia or greater. Young[40] found higher correlation between refractive error and reading achievement (-0.20) than with Stanford-Binet IQ scores (-0.12). The partial correlation between IQ and refractive error with reading achievement being held constant approached zero. These results indicate that the lack of precise control of IQ in Eames's studies was not likely to have distorted the results.

Eames[41] divided 57 third and fourth graders passing in reading and 64 reading disabled into three groups according to refractive error; emmetropes, myopes, and hyperopes. Reading level was determined by the Gates Silent Reading Test. Among the good readers, there were no differences in reading achievement across the three refractive groups. Among the poor readers however, the hyperopes had the lowest reading levels.

Young[40] compared refractive error and reading achievement with refractive error as the independent variable in 316 eyes. Hyperopia was defined as $> +0.75$ D, but myopia as any amount. There was a significant difference between hyperopes and myopes ($p < 0.05$ for the right eye, $p < 0.01$ for the left eye). The myopes were significantly better readers than the hyperopes and generally better readers than the emmetropes. Overall, these results provide an effective argument for hyperopia as a risk factor in reading disability.

More cases of significant levels of retinoscopic hyperopia (≥ 2.75 D) were found in a small group ($N = 23$) of male disabled readers with a mean age of 10.5 years, compared to a control group matched in age, sex and WISC performance scores ($p = 0.005$) by Drasdo.[42]

In two recent reports, the interactions between refractive status and visual-perceptual-motor development were reported.[43,44] Although not investigations of reading per se, children with visual-perceptual-motor delays are at risk for reading underachievement. In the first, of a sample of 712 children 6 to 12 years of age, only 18% of the children with significant hyperopia (>1.25) displayed age-appropriate visual-motor skills in contrast to 74% of the emmetropic and myopic children.[43] In a second and related study of 48 6- to 12-year-old hyperopes (>2.25 D), those children who were corrected before their fourth birthday fewer manifested visual-motor delays than those who were corrected later.[44] The importance of visual efficiency on visual-perceptual development is also evident in a study by Hoffman.[45] He has provided evidence for the positive effects of vision therapy on the perceptual skills discrimination and visual-motor integration in young school-aged children with demonstrable accommodative dysfunction.

Eames[36] found the prevalence of anisometropia of one diopter or greater among his group of 1000 nominal reading disabled of 13%, in contrast to the control group prevalence of 6% ($p = 0.0001$). In a later study looking specifically at the effect of anisometropia on reading achievement, Eames[46] found supporting data. A sample of 50 children was divided into control and experimental groups of 25 each. The controls had isometropia, the experimental group anisometropia, but the defining level of anisometropia was not reported. The subjects were matched for age, sex, and IQ. The Gates Silent Reading Test was subsequently administered to all subjects. The anisometropic group contained a significantly higher percentage (65% versus 24%) of children who were found to be 3 months or greater below expected reading level ($p = 0.0018$). Of additional importance, after refractive correction, the anisometropic group demonstrated greater relative gains in reading achievement over a 6-month period. The efficacy of refractive correction, particularly hyperopia, on reading progress was also noted by Farris.[47] Seventh-grade students wearing a spectacle correction for hyperopia made more substantial gains in reading over a 1-year period than an uncorrected hyperopic control group.

In the above described Swedish study, however, Ygge et al.[33] found no significant refractive differences between reading-disabled and control groups.

BINOCULAR VISION

Monocular reading

The capacity to read better under monocular conditions would argue that binocular vision has some negative effect on reading efficiency. Birnbaum and Birnbaum[48] found that second- and fourth-grade children read somewhat faster and with reduced error rate monocularly when compared to binocular reading. The authors noted difficulties with practice effects and test-retest reliability. Stein and Fowler[49] found improved reading ability relative to change in age after a 6-month period of monocular occlusion for all reading and close work in a group of children with poor synoptophore divergence ranges.

Overall, these results lend some support for the viewpoint that both visually unselected subjects and children with divergence limitations perform in a superior fashion when reading in the absence of binocular vision.

Heterophoria

Eames's 1935 study[35] found the prevalence of exophoria to be nearly four times greater in the nominal reading-disabled group than in the control group. In his latter large-sample 1948 study, Eames[36] found a somewhat greater prevalence of near-point exophoria in the nominally reading-disabled group (33% versus 22%, $p = 0.007$), as well as a greater median magnitude of exophoria. Unfortunately, no heterophoria testing method was described in these studies.

In a generally well-constructed research study, Good[50] used a case-control paradigm. Each case in the control group matched one case of the experimental group in age, sex, school experience, and IQ. The experimental group consisted of 25 elementary school children selected by teacher observation and whose reading level was confirmed by a reading test. The children were professionally examined. None of the control group had a lateral imbalance of 3 pd or greater; whereas 40% of the reading disabled did.

Evans, Efron, and Hodge[51] used a somewhat unorthodox but valid method, the Keystone Basic Binocular Test Number 2, for determining lateral imbalance. This anaglyphic procedure presents two drawings of rocket ships, one red and one green, vertically aligned. If the rockets are not seen aligned, a heterophoria is present. The prevalence of horizontal phoria was nearly twice as frequent in a sample of nominal reading disabled than in a larger sample of second- to fifth-grade normal readers ($p < 0.02$).

Others authors (Fendrick,[32] Park[52]) however have found no significant differences in heterophoria between reading disabled and controls with professional testing. In the above described Swedish study, Ygge et al.[33] found no significant heterophoria differences between reading disabled and control groups using the cover test.

Vergence

Eames[53] measured stereoscopic positive disparity vergence range in 88 nominal reading-disabled second, third and fourth graders and an age-matched control group. The test stimulus was a stereogram composed of the letters ON on the left half of the stereogram and NE on the right. When fused, they formed the word ONE. The median vergence range was 3 pd lower in the reading disabled group. Furthermore, more than 75% of the reading disabled fell below the level of the control-group median in the distribution of test results.

Good[50] also reported reduced positive and negative vergence ranges. Of particular interest, none of the control group had a positive fusional vergence range of less than 8 pd. Nearly all (92%) of the reading-disabled group failed to reach this level.

In a study with a negative result, Park[52] professionally tested 100 nominal reading disabled and 50 controls and found nearly identical near-point phoria and vergence ranges between the two groups. Although performance criteria were arbitrarily selected, they were close to expected optometric levels. However, no details of testing or subject-selection procedures were provided.

Likewise, Bedwell, Grant, and McKeown[54] found no differences in the frequency that good and poor readers exhibited abnormal vergence ranges assessed with vectograms. However, the performance standard was arbitrary and not stated in the paper. Bettman et al.[55] concluded that vergence ranges measured with the synoptophore were similar in reading disabled and control children, though the specifics of the testing were not provided.

Three recent investigations, both clinical and laboratory in nature, lend support to the idea that the reading disabled have disordered vergence. Stein, Riddell, and Fowler[56] measured vergence with 2.5-degree and 7-degree targets presented in a synoptophore. Vergence eye movements were recorded by the infrared photoelectric method. The 44 reading disabled had a reading level 2 standard deviations below that expected for age. The control group of 24 were matched in age and IQ with the reading-disabled group. The synoptophore tubes were altered at the rate of 0.5 deg/sec until diplopia was observed. All the controls but only 36% of the disabled readers achieved at least a 20-degree amplitude of positive disparity vergence and a 5-degree amplitude of negative disparity vergence. The differences were most obvious with the smaller targets. Rather than making disjunctive eye movements, the reading-disabled subjects tended to respond with conjugate (versional) eye movements. Using similar-sized synoptophore targets, Ygge et al.[33] found no such vergence differences. However, they did not provide information about the rate of disparity change, other than it was "slowly" changed.

Hung[11] compared the vergence responses of two young adult subjects with a documented history of reading disability with two control subjects. Eye movements were recorded by the infrared photoelectric method. Disparity was induced with ramp velocities of 1.33 to 32.0 deg/sec. Step displacements of a maximum of 4 degrees were also presented. The two reading-disabled subjects showed generally slower peak-velocity vergence movements than the controls did. They also had slower responses (peak velocity) to convergent and divergent step stimuli.

In a recent clinical study, the time required to complete 20 cycles of vergence facility with 16 pd base-out and 4 base-in prisms was significantly longer for a group of disabled readers versus controls.[57]

ACCOMMODATION

Not surprisingly, over the years accommodation has been studied much less frequently than other visual skills. Within optometric circles, it is widely believed that within the reading-disabled population there is a high prevalence rate of accommodative disorders, particularly accommodative infacility. This opinion has been based on results from both reading- and learning-disabled samples, unfortunately without accompanying control groups and well-defined performance criteria.[58-63] For example, in a sample of children drawn from a clinical population, Hoffman[59] found that 83% had reduced accommodative facility and 64% had either a reduced amplitude of accommodation or relative accommodation ranges. As expected from a population-based survey of only the push-up amplitude of accommodation, there were fewer disabled readers with reduced accommodation, though still significant (27%).[58] Other larger studies of a variety of visual functions using a control group have found no significant reductions in amplitude of accommodation among the reading disabled.[55,64]

It is obvious that the nature of accommodative function in reading-disabled children requires further investigation. Unfortunately, the only controlled studies have utilized measurements of push-up amplitude, a test notorious for its lack of sensitivity.

OCULAR MOTILITY

The subject of eye movements in reading converges on two important but distinct issues. The first is the nature of reading cyc movement patterns of disabled readers. When reading age-appropriate text, poor readers have eye movements characterized by an increased number of forward fixations per line of text, an increased number of regressions, longer fixation durations, and a greater prevalence of intraword scanning when compared to normal readers.[26] This pattern of eye movement activity is influenced greatly by the state of concurrent cognitive processing.[65]

The second major issue concerns the reading eye movement control. The programming and execution of saccadic eye movements impose an upper limit on reading rate and thus play an integral part of the reading process.[66] Two questions emerge, Do disabled readers have faulty eye movement skills, and ultimately can faulty eye movements contribute to poor reading? The answer is a qualified yes to both. Single and multiple saccadic intrusions have been recorded during reading, particularly in individuals with frank neurological impairments, making reading very difficult.[67,68] These have been found accompanying and corresponding to periods of perceptual disturbances of the text.[67] Other aspects of the necessity of precise oculomotor control for reading have been discussed earlier.

Pavlidis[69-71] has presented the most consistent argument that disabled readers have poor eye movement control. He required subjects to make saccades between a series of sequentially illuminated, equidistant targets. The reading-disabled subjects made significantly more inappropriate eye movements, especially regressions, and had longer and more variable fixations and longer reaction times than matched normal controls. His results however have not been successfully replicated; nor have others found significant differences in oculomotor skill (smooth pursuit, saccades) between controls and disabled readers.[72-75] The most plausible resolution of this discrepancy lies in the characteristics of Pavlidis's sample. Many were referred directly to his clinic from educational and clinical psychologists, remedial reading teachers, physicians, and child development clinics and may be overrepresented by individuals with visual or oculomotor deficits. Pavlidis defined his subjects as "unexpected reading failures," in that there were no negative health, socioeconomic, or environmental factors present to preclude normal reading achievement. These subjects also had several other interesting symptoms that Pavlidis suggested compose a dyslexia, (that is, reading disability) syndrome. This syndrome has a predominant component of visual-spatial deficits. Pirozzolo and Rayner[76] also have noted that disabled readers with visual-spatial deficits (low performance relative to verbal IQ, confusions of directionality, visual-motor integration delays, reading and spelling errors of a visual nature, with normal language abilities) have a pattern of eye movement abnormalities compared to those with auditory-linguistic deficits. These eye movement anomalies include increased saccade latency and return-sweep inaccuracies. Oculomotor dysfunction may be representative of an overall difficulty with analyzing space and spatial relationships. (See the box.)

Some case studies have reported a tendency for a reverse staircase (a series of consecutive regressions) in reading eye movement patterns of disabled readers.[20,77-79] These are not pathognomonic of reading disability, but they can be prevalent and indicate an abnormality in oculomotor control processes.[80]

Analysis of eye movement accuracy to relatively widely spaced targets, free of competing stimuli, may not fully represent the conditions normally

---

Pavlidis's dyslexia

Characteristics

IQ
Motivation
Emotional stability
Physical health
Socioeconomic background
Educational opportunities
Language spoken at home
Parent education
Teacher quality
Culture

Symptoms

Difficulty performing automated-sequential tasks
Reversals in ordering of letters
Transpositions of words
Omitting or repeating words when reading
Losing place or skipping lines when reading
Clumsy; hyperactive
Poor laterality, directionality
Familial pattern of reading disability

---

demanded of oculomotor control systems during reading. As discussed above, the oculomotor system must be programmed to locate and move the eye (fovea) to the optimum landing site (letter) for word recognition in the next word to be fixated. An oculomotor deficit of some subtlety may go undetected with currently available clinical tests or in experimental investigations up to now. This awaits further study.

EFFICACY OF VISION THERAPY

If visual conditions can have a deleterious effect on reading, improvement in visual efficiency should result in improved reading. There have been two noteworthy attempts to investigate the potential of visual efficiency enhancement by vision therapy to promote improved reading skill. Both studies were noteworthy because they were of good experimental design and manifestly interdisciplinary in nature.

In a study conducted at the University of Nebraska, 98 entering freshman were evenly divided into three groups, matched on reading and psychoeducational testing.[81] Group A received 6 weeks of vision therapy (3 half-hour sessions per week) followed by 3 weeks of reading instruction (2 hours per week). Group B received 6 weeks of similar reading instruction followed by 3 weeks of vision therapy. Group C received only reading instruction. Vision therapy emphasized instrument-based antisuppression, vergence, and ocular motility activities.

After the experiment, all groups improved in reading rate and comprehension. However, those receiving vision therapy made greater gains than those receiving reading instruction alone. Of particular interest, vision therapy made the most significant changes in those students with the highest scholastic aptitude potential determined by preadmissions tests relative to their initial reading levels. These subjects had a discrepancy between reading achievement and academic potential. It was concluded that in this group, vision therapy eliminated a visual deficiency that acted as a limiting factor in the development of reading ability. These results were reported in detail in the educational literature by Worcester.[82]

The second study was conducted by the Department of Psychology of North Carolina State University.[83] In this study, a sample of poorly achieving sophomore college students were placed into four groups matched for IQ and reading test scores. Group A received only vision therapy (three 45-minute sessions a week for 8 weeks), group B vision therapy and vocational counseling, group C counseling only. Group D served as the control group. Vision therapy emphasized instrument-based antisuppression, vergence, and ocular motility activities. Reading rate but not comprehension improved significantly (approximately 30% mean gain) for the vision therapy groups ($p = 0.01$).

These studies unfortunately have been conducted with adult subjects. Four more recent attempts to modify reading ability with vision therapy in children have appeared in the literature.[84-87] Unfortunately three of these are of limited value primarily because they lacked a control group.[84,86,87] Atzmon[84] used home vision therapy with a group of 146 children under 18 years of age with nominal reading disability. The visual characteristics of this sample were not individually specified, but it was noted that nearly all had reduced vergence ranges. Two or three daily sessions of 10 minutes over a period of a few weeks was sufficient to improve school performance in some area. However, specific achievement tests or other metrics of school performance were not stated. Haddad et al.[86] conducted vision therapy on a group of nominally reading-disabled children. Therapy emphasized antisuppression activities, physiological diplopia awareness, and vergence ranges. After therapy a majority of the children had increased time of uninterrupted reading and greater attentiveness and reading recall; all were evaluated subjectively. Masters[87] also reported success with vision therapy. These three studies can also be generally criticized because they did not rigorously establish the need for therapy and lacked specifics on the changes found in reading achievement.

The fourth recent study offers greater potential for evaluating the effects of vision therapy on reading achievement.[85] Atzmon et al.[85] randomized a group of 124 reading-disabled children into two groups. The experimental reading-disabled group received vision therapy but no remedial reading; the control group of reading disabled spent an identical amount of time receiving remedial reading instruction but no vision therapy (a no-treatment reading-disabled control group was lost because of the ethical and political issues necessary for denying treatment). Randomization occurred after the children were matched in IQ, reading rate and comprehension, and vergence ranges. Teachers and therapists were largely blind to a child's group placement. Each child in the experimental group received between 35 and 40 individual therapy sessions for a period of 2 to 3 months. Similar time was provided for remedial reading instruction for the control group. After this interval, both experimental and control groups showed significant increases in reading performance measured with the same standardized tests used initially. Both groups demonstrated approximately equal changes in reading; in other words, vision therapy and additional reading instruction produced the same results. Unfortunately there was not a no-treatment group to judge the true effectiveness of these interventions. The nature of the subjects' visual efficiency skills and hence the need for vision therapy were uncertain. There remains a compelling need to investigate similar effects of vision therapy in children, specifically, reading-disabled children diagnosed with visual efficiency problems.

SUMMARY

Visual skills are related to reading achievement. An analysis of the literature on the subject indicates that refractive error, in particular hyperopia and significant anisometropia, exophoria, and disordered vergence are associated with reading underachievement. Supporting evidence, though less persuasive, can also be found from studies considering overall indices of visual function, monocular versus binocular reading, correction of refractive error, the efficacy of vision therapy, and eye movement control.

Other visual functions have not been thoroughly investigated but have the potential for adversely influencing reading proficiency. For an intuitive example, accommodative infacility would make it difficult for classroom reading–related activities requiring rapid changes in fixation distance, from the chalkboard or teacher to the desktop. Any visual assessment of the child having difficulty learning must include not only tests of visual acuity and refractive status, but also tests of near-point visual skills that are associated with reading. The visual efficiency skills of accommodation, vergence, and ocular motility should be investigated in detail for the presence of any dysfunction that can not only induce visual signs or symptoms, but also have the potential for influencing reading achievement. Visual dysfunctions encountered should be managed aggressively with the goal of maximizing visual efficiency.

CHAPTER REVIEW

1. Describe the difficulty in evaluating the literature on the relationship between visual efficiency and reading.
2. What are the signs and symptoms of visual inefficiency that can occur during reading?
3. Discuss how a visual efficiency problem may influence reading skill.

4. Which visual skills show the strongest relationship to reading achievement?
5. Which visual skills should be evaluated in patients with a history of learning or reading difficulty?

REFERENCES

1. Meier JH: Prevalence and characteristics of learning disabilities found in second grade children, *J Learning Disabilities* 4:1-16, 1971.
2. Shaywitz SE, Shaywitz BA, Fletcher JM, Escobar MD: Prevalence of reading disability in boys and girls, *JAMA* 264:998-1002, 1990.
3. Leigh RJ, Zee DS: *The neurology of eye movements,* Philadelphia, 1991, FA Davis.
4. Lovegrove WJ, Garzia RP, Nicholson SB: Experimental evidence for a transient system deficit in specific reading disability, *J Am Optom Assoc* 61:137-146, 1990.
5. Grisham JD, Simons HD: Refractive error and the reading process: a literature analysis, *J Am Optom Assoc* 57:44-55, 1986.
6. Maples WC, Ficklin TW: Interrater and test-retest reliability of pursuits and saccades, *J Am Optom Assoc* 59:549-552, 1988.
7. Garzia RP, Richman JE, Nicholson SB, Gaines CS: A new visual-verbal saccade test: the Developmental Eye Movement Test (DEM), *J Am Optom Assoc* 61:124-135, 1990.
8. Borsting E: Measures of visual attention in children with and without visual efficiency problems, *J Behav Optom* 2:151-156, 1991.
9. Collewijn H, Erkelens CJ, Steinman RM: Binocular coordination of human horizontal saccadic eye movements, *J Physiol* 404:157-182, 1988.
10. Bahill AT, Ciuffreda KJ, Kenyon R, Stark L: Dynamic and static violations of Hering's law of equal innervation, *Am J Optom Physiol Opt* 53:786-796, 1977.
11. Hung GK: Reduced vergence response velocities in dyslexics: a preliminary report, *Ophthalmol Physiol Opt* 9:420-424, 1989.
12. Clark B: The effect of binocular imbalance on the behavior of the eyes during reading, *J Educ Psychol* 26:530-538, 1935.
13. Clark B: Additional data on binocular imbalance and reading, *J Educ Psychol* 27:473-475, 1936.
14. Walberg HJ, Tsai S: Matthew effects in education, *Am Educ Res J* 20:359-373, 1983.
15. LaBerge D, Samuels SJ: Toward a theory of automatic information processing in reading, *Cognit Psychol* 6:293-323, 1974.
16. Perfetti CA, Roth SF: Some of the interactive processes in reading and their roles in reading skill. In Lesgold AM, Perfetti CA, editors: *Interactive processes in reading,* Hillsdale, NJ, 1981, Lawrence Erlbaum.
17. Eames TH: The effect of glasses for the correction of hypermetropia and myopia on the speed of visual perception of objects and words, *J Educ Res* 42:534-540, 1949.
18. Rumelhart DE: Toward an interactive model of reading. In Dornic S, editor: *Attention and performance VI,* Hillsdale, NJ, 1977, Lawrence Erlbaum.
19. McConkie GW, Zola D, Grimes J, et al: Children's eye movements during reading. In Stein JF, editor: *Vision and visual dyslexia,* Boca Raton, Fla, 1991, CRC Press.
20. Pirozzolo FJ, Rayner K: Disorders of oculomotor scanning and graphic orientation in developmental Gerstmann syndrome, *Brain Lang* 5:119-126, 1978.
21. Park GE, Burri C: The effect of eye abnormalities on reading difficulties, *J Educ Psychol* 34:420-430, 1943.
22. Helveston EM, Weber JC, Miller K, Robertson K, et al: Visual function

and academic performance, *Am J Ophthalmol* 99:346-355, 1985.

23. Bond G, Tinker M, Wasson B, Wasson J: *Reading difficulties: their diagnosis and correction,* Englewood Cliffs, NJ, 1984, Prentice-Hall.

24. Norn MS, Rindziunski E, Skydsgaard H: Ophthalmologic and orthoptic examinations of dyslexics, *Acta Ophthalmol* 47:147-160, 1969.

25. Blika S: Ophthalmological findings in pupils of a primary school with particular reference to reading difficulties, *Acta Ophthalmol* 60:927-934, 1982.

26. Pirozzolo FJ: Eye movements and reading disability. In Rayner K, editor: *Eye movements in reading,* New York, 1983, Academic Press.

27. Simons HD, Gassler PA: Vision anomalies and reading skill: a meta-analysis of the literature, *Am J Optom Physiol Opt* 65:893-904, 1988.

28. Park GE, Burri C: The relationship of various eye conditions and reading achievement, *J Educ Psychol* 34:290-299, 1943.

29. O'Grady J: The relationship between vision and educational performance: a study of year 2 children in Tasmania, *Aust J Optom* 67:126-140, 1984.

30. Wilson WK, Wold RM: A report on vision-screening in the schools, *Acad Ther* 8:155-166, 1972-1973.

31. Edson WH, Bond GL, Cook WW: Relationships between visual characteristics and specific silent reading abilities, *J Educ Res* 46:451-457, 1953.

32. Fendrick P: Visual characteristics of poor readers, New York, 1935, Teachers College, Columbia University.

33. Ygge J, Lennerstrand G, Axelsson I, Rydberg A: Visual functions in a Swedish population of dyslexic and normally reading children, *Acta Ophthalmol* 71:1-9, 1993.

34. Eames TH: A comparison of the ocular characteristics of unselected and reading disability groups, *J Educ Res* 25:211-215, 1932.

35. Eames TH: A frequency of physical handicaps in reading in reading disability and unselected groups, *J Educ Res* 29:1-5, 1935.

36. Eames TH: Comparison of eye conditions among 1,000 reading failures, 500 ophthalmic patients, and 150 unselected children, *Am J Ophthalmol* 31:713-717, 1948.

37. Grosvenor T: Refractive state, intelligence test scores, and academic ability, *Am J Optom Arch Am Acad Optom* 47:355-361, 1970.

38. Nadell MC, Hirsch MJ: The relationship between intelligence and the refractive state in a selected school sample, *Am J Optom Arch Am Acad Optom* 35:321-326, 1958.

39. Hirsch MJ: The relationship between refractive state of the eye and intelligence test scores, *Am J Optom Arch Am Acad Optom* 36:12-21, 1959.

40. Young FA: Reading, measures of intelligence and refractive errors, *Am J Optom Arch Am Acad Optom* 49:257-264, 1963.

41. Eames TH: The influence of hypermetropia and myopia on reading achievement, *Am J Ophthalmol* 39:375-377, 1955.

42. Drasdo N: The ophthalmic correlates of reading disability, *Ophthalmic Optician* 30:948, 953-955, 1971.

43. Rosner J, Rosner J: Comparison of visual characteristics in children with and without learning difficulties, *Am J Optom Physiol Optics* 64:531-533, 1987.

44. Rosner J, Rosner J: Some observations of the relationship between the visual perceptual skills development of young hyperopes and age of first lens correction, *Clin Exp Optom* 69:166-168, 1986.

45. Hoffman LG: The effect of accommodative deficiencies on the developmental level of perceptual skills, *Am J Optom Physiol Optics* 59:524-529, 1982.

46. Eames TH: The effect of anisometropia on reading achievement, *Am J Optom Arch Am Acad Optom* 41:700-702, 1964.

47. Farris LP: *Visual defects as factors influencing achievement in reading,* Berkeley, Calif, 1934, University of California.

48. Birnbaum P, Birnbaum MH: Binocular coordination as a factor in reading achievement, *J Am Optom Assoc* 39:48-56, 1968.

49. Stein J, Fowler S: Effect of monocular occlusion on visuomotor perception and reading in dyslexic children, *Lancet* 2(8446):69-73, 1985.

50. Good GH: Relationship of fusion weakness to reading disability, *J Exp Educ* 8:115-121, 1939.

51. Evans JR, Efron M, Hodge C: Incidence of lateral phoria among SLD children, *Acad Ther* 11:431-433, 1976.

52. Park GE: Functional dyslexia (reading failures) vs. normal reading, *Eye Ear Nose Throat Mouth* 45:74-80, 1966.

53. Eames TH: Low fusion convergence as a factor in reading disability, *Am J Ophthalmol* 15:709-710, 1934.

54. Bedwell CH, Grant R, McKeown JR: Visual and ocular control anomalies in relation to reading difficulty, *Br J Educ Psychol* 50:61-70, 1980.

55. Bettman JW, Stern EL, Whitsell LJ, Gofman, HF: Cerebral dominance in developmental dyslexia, *Arch Ophthalmol* 78:722-729, 1967.

56. Stein JF, Riddell PM, Fowler S: Disordered vergence control in dyslexic children, *Br J Ophthalmol* 72:162-166, 1988.

57. Buzzelli AR: Stereopsis, accommodative and vergence facility: do they relate to dyslexia? *Optom Vision Sci* 68:842-846, 1991.

58. Hammerberg E, Norn MS: Defective dissociation of accommodation and convergence in dyslectic children, *Acta Ophthalmol* 50:651-654, 1972.

59. Hoffman LG: Incidence of vision dificulties in children with learning disabilities, *J Am Optom Assoc* 51:447-451, 1980.

60. Marcus SE: A syndrome of visual constrictions in the learning disabled child, *J Am Optom Assoc* 45:746-749, 1974.

61. Park GE: Reading difficulty (dyslexia) from the ophthalmic point of view, *Am J Ophthalmol* 31:28-34, 1948.

62. Sherman A: Relating vision disorders to learning disability, *J Am Optom Assoc* 44:140-141, 1973.

63. Wold RM, Pierce JR, Kennington J: Effectiveness of optometric vision therapy, *J Am Optom Assoc* 49:1047-1054, 1978.

64. Ygge J, Lennerstrand G, Rydberg A, et al: Oculomotor functions in a Swedish population of dyslexic and normally reading children, *Acta Ophthalmol* 71:10-21, 1993.

65. McConkie GW: Eye movements and perception during reading. In Rayner K, editor: *Eye movements in reading*, New York, 1983, Academic Press.

66. Rubin GS, Turano K: Reading without saccadic eye movements, *Vision Res* 32:895-902, 1992.

67. Ciuffreda KJ, Kenyon RV, Stark L: Saccadic intrusions contributing to reading disability, *Am J Optom Physiol Opt* 60:242-249, 1983.

68. Ciuffreda KJ, Kenyon RV, Stark L: Eye movements during reading: further case reports, *Am J Optom Physiol Opt* 62:844-852, 1985.

69. Pavlidis GTh: The "dyslexia syndrome" and its objective diagnosis by erratic eye movements. In Rayner K, editor: *Eye movements in reading*, New York, 1983, Academic Press.

70. Pavlidis G Th: Eye movement differences between dyslexia, normal, and retarded readers while sequentially fixating digits, *Am J Optom Physiol Opt* 62:820-832, 1985.

71. Pavlidis GTh: Diagnostic significance and relationship between dyslexia and erratic eye movements. In Stein JF, editor: *Vision and visual dyslexia*, Boca Raton, Fla, 1991, CRC Press.

72. Brown B, Haegerstrom-Portney G, Yingling CD, et al: Tracking eye movements are normal in dyslexic children, *Am J Optom Physiol Optics* 60:376-383, 1983.

73. Olson RK, Coners FA, Rack JP: Eye movements in dyslexic and normal readers. In Stein JF, editor: *Vision and visual dyslexia*, Boca Raton, Fla, 1991, CRC Press.

74. Olson RK, Kliegl R, Davidson BJ: Eye movements in reading disability. In Rayner K editor: *Eye move-

ments in reading, New York, 1983, Academic Press.

75. Stanley G, Smith GA, Howell EA: Eye movements and sequential tracking in dyslexic and control children, *Br J Psychol* 74:181-187, 1983.

76. Pirozzolo FJ, Rayner K: The neural control of eye movements in acquired and developmental reading disorders. In Avakian-Whitaker H, Whitaker HA, editors: *Advances in neurolinguistics and psycholinguistics,* New York, 1978, Academic Press.

77. Ciuffreda KJ, Bahill AT, Kenyon RV, Stark L: Eye movements during reading: case reports, *Am J Optom Physiol Optics* 53:389-395, 1976.

78. Elterman RD, Abel LA, Daroff RB, et al: Eye movement patterns in dyslexic children, *J Learning Disabilities* 13:16-21, 1980.

79. Zangwill OL, Blakemore C: Dyslexia: reversal of eye movements during reading, *Neuropsychologia* 10:371-373, 1972.

80. Jones A, Stark L: Abnormal patterns of normal eye movements in specific dyslexia. In Rayner K, editor: *Eye movements in reading,* New York, 1983, Academic Press.

81. Peters HB: The influence of orthop-

tic training on reading ability. Part 2: The problem, study and conclusions, *Am J Optom Arch Am Acad Optom* 19:152-176, 1942.

82. Worcester DA: The influence of orthoptic training on the reading ability of college freshman, *J Exp Educ* 9:167-174, 1940.

83. Olson HC, Mitchell CC, Westberg WC: The relationship between visual training and reading and academic achievement, *Am J Optom Arch Am Acad Optom 30:3-13, 1953.*

84. Atzmon D: Positive effect of improving relative fusional vergence on reading and learning disabilities, *Bino Vision* 1:39-43, 1985.

85. Atzmon D, Nemet P, Ishay A, Karni, E: A randomized prospective masked and matched comparative study of orthoptic treatment versus conventional reading tutoring treatment for reading disabilities in 62 children, *Bino Vision Eye Muscle Surg Q* 8:91-106, 1993.

86. Haddad HM, Isaacs NS, Onghena K, Mazor A: The use of orthoptics in dyslexia, *J Learning Disabilities* 17:142-144, 1984.

87. Masters MC: Orthoptic management of visual dyslexia, *Br Orthopt J* 45:40-48, 1988.

CHAPTER 7

The Relationship Between Visual Perception and Learning

SIDNEY GROFFMAN

KEY TERMS

learning disability	auditory-visual integration
visual perception	visual-motor integration
perceptual development	visual form perception
subtypes	visual memory
reading	spatial relations
spelling	reversals
mathematics	simultaneous processing
perceptual speed	sequential processing
automaticity	dyslexia

I find from my notebook that it was in January, 1903, just after the conclusion of the Boer War, that I had my visit from Mr. James M. Dodd, a big, fresh, sunburned upstanding Briton. The good Watson had at that time deserted me for a wife, the only selfish action which I can recall in our association. I was alone.

It is my habit to sit with my back to the window and to place my visitors in the opposite chair, where the full light falls upon them. Mr. James M. Dodd seemed somewhat at a loss how to begin the interview. I did not attempt to help him, for his silence gave me more time for observation. I have found it wise to impress clients with a sense of power, and so I gave him some of my conclusions.

"From South Africa, sir, I perceive."
"Yes, sir," he answered, with some surprise.
"Imperial Yeomanry, I fancy.
"Exactly."

"Middlesex Corps, no doubt."

"That is so. Mr. Holmes, you are a wizard."

I smiled at his bewildered expression.

"When a gentleman of virile appearance enters my room with such tan upon his face as an English sun could never give, and with his handkerchief in his sleeve instead of his pocket, it is not difficult to place him. You wear a short beard, which shows that you were not a regular. You have the cut of a riding man. As to Middlesex, your card has already shown me that you are a stockbroker from Throgmorton St. What other regiment would you join?"

"You see everything."

"I see no more than you, but I have trained myself to notice what I see. However, Mr. Dodd, it was not to discuss the science of observation that you called upon me this morning."

A. CONAN DOYLE: *THE ADVENTURE OF THE BLANCHED SOLDIER*

Sherlock Holmes devotees are rarely surprised by his remarkable reasoning powers. This excerpt shows us that his deductive ability is based on remarkable visual observational skills that he combines with stored information. Additionally his speed of information processing is unusually rapid so that the visitor is truly amazed at the quickness of Holmes's conclusion. These paragraphs provide an elegant illustration of the visual perception process in action.

VISUAL PERCEPTION: DEFINITIONS AND THEORIES

Perception is the active process of locating and extracting information from the environment. According to Forgus[1] perception is the core process in the acquisition of knowledge. He conceptualized perception "as the superset, with learning and thinking as subsets subsumed under the perceptual process." Although perception is the process of extracting information, learning is the process of acquiring information through experience and storing the information. Learning facilitates the perceptual process of extracting information, since the acquired and stored data are used as a model against which the environmental data are measured. Thinking, on the other hand, is the manipulation of information to solve problems. The easier it is for us to extract information (perceive), the easier our thinking process becomes. Perception steers us through our lives, and as a guide, perception proves itself creative and changeable. Perceptual knowledge is pervasive in our daily lives. As Bolles[2] puts it:

It is foremost in our dreams, our attentive examinations, our associations and our creative musings. Perception keeps us oriented, evaluates experiences, engages us with the day. . . . When we do turn to symbolic reasoning, be it verbal, scientific, or mathematical, we still have not done with perception, for reason's details and form come from perception.

Nobody has told Holmes, the great detective, who the man is or what his background has been. His perceptual skills are so highly developed that he sees a great number of things that ordinary mortals would overlook. He extracts information from the environment, such as a virile appearance, the tanned face, the beard, and the handkerchief in the sleeve. He is able to use his acquired knowledge and stored information (events in South Africa) to solve the problem with his cognitive processes because his visual perceptual skills are so efficient and instantly available for use. It is perception that is basic to learning and thinking.

Gibson's theory

Perceptual systems are the modalities utilized for the perceptual process. Gibson[3] describes five principal perceptual systems:

1. Basic orienting system
2. The haptic system
3. The taste-smell system
4. The auditory system
5. The visual system

A perceptual system must be differentiated from the passive, isolated activities of sense organs such as the nose, ear, eye, and skin because a perceptual system is integrated with the entire nervous system, motor activities, and the other perceptual systems. The perceptual systems actively seek to extract information from the environment using the sense organs as tools. Perception is an active, information-seeking process of searching ambient arrays of energy for information about the surrounding environment. This ambient array is rich in information that specifies layout, objects, and events in the world. Perception guides action, and actions inform perception.[4] Gregory[5] believes that perceptions are constructed, by complex brain processes, from fleeting fragmentary scraps of data signaled by the senses and drawn from the brain's memory banks. In his view all perceptions are based on past experiences selected by present sensory data.

Visual dominance

There is a partial equivalence, overlap, and interaction of the various perceptual systems in processing information, but in order to function at maximum capacity and efficiency, both Gesell[6] and Birch[7] observed that it is necessary for an individual to become visually dominant. Gesell wrote:

> Vision is the supreme sense of man. . . . Seeing is not a separate, independent function. It is profoundly integrated with the total action system of the child, his posture, his manual skills, his motor demeanors, his intelligence, and even his personality traits. When viewed in terms of the action system, the mechanisms of vision become a key to the understanding of behavior, both normal and deviate. To understand vision, we must know the child; to understand the child, we must know the nature of his vision.

The literature reveals a variety of theories, case studies, and experiments that tend to reinforce the concept of visual dominance over other modalities in perceptual tasks. Pick et al.[8] found that vision tended to dominate audition when the subjects were required to perform a location task. In a review of the literature Robinson[9] found that when visual and auditory signals are presented simultaneously subjects generally responded to the visual input and were often unaware that an auditory signal had occurred. Even when the subjects were told in advance that dual presentations could occur, visual dominance was still present. After a series of experiments, Posner, Nissen, and Klein[10] concluded that visual input tends to dominate other modalities in perception, memory, and speeded responses. Evidence for visual dominance was found in many different paradigms, some as a comparison of visual cues with auditory cues and others as a comparison of visual cues with proprioceptive cues.

The anthropologists Richard Leakey and Robert Lewin[11] consider the combination of stereoscopic vision and the ability to see the world in color as important evolutionary factors in the early development of the human brain. These visual skills enabled humans to perceive one object separable from among many others. They believe that:

> Ultimately, the ability to view objects as separate entities is an absolute prerequisite for the evolution of language, which is possibly the one unique human attribute. In a very real sense we owe our capacity for speech to the higher primate's reaching out to analyze their three dimensional world.

SPECIFIC RELATIONSHIPS BETWEEN VISUAL PERCEPTION AND LEARNING

The concept that perception is associated with learning disabilities developed out of the theories and research of many individuals such as Piaget,[12] Hebb,[13] Gesell,[6] Werner,[14] Strauss,[15] and many others. Researcher-clinicians such as Getman,[16] Kephart,[17] Ayres,[18] and Frostig[19] focused their attention on the deleterious consequences that perceptual disabilities had upon the learning abilities of children. They generally believed that adequate conceptual development is dependent on adequate perception.[20]

Kephart's theoretical construct

Kephart[17] developed a widely used perceptual-motor test and clinical therapy program based on several theoretical constructs. Kephart was associated with Strauss, and his work reflected Werner and Strauss's[21] assumption that perceptual and motor development form the basis for behavior, language, and conceptual learning. Kephart believed, as Piaget[12] claimed, that motor development preceded perceptual development. The earliest manifestations of intelligent behavior are motor in nature, and they predate the appearance of language. There must be a sound motor foundation for cognitive development. Kephart worked closely with Getman, and optometric influence is seen in his emphasis on eye movements, eye-hand coordination, and visual perception.

Kephart[22] conceptualized seven developmental stages that a normal child progresses through as the child develops increasingly effective and efficient strategies for information processing. The initial stage is at the level of proprioceptive or internal bodily awareness, and the final stage is thinking ability, which transcends motor or perceptual cues. His seven developmental stages include: motor stage, motor-perceptual stage, perceptual-motor stage, perceptual stage, perceptual-conceptual stage, conceptual stage, conceptual-perceptual stage

Motor stage. The child is "learning how to experience his environment" in the motor stage.[23] Kinesthetic information, that is, sensory feedback from the muscles and joints, enables the baby to learn control. Although the motoric activity in the crib appears to be without purpose, the child develops increased skill and control, and coordination begins to develop. An internal system of a body schema begins to emerge, and this body schema will provide a frame of reference from which the child will explore the world.

Motor-perceptual stage. In the motor stage the child is learning about space and objects through grasp and manual exploration. This information is mainly kinesthetic, and there is a very close relationship between kinesthesis and the motor response. During this activity all the other perceptual sense systems are detecting and transmitting information. The child uses the sense of kinesthesia as the standard by which all other perceptual data are evaluated. Eventually the child develops a body of perceptual data that is consistent, and intersensory integration will develop. Kephart calls this "establishing a perceptual-motor match." He says that it is best exemplified by eye-hand coordination. In the first step, the hand leads the eye and generates most of the information. It is hand-eye—the hand leading and the visual information secondary. In this stage the visual information is secondary and essentially meaningless.

Perceptual-motor stage. In the next step the child employs vision as the major source of information, and the hand is used to confirm. This is eye-hand—the eye leading and the kinesthetic information from the hand matching the visual data. Vision can allow the child to explore the environment much more rapidly and efficiently than the hand can, and it can process information in greater quantities. The eye soon becomes the primary sense system and perception takes the lead in the perceptual-motor match. Kephart, however, emphasized that it is important that the child develop the perceptual-motor match in the correct order: perception matched to motor. He believed that children who make the match in the wrong direction: motor matched to perception have perceptual distortions that create difficulties in future learning. In the perceptual-motor stage vision is still working in concert with the established bodily coordinate system.

Perceptual stage. Upon attaining the perceptual stage the child can begin to make discriminations and comparisons between objects in the environment, independent of motoric activity. Visual perception, however, is still dependent on a prior established kinesthetic frame of reference. Without such a foundation, visual perception remains fragmentary. Copying tasks are difficult for the child who is at a lower stage even though the ability to match a model is present. Language begins to assume importance in the perceptual stage.

Perceptual-conceptual stage. A major improvement in information processing occurs when the child attains the perceptual-conceptual stage. Now the child can conceive of a class of objects through perceptual constancy. All furry animals with four legs who bark can be identified as "dog" despite the various sizes, colors, shapes, and breeds. The concept of "dog" or "shoe" or "chair" or "A" can be perceived from the common perceptual properties common to these things.

Conceptual stage. The conceptual stage is a further elaboration of the integration of past and present perceptual information. The contribution of language becomes even more important and the child can abstract more information. Just as "dog" summarized the characteristics of all dogs, the still more abstract word "animal" includes more classes.

Conceptual-perceptual stage. Conceptual development now begins to dominate perception. At this level the child may shortcut the perceptual process and seemingly process only a few elements by filling in the gaps and perceptually constructing the organized whole with only a sampling of its features. The individual can now make predictions about events with little relevant information available.

Kephart believed that motor activity preceded the development of perception. This was consistent with the views of Hebb, Piaget, and Gesell. Hebb[13] expressed the view that it is learning that is based on repeated sequences of eye movements, and such repetition underlies the growth of the perception of form. Piaget[24] believed that motor action becomes changed into perception and cognition through a complex series of stages in which experience at the sensorimotor stage plays a great part. Vision is presumed to be reflexive, passive, and receptive only of light intensity until the development of "vision schemas" through repetitive actions. Gesell[6] set development norms for skill in fixating, following, and reaching for objects at successive ages, but these skills do not tell us very much about perceptual abilities. The ability to localize a dangling ring is not the same as discriminating the dangling ring from another object.

Salapatek's research[25] contradict the notion that the very young infant sees only an undifferentiated blur. He determined that at 7 to 8 weeks of life sustained binocular fusion is the rule, smiling to specific simple configurations is apparent, variable accommodation to objects at varying distance begins, oculomotor anticipation of visual trajectories is present, visual acuity is improving considerably, and discrimination of form can be measured. The experiments of Bower[26] indicate many surprising complex properties of the 2-month-old infant's visual processing capacities including visual memory, shape and size constancy, and visual organization. Bowers contends that the mechanisms underlying such abilities are largely not developed through experience and are probably present before 50 to 60 days of age in most infants. Fantz[27] maintains that various aspects of the visual system are functioning, at least to some degree, soon after birth. For example, infants under 5 days of age show far greater attention to a white face with black features than they do to colored disks. He concludes that babies can, from birth, discriminate patterns as the basis for form perception and that vision perception comes before action. Early perceptual experience is essential for the growth of coordinated and visually directed behavior. The growth of sensorimotor coordination will then in turn increase the efficiency of the perceptual process. In light of this research Kephart's developmental stages should perhaps begin with his third step, the perceptual-motor stage.

The viewpoint that perception precedes motor activity is significant for those of us involved in vision perception therapy, since it negates the concept that motoric training is a necessary first step for the development of perceptual abilities. In practice, of course, a combination of modalities should be utilized.

EXPERIMENTAL EVIDENCE RELATING VISUAL PERCEPTION TO LEARNING

Other researchers have concerned themselves with experimental evidence relating visual perception to learning disability. The following is a review of several research studies that are relevant.

Single-factor research

The single-factor approach to the study of learning and reading disability dominated much of the early research in the field. The single-factor paradigm is an attempt to locate the primary cause of the dysfunction. This approach is under the assumption that the population being studied is a homogeneous entity. As we shall see, this is an erroneous assumption, since heterogeneity is a hallmark of learning disability. All single-factor studies compare the abilities of a control group to a disabled group with specific tests that are hypothesized to be related to reading or some other aspect of learning. Single-factor research studies are valuable in pointing out specific deficit areas that may be a contributing factor to learning disability. Many of the single-factor studies are deficient in one or more aspects, and as a result the data may be suspect. Metanalysis is a method of improving the interpretation of many studies.

Metanalysis

Kavale[28] published a metanalysis of the relationship between visual perceptual skills and reading achievement. Metanalysis[29] refers to the statistical integration of the results of independent studies. Metanalytic statistics provide a single set of numbers that describe and summarize the results of many single-factor research studies. In coining the term metanalysis, Glass[30] identified three levels of analysis and thereby established a meaningful context for metanalytical statistical procedures. Primary analysis is the original analysis of data in a research study. Secondary analysis is the reanalysis of data for the purpose of answering the original research question with better statistical techniques, or answering new questions with old data. Finally, metanalysis refers to analysis of the results from a large number of studies for the purpose of integrating the findings. It is an analysis of analyses. In a sense then, metanalysis is a method of statistical analysis wherein the units of analysis are the results of independent studies, rather than the responses of individual subjects. The data from the studies provides an empirical statement about the magnitude of the relationship between the variables. Kavale's[28] review of the research included 161 studies and he then used metanalysis to statistically integrate the results from these studies. A total of 1571 correlation coefficients were collected and aggregated across eight visual perceptual factors, six reading abilities, three grade levels, and three subject groups. The findings indicated that visual perception is an important correlate of reading achievement and that visual perceptual skills should be included in the complex of factors predictive of reading achievement. The 161 studies investigated a variety of visual perceptual skills including:

visual discrimination The ability to perceive dominant features in different stimuli.
visual memory Either the ability to recall a dominant feature of a stimulus or the ability to recall the sequence of visually presented stimuli.
visual closure The ability to recognize a complete feature from fragmented stimuli.
visual-spatial relationships The ability to perceive the position of objects in space.
visual-motor integration The ability to integrate vision with body movements.
visual association The ability to conceptually relate visually presented data.
figure-ground discrimination The ability to distinguish an object from irrelevant background stimuli.
visual-auditory integration The ability to match serially presented visual stimuli with auditory counterparts.

Each of these perceptual skills was significantly related to reading achievement with the magnitude of association accounting for 6% to 20% of the variance in reading ability. Significant differences ($p < 0.001$) emerged among average correlations for visual perception skills. Visual memory and visual discrimination showed a larger association with reading ability than the other perceptual skills. Kavale included other analyses in his paper, but they all support his main conclusion that:

> Visual perceptual skills, when considered both individually and in combination, accounted for moderate proportions of the total variance in reading ability. Thus visual perceptual skills appear sufficiently associated with reading achievement to be considered among the complex of factors related to the prediction of reading ability.

This study is particularly significant because it contradicts and refutes with rigorously precise statistical analysis those who claim that reading disability is solely a language problem[31] or those who believe that visual perception skills are not significant enough to be related to academic achievement.[32]

Cluster analysis

The single-factor research studies in learning disability reveal that a wide array of deficits are found in learning-disabled students in addition to visual perception disabilities. They demonstrate linguistic, attentional, cultural, motoric, cognitive, emotional, as well as basic academic deficiencies.[28] This diversity negates the theory that learning disability is a homogeneous disorder with a single cause but is obviously a heterogeneous disorder characterized by considerable variability. In recent years researchers have been concerned with classifying learning disabled students into more homogeneous subgroups or subtypes.[29] "Cluster analysis"[30] is the generic name for a wide variety of procedures that can be used to create subtypes. These procedures empirically form "clusters," or groups of highly similar entities. It is a multivariate statistical procedure that reduces a large amount of data about a sample into relatively homogenous groups.

Early subtype studies used descriptive or subjective means to define the groups.[36] These clinical-inferential studies used predetermined criteria based on apparent patterns of performance on various tests to establish subtypes. Based on test results, subjects were then classified into the subtypes. More recent studies have used objective, statistical analysis (Q factor analysis and cluster analysis) to discover the nature of the subtypes. In this method the clusters describe groups of subjects rather than groups of tests.

A frequently cited clinical-inferential study of subtypes in learning disability was conducted by Mattis, French, and Rapin.[37] Their research was based on the neuropsychological concepts promulgated by A.R. Luria.[38] Mattis et al. studied 82 dyslexic children and isolated three independent syndromes: (1) language disorder, (2) articulatory and graphomotor dyscoordination, (3) visuospatial perceptual disorder. The articulatory and graphomotor cluster was identified in part by a test of visual motor skill, and 37% of the group were classified into this subtype. The third cluster, a pure visual processing group, had 16% of the children; therefore 53% could be considered as having a visual perception disability. The three syndromes were based on 10 tests that probed speech, language, visual perception, visual motor, eye-hand coordination, and spatial abilities.

Another landmark clinical-inferential study by Boder[39] identified three subtypes based on language disability. Boder claims that reading requires visual perception, auditory perception, and visual-auditory integration. The Boder test classifies dyslexic children into one of three distinctive subtypes, whereas normal readers cannot be classified into any of the patterns.

Group 1. Dysphonetic. Reading-spelling pattern reflects a primary deficit in symbol-sound integration and in the ability to develop skills in phonetic word analysis-synthesis. This child develops a limited sight vocabulary that can be read fluently as visual gestalts. The dysphonetic child spells by sight not by ear.

Group 2. Dyseidetic. Reading-spelling pattern reflects a primary deficit in the ability to perceive letters and whole words as configurations, or visual gestalts. The children in the dyseidetic group read laboriously as if seeing each word for the first time. The dysphonetic children have difficulty in learning what the letters sound like and the dyseidetic children have difficulty in learning what the letters look like. The dyseidetic child spells by ear not by sight.

Group 3. Mixed dysphonetic-dyseidetic. Reading-spelling pattern reflects a primary deficit both in ability to develop phonetic word-analysis skills and ability to perceive letters and whole words as visual gestalts. The children in the mixed group have the most severe reading problems, since they combine the deficits in groups 1 and 2. The response of these children to standard remediation is poor. The mixed dysphonetic-dyseidetic child cannot spell by either ear or sight. In her study of 107 children, Boder was able to place 94% of the sample in one of the three groups. Of this 94%, 63% fell into group 1 (dysphonetic), 9% into group 2 (dyseidetic), and 22% into group 3 (mixed dysphonetic-dyseidetic). In other words, 31% of the sample had visual perception dysfunction associated with their reading disability.

· · ·

Watson and Goldgar[40] used cluster analysis to derive a typology of reading disability from a sample of 63 moderately to severely reading-disabled children. Four clusters were derived from the administered tests: (1) auditory processing; (2) a mixed disorder of short-term memory, auditory processing, and visual processing; (3) language disorder; (4) another mixed disorder of auditory, memory, and visual processing. The authors noted that poor visual-motor skill is a "ubiquitous finding in this sample." A visual processing deficit was also found in a substantial number of the subjects, a confirmation that visual-motor skills and visual-perceptual skills contribute to reading disabilities even though a pure visual processing subtype was not isolated, as was found in a previous study.[41] The authors speculate that the reason for this finding may be that this sample contained severely retarded readers whereas the earlier study may have contained children who were not actually learning or reading disabled but who were below average intellectually and academically. In the earlier study[41] a similar battery of 23 measures was administered to 65 reading-disabled children. The cluster analysis revealed three clusters rather than four as found in the later experiment: (1) a visual processing deficit containing 31% of the sample; (2) a generalized language disorder subtype; (3) a minimal deficit subtype with relatively few impairments evident.

Many researchers believe that learning disabilities may be manifested in areas other than reading and arithmetic. In addition to the various academic areas affected by learning disabilities, such areas as fine-motor coordination, memory, speed of information processing, social skills, self-concept, and behavior are often influenced adversely. In an excellently designed study, Bender and Golden[42] derived five behavioral clusters from their data with some interesting conclusions for those of us concerned with visual processing. The five distinct clusters were no notable deficits, a visual deficit, a language deficit, poor reading with high self-concept, and behaviorally disordered.

A no notable deficits cluster included 37% of the students and was not particularly distinct from the others in the group and must be considered nondescript.

A visual deficit cluster included 25% of the group, and they demonstrated deficiencies in visually based cognitive skill. Acting-out behaviors were relatively high. Bender and Golden believed that some intervention such as reinforcement of on-task behavior may be indicated in order to deal with the behavior problems. Many of our vision therapy patients exhibit this type of behavior at the outset of therapy. It is not unusual to see behavioral improvements as a result of vision therapy, and this study tends to confirm our belief that there is a correlation between behavioral anomalies and visual disorders.

A language-deficit cluster included 23% of the subjects. They showed deficits in language-based cognitive abilities. The language-impaired students demonstrated very low scores on self-perception of intellectual status and popularity. The authors believed that visualization and imagery methods for reading comprehension might be appropriate since they have relative strength in visual processing. It is interesting to note that more subjects were found in the visual-deficit cluster (25%) than in the language- deficit cluster (23%). This is contrary to many other studies and the conventional wisdom that language deficits are presumed to be far more numerous than visual perception deficits.

A poor reading with high self-concept cluster included only 6% of the subjects. The authors characterized this group as the "I'm OK Kids" because despite their poor scores on the reading achievement tests they scored very high on the self-concept and personality measures.

A behaviorally disordered cluster included 10% of the group and showed major problems on every behavior variable and the two self-concept variables. They were also superior to every other cluster on the cognitive and reading scores. They believed that this group was incorrectly labeled as learning disabled and should be considered as behaviorally disordered.

The conclusions we can draw from this study is that a visual deficit subtype of significant numbers is present among learning-disabled youngsters and that it may be associated with a behavioral disorder characterized by acting out.

A recent study[43] was designed to extend the Mattis, French, and Rapin[37] study on subtypes, which was discussed previously. They believed the earlier research had several flaws that limited its usefulness. Lyon and Watson[43] used 100 subjects from public school classrooms rather than neurology clinics and used a quantitative empirical classification technique (cluster analysis) rather than a clinical-inferential procedure to define the subtypes. The group was limited to 11- and 12-year-old students as opposed to a wide scatter of ages. Six homogeneous subgroups of the reading-disabled group were identified, with two of them being mixed disorders including a visual perception factor. The largest cluster (34%) was surprisingly composed of children with a pure visual perception disability. They had deficits in visual memory, visual-motor integration, and spatial relations–visual reasoning. This finding is particularly significant because of the older age of the participants. Many have claimed that visual perception disability is found only in young children and affects learning in grades 1 and 2. Here, we see that 12-year-old students have significant visual perception disorders that are associated with their learning disability.

Not only did the visual perception disability subtype have the largest representation, but also, if we consider the perceptual disabilities from the other clusters, 58% of the children in this study have some form of visual perception dysfunction associated with their learning disability.

Satz and Morris[44] used cluster analysis in a very clever and unique manner to determine homogeneous subtypes of learning-disabled children. They then used two of the learning-disabled clusters, who were severely impaired in all three areas (reading, spelling, arithmetic) of the Wide Range Achievement Test for a subtype analysis of learning disability. Five distinct subtypes emerged including a visual perception cluster with 27% of the children and a mixed group with 12% of the sample. Thirty-nine percent of the subjects had a visual perceptual disability, which adds further evidence to our thesis that visual perception deficits are a significant factor in learning disability. Those who hold that language deficits are the sole factor in learning deficits should heed the words of the authors who emphasized that over 40% of the group showed no language impairment. This study also tends to contradict the concept that spatial-perceptual deficits are seen only in young children up to 8 years of age. The age of the children in this study was 11, and as Satz and Morris[44] advise:

> . . . most subtype studies have identified a subgroup of learning disabled children who continue to show selective cognitive differences in processing visual information—even at older ages (11-12 years). To ignore this subgroup of learning disabled children could retard progress in the search

for differential causes as well as to subject these children to inappropriate methods of remediation.

The results of these subtype studies, as well as Kavale's metanalysis, refute the group of educators who claim that mastering the sound-symbol code is the only requirement for learning to read. These people tend to view reading as primarily a process of "translating" print into sound so that already learned language processing skills can be applied.[45] Without negating the importance of the print-sound code in reading disability, many clinicians have noted that children with adequate phonological skills often have reading-comprehension problems. For these children a unitary, phonics-only approach to remediation may be counterproductive. The cause and characteristics of learning and reading disability cannot be attributed to a unidimensional factor. Most dysfunctional individuals have multiple needs that must be considered diagnostically and when patient management is planned.

Table 7.1 summarizes the percentage, in the analyses of subtypes reviewed, of pure visual perception disabilities and visual perception disabilities mixed with other deficit areas. As indicated in this table, there is a pure visual perception subtype of over 20% and a mixed subtype of almost 20%. Over 40% of the subjects in these studies have a visual perception deficit, thus validating the optometric thesis that stresses the importance of visual perception deficits in learning disabilities.

SPECIFIC RELATIONSHIPS BETWEEN VISUAL PERCEPTION AND READING

One in five learning-disabled subjects have a pure visual perception disorder, and another one in five have a visual perception disorder mixed with other factors. Can we identify the specific perceptual factors associated with reading disability? A review of the literature indicates many conflicting studies, and it is difficult to draw strong conclusions. Much of this confusion is attributable to poor research methodology and inaccurate definitions of vision perception, dyslexia, nonspecific reading disability,

TABLE 7.1   Summary of cluster analysis studies

Name of study	Visual perception subtype (%)	Mixed subtype (%)	Total (%)
Mattis, French, Rapin	16	37	53
Boder	9	22	31
Watson, Goldgar	31	31	31
Watson, Goldgar	44	44	44
Bender, Golden	25	25	25
Lyon, Watson	34	24	58
Satz, Morris	27	12	39
Average percent	20	20	40

and learning disability. With this caveat in mind let us see if we can identify the relevant perceptual factors associated with reading disability.

Perceptual speed

It is a common observation that many learning disabled children can successfully complete visual perception tasks if given enough time but do poorly if time limits are imposed. Inferior processing speed is one of the major characteristics of learning disability, not only in perceptual tasks, but also in most learning situations. Automaticity is an important phenomenon in skill acquisition. Skills are believed to consist largely of collections of automatic processes and procedures. There is evidence that automatic processing differs qualitatively from nonautomatic processing in several respects, including the fact that automatic processing is fast and effortless.[46]

LaBerge and Samuels[47] described a model of automatic information processing to explain some aspects of reading disorder. They claimed that beginning readers may not be able to learn to read for meaning until they have learned to identify words and letters automatically. Their model contained four key elements; attention, visual memory, phonological memory, and semantic memory.

Poor readers are said to have a common problem in speed of naming words, digits, and figures. Denkla and Rudel[48] devised a Rapid Automatized Naming (RAN) test for colors, numbers, pictures, and words. On all these naming tasks dyslexic children were slower than normals and learning-disabled children who were not dyslexic. Among the several components involved in rapid automatized naming, visual scanning and sequential processing are significant.

Wolff, Michel, and Ovrut[49] suggest that an abnormally long visual-stimulus registration time contributes significantly to the impaired rapid automatized naming performance of dyslexic subjects. The importance of testing for processing speed was emphasized by Jarman and Krywaniuk,[50] who used a set of perceptual tasks to measure different types of speed of information processing. Their results indicated two varieties that were interpreted as simultaneous and successive cognitive processing speed.

Perceptual speed in poor readers was examined by Spring,[51] who found that the poor readers were substantially slower than the good readers on the task and additionally the central processing speed of the poor readers deteriorated significantly during a period of 10 minutes of intensive testing. Lyle and Goyen[52,53] in a series of studies comparing good readers with poor readers on tachistoscopic recognition tasks found that poor readers were much worse than the good readers. They eliminated factors such as motivation, impulsivity, short-term memory, and discrimination difficulty and concluded that speed of perceptual processing was the perceptual deficit manifested by the disabled readers. Steinhauser and Rick[54] found that perceptual and linguistic processing was significantly slower for disabled readers and are a primary source of deficiency in disabled readers. The rate of visual information pickup was found to be slower for learning-disabled subjects in a span of apprehension (see Bryant et al.[55]). The coding subtest of the Wechsler Intelligence Scale for Children (WISC) was found to be a sequential speed-of-processing task[50] and Whitehouse[56] found that dyslexic readers performed significantly poorer than normal readers on the coding task. Koslowe,[57] an optometrist and educational psychologist found a relationship between reading difficulties, binocular vision disability and low scores on the coding subtest of the WISC-R. He claims that the coding test requires rapid shifts of gaze, focusing, and fixation and recommends that a low coding score may be an adequate reason for referral for a full visual evaluation, especially in the area of binocular vision.

Solan and Ficarra[58] found that the perceptual speed subtest of the Primary Mental Abilities battery correlated significantly with reading disability in fourth, fifth, and sixth graders. They believed that the perceptual speed test evaluates the rate of visual processing and is an important factor in distinguishing accuracy from automaticity in perceptual testing and in planning the treatment of learning- and reading-disabled children.

Integrative factors

The ability to integrate information arriving as input from different sensory modalities may be deficient in individuals with perceptual disability. The forms of integration that are significant in learning disability are intramodal and intermodal. Intramodal integration is the input, organization, and output of stimuli received in one perceptual modality. Examples would be visual-visual or auditory-auditory pattern matching. Intermodal integration is the input, organization, and output of stimuli received in different perceptual modalities. Examples of cross-modal integration are visual-motor, auditory-visual, auditory-motor pattern matching. Learning is facilitated when intermodal skills are utilized. When a new word is being learned, good pedagogical technique involves matching the word with a picture (visual-visual integration) and then saying or spelling the word orally (auditory-visual integration), and finally writing the word (visual-motor integration). Learning-disabled children are generally less efficient in both intermodal and intramodal integration, but the intermodal skills of visual-motor integration and auditory-visual integration appear to be most important.

Visual-motor integration

The Gesell Copy Forms test of visual-motor integration is a commonly utilized developmental probe by optometrists. The basic test of copying six geometric forms—circle, square, triangle, divided rectangle, vertical diamond, and horizontal diamond—reveals much about the child. Ilg and Ames[59] ask:

How does the child begin to show us his own experiencing of these forms? Is it not from this matrix of his own inner experiences that he is finally capable of projecting into them, first with the visual recognition of his own eyes and then with the capacity to reproduce them with the movement of his own hands?

To show that reproduction of geometric forms is an integrative task Mattison et al.[60] analyzed the visual-motor problems in learning-disabled children and concluded that the visual-perceptual and the perceptual-conceptual components of the visual-motor system were intact for the learning disabled children but the motor-coordination component and the integration between the visual-perceptual and the motor-coordination components were disturbed. Leonard et al.[61] asked: "Are visual-perceptual and visual-motor skills separate abilities?" They answered their question by correlating scores on a motor-free visual perception test, a visual-motor integration test, and two motor ability tests. A small but significant correlation was found between scores on the motor-free test and the visual-motor integration test but neither of the motoric tests were correlated. They believed that visual perception and motor skills are separate abilities. Their results do not support the notion that impaired visual perception is a major contributor to visual-motor disability. The correlation found is probably attributable to a defect in integrative ability. A possible cause of this integrative deficit may be found in a very clever study by Gladstone, Best, and Davidson,[62] who assessed bimanual coordination in dyslexic and normal boys using a task like Etch-a-Sketch. Group performance was equivalent for parallel hand movements (both clockwise), but the dyslexics showed significant impairments on mirror movements and often reverted to parallel movements. Differences were apparent on both speed and accuracy measures. They concluded that the impaired performances of the dyslexics were possibly attributable to deficient interhemispheric processes and anomalous organization of the ipsilateral motor pathways.

Visual-motor tests have been widely used, usually in concert with other tests, as a predictor of academic achievement. Beery[63] in a discussion of his visual-motor integration test (VMI) says that researchers have found the VMI to be a valuable predictor when used in combination with other measures. It is particularly sensitive in identifying high-risk boys who subsequently had reading difficulty. The inclusion of the VMI with three other tests correctly predicted 85% of kindergarten children who were problem readers 7 years later.[64] Keogh and Smith[65] showed that the Bender Visual Motor Gestalt test administered in kindergarten was a good predictor of school achievement in third and sixth grades. Children who performed poorly in visual-motor integration in kindergarten did less well academically in later grades. Koppitz[66] used the Bender gestalt test in the beginning of first grade and the scores correlated significantly with school achievement in first, second, and third grades. Koppitz claims that a certain degree of maturity in visual-motor perception is necessary before a child can learn to read. She found that children with above-average Bender scores are unlikely to have difficulty in reading if other conditions are favorable. A suggestion that the Bender gestalt test is a reasonable predictor of reading achievement was made by Olson.[67] Learning-disabled children made more spacing, visual-motor mistakes, reversals, and transpositions as compared to average readers in a recent study on early writing.[68] Solan and Ficarra[58] determined that the VMI was correlated with verbal tasks in grades 4 to 6. A form discrimination and a form copying test were used[69] to demonstrate the relevance of visual-perceptual factors to academic achievement at different age levels. The instrument used in this study, the Kent Perceptual Processing Inventory (KPPI), uses designs in its visual perception sections based on the structural characteristics of the forms involved in written language. KPPI results were significantly correlated with concurrent as well as with follow-up achievement scores. The authors conclude that perceptual processing skills are critically important in early achievement and can predict concurrent and future achievement in the early elementary grades. The therapeutic implications of this study is that developmental considerations must be paramount when designing a visual therapy program for perceptual deficits in visual-form discrimination and visual-motor integration.

Auditory-visual integration

Children with reading deficits have a less efficient capacity to integrate information from auditory and visual channels than normal readers have. Birch and Belmont[70] were the first to find auditory-visual deficits in poor readers. They devised a task that required that the child match the sound patterns made by pencil taps to corresponding dot patterns. In other words, the child had to integrate and regard as equivalent an auditorily presented and temporally distributed stimulus pattern with a visually presented and spatially distributed stimulus pattern. The data indicated that the function improves with age with the most rapid period of development occurring between 5 and 7 years of age. There was also high correlations between auditory-visual integration performance and reading skills in younger children. They concluded that the acquisition of auditory-visual integration may be viewed as learning to learn to read and may well represent a primary competence requisite to reading. They did not find a correlation between auditory-visual skill and reading after 8 years of age. They believed that the demands of the task, which included only 10 items, could have created an age plateau. Beery[71] proved that this was the case by testing normal and reading-disabled children, who ranged in age from 8 years and 9 months to 13 years and 3 months, on three tasks: the original Birch and Belmont task, a 20-item version of the same test, and a third test, which employed the same configurations but interchanged the stimulus presentations. That is, a visual stimulus was exposed before the auditory stimuli were heard. Her findings were consistent in that, regardless of the length of the test and whether the standard was auditory or visual, the ability of the poor readers at all ages was significantly inferior to that of average readers.

The relation of auditory-visual integration and tactual-visual integration to intelligence and reading achievement was studied by Ford[72] in a sample of fourth-grade boys. Results showed that auditory-visual integrative skills, but not tactual-visual integrative skills, were significantly related to intelligence and reading achievement. Sterrit and Rudnick[73] found that auditory-visual integration, but not visual-visual integration, was related to reading and speculated that auditory pattern perception is the primary function related to reading rather than an integrative function. Memory and attention factors were cited as possible sources of deficient performance on a simultaneous visual-auditory recall of letters test[74] rather than integrative functioning. Short-term auditory sequential memory deficit was the major factor in the inferior auditory-visual integration performance of the retarded readers in a study by Badian.[75] She found that as the memory demands increased the performance of the retarded readers decreased in contrast to the adequate readers. Memory factors were not supported by the research of Vande Voort, Senf, and Benton.[76] They suggested that deficiencies in attentional or encoding processes are implicated, since their poor readers did badly on two intramodal tasks as well as intermodal tasks. Blank and Bridger[77] not only required their subjects to match both auditory and visual sequences to dot patterns but also asked their subjects to describe the patterns. They found that poor readers described the patterns poorly and argued that the poor readers are deficient in their ability to encode temporal sequences verbally. Bryden[78] also found poor verbal coding contributing to reading-disabled children's poor performance on a variety of intermodal and intramodal tasks. It was found that cross-modal matches and that matches involving a shift from sequential to spatial display were even more difficult for the disabled readers. Kahn and Birch[79] studied 350 elementary school–aged boys from grades 2 through 6. Visual and auditory discrimination skills, auditory memory, verbal mediation, and intelligence were investigated as possible factors in the relation of auditory-visual integration to reading. They found that auditory-visual integration was correlated to reading achievement at all grade levels. Even when the effects of intelligence were considered, auditory-visual integration continued to be related to reading skill, especially word knowledge. None of the strategies postulated as effective mediators for auditory-visual integration—visual discrimination, auditory discrimination, auditory memory, and verbal mediation—satisfactorily accounted for individual differences in auditory-visual integrative ability. The ability to apply verbal labels to the auditory and visual physical stimuli, verbal mediation, was the least effective technique for success at the task.

What does this research mean for the practicing optometrist? It is clear that a test of auditory-visual integration is essential in our diagnostic battery. The underlying skills involved in cross-modal integrative ability may involve many important factors associated with learning disability. This makes it a valuable target area for therapy, since improvements in auditory-visual integration may have a positive effect on several dysfunctions.

Transient visual deficit

There is increasing evidence[80] that indicates that as many as 70% of children with reading disability may have an impairment in the visual mechanisms that transmit information about stimulus movement and stimulus change, called a "transient visual deficit" (Chapter 4). Williams and LeClyse[81] claim that reading-disabled children with this type of visual problem will exhibit visual perceptual disabilities. In a substantial number of patients it is found that the transient mechanism deficit results in weak inhibition, giving rise to longer visual persistence at low-level spatial frequencies. Afterimages seem to persist too long, and so an image is still being processed when a subsequent image overlaps with it and causes confusion. These individuals need a longer period without any interference from a new stimulus in order to interpret what they have seen. It is these problems that are believed to create perceptual deficits and reading difficulty. It is also possible, according to Lovegrove[82] that there is some relationship between phonological coding disability and transient visual deficit in specific reading disability. It was found that certain phonological coding measures (nonsense-word performance and sentence verification) loaded on the same factor as transient visual processing.

Winters et al.[83] found that the adults with reading problems showed the increased visual persistence that is found in children with reading disability. This finding indicates that untreated learning and perceptual problems found in childhood are carried forward into later life. This is confirmed by social workers Kaplan and Schater,[84] who find that for a variety of reasons many persons reach adulthood with undiagnosed learning disabilities, which may have had a profound, if poorly understood, influence on their lives. They claim that virtually no research has been done on adults with undiagnosed learning disabilities, and they often go unrecognized by therapists.

Reversals and reading

> Pooh looked at his two paws. He knew that one of them was the right, and he knew that when you had decided which one of them was the right, then the other was the left, but he could never remember how to begin.
>
> A.A MILNE: HOUSE AT POOH CORNER

There is no doubt that poor readers reverse letters, sequences, and words while reading, spelling, and writing. This has been amply demonstrated by Mann,[85] who found poor readers making more reversals than good readers. Reversals were cited by Ginsberg and Hartwick[86] and also Bryant[87] as one of the major errors linked with dyslexia.

Does directional orientation disability as manifested by our friend Winnie the Pooh cause reading reversals? Some authorities believe this, but the cause of reversals has intrigued many researchers, and there is still no definitive answer. The neurologist, S.T. Orton[88] believed that reversals were the consequence of a delay in the development of cerebral dominance. He suggested that insecure directional orientation in the visual perception of symbols accounted for reading disability and coined the term "strephosymbolia" ('twisted-symbols condition') to describe reading reversals in poor readers. He presumed that left-handedness or mixed eye-hand preference was related to language laterality and used handedness as a measure of hemispheric dominance. Orton's theory does not explain many of the phenomena associated with reversals, and physiologically his concepts are incorrect. Gardner[89] says that the evidence against the Orton theory of reversals is so compelling that the theory should best be discarded.

Gibson[90] postulates that perceptual learning and development occurs as children develop increased sensitivity to visual stimuli. The ability to recognize letters develops in two stages. First the child learns to look for the individual parts of letters that enable him to identify and name them. This works well for many letters but not so well for **d, b, p,** and **q.** The second stage, therefore, requires attention to directional orientation. In Gibson's view, reversals are normal for young children and should disappear without special remediation during first or second grade. Reversal tendencies do diminish with age as Gibson demonstrated that 4-year-olds show a 45% error rate and 5-year-olds a 31% error rate and at 6 it is down to 19% but almost zero at age 8. Ilg and Ames[91] similarly found reversals of letters and words common for 5½-year-old children but almost nonexistent at 8. Recently Jordan and Jordan[92] revised the norms for their left-right reversal test and again confirmed that younger readers made more errors than older readers. They also found that girls made fewer errors than boys. Their study also supported the connection between visual reversals and reading.

Lyle[93] equated two groups of boys for cultural background, intelligence, academic opportunities, and physical condition. A major hypothesis of the study, which was proved, was that there are two distinct factors in reading retardation, one verbal and the other nonverbal (perceptual). The results of an extensive battery of tests revealed that all types of reversals were associated with reading retardation but they were attributed to verbal factors rather than perceptual factors. Mixed laterality, crossed eye-hand dominance, and finger agnosia were unrelated to reading reversals. An optometrist[94] reported the case of an 8-year, 11-month-old boy in whom the chief complaint of letter reversals and poor reading achievement was suggestive of a visual-perceptual problem. Analysis of the history, refraction, visual skills, and visual-perceptual test results indicated that a visual system dysfunction was not a significant factor. Rather, a linguistic skills deficit was suggested by the author.

Kephart[17] defined the internal sense of "sidedness" from which directional judgments are made as laterality and the act of projecting that sense into the physical world as directionality. He believed that the older child who has persistent reversal difficulty is still struggling with the establishment of directionality and that directionality must rest upon a sound and stable motor awareness. If laterality has been well established, the child needs to work with the haptic-motor match and then in turn stabilize his visual world by perceptual-motor matching. The intermediary step in transferring laterality to directionality is supplied by the eye and its kinesthetic information. It is necessary, therefore, to emphasize hand-eye tasks in the learning of directionality so that we can control the eye with accuracy and know where the eye is pointed. Some support for this is supplied by Greenspan,[95] who matched two groups with reversal tendencies and gave one group perceptual-motor training involving gross and fine motor skills, spatial directionality, and form perception. The other group received orthoptic visual training. Only the perceptual-motor group showed significant improvement as manifested by decreased reversals on test measures. Further confirmation of this approach was supplied by Heydorn,[96] who found that reversals could be remediated with a visual-motor training program. Ludlam[97] recommends that if a patient manifests reversals of short words and individual letters, such as *god* for *dog* or *bat* for *pat,* train to replace habitual head movements with eye scanning movements. If, on the other hand, a patient confuses long words, such as *cloud* for *could,* train to replace habitual eye scanning movements with head movements.

In a long review of the etiology of reversals Gardner[89] criticizes most theories and considers an impairment in visual memory to be central to the problem. He considers reversals as "organic" in nature and when found diagnostically they indicate a neuropsychological learning disability as differentiated from a psychogenic learning disability. He has developed a useful test, the Reversals Frequency Test (RFT),[89] which can be used to obtain an objective evaluation of the frequency of reversals. The Reversals Frequency Test was employed, along with other tests, in a effort to determine the neuropsychological underpinnings of the cognitive processing deficits in reading disability.[98] The RFT, which is said to measure left and right parietal and occipitoparietal brain functions, was significantly correlated with poor reading scores. Posterior cortical disabilities therefore appear to account for the reversal and sequence errors noted in the oral reading and spelling of some reading disabled youngsters.

Can tests of reversal tendencies allow prediction of reading disability?

Bannatyne[99] used the Horst Reversals Test as a diagnostic measure for dyslexia with success. Goins[100] administered 14 perceptual tests along with reading tests to 120 first-grade children. One of the tests, Reversals, presented pairs of identical figures and pairs that are identical except that one item of the pair is a reversed drawing. The child was required to identify the identical pair. Her results showed that the reversals test correlated with the scores on the reading test. It was the second best predictor of reading ability. Barrett[101] replicated Goins study and also found that the reversals test was a good predictor of reading achievement.

It is clear that reversals are present in poor readers and tests of reversals are useful in a diagnostic battery. When perceptual disabilities are found, vision perception therapy is indicated.

Visual memory and reading

There are two distinct types of visual memory associated with reading disability: visual sequential memory and visual spatial memory. Visual sequential memory is the ability to perceive and remember a sequence of objects, letters, words, or other symbols in the same order as originally seen. Visual spatial memory is the ability to remember the spatial location of stimuli or to remember, identify, or reproduce a design or form.

Visual sequential memory is strongly tied to the use of language to label the stimuli. These labels help in organizing, storing, rehearsing, and recalling the visual information. This labeling process is called "verbal mediation," and those persons who are efficient in verbal mediation are usually better students. Learning-disabled students are either poor at verbal mediation or fail to use the skill efficiently. Retarded readers have poorer visual sequential memory than children with similar intelligence who are good readers.[102] Amoriell[103] tested retarded and normal readers in the third grade on a battery of intrasensory and intersensory tests. The variable that yielded a significant difference in the performance of the poor and average readers was visual sequential memory for letters. He recommends that an organized program of therapy for visual sequential memory should be part of reading programs. Stanley and Hall[104] compared two measures of visual information processing for dyslexic and control samples of children. With the first measure 2 parts of a stimulus were exposed sequentially for 20 msec each at increasing interstimulus intervals. Both separation and identification thresholds were longer for dyslexics than normals. With the second measure, letters presented for 20 msec were masked by dots, with the interstimulus interval being incremented over trials. Dyslexics again required longer intervals for identification. These experiments provide evidence that significant differences exist between dyslexics and normals at early stages of visual information processing and involve memory for visual information. The masking task also indicates that dyslexics have a slower processing time than normals. The Visual Sequential Memory Subtest of the Test of Visual Perceptual Skills was one of two subtests that best discriminated between a learning-disabled and a normal group of young men.[105]

Other researchers believe that specific reading disability is not attributable to inadequate visual memory. Vellutino et al.[106] presented randomly arranged Hebrew letters to poor and normal readers unfamiliar with Hebrew, and both groups were asked to demonstrate retention for these stimuli on three separate occasions: immediately after presentation, 24 hours later, and 6 months later. It was found that retention in both groups was equivalent under all the temporal conditions, and they concluded that deficient visual memory is an unlikely source of specific reading disability. Swanson[107] used a serial memory task in which the normal readers and disabled readers were compared on memory performance after pretraining of named and unnamed stimulus conditions. The named condition for normal readers was superior in terms of recall performance, but no difference was found in recall of nonverbal stimuli. These data indicate that primary reading deficits are not related to deficiencies of visual memory.

Fletcher and Satz[108] have criticized Vellutino's research on methodological grounds and argue that his conception of a lack of a perceptual process in reading is incorrect. Farnham-Diggory and Gregg[109] found that short-term memory span, both visual and auditory, deteriorated over time in poor readers as compared to good readers. Morrison et al.[110] found that 12-year-old reading-disabled youngsters exhibited major deficiencies in memory skills for both labelable and nonlabelable visual information. Kavale[28] in his metanalysis study showed that visual memory and visual discrimination have a larger association with reading ability than the other perceptual skills. The dyseidetic (visuospatial) group identified by Boder[39] has a primary deficit in remembering whole words as configurations or visual gestalts. The subtype analysis by Lyon and Watson[43] produced a visual perception cluster that contained more subjects than any other. Visual spatial memory deficits were prominent in this cluster. In a very significant experiment, Willows et al.[111] used Hebrew letters to study visual recognition memory. In contrast to Vellutino and his colleagues[106] they found a significant difference in performance between reading-disabled children and normal readers. They attribute the difference in findings to the speed of exposure of the stimuli. Vellutino et al. used long stimulus-exposure times, whereas Willows et al. used brief exposure times. They conclude that visual processing factors are implicated, to some degree, in both word recognition and reading comprehension.

A fascinating single-case study[112] provides an explanation of the mechanism involved in how a visual spatial memory disability can produce severe reading and spelling disability. The subject was a developmental dyslexic who had largely resolved her reading problems as a college student even though testing revealed subtle reading deficits and severe spelling problems. She could spell only phonologically, and her reading and spelling difficulties were accompanied by severe visual memory impairments. Of the five visual memory tests administered, three were visual spatial tests and two were visual sequential. However, the two visual sequential memory tests used Greek letters and abstracts letter shapes for stimuli, and even though she attempted to use verbal mediation, it was of limited value. The authors concluded that visual memory deficits were central to her disorder and offered the following explanation:

Since there is a specific relationship between phonological awareness and learning to read, it seems likely that during the acquisition of reading, children set up expectations as to how the sound components of spoken words map onto the letters and letter groups within printed words. After children acquire phonological awareness and knowledge of letter-sound correspondences, their reading errors change. Rather than making random errors, children start to attend to beginning and end letters in words. This might account for the expansion of sight vocabulary, but such expansion depends on the child's ability to memorize the graphemic information that corresponds to the phonological markers. They speculate that children with visual memory deficits are unlikely to be able to establish detailed lexical representations for printed words even though they can use phonemes to structure their attempts to do so. A child who fails to establish a store of orthographic information because of an inability to memorize graphemic information would fail to abstract spelling patterns comprising morphemes, common letter strings, and syllables. This would constitute a failure to pass to the orthographic phase of literacy development. Visual memory is of fundamental importance for the acquisition of orthographic competence over and above phonological awareness. This might also validate Gardner's[89] concept that reversals are basically a problem in visual memory.

Clinically the existence and importance of two types of visual memory means that we must both test and train for visual sequential memory and visual spatial memory. This requires separate and distinct tests and therapeutic modalities.

Simultaneous-sequential information processing and reading

In recent years the concept of a dual system of perceptuocognitive information processing has become popular in psychological and educational circles. This theory, based on ideas originally developed by Luria[38] and expanded by Das and his associates,[113] maintains that humans process information in two qualitatively different ways, which are labeled simultaneous and successive. Simultaneous processing is defined as the integration of separate elements into a whole. Its essential characteristic is that information is handled in a holistic fashion with a gestalt-like integration of information. Strength in simultaneous processing indicates a strong visuospatial capability. A simple illustration of simultaneous processing is in locating the Big Dipper in the night sky. To accomplish this task you would need to locate and identify the spatial configuration of the constellation.

Successive, or as it is also called, sequential processing involves information arriving in the brain in a serial order. The stimuli are temporal in nature and not totally surveyable at any one point in time. When sequential data are being processed, each stimulus is related to the previous one, either temporally or cognitively, and the information is processed in a linear, step-by-step fashion. Counting the number of stars in the Big Dipper would be an example of sequential information processing. However, there is no hierarchy of these systems. A deficit in either modality can produce academic, behavioral, vocational, and other areas of dysfunction. It is desirable that both simultaneous and sequential processing be at adequate levels. Das,[113] Kaufman and Kaufman,[114] and Hammill[115] have batteries of perceptuocognitive tests that can be used to determine simultaneous and sequential processing ability. Many of the tests are identical or similar to the tests utilized by behavioral optometrists, but they are interpreted according to the perceptuocognitive processing paradigm.

Das and his associates[116,117] have reported on experimental studies in which reading achievement and simultaneous-successive processing were related. They studied normal groups, retarded groups, various grade levels, and children with learning disabilities. In all the experiments factor analysis of the test data confirmed two clear factors labeled as simultaneous and successive. They then divided the subjects into four contrasting groups: high simultaneous and high successive; high simultaneous and low successive; low simultaneous and high successive; low simultaneous and low successive. Reading scores for decoding and comprehension were then analyzed for the four groups. The essence of the findings is that successive processing is critical for reading achievement in the beginning grades, whereas at advanced levels of reading skill simultaneous processing is essential for comprehension. Table 7.2 summarizes their analysis of the relationship between simultaneous-successive processing and reading ability.

Kirby and Robinson[118] administered the same battery of tests to 105 reading-disabled children, and the results provided further evidence that simultaneous processing is involved in direct lexical access, text organization, and semantic processing whereas successive processing is concerned

TABLE 7.2 Relationship between simultaneous successive processing and reading ability

Processing pattern	Comprehension	Decoding
High simultaneous–high successive	high	high
High simultaneous–low successive	high	low
Low simultaneous–low successive	low	low
Low simultaneous–high successive	low	high

with decoding and syntactic analysis. They also point out that many reading-disabled youngsters use simultaneous processing techniques in the early stages of reading, which is inappropriate for success in decoding. Simultaneous processing is useful in early reading only for letter identification and recognition of sight words. Several studies using the Kaufman Assessment Battery for Children (KABC)[114] tend to confirm the conclusions of the Das group. Hooper and Hynd[119] used the KABC to differentiate between normal and dyslexic readers. They found that the dyslexics had significantly poorer scores on the sequential tests. McRae[120] used the KABC to investigate the relationships between processing skills and two types of reading skills: word recognition and comprehension. Second and third graders were divided into four groups: high word recognition–high comprehension, high word recognition–low comprehension, low word recognition–high comprehension, low word recognition–low comprehension. She found that the low comprehension groups were associated with poor simultaneous ability. Solan[121] found that vocabulary and comprehension are dependent on both forms of processing in normally achieving children in grades 4 and 5. This is similar to the findings of Kirby and Das,[117] who reported that both simultaneous and successive processing is related to four measures of school achievement and that both forms of processing are necessary. Aaron[122] divided his reading-disabled group on the basis of errors made in a writing-from-dictation task. The groups were either analytic-sequential deficient or holistic-simultaneous deficient. Testing showed that the first group was poor in sequential processing tests and the second group poor in simultaneous tasks thus confirming that an imbalance in processing strategies will result in reading disability and that both processes are required for normal reading achievement. We have found that utilizing the simultaneous-sequential information processing concepts is a convenient, practical, and efficient method for organizing the data from a variety of perceptual tests. In addition it provides a guide for specific therapeutic intervention with individual patients.

SPECIFIC RELATIONSHIPS BETWEEN VISUAL PERCEPTION AND MATHEMATICS

Students with arithmetic learning disorders are rarely referred for evaluation, despite the fact that children with learning disabilities often are delayed in mathematical skills. Arithmetic problems are as common and widespread as many other learning disabilities[123] but are not considered as important as reading disabilities. Learning disabilities in mathematics have often been related to deficiencies in visuospatial organization and visuomotor association.[124] Wheatley[125] claims that current thinking views mathematics as an activity of constructing patterns and relationships that requires a good spatial sense. Spatial sense refers to a variety of skills such as spatial visualization, spatial reasoning, spatial perception, visual imagery, and visual thinking and includes such visual perceptual abilities as visual-motor integration, visual closure, figure-ground perception, perceptual constancy, visual discrimination, and visual memory. Spatial sense is important "for its relationship to most technical-scientific occupations and especially to the study of mathematics, science, art and engineering."[116] Das[127] says that logicomathematical and spatial abilities share the same underlying simultaneous cognitive process. He describes two different projects in Canada and India in which the grade levels ranged from kindergarten to fifth grade. They were divided into the four groups of high simultaneous–high successive, high simultaneous–low successive, low simultaneous–high successive, low simultaneous–low successive as in their previous research with reading groups. Statistical analysis indicated a strong level of significance for simultaneous processing and arithmetic and no significance for successive processing. The conclusion was that simultaneous processing is a major contributor to proficiency in arithmetic. A similar study[127] with fourth- and sixth-grade children in Hong Kong found quite clearly that simultaneous processing was the best predictor of mathematics achievement. In the sixth-grade students it accounted for 18.6% out of a total variance of 21% whereas in the fourth grade it accounted for 16.7% out of a total variance of 25%. Pennington[128] believes that we must differentiate between math problems found in dyslexics and math problems found in nondyslexics. The dyslexics have problems memorizing math facts, such as the multiplication tables, doing multistep calculations, and of course understanding word problems. The nondyslexics, on the other hand, have difficulty in conceptualizing mathematical concepts, and their specific math deficits are related to visuospatial problems. Mcleod[124] found that visuospatial skills, spatial relations, and spatial orientation were moderately to highly related to mathematics achievement but also found verbal ability to be of equal importance. Rourke and his associates[129] completed subtype analyses of arithmetic-impaired children. The children ranged from 9 to 14 years old with WISC-R Full Scale IQ's between 86 and 114. Three groups of children were obtained on the basis of their scores on the Wide Range Achievement Test.

Group 1 students were deficient in reading, spelling, and arithmetic. They were at least 2 years behind grade level in all three areas with very little scatter between the scores.

Group 2 students were relatively better in arithmetic than in reading and spelling. The reading and spelling scores were at least 1.8 years below the arithmetic scores.

Group 3 students were average or above average in reading and spelling but deficient in arithmetic. The reading and spelling scores were at least 2.0 years above the arithmetic scores.

These groups were then analyzed on the basis of their performance on a battery of auditory perceptual, visual perceptual, verbal, motor, psychomotor, and tactile perceptual tests, The results indicated that the children in group 2 had good scores on the visual perception, psychomotor, and tactile perception tests but poor scores on verbal tests and very poor scores on the auditory perceptual tests. The group 3 children, however, had good verbal and auditory perception test scores but poor visual perception, psychomotor, and tactile perception test scores. The group 3 children, those with poor arithmetic skills but average reading and spelling skills, exhibited poor visuospatial skills. Batchelor et al.[130] examined 989 learning-disabled students with a wide-ranging neuropsychological battery, and their results confirmed and extended Rourkes findings.

Visual perception is an important factor in mathematics, and optometrists should ascertain if patients have a math deficiency and visuospatial disabilities. This combination of dysfunctions is an excellent indication for vision therapy.

SPECIFIC RELATIONSHIPS BETWEEN VISUAL PERCEPTION AND SPELLING

Frith[131] claims that more and more value has been put on reading achievement and word recognition, with an increasing tendency to belittle spelling achievement. Spelling is of minor importance compared with recognizing what words mean, in our schools. She believes that this imbalance is wrong, since it does not correspond to the relative difficulty or practical importance of the skills. Spelling is a skill that is a much more difficult task for most children than reading. Spelling problems can persist long after reading problems are resolved. It is a confusing area to study, since there are good readers who are good spellers, there are good readers who spell poorly, there are poor readers who are good spellers, and there are poor readers who spell poorly. Frith[131] claims that those children who are poor spellers and good readers show a failure of the lexical "visual" route in their spelling. They tend to pay attention to some letters but not to others, which of course results in spelling errors. It is, however, generally true that children's spelling reflects what they have been able to organize, store, and recall about the words they can read.[132] In the case study reported by Goulandris and Snowling[112] the patients' reading deficit was accompanied by serious spelling problems. She showed a pronounced tendency to spell phonetically, which the authors attributed to her significant visual memory disability. Levine[133] believes that students with a visual spatial or simultaneous processing deficiency will have spelling problems because they will have difficulty developing the "whole-word" awareness that requires simultaneous processing of the spatial, directional, and configurational attributes of words. These children, who are comparable to Boder's[39] dyseidetic classification, will have a poor sight vocabulary and will tend to spell unknown words phonetically. Their incorrect spellings will be phonetically accurate and readable. A recent patient with simultaneous processing disability produced the following spellings: *flie* for *fly; spaship* for *spaceship; ritin* for *written;* and *dron* for *drawn.*

They will also show letter and word reversals such as *god* for *dog, big* for *dig*.

Levine[133] does not believe that sequential processing disability produces clear-cut spelling difficulty. He claims that recognition of the sequential order of the letters is less important than visualization of a gestalt, language awareness, and grapheme-phoneme correspondence. Boder[39] says that the dysphonetic spellers make errors that are phonetically inaccurate (PI) such as *cottegt* for *cottage* or *diter* for *doubt* and that dyseidetic spellers make errors that are phonetically accurate (PA).

Rourke and his associates[38] used subtype analysis on a series of phonetically accurate and phonetically inaccurate spellers and determined that the phonetically accurate spellers had superior visuospatial skills as compared to the phonetically inaccurate, who had poor language skills.

Table 7.3 summarizes the relationship between simultaneous (visual spatial) processing and sequential (language) processing and phonetically accurate (PA) and phonetically inaccurate (PI) spelling errors.

It should be noted that some researchers believe that these perceived or measured differences in spelling errors are simply a function of the subject's level of spelling achievement. Moats[134] claims that this type of analysis has little value since the qualitative aspects of spelling errors are not reliable and phonetic spelling ability is not independent of the child's instructional history, and this ability appears to be a function of achievement level and verbal intelligence. She does say, however, that graphomotor development should be studied to illuminate the role that transcription plays in learning to spell. This coincides with Frith's[131] concerns, in that dysgraphia is a significant problem for poor spellers. It is important not to overlook the good reader who might have poor spelling. If they have perceptual disabilities, vision therapy is indicated.

SUMMARY

Perception is the basic process in cognitive development. Perceptual development proceeds, in stages, from a sensorimotor base to conceptualization. There are five principal perceptual sense systems, but vision must become the dominant perceptual modality. Learning disability is a heterogeneous disorder that has been associated with language, speech, audi-

TABLE 7.3 Relationship between simultaneous and sequential processing and accuracy errors

Processing pattern	Phonetically accurate errors	Phonetically inaccurate errors
High simultaneous–high sequential	No	No
High simultaneous–low sequential	No	Yes
Low simultaneous–high sequential	Yes	No
Low simultaneous–low sequential	Yes	Yes

tory perception, motoric skills, and visual perception. Metanalysis of single factor experimental studies showed that reading achievement was significantly related to visual perception. Analyses of subtypes of learning-disabled children are used to classify the children into homogeneous clusters. These studies indicate that 20% of the children can be identified in a pure visual perception cluster whereas an additional 20% are in a mixed cluster, with visual perception deficits as a significant factor.

Deficits in perceptual speed, visual memory, visual-motor integration, auditory-visual integration, visual-spatial skills, spatial orientation, transient visual deficits, simultaneous processing, sequential processing, and other perceptual abilities have been shown to have an effect on reading, spelling, arithmetic, and all aspects of learning disability.

The information in this chapter clearly demonstrates the relationship between visual information processing and learning and forms the basis for the important role optometry must play in this area. When a child presents with school-related problems, optometrists must consider the issue of visual information processing skills. The primary care optometrist should modify the case history to probe for signs and symptoms related to visual information processing. If such problems are suspected, a screening battery should be performed to detect visual information processing disorders. Once such problems are detected these children should be referred to optometric specialists who can develop appropriate management strategies to deal with these problems.

CHAPTER REVIEW

1. Perceptual skills are significant only at early ages. Is this a myth or a fact? Cite studies to support your answer.
2. Describe Kephart's seven stages of perceptual development. Discuss recent research that contradicts part of Kephart's thesis.
3. What are the major perceptual abilities that affect spelling and mathematics?
4. What does Kavale's metanalysis show regarding the relationship between visual perception and reading?
5. Compare Boder's subtypes of dyslexic children with the simultaneous and sequential information processing subtypes.
6. How important are reversals in learning disability?
7. Discuss the clinical significance of the two types of visual memory.

REFERENCES

1. Forgus RH: *Perception—the basic process in cognitive development,* New York, 1966, McGraw-Hill.
2. Bolles EB: *A second way of knowing: the riddle of human perception,* New York, 1991, Prentice Hall.
3. Gibson JJ: *The senses considered as perceptual systems,* Boston, 1966, Houghton Mifflin.

4. Gibson E, Gibson JJ: The senses as information seeking systems. In Gibson E: *An odyssey in learning and perception,* Cambridge, Mass., 1991, MIT Press.

5. Gregory R: Seeing as thinking: an active theory of perception. In Gibson E: *An odyssey in learning and perception,* Cambridge, Mass., 1991, MIT Press.

6. Gesell AL, Ilg FL, Bullis GE: *Vision—its development in infant and child,* New York, 1949, Hoeber.

7. Birch HG: Dyslexia and the maturation of visual function. In Money J, editor: *Reading disability,* Baltimore, 1962, Johns Hopkins Press.

8. Pick HL, Warren DH, Hay JC: Sensory conflict in judgments of spatial direction, *Perception and Psychophysics* 6:203-205, 1969.

9. Robinson K: *Visual and auditory modalities and reading recall: a review of the research,* ERIC report no. ED 272 840, Washington, 1985, US Dept of Education.

10. Posner M, Nissen MJ, Klein RM: Visual dominance: an information processing account of its origins and significance, *Psychol Rev* 83: 157-171, 1976.

11. Leakey R, Lewin R: *Origins,* New York, 1977, Dutton.

12. Fakouri ME: Learning disabilities: a piagetian perspective, *Psychology in the Schools,* 28:70-76, 1991.

13. Hebb DO: *The organization of behavior: a neuropsychological theory,* New York, 1949, John Wiley.

14. Werner H: *Comparative psychology of mental development,* New York, 1948, Science Editions Inc.

15. Strauss AA, Lehtinen LE: *Psychopathology and education of the brain-injured child,* New York, 1947, Grune & Stratton.

16. Getman GN: *How to develop your child's intelligence,* Luverne, Minn., 1962, self-published.

17. Kephart NC: *The slow learner in the classroom,* ed 2, Columbus, Ohio, 1971, Charles E. Merrill.

18. Ayres AJ: Patterns of perceptual-motor dysfunction in children: a factor analytic study, *Percept Mot Skills,* 20:335-368, 1965.

19. Frostig M: Education for children with learning disabilities. In Mykleburst HM, editor: *Progress in learning disabilities,* New York, 1969, Grune & Stratton.

20. Hallahan DP, Cruickshank WM: *Psychoeducational foundations of learning disabilities,* Englewood Cliffs, NJ, 1973, Prentice Hall.

21. Strauss AA, Kephart NC: *Psychopathology and education of the brain injured child.* II: *Progress in theory and clinic,* New York, 1955, Grune & Stratton.

22. Ball TS, Itard JMG, Sequin E, and Kephart NC: *Sensory education—a learning interpretation,* Columbus, Ohio, 1971, Charles E Merrill.

23. Kephart NC: Perceptual-motor aspects of learning disabilities, *Except Child* 31:201-206, 1964.

24. Flavell JH: *The developmental psychology of Jean Piaget,* Princeton, NJ, 1963, Van Nostrand.

25. Salapatek P: Visual scanning of geometric figures by the human newborn, *J Comp Physiological Psychol* 66:247-258, 1968.

26. Bower TGR: The visual world of infants, *Sci Am* 215:80-84, 1966.

27. Fantz RL: Pattern discrimination and selective attention as determinants of perceptual development from birth. In Kidd AK, Rivoire JL, editors: *Perceptual development in children,* New York, 1066, International Universities Press.

28. Kavale K: Meta-analysis of the relationship between visual perceptual skills and reading achievement, *J Learning Disabilities* 15:42-51, 1982.

29. Wolf FM: *Meta-analysis,* Newbury Park, Calif, and London, 1986, Sage Publications.

30. Glass GV: Primary, secondary and meta-analysis of research, *Educational Researcher* 5:3-8, 1976.

31. Vellutino FR: *Dyslexia: theory and research,* Cambridge, Mass., 1979, MIT Press.

32. Larsen SC, Hammill DD: *The relationship of selected visual percep-*

tual abilities to school learning, J Special Educ 9:281-291, 1975.

33. Kavale KA, Forness SR: The far side of heterogeneity: a critical analysis of empirical subtyping research in learning disabilities, *J Learning Disabilities* 20:374-382, 1987.

34. Rourke BP: *Neuropsychology of learning disabilities: essentials of subtype analysis,* New York, 1988, Plenum Press.

35. Aldenderfer MS, Blashfield RK: *Cluster analysis,* Beverly Hills, Calif, 1984, Sage Publications.

36. Gordon HW: The effect of "right brain/left brain" cognitive profiles on school achievement. In Molfese DL, Segalowitz SJ: *Brain lateralization in children: developmental implications,* New York, 1988, Guilford Press.

37. Mattis S, French JH, Rapin I: Dyslexia in children and adults: three independent neuropsychological syndromes, *Dev Med Child Neurol* 17:150-163, 1975.

38. Luria AR: *Higher cortical functions in man,* New York, 1966, Guilford Press.

39. Boder E: Developmental dyslexia: a diagnostic approach based on three atypical reading-spelling patterns, *Dev Med Child Neurol* 15: 663-687, 1973.

40. Watson BU, Goldgar DE: Evaluation of a typology of reading disability, *J Clin Exp Neuropsychol* 10:432-450, 1988.

41. Watson BU, Goldgar DE: Subtypes of reading disability, *J Clin Neuropsychol* 5:377-399, 1983.

42. Bender WN, Golden LB: Subtypes of students with learning disabilities as derived from cognitive, academic behavioral, and self-concept measures, *Learning Disabilities Q* 13:183-194, 1990.

43. Lyon GR, Watson B: Empirically derived subgroups of learning disabled readers: diagnostic characteristics, *J Learning Disabilities* 14:256-261, 1981.

44. Satz P, Morris R: Learning disability subtypes: a review. In Pirozzolo FJ, Wittrock MC, editors: *Neuro-*

psychological and cognitive processes in reading, New York, 1981, Academic Press.

45. Lesgold AM, Resnick LB: How reading difficulties develop: perspectives from a longitudinal study. In Das JP, Muchay RF, Wall AE, editors: *Theory and research in learning disabilities,* New York, 1983, Plenum Press.

46. Logan GD: Toward a theory of automatization, *Psychol Rev* 95(4): 492-527, 1988.

47. Laberge D, Samuels SJ: Toward a theory of automatic information processing in reading, *Cognitive Psychology* 6:293-323, 1974.

48. Denckla MB, Rudel RG: Rapid automated naming: dyslexia differentiated from other learning disabilities, *Neuropsychologia* 14:471-480, 1976.

49. Wolff PH, Michel GF, Ovrut M: Rate variables and automatized naming in developmental dyslexia, *Brain Lang* 39:556-575, 1990.

50. Jarman RF, Krywaniuk LW: Simultaneous and successive syntheses: a factor analysis of speed of information processing, *Percept Mot Skills* 46:1167-1172, 1978.

51. Spring C: Perceptual speed in poor readers, *J Educ Psychol* 62:492-500, 1971.

52. Lyle JG, Goyen JD: Effect of speed of exposure and difficulty of discrimination on visual recognition of retarded readers, *J Abnorm Psychol* 84:673-676, 1975.

53. Goyen JD, Lyle JG: Short term memory and visual discrimination in retarded readers, *Percept Mot Skills* 36:403-408, 1973.

54. Steinhauser R, Guthrie JT: Perceptual and linguistic processing of letters and words by normal and disabled readers, *J Reading Behav* 9(3):217-225, 1977.

55. Bryant SK et al: Rate of visual information pick-up in learning disabled and normal boys, *Learning Disability Q* 6(2):166-171, 1983.

56. Whitehouse CC: Analysis of WISC-R coding performance of normal and dyslexic readers, *Percept Mot Skills* 57:951-960, 1983.

57. Koslow KC: Binocular vision, coding tests and classroom achievement, *J Behav Optom* 2:16-19, 1991.

58. Solan HA, Ficarra AP: A study of perceptual and verbal skills of disabled readers in grades 4, 5, and 6, *J Am Optom Assoc* 61:628-634, 1990.

59. Ilg FL, Ames LB: School readiness: behavior tests used at the Gesell Institute, New York, 1964, Harper & Row.

60. Mattison RE, McIntyre CW, Brown AS, Murray ME: An analysis of visual-motor problems in learning disabled children, *Bull Psychonomic Soc* 24(1):51-54, 1986.

61. Leonard P, Foxcroft C, Kroukamp T: Are visual-perceptual and visual-motor skills separate abilities? *Percept Mot Skills* 67:423-426, 1988.

62. Gladstone M, Best CT, Davidson RJ: Anomalous bimanual coordination among dyslexic boys, *Dev Psychol* 25(2):236-246, 1989.

63. Beery KE: *The VMI-developmental test of visual-motor integration—administration, scoring, and teaching manual,* ed 3, Cleveland, 1989, Modern Curriculum Press.

64. Fletcher JM, Satz P: Developmental change in the neuropsychological correlates of reading achievement: a six year longitudinal followup, *J Clin Neuropsychol* 2:23-37, 1980.

65. Keogh BF, Smith CE: Visual motor ability and school prediction: a seven year study, *Percept Mot Skills* 25:101-110, 1967.

66. Koppitz EM: *The Bender-Gestalt Test for Young Children,* New York, 1964, Grune & Stratton.

67. Olson AV: The questionable value of perceptual tests in diagnosing reading disabilities, *J Res Reading* 3(2):129-139, 1980.

68. Johnson DJ, Grant JO: Written narrative of normal and learning disabled children, *Ann Dyslexia* 39:140-158, 1989.

69. Melamed LE, Rugle L: Neuropsychological correlates of school achievement in young children: longitudinal findings with a construct valid perceptual processing instrument, *J Clin Exp Neuropsychol* 11:745-762, 1989.

70. Birch HG, Belmont L: Auditory-visual integration, intelligence, and reading ability in school children, *Percept Mot Skills* 20:295-305, 1965.

71. Berry JW: Matching of auditory and visual stimuli by average and retarded readers, *Child Dev* 38:827-833, 1967.

72. Ford MP: Auditory-visual and tactual-visual integration in relation to reading ability, *Percept Mot Skills* 24:831-841, 1967.

73. Sterritt GM, Rudnick M: Auditory and visual rhythm perception in relation to reading ability in fourth grade boys, *Percept Mot Skills* 22:859-864, 1966.

74. Senf GM, Freundl PC: Memory and attention factors in specific learning disabilities, *J Learning Disabilities* 4:94-106, 1971.

75. Badian NA: Auditory-visual integration, auditory memory, and reading in retarded and adequate readers, *J Learning Disabilities* 10:108-114, 1977.

76. Vande Voort L, Senf GM, Benton AL: Development of audiovisual integration in normal and retarded readers, *Child Dev* 43:1260-1272, 1972.

77. Blank M, Bridger W: Deficiencies in verbal labeling in retarded readers, *Am J Orthopsychiatry* 36:840-847, 1966.

78. Bruden MP: Auditory-visual and sequential spatial matching in relation to reading ability, *Child Dev* 43:824-832, 1972.

79. Kahn D, Birch HG: Development of auditory-visual integration and reading achievement, *Percept Mot Skills* 27:459-468, 1968.

80. Lovegrove W, Martin F, Slaghius W: A theoretical and experimental case for a specific visual deficit in specific reading disability, *Cognitive Neuropsychol* 3:225-267, 1986.

81. Williams MC, LeCluyse K: Perceptual consequences of a temporal processing deficit in reading dis-

abled children, *J Am Optom Assoc* 61:124-135, 1990.

82. Lovegrove W: Spatial frequency processing in dyslexic and normal readers. In Stein JF, editor: *Vision and visual dyslexia,* Boca Raton, Fla., 1991, CRC Press.

83. Winters RL, Patterson R, Shontz W: Visual persistence and adult dyslexia, *J Learning Disabilities* 22:641-645, 1989.

84. Kaplan CP, Schacter E: Adults with undiagnosed learning disabilities: practice considerations, *Families in Society* 72(4):195-201, 1991.

85. Mann GH: Reversal reading errors in children trained in dual directionality, *Reading Teacher* 22:646-649, 1969.

86. Ginsburg GP, Hartwick A: Directional confusion as a sign of dyslexia, *Percept Mot Skills* 32:535-543, 1971.

87. Bryant ND: Characteristics of dyslexia and their remedial implications, *Except Child* 31:195-200, 1964.

88. Orton ST: Specific reading disability—strephosymbolia, *JAMA* 90:1090-1099, 1928.

89. Gardner RA: The objective diagnosis of minimal brain dysfunction, Cresskill, NJ, 1979, Creative Therapeutics.

90. Gibson EJ: Principles of perceptual learning and development, New York, 1969, Prentice-Hall.

91. Ilg FL, Ames LB: Developmental trends in reading behavior, *J Genet Psychol* 76:291-312, 1950.

92. Jordan BT, Jordan SG: Jordan left-right reversal test: an analysis of visual reversals in children and significance for reading problems, *Child Psychiatry Hum Dev* 21(1):65-73, 1990.

93. Lyle JG: Reading retardation and reversal tendency: a factorial study, *Child Dev* 40:833-843, 1969.

94. Worral RS: Reading disability: a discussion of visual, auditory, and linguistic factors, *J Am Optom Assoc* 57:60-64, 1986.

95. Greenspan SB: Effectiveness of therapy for children's reversal con-

fusions, *Acad Ther* 11(2):169-178, 1975-1976.

96. Heydorn BL: Visual-motor training program and symbol reversal errors, *Reading Horizons* 24(4):249-252, 1984.

97. Ludlam WM, quoted by Margach CB: *Reversals—II, Optometric Extension Program (OEP) Curriculum II* 59(9):57-62, 1987.

98. Kelly MS, Best CT, Kirk U: Cognitive processing deficits in reading disabilities: a prefrontal cortical hypothesis, *Brain Cogn* 11:275-293, 1989.

99. Bannatyne A: Mirror-images and reversals, *Acad Ther* 8:87-92, 1972.

100. Goins JT: *Visual perceptual abilities and early reading progress,* University of Chicago Press, Supplementary Educational Monographs 87, 1958.

101. Barrett TC: Visual discrimination tasks as predictors of first grade reading achievement, *Reading Teacher* 18:276-282, 1965.

102. Kass CE: Psycholinguistic disabilities of children with reading problems, *Except Child* 32:533-539, 1966.

103. Amoriell WJ: Reading achievement and the ability to manipulate visual and auditory stimuli, *J Learning Disabilities* 12:562-566, 1979.

104. Stanley G, Hall R: Short-term visual information processing in dyslexia, *Child Dev* 44:841-844, 1973.

105. Hung SS, Fisher AG, Cermak AC: The performance of learning disabled and normal young men on the test of visual perceptual skills, *Am J Occup Ther* 41:790-797, 1987.

106. Vellutino FR, Steger JA, DeSetto L, Phillips F: Immediate and delayed recognition of visual stimuli in poor and normal readers, *J Exp Child Psychol* 19:223-232, 1975.

107. Swanson L: Verbal encoding effects on the short term memory of learning disabled and normal readers, *J Educ Psych* 70:539-544, 1978.

108. Fletcher JM, Satz P: Has Vellutino led us astray? *J Learning Disabilities* 12:168-171, 1979.

109. Farnham-Diggory S, Gregg LW: Short term memory function in

young readers, *J Exp Child Psychol* 19:279-298, 1975.

110. Morrison FJ, Giordano B, Nagy J: Reading disability: an information processing analysis, *Science* 196(4): 77-79, 1977.

111. Willows DM, Corcos E, Kershner JR: Perceptual and cognitive factors in disabled and normal readers' perception and memory of unfamiliar visual symbols. In Wright SF, Groner R, editors: *Facets of dyslexia and its remediation,* Amsterdam, 1993, Elsevier Science Publishers.

112. Goulandris NK, Snowling M: Visual memory deficits: a plausible cause of developmental dyslexia? Evidence from a single case study, *Cognitive Neuropsychol* 8:127-154, 1919.

113. Das JP, Kirby JR, Jarman RF: Simultaneous and successive cognitive processes, New York, 1979, Academic Press.

114. Kaufman AS, Kaufman NL: *Administration and scoring manual for the Kaufman assessment battery for children,* Circle Pines, Minn, 1983, American Guidance Service.

115. Hammill DD: Detroit tests of learning aptitude, ed 3, Austin, Tex, 1991, Pro-Ed.

116. Cummins J, Das JP: Cognitive processing and reading difficulties: a framework for research, *Alberta J Educ Res* 23:245-256, 1977.

117. Kirby JR, Das JP: Reading achievement, IQ and simultaneous-successive processing, *J Educ Psychol* 69:564-570, 1977.

118. Kirby JR, Robinson GLW: Simultaneous and successive in reading disabled children, *J Learning Disabilities* 20:243-252, 1987.

119. Hooper SR, Hynd GW: Performance of normal and dyslexic readers on the Kaufman assessment battery for children (KABC): a discrimination analysis, *J Learning Disabilities* 19:206-210, 1986.

120. McRae SG: Sequential-simultaneous processing and reading skills in primary grade children, *J Learning Disabilities* 19:509-511, 1986.

121. Solan H: A comparison of the influences of verbal-successive and spatial-simultaneous factors on achieving readers in fourth and fifth grade: a multivariate study, *J Learning Disabilities* 20:237-242, 1987.

122. Aaron PG: Dyslexia, an imbalance in cerebral information processing strategies, *Percept Mot Skills* 47: 699-706, 1978.

123. Kavale KA, Forness SR, Beneder M: *Handbook of learning disabilities,* Vol I: *Dimensions and diagnosis,* Boston, 1987, Little, Brown.

124. McLeod TM, Crump DW: The relationship of visuospatial skills and verbal ability to learning disabilities in mathematics, *J Learning Disabilities* 11:237-241, 1978.

125. Whatley GH: Spatial sense and mathematics learning, *Arithmetic Teacher* 37(6):10-11, 1910.

126. Ben-Chaim D, Lappan GL, Houang R: The role of visualization in middle school mathematics curriculum, *Focus on Learning Problems in Mathematics* 11:49-60, 1989.

127. Das JP: Simultaneous-successive processing and planning: implications for school learning. In Schmeck RR, editor: *Learning strategies and learning styles,* New York, 1988, Plenum Press.

128. Pennington BF: Diagnosing learning disorders: a neuropsychological framework, New York, 1991, Guilford Press.

129. Rourke BP, Fisk J: Subtypes of learning disabled children: implications for a neurodevelopmental model of differential hemispheric processing. In Molfese DL, Segalowitz SJ: *Brain lateralization in children: developmental implications,* New York, 1988, Guilford Press.

130. Batchelor ES et al: Empirical testing of a cognitive model to account for neuropsychological functioning underlying arithmetic problem solving, *J Learning Disabilities* 23:38-42, 1990.

131. Frith U: The similarities and differences between reading and spelling

problems. In Rutter M: *Developmental neuropsychiatry,* New York, 1983, Guilford Press.

132. Smith CR: Learning disabilities: the interaction of learner, task and setting, ed 2, Boston, 1991, Allyn & Bacon.

133. Levine MD: Developmental varia-

tion and learning disorders, Cambridge, Mass, 1987, Educators Publishing Service.

134. Moats LC: A comparison of the spelling errors of older dyslexic and second-grade normal children, *Ann Dyslexia* 33;121-139, 1983.

PART THREE

ASSESSMENT

CHAPTER 8

The Role of the Optomertrist in the Diagnosis and Management of Learning-Related Vision Problems

LOUIS G. HOFFMAN

KEY TERMS

vision

multidisciplinary

perception

development

psychoeducational testing

occupational therapist

developmental milestones

school consultant

Optometrists do not treat learning problems. The optometrist's primary role is the diagnosis and treatment of vision problems, which may prevent or interfere with the normal learning process. Remediating these vision problems allows children and adults to benefit more fully from educational instruction. Optometrists fulfill this role as a member of the multidisciplinary team involved in the evaluation and management of children presenting with learning problems. To define the role or roles of an optometrist within this multidisciplinary team it is necessary to define certain terminology.

First, what is the scope of professional responsibility of an optometrist? Although the specific legal definitions vary from state to state, the American Optometric Association (St. Louis, 1993) presents the following definition of an optometrist: "Doctors of optometry are independent primary health care providers who specialize in the examination, diagnosis and management of diseases and disorders of the visual system, the eye and associated structures as well as the diagnosis of related systemic conditions." It is important to note that the optometrist is legally responsible for both the diagnosis and management of disorders of the visual system.

217

Second, how do we define vision? The *Dictionary of Visual Science* defines vision as "the special sense by which objects, their form, color, position, etc., in the external environment are perceived, the exciting stimulus being light from the objects striking the retina in the eye; the act, function, process, or power of seeing. . . ."[1] Vision includes development, visual perceptual motor skills, and the ability to integrate vision with other sensory motor skills.[2] Perception is an integral part of vision, since vision leads to some action on the part of the individual. Vision cannot be considered, as it appears to be, by much of the public and many eye care practitioners, a simple measure of visual acuity. Vision is an extremely complex act that changes with growth, maturation, development, and learned experiences.

The definition of vision that is utilized by a particular eye care professional will have a significant effect on his or her approach to patient care. Also, the conclusions drawn from research investigating the relationship between vision and learning problems is not only dependent on appropriate research methodology, but also contingent on the definition of vision used by the researcher. In addition to professional biases and the political agendas that often interfere with professional communication, the ability to communicate between professionals within the eye care field and other multidisciplinary team professionals will be influenced by their conceptual framework. Some tend to emphasize optical and anatomical considerations, whereas others are more concerned with functional aspects of vision.[3]

The definition of the continuous and integrative process known as vision that is used in this text may be divided into three major components:

1. Visual acuity, which is largely dependent on eye health, refractive status, and the normal development of the visual system.
2. Visual skills efficiency, which is composed of oculomotor, accommodative, and binocular skills.
3. Visual perceptual-motor development, which is what we are referring to in this text as visual information processing. This represents the ability to recognize and discriminate visual stimuli and interpret them correctly in light of previous experiences.

These categories will help the reader in realizing that no one specific component defines "vision." Furthermore, no component can be thoroughly assessed by a single test measurement. The complexity of vision requires extensive optometric evaluation, particularly if vision's relationship to learning difficulties are considered.[4]

With a conceptual framework of knowing the scope of optometric responsibilities and how vision is comprehensively defined, we can consider the roles of the optometrist in the diagnosis and management of patients with vision problems and concurrent learning problems. Based on their education and training, optometrists diagnose, manage, and treat visual deficiencies, not educational problems. The inability to learn in the academic situation is an educational problem. However, as a member of the multidisciplinary team working with children and adults with learning problems, the optometrist must always keep in mind that disorders of the visual system often result in a variety of signs and symptoms that may affect performance in many situations, learning being only one.

THE VISION CARE ROLE OF THE OPTOMETRIST

Depending on the optometrist's clinical and post-graduate education, practice setting, and personal interests, there are many levels of involvement in this area, from comprehensive care to woeful neglect. For the primary care optometrist seeing children and adults with learning problems it would be helpful to have a clinical strategy for evaluating these patients that would fulfill the ethical and moral obligations suggested in the definition put forth by the American Optometric Association. We would like to propose a realistic and practical role for the primary care optometrist in the evaluation of children and adults presenting with learning problems. If the primary care practitioner does not provide comprehensive care in this area, he or she should be able to screen for and detect signs and symptoms that indicate the possibility of learning related vision problems (see Chapter 9 for a modified case history and preexamination checklist). He or she should conduct the primary care vision examination and address visual acuity, ocular health, and refractive conditions that may have an influence on the patient's learning problem (see Chapters 6 for a review). He or she should complete additional screening of visual efficiency and visual information processing (see Chapters 10 and 11 for screening strategies that can be done in a primary care setting) to determine if referral is necessary, or immediately refer a patient with a history of learning-related visual problems.

The role of the optometrist providing comprehensive care to patients with learning-related visual problems is similar to the care necessary for other visual problems, with some slight modification. There are three components to the role of the optometrist with this type of patient. The optometrist providing comprehensive care should provide:

1. Comprehensive diagnostic services, including those areas evaluated in a primary care setting, in addition to a complete evaluation of visual efficiency and visual information processing abilities. The goal is to identify and quantify any visual disorders and correlate this information with the patient's entering complaints.
2. Management or treatment services, including the correction or remediation of decreased visual acuity, refractive anomalies, visual efficiency, and visual information processing disorders.
3. Information to assist the educator in devising a more suitable educational program for the individual student, relative to his or her visual problems. This information would identify the patient's strengths and weaknesses, the effect on classroom performance, and

possible ways that the teacher can accommodate the patient's visual problems in the classroom.

ROLE OF THE OPTOMETRIST WITH THE PATIENT OR PARENTS

A complete vision evaluation should be provided for the purpose of ruling out and quantifying visual disorders. Not only should a diagnosis of vision deficiencies be made, but also strengths and weaknesses should be ascertained by the optometrist and explained to the patient or parents.

If vision care is required, the patient or parents should be informed of the diagnosis, the relationship of the diagnosis to entering signs and symptoms, the purpose of a refractive correction and when it is to be worn, the purpose and goals of vision therapy, the estimated length of time of therapy, the role of the patient and parent during a therapy program, and the cost of materials and services. Should questions relative to insurance coverage for these services arise, the optometrist is obligated to assist the patient in every way possible.

Parents will frequently question the optometrist relative to the educational placement of their child. They may wish to know whether the child should be retained in his or her present grade as recommended by the teacher or the school psychologist, promoted to the next grade, or placed in a special class. The optometrist can and should provide information relative to the child's visual status that may be helpful to the educator, school psychologist, and the parents in reaching conclusions relative to these areas of concern. However, the optometrist should under no circumstances make suggestions of retention or special class placement unilaterally. It is imperative that the optometrist function as a member of the multidisciplinary team and be in contact with the educators and the school psychologist to ensure that consistent information is provided to the patient and the parents.

The optometrist also has a responsibility to recommend additional referrals if they are necessary. Information obtained in the case history or during the evaluation may indicate referral for additional diagnostic or treatment services. Such services might include psychoeducational testing, psychological counseling, speech and hearing evaluation, occupational therapy, nutritional counseling, or medical evaluation.

Solan stated that the role of the optometrist in treating children with learning problems includes management and guidance. He goes on to say that although teaching reading is primarily the responsibility of the educator the optometrist (and other professionals) often assist in defining and clarifying the nature of certain disorders that are contributing to a child's reading difficulty.[5] Solan has also suggested that the optometrist can be helpful in providing the parents with simple rules that can assist them in parenting.[5] He believes that (1) parents could be helped in establishing a hierarchy of importance—what is trivial, important, and essential; (2) parents must determine in advance a plan for reward and punishment, which must be commensurate with the behavior; (3) the child must be provided with a predictable environment; and finally (4) both parents must agree upon and carry out a prescribed course of action. It is extremely important to be aware of the limitations of the patient or parents in solving their own problems, and in such cases, appropriate referrals should be made.

ROLE OF THE OPTOMETRIST WITH OTHER MULTIDISCIPLINARY TEAM PROFESSIONALS

The optometrist has a responsibility to communicate and interact with the other multidisciplinary professionals in the best interest of the child. One of the major responsibilities is establishing this relationship with the patient's educator. If this communication is based on a mutual understanding of each professional's role, the patient will receive the greatest benefit from this cooperative effort.

Role with educators

Optometrists do not teach reading, writing, and arithmetic. This is the educator's primary role. It is the optometrist's responsibility to provide the educator with pertinent information relative to the visual processes to assist them in developing an educational program that will more effectively allow the child to learn. It is beneficial for the educator to make the optometrist aware of behaviors noted in the classroom that might be attributable to vision disorders (see Appendix D, for a sample teacher questionnaire). Close communication between the educator, the optometrist, and other professionals can be of great benefit to the patient. Therefore the optometrist has two obligations to the educator: first, to provide general information relative to the effect of vision disorders on learning and, second, to provide specific information about the vision disorders of the educator's student. This might include the patient's particular strengths and weaknesses, the suspected relationship with teacher observations, the mode of treatment, and the estimated time of treatment. It also should include recommendations for classroom accommodations that the educator can make in the short term until the vision disorder is resolved, or for the long term if the vision disorder cannot be resolved.

The educator should be made aware of any therapeutic intervention the optometrist may be providing for the patient for the purpose of remediating visual deficiencies. As an example, if spectacles are prescribed, the educator should know when these are to be worn and when the child is to be reexamined.

Because the optometrist is aware of the specific visual capabilities of the patient, he or she should provide the classroom teacher with recommendations for special seating, lighting, materials, and compensations that would be of benefit to the child in the educational setting until the problem or problems are treated. These might include, for example, large-print materials, line markers, and shortened time on tasks.[6] A major problem to the educator and in many cases the parents is the inability of the patient to learn adequately in the academic situation. It is important also for the educator to be made aware of any recommendations made by the optometrist for additional testing or treatment. All these issues should be communicated in a summary letter explaining the results of the optometric evaluation, correlation of findings to the patient and especially the teacher's entering complaints, and finally the recommendations (see Appendix G for examples). It is helpful to follow up the letter with an oral communication with the teacher.

Role with other professionals

Optometry has been and continues to be a strong supporter of a multidisciplinary approach to the problem of learning problems.[7,8] The importance of a multidisciplinary team concept is supported by researchers such as Fletcher and Satz. They concluded that reading disabilities are so complex that no theory proposing a unitary deficit hypothesis is acceptable.[9] The importance of a broad-based evaluation of the child's strengths and weaknesses would appear to be critical for developing the most efficacious management plan.

In many cases, the patient has been referred to the optometrist for a complete vision evaluation. In all such cases, a written report with a summary of test results and recommendations should be sent to the referring professional. The report should include significant case history information, a summary of test results, a diagnosis, recommendations for management, any proposed treatment plan, and any other information deemed pertinent by the optometrist.

Patients with learning difficulties may have multiple problems contributing to their overall learning difficulty. As an example, the patient may have emotional, physical, and visual problems that are believed by the involved professionals to be contributing to the learning difficulty. Therapeutic intervention may have been recommended by all the professionals on the multidisciplinary team. It is important therefore that any treatment recommended by the optometrist should be coordinated with other recommended professional care.

If the patient is seen first by the optometrist, appropriate referrals to other professionals may be deemed necessary. If so, they should be made as soon as possible. When making such referrals, the optometrist should send a summary of his or her findings and recommendations including the reason or reasons for the referral.

ROLE OF THE OPTOMETRIST IN THE EDUCATIONAL SETTING

In many cases, optometrists act as consultants within the educational setting. The optometrist may provide or supervise vision screening programs. The optometrist may also make visual recommendations for the visually impaired and exceptional or learning-disabled children. When optometrists provide vision screenings within the school setting, it is imperative that educators, school nurses, school administrators, and especially parents understand that a screening is not comparable to a complete vision evaluation. When the optometrist is personally involved in the screening, the vision screenings are generally more comprehensive than those normally provided. As an example, the optometrist might perform ophthalmoscopy or screen for visual efficiency or visual information processing deficiencies, whereas in a screening performed by lay people under the direction of an optometrist, such specialized testing would not be done.

Optometrists may also act as consultants to special programs within the academic setting for low-vision (partially sighted) children, exceptional children, and children with learning problems. Their role within this setting is to make recommendations to educators relative to the visual system in order to assist them in the educational process. These recommendations may stem from the reports of the patient's personal eye care practitioner. The optometric consultant frequently acts as a communicator between the patient's personal eye care practitioner and the educator to ensure effective communication. The optometric consultant may also assist the educator in carrying out some form of treatment recommended by the patient's personal eye care practitioner when this practitioner believes such treatment might best be carried out in the school setting.

In today's educational environment, there appears to be a constant influx of new instructional materials designed to assist the educator. The optometric consultant might assist the educator in evaluating the influence of such materials on the visual system of a specific student or an entire classroom.

ROLE OF THE OPTOMETRIST IN THE PREVENTION OF VISION PROBLEMS

Early childhood experiences are extremely important in the development of the visual system. Research has demonstrated that both animals and human beings require actual movement if the visual system is to learn from the activity.[10,11] If perceptual skills are to develop normally, children must be given the opportunity to acquire multisensory experiences. Appropriate guidance should be given to parents for the development of their children's vision including recommendations for toys for different ages as well as the safety of such toys. Optometrists should be aware of the age ranges of important developmental milestones, as when a child sits upright, walks, uses language to communicate, and draws different shapes. Deficiencies in normal childhood development in one area may relate to deficiencies in vision development.

The optometrist may recommend treatment for a detected visual problem even though currently there are no apparent signs and symptoms. This may be done to address anticipated increases in visual demand. For example, the correction of a moderate amount of hyperopia may be indicated because the child is entering second grade where the need for sustained visual attention is increased over first grade needs. If the problem was not addressed, the child might go through a cycle of symptoms and avoidance before the teacher or parent recognized the problem as visually related. At a minimum the optometrist's role is to identify potential visual problems for the patient or parent and to alert them to the potential signs and symptoms. This strategy will increase the likelihood that the patient will return for vision care if signs and symptoms are noticed in the future.

Good visual health habits are as important for the individual with learning problems as they are for the general population. Good lighting, appropriate posture, and a normal working distance are all necessary to avoid unnecessary stress on the visual system. Such stress can lead to possible adaptations, such as closing one eye or avoidance, to allow the completion of the particular school task. These adaptations, repeated on a daily basis, may lead to future visual problems.

SUMMARY

The optometrist is responsible for the evaluation, diagnosis, and management of visual acuity, visual efficiency, and visual information processing deficiencies. The teaching and remediation of educational deficiencies is the responsibility of the educator. Vision is a complex act that includes more than simply visual acuity. Assessment of the effect of vision on learning requires a comprehensive evaluation by the optometric practitioner. The total process of vision is affected by growth, development, maturation, and learned experiences and therefore requires a broad background and understanding in these areas. In the management of patients with these deficiencies and accompanying learning problems, optometrists must understand and appreciate the importance of their role. Optometric vision therapy is one method of management designed to remediate the signs and symptoms of vision deficiencies. At the same time, the optometrist, as a member of the multidisciplinary team, must work closely with educators, psychologists, school administrators, other health care professionals, and parents to ensure a coordinated management plan. The goal is to detect and remediate any problems that might interfere with the patient's ability to benefit from teacher instruction.

CHAPTER REVIEW

1. Define the comprehensive term "vision" and describe the three major components as used in this text.
2. Describe the appropriate vision care role of the primary care optometrist when evaluating children and adults with learning problems.

3. Describe the role of the optometrist providing comprehensive vision care to patients with learning-related visual problems.

4. Discuss what the patient or parents of a child with learning-related visual problems should be informed of by the optometrist providing comprehensive care.

5. Describe the role of the optometrist providing comprehensive vision care to patients with learning-related visual problems when working with other multidisciplinary team professionals.

6. Describe the role of an optometrist providing comprehensive vision care to patients with learning-related visual problems when working with educators.

7. Describe the role of the optometrist as a consultant within the educational setting.

8. Describe the role of the optometrist in the prevention of vision problems.

REFERENCES

1. Cline D, Hofstetter HW, and Griffin JR: *Dictionary of visual science*, ed 3, Radnor, Penn, 1980, Chilton Book Co.

2. Flax N: Visual function in dyslexia, *Am J Optom* 45:574-586, 1968.

3. Spache GD: Children's vision and their reading success, *J Calif Optom Assoc* 29(5):227-228, 1968.

4. Rouse MW, Hoffman LG: Vision: its evaluation, treatment and relationship to academic performance, Fullerton, 1984, the Southern California College of Optometry. (This project was partially funded by a grant from the California Optometric Association.)

5. Solan HA: Learning disabilities: the role of the developmental optometrist, *J Am Optom Assoc* 50(11): 1259-1265, 1979.

6. Rouse MW, Ryan JB: Teachers' guide to vision problems, *The Reading Teacher* 38:306-318, 1984.

7. Wold RM: Vision and learning: the great puzzle, part II, *Optometric Weekly*, Oct 14 to 21, 1971.

8. Grosvenor T: Are visual anomalies related to reading ability? *J Am Optom Assoc* 48(4):510-517, April 1979.

9. Fletcher JM, Satz P: Unitary deficit hypothesis of reading disabilities: Has Velutino led us astray? *J Learning Disabilities* 12:155, 1979.

10. Held R, Hein A: Movement produced stimulation in the development of visually guided behavior, *J Comparative and Physiological Psychol* 56(5):872-876, Oct 1963.

11. Gibson EJ, Walk RD: The visual cliff. In *Readings from Scientific American: Perception mechanisms and models*, pp 341-348, April 1960.

CHAPTER **9**

Optometric Assessment: Case History

Susan A. Cotter
Janice Emigh Scharre

The free practitioner . . . treats their diseases by going into things thor-
oughly from the beginning in a scientific way, and takes the patient and
his family into confidence.

PLATO: *THE LAWS*

KEY TERMS

interview	otitis media
risk factors	lead exposure
symptoms	psychostimulant medication
signs	developmental milestones
asthma	auditory processing
allergies	soft neurological signs
theophylline	prenatal
low birthweight	intranatal

The optometric assessment of a child who is suspected of having learning-related vision problems begins with the case history or interview. The case history is the formalized process of asking relevant questions to elicit information that will contribute to an accurate diagnosis and appropriate treatment. As a diagnostic tool, the case history has an importance that cannot be underestimated. An integral part of the evaluation, the case history offers a rich source of data for case formulation that is not available from other forms of assessment. From the information gained, the optometrist will develop hypotheses regarding the basis for the chief complaint and identify areas that warrant further investigation. The case history will shape the examination strategy, thereby affecting the accuracy of the diagnosis, development of the management plan, and the formulation of the prognosis. In addition to contributing to better diagnostic and therapeutic decisions, the foundation for a good patient-doctor and parent-doctor relationship is established during this time.

THE INTERVIEW PROCESS

A history questionnaire (see Appendix C) should be given to the child's parents. If an appointment for a visual information processing evaluation is made by phone or the receptionist is aware that one is likely to be scheduled, the questionnaire can be sent to the parents in the mail before the first office visit. If the child is initially in the office for a routine eye exam and it is determined at this visit that a visual information processing evaluation is warranted, the form can be sent home with the parents. The parents may use this opportunity to refer to "baby books" or logs to provide a more accurate developmental and medical history. In either case, the parents are asked to bring the completed form with them to the next office visit. If the parents did not receive the questionnaire before the evaluation, it can be filled out by the parents as the child is examined. History questionnaires serve to provide the doctor with a quick overview, so that he or she may elaborate on pertinent issues raised by the responses on the questionnaire. Although these forms are helpful in eliciting information with an economy of time, they are not a substitute for the interview with the parents and child.

Doctors make most of their diagnostic hypotheses on the basis of the case history. In terms of relative importance, the case history frequently "is the most important and the most revealing portion of the data base."[1] Consequently, the interview process should be given serious consideration and should be planned carefully. As a clinical skill, case history taking can be learned and improved with practice. Helpful hints for a successful interview are listed in Box 9.1.

The setting

The case history interview is an excellent time to establish rapport with the parents and patient, to demonstrate interest in the patient as a person, and thereby to establish a basis for effective communication. The beginning of the interview sets the atmosphere for the remainder of the evaluation process. Therefore the setting of the interview should be considered first.

The case history should be taken in a private area. Generally, this is the examination room; the interview should not take place in the waiting room where the conversation can be overheard by other patients or ancillary office personnel. Adequate space and seating for all parties should be provided. The parents and child should be seated comfortably, and the doctor seated in a position where all participants are visible and in such a way to facilitate communication. Nonverbal behaviors, including the is-

Box 9.1 The Do's and Don'ts for a Successful Interview

Things to do

- Use a private setting
- Frequently address patient and parents by name
- Maintain an attentive body position and good eye contact
- Demonstrate a willingness to listen
- Use open-ended questions
- Structure questions from general to specific
- Show interest and empathetic concern
- Interview the child and parents separately when appropriate
- Give patient or parent enough time to answer in his or her own words

Things NOT to do

- Appear hurried or indifferent
- Moralize or make judgmental comments
- Accept phone interruptions
- Take copious notes thereby maintaining little or no eye contact
- Use optometric jargon
- Ask leading questions

sue of personal space, should be considered. If possible, the doctor should not sit behind a desk. Instead, he or she should sit in a chair that is located close enough for person-to-person interaction but not so close as to intrude on the interviewee's personal space. Sitting at the same eye level as the parents helps to establish good eye contact and to diminish any perceived power differential that might prevent open communication. By leaning slightly toward the person being spoken to rather than lounging back in a chair, the doctor will convey a sense of interest and involvement.[2]

Interviewing the parents

The rapport established between the doctor and parents will influence the accuracy of the information obtained during the interview as well as the parent's confidence in the assessment and their response to later recommendations. Therefore the doctor's attitude should be one of interest, willingness to listen, and empathetic concern. A manner that is friendly and informal will lessen any anxiety associated with the visit. A hurried, indifferent, detached, or unempathetic presence is a barrier to effective communication, which in turn may have a deleterious effect on the interview process. Breakdowns in communication frequently result in failure to comply with a doctor's recommendations.[3]

Parents should be allowed to speak freely and express concerns in their own words. Parents often feel inhibited, however, by the presence of their child. Common concerns are that the child will be embarrassed or have hurt feelings because of what is said, or that there will be a negative effect on the child's self-esteem. Consequently, doctors often choose to interview the parents separately from the child. When the interview begins with both the parents and the child present for the history, it is often easy to tell when the parents do not feel comfortable in speaking in front of the child. Hesitancy in responding to questions is often observed. If the doctor suspects that the parents are not speaking frankly or are reluctant to voice their concerns, the doctor may ask the child to wait with a technician or a relative in the reception room. Alternatively, the doctor can wait until the end of the examination. After the child has left the room (perhaps to go to the "treasure chest" to choose a reward), the parents may be asked whether they would like to elaborate or impart additional information now that the child is no longer present.

Broad-based questions should be asked first with a progression to more focused inquiries. The strategy is to scan potentially important areas and focus in when appropriate, while maintaining sensitivity and flexibility in listening and pursuing. Leading questions should be avoided because they may result in inaccurate information. Clues regarding family concerns and the parent-child relationship can be gathered by observation of the interactions, facial expressions, and body language of the parents and child. Careful observation of the parents and child may uncover concerns that may not be verbalized. When the child is present for the interview, it is important that the doctor be sensitive to the child's feelings and refrain from ignoring the child or implying that he or she is a "condition."

The case history information should be recorded carefully and in an abbreviated form as it is elicited. The doctor should avoid, however, looking solely at his or her writing tools; good eye contact is essential for good communication. Frequently addressing the child and parents by name will personalize the interview and facilitate communication. Care should be taken to allow the parent or patient to answer each question fully before proceeding to another question. Repeating questions for information that was already given spontaneously should be avoided so that the doctor does not imply that he or she is impatient, disrespectful, not interested in, or not listening to what was said.

Optometric jargon, theories, and moralistic or judgmental comments are not appropriate. The doctor should avoid making the parents feel anxious or guilty by lines of questioning that imply that the parents were neglectful or that the child's problems resulted from something the parents did or did not do. In addition, it is inappropriate to make any conclusions or suggestions regarding a genetic link because this may result in one parent blaming the other parent for the child's difficulties. Potentially adverse situations may result when the doctor is not sensitive to these issues.

The doctor should not respond to parental distress by false reassurance or by changing the subject but instead should demonstrate empathy and express in words what the parents are experiencing (for example, "This must be very frustrating for you"). It is important to convey to the parents that one is listening and understands what they are saying. This type of response encourages the parents to elaborate and to realize that they are not alone and that their response to their child's problem is normal, accepted, and understood. The empathetic doctor will be the most likely to obtain a thorough and accurate history.

Interviewing the patient

A case history should always be obtained from the patient in addition to the parents, especially in the areas of chief complaint and symptoms. The doctor's technique and approach will influence the child's willingness to respond. To put the patient at ease, one can first ask nonthreatening demographic questions such as age, date of birth, name of school, and present grade. Additional questions concerning number of siblings, pets, and hobbies also serve to break the ice.

The doctor has the choice of interviewing the child together with the parents or alone (either before or after talking with the parents). There is no absolute rule as to which is best; circumstances and the clinician's judgment will determine the most appropriate approach for the individual case. In all cases, the child's account should be received and treated in a serious manner. Doctor-patient rapport will be strengthened when the child is treated as a person whose opinion matters.

Interviewing an adolescent is often a particular challenge. Adolescents frequently feel self-conscious about the visit and are usually reluctant to discuss their shortcomings. They may deliberately withhold information from their parents. Consequently, it may be helpful to interview adolescent patients alone. A private interview has the advantage of giving the patient an opportunity to describe the problem and his or her perception of it. Once again, circumstances and the clinician's judgment will determine when the child should be interviewed separately.

COMPREHENSIVE CASE HISTORY

The case history portion of the optometric assessment of a child with suspected learning-related vision problems is a systematic inquiry that encompasses several areas. A general outline is presented in Box 9.2. The emphasis of the investigation is to identify the chief concerns of the parents and patient, to obtain a clear understanding of the child's academic performance, and then to evaluate possible contributions that the visual system may have on the child's success or failure in learning. Developmental, medical, behavioral, and educational histories are reviewed as possible contributors to the learning difficulty.

Gathering enough information to enable the doctor to develop clinical hypotheses is the primary objective. The optometrist is interested mainly in whether there is a visual component to the learning problem (that is, whether the patient suffers from a visual efficiency or visual information processing deficiency that might adversely affect academic performance). Based on a well-taken case history alone, the doctor should be able to pre-

---

Box 9.2 Case History Format for a Child with Learning-Related Vision Problems

Chief complaint or concern
Educational history
Medical history
   Prenatal and intranatal history
   Childhood medical history
Developmental history
Previous assessments and treatment
   Visual
   Psychoeducational evaluation
   Audiological, speech and language
   Occupational and physical therapy
   Neurological evaluation
   Other assessments and treatment
Behavior and attention
Family history

Box 9.3 Chief Complaints Frequently Reported by Parents and Teachers

Not performing up to potential
Frequent reversal errors
Poor reading performance
Frequent loss of place when reading
Unable to finish written work in time allotted
Distractibility or short attention span
Difficulty copying from the blackboard

---

dict whether the child has a vision problem and if the problem is related to a deficit in visual efficiency or visual information processing skills or both. A thorough case history not only allows the doctor to develop clinical hypotheses, but also shapes the diagnostic strategy of the examination and ultimately contributes to an accurate diagnosis and appropriate management plan.

Chief complaint or concern

The chief complaint is the reason for the visit, and the interview process is based initially on this concern. The stated complaint may be very specific (for example, the child demonstrates letter reversals) or described in general terms (for example, the child is experiencing difficulty in school). Box 9.3 is a list of chief complaints that are commonly reported by parents and teachers of children with learning difficulties.

The chief complaint as expressed by the parents, the school, and the child should be defined as precisely as possible. It is important that the

---

Box 9.4 Representative Behavioral Signs and Symptoms Related to Visual-Efficiency Deficits

Accommodative deficiencies

Blur or fluctuating vision at near point
Eyes hurt, burn, or tire while reading
Asthenopia, headaches, or ocular fatigue with near work
Excessive rubbing, blinking, or tearing of eyes
Intermittent blur of distance vision after near-point activities

Vergence deficiencies

Asthenopia
Intermittent diplopia
Closing or covering one eye
Difficulty aligning columns of numbers
Letters or words appear to jump, float, or move around
Asthenopia, headaches, or ocular fatigue with near work

Ocular motility deficiencies

Excessive head movement when reading
Frequent loss of place when reading
Omission of words or skipping of lines when reading
Use of a finger or a marker when reading
Lack of comprehension when reading

---

child and parents be given the opportunity to explain completely and in their own words what is believed to be the most important presenting problem. The reason for the visit should be recorded in the parents' and child's own words. If the stated complaint is described in global or abstract terms, the interviewer may request anecdotal accounts or examples for further clarification. Specifically, the interviewer should determine the presenting symptoms and signs. Once these are identified, they should be investigated fully.

Symptoms refer to the child's subjective complaints (for example, the print is blurry; the words go double), whereas *signs* describe objective evidence or observations, which in a child's case are usually made by the parents or teacher (for example, uses a finger as a pointer when reading; has difficulty completing assignments on time). Boxes 9.4 and 9.5 list common signs and symptoms for visual efficiency and visual information processing problems; more complete listings can be found in Chapters 10 and 11. One should investigate further each symptom and sign by noting its onset, nature, manifestations, severity, and duration. The parents' and child's perception of whether the problem is getting better or worse and what has been done for it should also be established.

It is wise to determine whether the parents initiated the optometric assessment on their own or after consultation with the school or with another professional. If it is on the advice of the school, it is critical to de-

Box 9.5 Representative Behavioral Signs and Symptoms Related to Visual Information Processing Deficits

Bilateral integration

Lack of coordination and balance
Difficulty sitting or standing still
Clumsy; falls and bumps into things often
Poor athletic performance

Laterality and directionality

Difficulty learning right and left
Reverses letters or words
Reads from right to left
Confuses directions

Visual discrimination

Confuses likenesses and differences
Mistakes words with similar beginnings or endings
Difficulty with alphabet recognition
Overgeneralizes when classifying objects

Visual figure-ground

Difficulty completing work
Difficulty discriminating relevant from irrelevant
Works slowly compared to peers
Perseverates on details with written work

Visual closure

Ignores details of visual tasks
Incomplete work
Works slowly compared to peers
Poor comprehension during visual tasks

Visual memory and sequencing

Poor spelling skills
Difficulty with math concepts
Difficulty visualizing what is read
Whispers to self during reading
Poor recall of visually presented tasks

Visual-motor integration

Sloppy writing or drawing skills
Poor spacing and inability to stay on lines
Can respond orally but has difficulty producing answers on paper
Difficulty completing written work in time allotted

Auditory-visual integration

Poor spelling ability
Difficulty learning to read phonetically
Difficulty relating symbols to their sounds

termine the parents' interest, willingness, or resistance to the assessment because it is likely to influence the interview. The majority of the time the parents are very concerned about their child's academic difficulties, regardless of who initiated the optometric assessment. In some instances, however, resistance can be present. The parents may feel the child "will grow out of it," "just needs more discipline," or may even believe that they or the school are in some way at fault. In some situations, one parent may feel differently from the other. For example, the mother may be very concerned about her child's academic achievement, yet the father may believe that his son is doing just fine, pointing out that "after all, boys will be boys."

Parents may believe that the school is abdicating its educational responsibilities in some way by seeking additional testing. Eliciting feelings such as these early in the interview is helpful in understanding and directing the rest of the discussion. In addition, it is advantageous for the doctor to know exactly what the parents or school expect or would like to achieve from the optometric assessment. The parents may be advocating that the school provide special services or the school may be hoping to find a visual problem in order to clarify the need for special services. The stated complaint may not be the primary reason that the parents are seeking an evaluation. The interpretation of the problem and anticipated results from the assessment must be identified; it is important to know whether there is a hidden agenda. With experience, the doctor can sense when the parents have concerns other than those they are disclosing during the interview. Questions that are often helpful in identifying parents' true concerns and expectations include the following: (1) What worries you the most? (2) What do you think the problem is? (3) What are your suspicions about the cause of your child's difficulties? (4) How do you think that this problem has affected your child thus far and how do you expect that it will affect your child in the future? In addition, it is often helpful to say something such as, "I want to be sure to answer all your questions and concerns. Can you tell me what you expect or would like to achieve from this evaluation today?"

After carefully investigating the chief complaint, the other areas of the history should be addressed. Although there is no specific order in which to progress, it is likely that school performance was touched upon and thus would be a natural area with which to continue questioning.

Educational history

The optometrist should inquire about the child's present educational placement and functioning, in addition to the child's past educational history. Information regarding the child's current grade placement and the grade level that he or she is functioning at, specifically in reading and math, give the doctor a general feel for the child's overall academic functioning. Inquiries concerning specific areas of strengths and weaknesses, the grades the child received on his or her last report card, and whether the child is graded on individual effort or on the basis of comparison with classmates supply the doctor with more specific academic information. Repetition of any grades, periods of excessive absence, and the age at which formal schooling (including preschool) was initiated provide a historical perspective of the child's academic achievement.

Past or present special educational services and copies of individualized educational plans give the doctor insight regarding the school's perception of areas of difficulty and the severity of the academic problem. Types of classroom settings (that is, mainstreamed, resource, or self-contained) and an account of the remedial approaches that have been tried, including how consistently, for what length of time, and with what effect, should be identified. The results (a copy of the actual reports, if possible) of psychoeducational testing, speech and language evaluations and therapy, occupational therapy, and other services furnish the doctor with valuable data (see Chapter 12).

Although many parents can provide accurate data concerning the above areas, the classroom and resource teachers should also be contacted. A teacher questionnaire (see Appendix D) or personal interview should be used. When possible, the teacher should be sent a questionnaire (with the parents' permission) before the evaluation. Ordinarily, teachers contribute a great deal of helpful information. They usually respond positively when asked for their help and their opinions and are eager to provide any information that might help the child. In addition, a working relationship between the optometrist and the teacher can be established. Not only will the child benefit from this cooperative effort during any remedial efforts, but also this working relationship will allow the doctor and the teacher to learn from each other and serve as a vehicle for future endeavors.

The doctor should contact the teacher by phone after the questionnaire has been returned and the evaluation has been completed. We recommend that the doctor first thank the teacher for responding to the questionnaire and then ask a general question such as, "What is your opinion regarding this child's academic performance in school?" Usually no more than this needs to be said, and the teacher will outline all his or her concerns, observations, hypotheses, any testing results, and other pertinent information. One then can ask more detailed questions in specific areas of concern. This personal communication provides the teacher with an opportunity to elaborate on responses and comments written on the teacher questionnaire and to say things that he or she would not feel comfortable writing down. Of course, one must obtain the parents' permission to exchange information with the teacher and the school.

The teacher can provide both quantitative (such as standardized test scores) and qualitative information regarding the child's academic functioning. Teachers have informally observed many children over a long period of time and have seen a wide range of performance, thereby providing them with a good basis of comparison. Teachers' observations are very helpful in giving the doctor an indication of how the child compares to his or her peers.

General academic achievement and perceived strengths and weaknesses in academic performance as reported by the teacher should be compared to those reported by the parents. Any areas of contradiction should be analyzed. The possibility of unrealistic parental standards or internal school policies leading to denial by the school should be considered if the school sees the child functioning well and the parents report that the child is failing or having academic difficulty. The opposite scenario, when the school reports that the child is having academic problems and the parents believe that the child is performing adequately, should also be evaluated carefully.

Medical history

A child "at risk" is one who has a greater than average chance of developing a sensorimotor deficit or a mental handicap in childhood.[4] "Risk" is not a condition in itself, but a particular circumstance that increases the probability that a certain disorder will occur. Because it is a statistical concept, it cannot be treated. However, when factors that are known to place a child at risk are present, the child can be monitored closely, so that early identification can occur and appropriate intervention can be prescribed. In some cases, it may actually be possible to reduce the risk to which the child is exposed. Early identification, appropriate intervention, and reduction of risk will increase the probability that the child will develop to his or her fullest potential.

Being "at risk" begins at the moment of conception and continues throughout childhood. Many variables are known to contribute to risk status. Research has focused primarily on factors in two areas—medicobiological and environmental-psychosocial. Medicobiological factors include hereditary and genetic conditions, prenatal factors such as maternal drug use or infection, prematurity and low birthweight, complications during birth and delivery, postnatal medical events, and nutrition. Variables such as socioeconomic status, parental education and intelligence, and mother-child interactive behaviors are considered to be environmental-psychosocial risk factors.

At one time, the various risk factors were viewed in isolation and emphasis was placed on prenatal and intranatal (during or at time of birth) factors. The presence of a single risk factor (especially medicobiological) was considered sufficient to place the child at risk for a compromised developmental outcome. However, the prediction of later childhood outcome (including school-age functioning) from prenatal or intranatal factors, especially for isolated events (such as intranatal hypoxia, low APGAR scores) has proved to be weak.[5-7] Prediction of impairment is improved if clusters of measures or events are used rather than single events.[6,8,9] Medicobiological variables are more influential when the outcome measure is taken at an early age, as opposed to environmental influences, which are stronger when the outcome measure is taken at a later age.[10,11]

Even in instances of very early occurring medicobiological events, the outcome measure has been found to be influenced strongly by circumstances of the environment.[6,10] Environmental variables can exacerbate or ameliorate the effects of a medicobiological event that placed the child at risk.[10,12,13] In fact, environmental factors can be stronger and actually override biological events in some cases. Therefore, risk is now conceptualized as the interaction between the function of child's biological status and the environment.[14]

Who then is "at risk" for developmental and learning problems? From a medicobiological standpoint, there is a variety of exogenous influences that are potentially damaging. The major categories of insult are the introduction of neurotoxins in the body, the withholding of essential nutrients, and oxygen deprivation, all of which may have deleterious effects on the developing child's central nervous system. These insults can occur prenatally and reach the fetus indirectly (such as medication or a noxious substance such as alcohol reaching the fetus by way of the mother's bloodstream) or in the postnatal period and affect the infant directly (such as an infant directly ingesting a noxious substance such as lead). Most of the research evaluating the relationship between medicobiological factors and subsequent developmental problems focuses on the prenatal and intranatal period. Medical events and environmental conditions present during infancy and childhood, however, may also place the child at risk. The medical history allows the doctor the opportunity to identify particular circumstances that may have contributed to the child's learning difficulties or that currently place the child at risk for future academic problems. In addition, this information may identify an event or condition that warrants a referral to another professional for further assessment.

Prenatal and intranatal history. It is important to start at the beginning, with a review of the prenatal and intranatal periods. The parent questionnaire (see Appendix C) usually contains a survey of pregnancy, labor, delivery, and the immediate newborn period. The doctor should scan the responses, searching for prenatal and intranatal stresses that may predispose the child to later learning difficulties. Any potentially significant responses can be investigated more fully.

The prenatal period is surveyed first. Maternal health and nutrition may be significant. A history of maternal illness during pregnancy can cause severe or subtle fetal damage. Likewise, some infections, if contracted during pregnancy, may damage the central nervous system; some of these have been associated with subsequent learning disabilities.[15] Box 9.6 lists many prenatal and intranatal conditions that have been associated with later learning difficulties.

Maternal nutrition before and during pregnancy may play a role in placing the child at risk for later developmental handicaps.[16] Poor maternal nutrition may negatively influence fetal growth and birthweight. A classic study by Penrose[17] partitioned birthweight variance into its components and reported that 18% of the variation among infants with differing birthweights was attributable to the mother's general health and nutritional status. Young mothers and mothers from lower socioeconomic backgrounds often have inadequate prenatal care and therefore may suffer from nutritional deficiencies. A frequent sequel of fetal malnutrition is an infant who is small for gestational age (SGA), even if born at term.[16]

Maternal exposure to toxins, drugs, alcohol, cigarette smoking, and medication may also contribute to a child's later learning problems. The placenta acts more like a sieve than a wall, with most drugs crossing the placenta readily. There is a growing body of knowledge indicating that a connection between fetal exposure to cocaine, alcohol, and other drugs

Box 9.6 Examples of Prenatal and Intranatal Risk Factors Associated with Subsequent Learning Problems

Pregnancy	Labor and delivery
Poor maternal nutrition	Obstetric medications
Toxemia	Inhalation anesthetics
Maternal infections	Oxytocin-induced labor
Rubella	Scopolamine sedative-hypnotic
Cytomegalovirus	Vaginal breech delivery
Tuberculosis	Obstetrical trauma
Toxoplasmosis	Prematurity or low birthweight
Inborn errors of metabolism	Toxemia
Phenylketonuria	Failure of labor to progress
Galactosemia	Hypoxia
Preeclampsia	Abnormal bleeding
Maternal lead ingestion	
Maternal alcohol intake	
Maternal smoking	
Maternal drug use	
Irradiation	

and later developmental deficiencies and learning problems exists.[18] Prenatal implications of cocaine exposure include shorter gestational ages, low birthweights, and delivery of SGA infants[19,20] as well as other deleterious effects.[21] Infants exposed to cocaine and crack may suffer from many pernicious conditions, including shorter gestational age, lower birthweight, prenatal cerebral infarctions, central nervous system malformations, and respiratory abnormalities. A strong correlation between fetal exposure to alcohol and later hyperactivity,[22] distractibility,[22] and learning disabilities[23] in school-aged children has been reported. Subsequent fine-motor and gross-motor deficits have been associated with moderate levels of prenatal alcohol exposure.[24] Fetal exposure to multiple agents (such as tobacco, alcohol, marijuana, cocaine) may be more significant than a single-agent exposure.[19,21] Obviously, inquiries into this area should be discreet.

Any report of obstetrical complications or trauma associated with labor and delivery should be clarified. Prolonged labor as well as extensive length and difficulty of delivery are associated with an increased risk of damage to the fetal nervous system or asphyxia of the fetus (leading to hypoxia of the nervous system) (see Box 9.6). Infants who sustain mild intranatal brain injuries such as intraventricular hemorrhages may show a delay in expressive language and those with birth asphyxia may demonstrate a delay in both expressive and receptive language milestones,[25] as well as a delay in visual-motor integration and school-readiness.[26]

There are some indications that low birthweight (LBW) infants are at an increased risk for learning disabilities or for behaviors related to learning disabilities.[27] On average, performance later in childhood on intellectual, academic, and behavioral measures is slightly less (though many perform at normal or higher levels) than infants of normal birthweight.[27] Although commonly defined as having a birthweight of less than 2500 grams, the LBW category is often used to include both preterm infants (born before 37 weeks of gestation) and infants born SGA, regardless of whether they were born early or at term. Very low birthweight (VLBW) (that is, <1500-gram) infants may also be included in this heterogeneous group of LBW infants.

LBW infants may be at risk for perceptual, language, and motor deficits whether born SGA or appropriate for gestational age (AGA).[28] SGA infants with slow intrauterine head growth are more prone to have later cognitive, perceptual, and motor defects.[29] Although there is a general consensus that children who were LBW or VLBW infants are at risk for a variety of cognitive and behavioral tasks, the association between these children and learning disabilities is somewhat less clear.[27] Deficits in visual-motor integration and perceptual organization, however, are commonly found in school-aged children with a history of VLBW or LBW.[27,30-32]

Hunt and colleagues[33] reported that learning disabilities constitute the majority of intellectual deficits found in VLBW survivors. They described a group of VLBW children who were followed and tested longitudinally. Delays in language comprehension or visual-motor integration skills were found in 49% of those tested at 6 years of age. Of particular interest is their description of a subgroup of children who did not demonstrate any cognitive abnormalities at school entry but who were later diagnosed as having learning disabilities in middle childhood.[33] Consequently, the researchers recommended that high-risk infants who originally appear and test as unimpaired should be monitored well into childhood because a learning problem may not be readily apparent until later in life. In a later study, Hunt et al.[32] reported that a subsequent visual-motor disability was found in 21.4% of 8- and 11-year-old children who were formerly VLBW infants.

It should be noted and emphasized that the relationship between specific prenatal and intranatal events and learning disorders is still controversial. The majority of research has attempted to correlate one or more events with the presence of learning disorders. Although prenatal and intranatal complications are found more frequently in the case histories of children with learning disabilities, this does not provide proof of cause, however. In other words, correlation does not imply causation. A clear causal relationship between prenatal and intranatal factors and the subsequent development of learning disabilities has yet to be proved. Single prenatal and intranatal risk factors should be viewed in relation to concurrent risk factors and environmental variables. For example, prematurity is related to delivery complications and respiratory distress; however, prematurity also is more likely to occur in the context of socioeconomic disadvantage (a risk factor itself). Therefore it is difficult to extricate this single intranatal event and to determine the exact role it plays (if at all) in a child's later learning difficulties. Furthermore, it has been shown that prenatal and intranatal stress superimposed on an environment of economic deprivation or social disorganization is more likely to result in later academic difficulties than when the same events occur under optimal environmental conditions.[13]

One then may ask, Why should the doctor even inquire about prenatal and intranatal stresses if their exact role in the causes of learning problems is uncertain? Furthermore, because we cannot turn back the clock of time and undo an event that has occurred already, why spend time discussing it? The reason that eliciting this type of history information is pertinent is that it allows the doctor to weigh the cumulative effects of a combination of potentially detrimental factors and gives the examiner a better understanding of how the child may have become the person (with attendant problems) that he or she is. From a prognostic standpoint, some indication of how heavily the deck may be stacked against the child may be obtained. Furthermore, the case history information may lead to a suspicion that the child's academic difficulties may be related to more than just a learning-related vision problem and a referral to another professional (such as a neurologist) may be warranted.

Childhood medical history. The child's general health is surveyed as part of a complete history. A health inventory regarding illnesses, metabolic disturbances, injuries, hospitalizations, allergies, and medications is usually included on the parent questionnaire (see Appendix C). After reviewing the questionnaire form, the doctor can delve deeper into areas of the child's medical history that might be significant.

Health events that are most likely to have later educational influence are stressed. Childhood illnesses, metabolic disturbances, environmental contaminants, and various medical events have been associated with learning problems (see Box 9.7 for a representative listing). Any condition resulting in hypoxia or cerebral trauma deserves special attention because of the increased risk of learning disabilities. In addition, a report of a sustained high fever (>103° F or 39° C) or hospitalization may be significant.

A history of a high fever may be significant in that the fever may have been associated with an infectious disease that affects the central nervous system (such as meningitis, encephalitis, collagen-vascular diseases).[34] For example, central nervous system sequelae from encephalitis can be intellectual, motor, epileptic, psychiatric, visual, or auditory. Children with a history of acute bacterial meningitis are at risk for sequelae that include hearing impairments, permanent seizure disorders, and learning disabilities.[34] Although many of the resulting complications may be readily apparent, less obvious may be the child who is reported to be inattentive and to daydream in the classroom. The periods in which the child is noted

---

Box 9.7 Adverse Postnatal Factors Associated with Learning Disabilities

Infections
Reye's syndrome
Meningitis
Encephalitis
Otitis media

Metabolic disturbances
Phenylketonuria (PKU)
Histidinemia
Leucine metabolism abnormalities
Diabetes
Galactosemia

Chronic diseases
Acute lymphocytic leukemia
Otitis media
Neurofibromatosis
Chronic renal failure

Environmental contaminants
Lead
Aluminum
Carbon monoxide

Hazardous medical events
Seizures
Hospitalization
Abuse or neglect
Head injury

---

to be staring into space may actually be related to an undiagnosed postinfectious convulsive disorder (such as petit mal epileptic seizure).

Long periods of hospitalization or illness during important developmental periods in a young child's life may account for developmental delays. For example, the child may have been too ill to participate in activities that were essential for the development of visual information processing skills. The school-aged child might have missed instruction in important subject matter (such as phonics), which could negatively influence subsequent academic achievement. It is also possible that there may be consequences related to learning that are beyond the actual illness or accident. For example, a child suffering from a chronic illness (such as leukemia or kidney failure) may be so physically or emotionally incapacitated by the medical problem that optimum intellectual and perceptual growth are not achieved. Other medical conditions that have been reported to affect a child's normal development or have been associated with learning problems include lead intoxication, malnutrition, allergies, and chronic ear infections.

The relationship of lead exposure to cognitive development and learning potential has received considerable attention. A prospective study of child development and low-level lead exposure found that increased blood-lead levels at 24 months of age are associated with lowered cognitive development at 57 months of age.[35] This inverse relationship is especially prominent in the areas of visual-spatial and visual-motor integration skills. Needleman et al.[36] reported that elevated levels of lead as measured in first and second graders' teeth correlated with lower IQ scores, decreased speech and language processing, and impaired attention. When these children were retested in the fifth grade,[37] decreased IQ scores, a greater need for special educational services, and a greater rate of grade retention were found. An extended follow-up study,[38] demonstrated that the deficits associated with early lead exposure persisted into young adulthood and resulted in significant impairment of academic success. Specifically, these individuals were seven times less likely to graduate from high school and six times more likely to have a reading disability. Other findings included a lower class ranking in high school, poorer hand-eye coordination, lower vocabulary scores, impaired fine-motor skills, and slower reaction times.

Frequent bouts of otitis media (middle ear infections) during the first 3 years of life (critical period for speech and language development) may result in substantial auditory processing problems, disturbances in auditory-visual integration, speech and language delays, reading disorders, and poor spelling skills.[39] In addition, children with a history of chronic otitis media have been found to have a decline in verbal IQ and to be slower in developing word combinations.[40] It is important to ask the parent at what age the otitis media began and to determine the frequency of the infections. The younger the child and the more frequent the ear infections, the greater the risk for auditory and speech and language problems.[41] Data presented by Bennett at al.[41] showed recurrent otitis media to be more common in their group of learning-disabled children than in the control group of children without academic difficulties; only 9% of the control children had a history of chronic otitis media compared to 23% of the learning-disabled children. In addition to being linked with later language deficits, chronic otitis media has been associated with hyperactivity or inattention, independent of a learning disability.[42]

Eliciting a history of frequent or severe ear infections is important for reasons other than identifying a child at risk for future learning problems. An undiagnosed hearing defect or auditory processing deficiency should be considered when a child with a history of significant ear infections constantly asks for directions to be repeated, does not appear to pay attention, or does not appear to understand oral directions. In addition, one should consider that any previous diagnostic testing using oral directions (including visual information processing testing) could have been affected adversely by an undiagnosed auditory deficit. If a significant auditory processing deficit is diagnosed, the results of the visual information processing assessment should be reviewed carefully.

Cravioto and DeLicardie[43] cite several studies that found children with a history of severe malnutrition to be at risk for a lowered IQ and developmental lags in hearing, speech, eye-hand coordination, categorization skills, and language acquisition, even long after clinical recovery. In addition, their report included studies demonstrating impairment in intersensory organization, particularly visual-kinesthetic development and auditory-visual performance, as well as visual form perception and discrimination. In a series of reports, Galler and colleagues provided evidence that a group of children with a history of early malnutrition demonstrated a reduction in IQ,[44] impaired classroom behavior,[45] and reduced academic performance.[46]

Although it is generally agreed upon that severe malnutrition interferes with normal physiological and neurological development, the influence of poor nutrition and vitamin or mineral deficiencies is less clear. The American Academy of Pediatrics Committee on Nutrition[47] has taken the stand that healthy children with a normal diet meet the recommended dietary allowances of common vitamins and therefore do not need to take supplements. However, Greenwood and Richardson's[48] review of published work on adolescent nutrition found that specific nutritional deficiencies occur commonly, even in socially advantaged populations. Benton and Roberts[49] and Schoenthaler et al.[50] reported that nonverbal intelligence was found to increase significantly in schoolchildren who began taking multivitamin and mineral supplements as compared to children in control groups. Although the role of nutrition, diet, and supplements is not entirely clear, nutritional counseling may be appropriate for children suspected of having a deficient diet.

A variety of other medical conditions have been associated with decreased cognitive functioning or learning disorders. A high rate (56%) of visual-perceptual disability has been found in children with neurofibromatosis and learning problems.[51] Visual-spatial orientation and integration deficits[52,53] as well as visual-motor integration delays[51] have been identified and believed to contribute to the development of learning disabilities in these children.[52] Children with acute lymphocytic leukemia who have received cranial irradiation have been shown to be at high risk for learning disorders.[54,55] Galactosemia, even when treated early, predisposes the child to speech and language difficulties, especially in the area of expressive language.[56] Language delays and short-term auditory-memory deficits have been found in children with phenylketonuria and normal intelligence.[57] Infants and preschoolers who sustain severe closed-head injury have been found to have impairments on measures of intelligence and with expressive and receptive language functions.[58] Although most of these medical conditions are somewhat uncommon, the doctor should be aware that they place a child at risk for learning difficulties.

In addition to past illnesses, it is important to ascertain whether the child is suffering from any chronic illnesses or allergies or is taking any medications. Asthma, the most common chronic illness[59,60] and cause of school absenteeism in childhood[61,62] is often treated with antiasthmatic medication. Sold under several brand names (Box 9.8), the bronchodilator theophylline is a xanthine derivative closely related to caffeine; it is the pharmacological agent used most often for the maintenance of asthmatic children.[63]

Box 9.8 Commonly Prescribed Brand Names for Theophylline Preparations

K-Dur   Bronkodyl
Slo-Bid   Slo-Phyllin
Theo-Dur   Theophyl
Thoelair   Theo-Dur Sprinkle

This popular agent has received considerable attention regarding its effects on the central nervous system, particularly related to behavior and learning. There have been numerous reports stating that theophylline may be linked to behavior problems and poor school performance.[64-66] Hyperactive behavior,[67] distractibility or inattentiveness,[66-68] and sleeplessness[68] have been reported to characterize the behavior of asthmatic children taking theophylline.

In addition to the behavior changes attributed to theophylline, other potentially adverse effects have been reported. Using a crossover, repeated-measures design, Kasenberg et al.[65] found a decline in verbal concentration and visual skills (perception, memory, construction) during the time period the child was medicated. Memory and concentration were reported to increase after a group of children taking theophylline were switched to an alternative medication, cromolyn sodium.[64] Visual-spatial planning deficits have also been reported in a small group of asthmatic children medicated with theophylline.[69]

There is not overall agreement that theophylline may contribute to learning disabilities or behavioral disorders such as hyperactivity.[70,71] Schlieper et al.[72] reported that no statistically significant difference was found in the cognitive functioning of asthmatic children when they were taking theophylline as compared to when they were not. Their conclusion was tempered, however, with a qualification that a wide variability of individual responses were found and that some children did indeed suffer adverse effects. The study suggested that children already demonstrating attentional problems and academic difficulties appeared to be most vulnerable to the adverse effects of theophylline.

Indeed, there appears to be a subgroup of individuals who have a heightened central nervous system response to the ingestion of theophylline or other xanthine derivatives such as coffee, tea, cola, and chocolate. Sensitive individuals who are already taking theophylline may be adversely affected by consuming foods and beverages high in caffeine content.[70] Considering that a couple of soft drinks and one or two chocolate candy bars can add about 120 mg of caffeine to the bloodstream,[70] one can readily understand that this could be potentially harmful for the child who is already taking theophylline. Therefore the doctor should consider inquiring about the caffeine intake (coffee, tea, soft drinks, and chocolate, in particular) of asthmatic patients medicated with theophylline.

Box 9.9 Common Allergic Signs and Symptoms

Skin

Rash
Itchiness

Ears

Itchiness
Feeling of clogged ears
Sensation of dripping within the ear

Eyes

Conjunctival hyperemia
Tearing
Itching
Lid swelling
Mucus

Chest

Recurrent cough
Shortness of breath
Sensation of tightness
Whistling wheeze when breathes out

Nose

Runny nose with clear, watery discharge
Sneezing
Cannot breath well
Constantly sniffs and wipes nose
Breathes through mouth

Gastrointestinal tract

Nausea
Vomiting
Diarrhea
Stomachaches or cramps

Mouth

Roof of mouth itches
Postnasal drip
Frequent clearing of throat
Sore throat

In addition to asthma, the doctor should inquire about the presence of allergies (both environmental and food). Ten percent to 20% of all children in the United States suffer from some type of allergic problem.[73] Many parents have already had their child tested for allergies and know exactly what substances the child is allergic to. Other parents are fairly certain that allergies to specific substances exist but have not taken the child to an allergist. There are also parents who have never considered that their child might suffer from allergies.

What should make one suspicious that allergies might be present? First, a pattern of signs and symptoms (Box 9.9) that occur at regular intervals or under identical circumstances may be indicative of allergies. For example, every time the child visits her friend's house (who has two cats), she comes back with red, itchy, and watery eyes, or each time a certain food is eaten, she starts to wheeze. Second, the chronicity of symptoms such as sneezing, wheezing, coughing, nasal congestion, or what appears to be a cold that hangs on for a long period of time are suggestive of allergies.

The most common form of allergy is chronic rhinitis. It can be seasonal (such as allergies to pollen or ragweed) and then is commonly referred to as "hay fever" or it can be active year round (such as allergies to dust, cat dander). In addition to exhibiting the typical allergic symptoms, children suffering from allergic rhinitis tend to be listless, moody, irritable, and cranky.[73]

Food allergies are usually more difficult to recognize than environmental allergies because there is often no obvious pattern of symptoms. Although gastrointestinal difficulties (such as stomachaches, nausea, vomiting, diarrhea) or skin reactions (such as itching, redness, hives) that occur whenever a certain food is ingested clearly signal an allergic problem, other allergic manifestations such as sneezing, congestion, and a runny nose are less obvious. A variety of other symptoms may result from food allergies; these include hyperactivity, fatigue, migraine headaches, anxiety, and depression. The foods that most often cause allergic reactions are milk, cereal grains (especially wheat and corn), fresh fruits (especially berries), chocolate, eggs, fish, nuts, pork, shellfish, and tomato products.[73]

Allergic children have significantly more school absences than nonallergic children. Data are not available, however, to support an etiological role for allergies in the pathogenesis of learning disorders.[67] Nonetheless, there are various ways in which the presence of allergies can affect school performance indirectly. For example, upper and lower respiratory problems caused by allergies may affect an allergic child's ability to attend to auditory information or to express himself or herself. This would be especially significant during the time period in which speech and language skills are developing. Furthermore, allergic symptoms may distract the child from the teacher's instructions and the task at hand. Conditions such as upper respiratory congestion, persistent rhinitis, coughing, tearing, and itching will interfere with a child's ability to sustain attention. Energy level and self-control may be affected. A chronically upset stomach or the general feeling of illness often associated with allergies may deter a child from normal behavior and may cause the child to become hyperactive or even withdrawn.[67] This could be an added burden for a child already experiencing academic difficulties.

A substantial number of children with "hyperactive" behavior or diagnosed as having attention deficit disorder (ADD) are treated with psychostimulant medications. The most popular of these stimulant medications are methylphenidate (Ritalin), pemoline (Cylert), and dextroamphetamine (Dexedrine). Although psychostimulants are usually prescribed for hyperactive children with learning difficulties, they are also prescribed for children who display excessive distractibility or impulsiveness in the classroom. Paradoxically, these stimulant drugs alter behavior by strengthening selective attention and reducing distractibility and impulsivity in some children. Academic underachievement alone does not warrant psychostimulant use. Stimulant medications have been found to improve classroom manageability and attentiveness in terms of time on a task in children diagnosed with attention deficit disorder.[74,75] It is not clear, however, if the medication actually improves learning or long-term academic achievement.[76]

The optometrist should be familiar with the clinical and behavioral effects as well as the most common side effects of these medications (see Table 9.1). Furthermore, he or she should determine who prescribed the medication (such as pediatrician, neurologist), how long the child has been taking the medication, whether any changes in behavior or academic performance have been demonstrated, and if any adverse side effects have been noted.

The most commonly reported side effects of psychostimulants, insomnia and decreased appetite, can occur even with the optimum dosage. They are often transient, however, and decrease as tolerance to the medication develops.[77] Headaches, nausea, dizziness, and abdominal pains may also occur. Visual disturbances associated with Ritalin and Dexedrine may include mydriasis, decreased accommodation, and blurring of vision,[78,79] and strabismus, diplopia, and nystagmus may result from Cylert.[78]

The medical history can supply information that is significant now or at a later date. Past medical history may account for present academic difficulties or provide evidence that the child is at risk for learning problems. Determining that a child has a particular chronic illness, suffers from allergies, or is taking certain medications alerts the optometrist to the possibility that school performance and behavior might be affected. Medications, in particular, may be related to certain symptoms or ocular findings (see Table 9.1). For example, chronic antihistamine use for allergies may cause accommodative insufficiency and blurred vision, as well as drowsiness and diminished mental alertness; any of these potential side effects could decrease the child's ability to sustain attention in the classroom as well as for optometric testing. A child on antiseizure medication such as carbamazepine (Tegretol) may not be very alert in the classroom and may suffer from medication-induced strabismus and diplopia. The doctor should take note of any condition or medication that might interfere with visual behavior or divert physical energy and attention from educational endeavors and the ability to attend. As part of the multidisciplinary team, the optometrist should share any concerns with the physician responsible for the child's medical care.

Developmental history

Once the prenatal, intranatal, and postnatal medical histories are obtained, the next area to consider is the child's developmental attainments (that is, developmental milestones). The parent questionnaire (see Appendix C) usually contains a section regarding the age at which certain milestones were achieved. Any delays that are noted upon review of the questionnaire can be pursued during the interview. Because delays in achiev-

TABLE 9.1 A sampling of common pediatric medications and possible adverse reactions

Generic (brand) name	Primary indication	Ocular side effects	Systemic side effects
Methylphenidate (Ritalin)	Attention deficit disorder	Decreased accommodation, blurring of vision	Nervousness, insomnia, headache, anorexia, drowsiness, weight loss, loss of appetite, abdominal pain
Dextroamphetamine (Dexedrine)	Attention deficit disorder with hyperactivity	Decreased accommodation, decreased vision	Restlessness, dizziness, insomnia, headache, anorexia, weight loss
Pemoline (Cylert)	Attention deficit disorder with hyperactivity	Diplopia, decreased vision, nystagmus, strabismus	Insomnia, anorexia, weight loss, dizziness, drowsiness, headache, increased irritability
Phenytoin (Dilantin)	Anticonvulsant	Diplopia, decreased vision, decreased accommodation, decreased convergence, nystagmus	Mental confusion, slurred speech, ataxia, decreased coordination
Carbamazepam (Tegretol)	Anticonvulsant	Diplopia, blurred vision, heavy feeling in the eyes	Dizziness, drowsiness, nausea, unsteadiness
Theophylline preparations	Bronchodilator for asthma	None reported	Restlessness, irritability, nausea, headaches, hyperactive behavior,* distractibility,* sleeplessness,* inattentiveness*
Antihistamine preparations	Treatment of allergies	Blurred vision, diplopia, decreased accommodation	Sedation, sleepiness, drowsiness, dizziness, diminished mental alertness, disturbed coordination

*Information from references 66 to 68.

ing developmental milestones at the appropriate ages are reported to correlate with subsequent academic difficulties,[80-83] the developmental history is considered to be an integral part of the overall case history.

When investigating the child's developmental history, one is primarily interested in the temporal aspects of development in the areas of motor (gross and fine) and language (expressive and receptive). It is often difficult for parents to remember exactly at what age certain motor and language acquisitions were achieved. This is especially true when written records such as "baby books" were not kept or when there are several older siblings. (The age at which a third- or fourth-born child first walked or talked is not quite the same monumental event as when the first-born child did the same.) Nevertheless, a parent often will remember whether there was an overall delay in the development of language or motor skills and can often make a comparison between the child in question and his or her siblings in the acquisition of these skills.

Attainment of motor milestones is the major developmental focus for the child's first 18 months. Early gross-motor milestones (see Table 9.2 and Chapter 1), however, generally have the poorest correlation with later learning and reading disorders.[83,84] Later motor events such as learning to ride a bicycle or to tie one's shoes may be associated more highly with later academic difficulties.[85]

An indication of later (preschool and school age) gross-motor skills can be obtained when questions relating to participation in sports and bike riding are asked. If a gross-motor defect is suspected, it is helpful to determine the child's preference in sports and games, in addition to activities that he or she actively avoids. Children with gross motor difficulties have a tendency to avoid situations that require motor activity and often play with younger children (even though children their age are available) because they are unable to keep pace with their peers. These children often prefer to watch television rather than go to the park. The parents may report that they are always trying to send their child outdoors to play with the other children; however, soon after the child departs to play, he or she ends up in a fight and comes back crying.

A lag in fine-motor development is of particular concern because hand-

TABLE 9.2   A sampling of gross-motor milestones

Skill	Approximate age
Roll-over	4-5 months
Sit without support	6-7 months
Pull to standing	9-10 months
Walk independently	12-14 months
Run	18-24 months
Pedal tricycle	3 years
Walk up and down stairs (alternate feet)	3.5-4 years
Ride two-wheel bicycle without training wheels	6-7 years

written work is a major determinant of school performance in the early grades. Table 9.3 lists some developmental milestones related to fine-motor development. Later milestones include the ability to button clothing by 3 to 4 years of age and tying shoelaces at 5 to 6 years of age. (However, with the advent of Velcro, less children are learning to tie shoelaces.) Typically, the child with a fine-motor deficiency exhibits difficulty with jigsaw puzzles, block building, catching a ball, and coloring within the lines. When questioning the parents about the child's ability in construction tasks such as Lego blocks and models, the parent is apt to respond that the child is more likely to play with the box that the toy came in than the toy itself. (Activities requiring fine-motor skills may seem to the child to be more work than play.)

An association between early language delay, language disorders, and subsequent reading problems in primary grades has been reported.[83,86] Parents should be questioned as to when their child first began to speak and if any difficulty with speech development was noted. Representative developmental milestones related to expressive and receptive language acquisition can be found in Table 9.4 and Chapter 1. Nonsequential achievement and slower acquisition of several milestones are more likely to be associated with later difficulty than the developmental delay of a single

TABLE 9.3   A sampling of fine-motor milestones

Skill	Approximate age
Transfer of objects from hand to hand	3-5 months
Holds bottle	6 months
Pincer grasp	10-12 months
Throws objects to floor	12-15 months
Scribbling	18-24 months
Copies a circle	3 years
Buttons clothes	3.5 years
Catches a ball	4-5 year
Ties shoelaces	5-6 years

TABLE 9.4   A sampling of language (expressive and receptive) milestones

Skill	Approximate age
Pays attention to familiar voices	3-4 months
Babbling	5-6 months
"Ma-ma" and "da-da" used appropriately	12 months
Recognizes names of common objects	13-15 months
Follows simple commands	15-18 months
Two-word sentences	2 years
Simple "kernel sentences" (subjects, verb, and object)	3 years
Names primary colors accurately	4 years
Vocabulary of 2000 to 2500 words; asks "why?"; counts to 10	5 years

milestone.[83] During the case history and examination, the doctor should note whether the child's speech is easily understandable. Difficulty in expressive language is an indication that language development should be investigated thoroughly by a speech and language specialist. A report of prior speech therapy is usually an indication of a previously diagnosed speech delay or deficiency.

Although early language development (versus motor development) appears to be the best predictor of ultimate function in school[84,87] and behavioral functioning,[88] motor skills are also important. A young child's motor skills affect how he or she relates to other children during play. Just ask the uncoordinated and nonathletic child, who is always the last one to be picked for teams, about the importance of motor abilities in relationship to team sports and self-esteem. Academically, fine-motor ability is important because of its direct relationship to handwriting and the emphasis placed on neatly written work in the early primary grades.

Although developmental milestones are described in terms of age-expected performance, it should be noted that cut-off scores or norms must be used with caution. There is always a range of "normal" development and individual variations may be present. For example, if a child does not speak until 3 years of age, but then speaks clearly in full sentences, the delay is probably not very significant. On the other hand, the scenario of a child who first speaks at 2 years of age yet is still difficult to understand at 4 years would make one suspicious of a developmental lag or deficit in language skills. Because of the significant number of developmental milestones, the optometrist is initially encouraged to memorize two or three examples of age-expected performance in each area or to keep a list chairside as a helpful guide.

Previous assessments and treatment

In a search for a cause or some form of treatment, parents may consult a range of "specialists." Children with learning difficulties therefore are often evaluated by a multitude of other professionals, each delving into his or her own area of expertise. The types of evaluations that are often conducted include visual, audiological, speech and language, psychoeducational, neurological, medical, physical therapy, and occupational therapy. Information regarding previous testing and treatments can prove to be very helpful. For example, a child who has received an audiological or speech and language assessment may have been diagnosed with a hearing deficit or language delay. This information may modify the optometric test battery or later explain an area of deficiency. Parents do not always realize that one area of investigation may have an effect on another and might not volunteer previous testing information unless asked.

The doctor may develop an impression of the concerns of the parents and teachers by the type of evaluations and treatments that were recommended previously. Prior treatment points to a diagnosed deficiency that then can be investigated further. Associated problems that may affect the management plan may be uncovered. This information will assist the doctor in understanding the nature of the child's difficulties and will provide the doctor with a clearer view of the total picture. All available reports from other professionals should be read thoroughly and copies made for the patient's file if parental permission is obtained. In review of earlier management, one should determine the methods that were tried, for how long, and with what success.

In addition to the identification of underlying factors or clarification of the nature of the child's learning problems, knowledge of previous testing and treatment is valuable for other reasons. This information is essential to develop a comprehensive management plan; the doctor must decide whether referrals to other professionals are warranted. Moreover, this information is important in helping the doctor to set the stage for a successful case presentation. The results from the optometric assessment will be evaluated in relation to the results reported and recommendations made by the other professionals. The optometrist can better determine the significance and role in the overall picture that any visual dysfunctions play. The management strategy that the doctor suggests then can be discussed in relation to past recommendations and management. Embarrassment over recommending something that has already been tried can be avoided, and any differences in proposed treatment or philosophical approach can be addressed.

Visual. Inquiries should be made in regard to the child's previous visual care, including any treatment that was recommended or prescribed as a result of the evaluation. Determining whether the examination was performed by an optometrist or an ophthalmologist will help place the results and recommendations in perspective. Because parents frequently confuse vision screenings by school nurses and pediatricians with an eye examination, it is important to clarify who actually performed the testing and where the evaluation took place.

Previous vision care should be reviewed carefully. Pertinent questions include: (1) Was any visual problem detected? (2) Were prescription glasses recommended, and if so, why were they prescribed, what was the suggested wearing schedule, and were they worn as recommended? (3) Was any other treatment (such as occlusion, vision therapy, medication, surgery) recommended? (4) Was any other testing recommended, and if so, was it done? Compliance with the former doctors' recommendations and prescribed treatment should be determined. If there was noncompliance, one should ascertain why.

A thorough investigation of the child's previous vision care is important for numerous reasons. An indication of how important the parents perceive eye care can be determined based on the last time the child was seen for a visual examination. The age at which certain visual conditions were first identified can be determined, and a record of visual changes that may occur over time can be provided. If a history of prior trauma or ocular disease is identified through the history, it may save the doctor from pursuing unnecessary testing. Furthermore, an indication of compliance patterns can be determined. Once again, any treatment recommendations that the doctor will later recommend should be discussed in relation to past treatment, with any differences in approach addressed.

Psychoeducational evaluation. A psychoeducational evaluation for a child with academic difficulties is usually performed by a certified school psychologist or by a private psychologist who specializes in learning problems. The evaluation generally probes four areas: history, cognitive functioning, academic achievement, and emotional functioning. Various assessment inventories and diagnostic instruments are used to obtain an assessment of the child's intellectual abilities (usually in the form of an IQ score), academic achievement, and psychosocial status. The psychologist attempts to delineate the child's strengths and weakness in these areas. The optometrist may use the information contained within the psychoeducational report to further define his or her testing hypotheses and later to help form the prognosis and determine the final recommendations.

The optometrist will want to know the results of cognitive testing (that is, the child's IQ score). Three scores will be given for the commonly administered WISC-III (Wechsler Intelligence Scale for Children in its latest revision). The verbal IQ is a language-based score, and the performance IQ is based mainly on visual-spatial information. The full-scale score is a combination of the verbal and performance IQs and will give an indication of whether the child's achievement is consistent with other children of his or her chronological age. The WISC therefore determines (1) whether the child is expected to achieve at a rate comparable to other children of the same chronological age and (2) whether the child's verbal and nonverbal abilities are fairly consistent.

The WISC scores provide the optometrist with valuable information concerning the child's cognitive level, and the scores are particularly helpful when one is evaluating the results of the visual information processing evaluation. For example, a child may exhibit below-average results on the visual information processing evaluation. However, if the child's verbal and performance IQs both are also below average, visual information processing skills may not be weak but consistent with the child's mental age. (A very thorough discussion of the psychoeducational evaluation and its interpretation in relation to the vision assessment is found in Chapter 12.)

The educational portion of the psychoeducational assessment measures the child's abilities and achievement in basic academic areas such as reading, mathematics, and written language. Scores for specific subskills (as in reading—word-attack skills, passage comprehension, and sight vocabulary) are provided. Again, strengths and weakness should be identified. Academic achievement scores can be compared to measures of intelligence obtained from the cognitive portion of the assessment. The social information contained in the report will forewarn the doctor of any nonadaptive behaviors and pertinent information concerning family relations, self-esteem, behavioral issues, and emotional problems.

It is more valuable to obtain a copy of the report rather than a verbal summary from the parents. First, because of the significant amount of data contained within the report, the parents will not possibly be able to recall all the information accurately. Furthermore, there may be information (on, for example, testing style or responsiveness) that the parents might not consider to be important, but the optometrist will find valuable. Occasionally, parents are reluctant to provide a copy of the psychoeducational report because it contains sensitive information on the child's intellectual abilities and emotional state. If this occurs, it is best to explain to the parents the importance of this information and ask if they will allow the report to be reviewed.

Audiological, speech and language. Children suspected of having a speech delay or language dysfunction are frequently evaluated for auditory function as well as speech and language skills. The evaluations may be performed separately or completed as one.

The primary goal of an audiological assessment is to determine the presence and degree of a hearing impairment. A quantitative measure of hearing (auditory acuity) is conducted using an audiometer. If a deficit is found, a measure of the amount of hearing loss can be made. The tuning fork test helps differentiate whether a hearing loss is sensorineural or conductive in nature. Children with a conductive deafness (middle ear involvement) will understand speech if it is loud enough. Children with a sensorineural loss, however, may have difficulty even when speech is sufficiently loud. Otitis media with fluid accumulation is the most common cause of childhood hearing loss; it results in a mild-to-moderate conductive hearing loss.[89]

A formal speech and language assessment is usually performed by a speech pathologist or psycholinguist. The intention of the evaluation is to determine whether a speech or language problem exists and to characterize the problem if one is present. Standardized clinical tests are used to assess receptive (comprehension) aspects separately from expressive (production) aspects. Articulation impairment can also be evaluated separately from receptive and expressive language disorders. An auditory processing evaluation can rule out or identify auditory processing deficits in areas such as discrimination, figure-ground, memory, sequencing, and closure.

Speech and language disorders are commonly reported in children with reading and academic difficulties. Speech disorders (such as articulation difficulties) are more common than language disorders and their presence does not usually affect academic achievement to the degree that language disorders do. Generally the prognosis is poorer for children with impaired receptive language skills than expressive language skills.[90]

The doctor should keep in mind that deficient auditory or speech and language function may have a strong influence on the optometric test strategy or on the interpretation of the optometric test results. The child with a speech and language disorder may have difficulty in understanding or responding during the optometric evaluation, thereby biasing the data collected. A child with a hearing impairment or auditory processing deficit may appear inattentive, may frequently request repetition of spoken words, and may appear to be confused by auditory directions.

Occupational and physical therapy. Children with fine- and gross-motor problems may have received occupational or physical therapy evaluations and treatment. An occupational therapy assessment evaluates the child's fine- and gross-motor skills, motor-planning abilities, postural control, perceptual-motor skills, and sensory-integration abilities.[91] If a dysfunction is found, its influence on daily-life tasks (including academic performance) is assessed. A child may exhibit deficiencies in maintaining adequate posture when seated in a chair, crossing the midline, and writing legibly or at a speed sufficient to keep up with his or her classmates. Poor muscle tone or inadequate bilateral coordination may result in fine-motor difficulties. Deficiencies in any of these areas may influence the child's ability to attend or to perform adequately in the classroom. Likewise, the child's performance on visual information processing testing could be adversely affected. Therapy may address the development of a specific skill (such as handwriting) or basic, foundation skills (such as postural control). Fine-motor therapy is commonly prescribed for children with learning problems and poor printing or handwriting skills.

A physical therapy assessment provides evaluation of gross-motor (large muscle) coordination and the organization and execution of movement skills. Although gross-motor deficits may not be related to learning in itself, they may affect a child's already vulnerable self-concept. The child's selection of pastimes can be influenced, as well. Gross-motor deficits may contribute to the child's sense of failure and inability to participate positively in organized play or sport activities.

Occupational and physical therapy are educationally related services and are commonly provided within the school setting. Occupational therapists frequently work with children to improve tracking and fine-motor abilities, in addition to visual perceptual skills. Obviously, the optometrist would want to know whether deficiencies or remedial efforts in these areas have taken place. Of all the other professionals that a child with learning difficulties may encounter, the occupational therapist is the most likely (other than the optometrist) to be concerned with visual efficiency and visual information processing skills.

Neurological evaluation. The optometrist will want to know whether a pediatric neurological assessment was recommended or completed. Children who would be most likely to have undergone a neurological assessment are those with a history of significant developmental delays or of an injury with a subsequent change in developmental abilities, symptoms of a seizure disorder, or recurring headaches. In addition, a neurological examination is frequently recommended for children presenting with academic problems associated with behavioral characteristics of "hyperactivity" (that is, impulsivity, excessive motor activity, and distractibility). In fact, the neurologist may be the professional who makes the diagnosis of attention deficit disorder and who may prescribe psychostimulant medication in an effort to affect behavioral changes.

There are usually two components to the neurological evaluation of a child with a learning disorder—a standard neurological evaluation and an assessment for "soft neurological signs."[85] The standard pediatric neurological examination permits an assessment of the integrity of the central nervous system (CNS) by means of a history and examination that includes a cranial nerve examination; motor and sensory examination; evaluation of coordination, gait, and posture; assessment of deep tendon reflexes; and mental status.[92] Although rarely found in a learning-disabled child who is otherwise normal and healthy, muscular dystrophies, demyelinating diseases, tumors, and mild forms of cerebral palsy can be ruled out.

The examination for soft neurological signs is a search for mild neurological signs or indicators of CNS maturation and CNS efficiency. An indication of CNS maturation is obtained by evaluation of a series of neuromaturational markers (such as identification of right and left on self, repeated finger-to-thumb opposition). The presence of an age-dependent neurological marker beyond the age at which it normally should disappear is considered to be a soft neurological sign. Mild neurological abnormalities (such as reflex asymmetries, tremors, coordination deficits) that would be considered to be neurological inefficiencies in a patient of any age are also considered to be soft neurological signs. Soft neurological signs have been associated with learning disorders, but clusters of signs appear to be more meaningful than a single, isolated sign.[85,93] Soft neurological signs, however, are not diagnostic of learning disorders and are of little value in and by themselves.

Parents often have unrealistic expectations concerning neurological evaluations for children with academic difficulties. Many believe that the neurologist will unequivocally determine whether the child's learning difficulties are organic or emotional and then provide them with a definitive diagnosis. Although specific neurological dysfunctions, structural deficits, and pathological processes can be ruled out, it is rare that the results obtained from neurological evaluation will account entirely for a child's learning problems. The neurological evaluation, however, can contribute to the optometrist's understanding of the child's overall functional status, especially when the diagnosis of attention deficit disorder has been made.

Other assessments and treatments. After inquiry into any formal assessments or treatments that the child has received, it is important to determine whether or not the child has had any other type of intervention or treatment related to his or her learning difficulties. In some cases, a child may not have received a formal evaluation (such as a neurological evaluation) but may have received treatment through an early intervention or preschool program. For example, the child may have been identified in preschool as having motor delays and subsequently received physical or occupational therapy. This line of questioning may reveal that the parents have sought counseling or psychological therapy for the child and possibly for the entire family. In their search for a cause or cure, parents often explore multiple interventions, even some that the doctor may consider fairly unconventional. The parents may mention the use of such things as colored filters,[94,95] patterning,[96] hair analysis,[97] and megavitamins.[98]

It is important to remain neutral when previous treatments or forms of intervention are discussed. The parents may report that they suspected a problem in a specific area early on but were discouraged from seeking treatment because of reassurances from others (such as professionals, teachers, relatives) that the child would "outgrow it." Parents may feel guilty that they did not seek intervention sooner. The parents' perception of the effectiveness of any intervention needs to be explored. They may be angry that the treatment their child received was not so effective as they expected or were led to believe, or, alternatively, they may be under the impression that a particular treatment was more effective than it actually was. If the parents believe that a previous treatment was not efficacious, they may be reluctant to comply with subsequent treatment recommendations. All this information is important so that the doctor can set the stage for a successful case presentation at the completion of the evaluation process.

Behavior and attention

The parents should be questioned regarding the child's behavior and attention (particularly in school). Reports of hyperactivity, inattention, distractibility, impulsiveness, or overactivity may be indicative of attention deficit disorder. Alternatively, an increase in activity level may result from the child's reacting to the effects of anxiety, tension, and frustration, just as inattention and distractibility may be the child's attempt to leave the classroom situation mentally.

When behavior and attention are reported to be areas of concern, one should determine whether there have been any evaluations to assess behavior and, if so, whether any treatment (such as diet, medication, behavior modification program) was recommended. Psychoeducational and neurological evaluations usually address this area; pertinent information regarding behavior and attention is generally included in these reports. The diagnosis of attention deficit disorder may have resulted from the evaluations, and psychostimulant medication may have been prescribed (see Chapter 4 for further discussion).

Behavior information obtained from the parents may assist the doctor in modifying the optometric evaluation. For example, in the case of a child with a short attention span, frequent breaks and behavior modification techniques may be necessary. A child who is easily frustrated may need frequent reassurance of the correctness of his or her responses.

Family history

Inquiries should be made as to whether there is a family history of learning problems. Family members, particularly parents, grandparents, and siblings, who have had academic difficulties or were retained in school should be identified and specific areas of difficulty determined. The familial occurrence of learning disorders is well documented.[99,100] It should be noted, however, that familial occurrence by itself does not prove heritability because common environmental influences are present. Nevertheless, there is convincing evidence for the existence of genetic factors in some reading and learning disabilities.[100,101]

Immediate family members sometimes reveal patterns of reading or learning disabilities. For example, family studies have found predominancy of visual or auditory impairment[102] as well as similar types of spelling errors[103] to be present in families with dyslexia. An autosomal dominant mode of transmission for the dyseidetic type of dyslexia has also been suggested.[104] In most instances of reading and learning problems, however, the mode of transmission and the degree in which heritability contributes to familial occurrence is not firmly established.

It is not uncommon for a parent to report that he or she had difficulties in learning to read and in some instances to admit that he or she still is not a good reader. This may cause the parent to have a great deal of empathy for the child or may provide the parent who became successful, despite the reading problem, with reasons to diminish the significance of the child's problem.

Because the diagnosis of learning disabilities comprises heterogeneous disorders, with both genetic and environmental determinants, the exact role of genetics as a contributing factor is not clear cut. Therefore the doctor should think carefully before making any remarks or conclusions to the parents concerning a genetic link; this will prevent feelings of guilt or blame in the family.

The ocular and medical histories of family members should also be probed to alert the clinician to risk factors. The goal is to determine whether there are any ocular or systemic conditions that the child may be genetically predisposed to develop that will influence learning ability.

CONCLUDING THE INTERVIEW

At the end of the case history, it is prudent to return to the initially stated concerns. The doctor should briefly summarize the major concerns and ask further questions if needed. This indicates that the doctor listened to and understood the stated concerns and that he or she intends to treat the concerns seriously and will attempt to find answers to the parents' questions. At the close, it is often helpful to say something such as, "Is there anything else that we did not discuss that I might need to know or that might have some bearing on this child's difficulties?" This will decrease the chance that other pertinent information will be overlooked. In fact, it is not unusual for additional information to surface at this point, or even later after the evaluation process. The more comfortable the parents feel, the more likely they are to share their thoughts and concerns.

CASE HISTORY SCREENING FOR DETECTION AND REFERRAL

The comprehensive case history discussed in this chapter is just that—comprehensive. It is an in-depth interview that not only includes the patient's and parents' chief complaints, but also thoroughly investigates the patient's educational, medical, developmental, family, and behavioral histories, as well as previous assessments and treatments. Therefore this inclusive interview may be somewhat time consuming. This time is well spent for the doctor who plans on evaluating the child's visual efficiency and visual information processing skills to determine whether there is a visual component to the child's academic difficulties.

Most doctors in a primary care setting either do not have the time or the inclination to conduct the previously discussed comprehensive case history. In an effort to provide the best vision care, however, the doctor will want to at least identify the children likely to have visual efficiency or visual information processing deficits that might adversely affect academic performance. If these children are identified, they then can be referred to a colleague (if the practitioner chooses not to do the evaluation himself or herself) who can perform a thorough assessment of visual efficiency and visual information processing skills.

For this reason, we present a case history supplement for school-aged children (see Appendix E) to be used as a screening checklist. It is concerned primarily with school performance, and the signs and symptoms of visual efficiency and visual information processing deficits. Attention and distractibility in the classroom are included as well. This screening history is designed to be used in a primary care setting for the purpose of identifying those children most likely in need of further assessment of visual efficiency or visual information processing skills.

We suggest that this form be given to a parent when the family first arrives at the doctor's office and checks in at the reception desk. After greeting the patient, the receptionist can attach the form to a clipboard and give it to the parent requesting that it be completed before the patient is seen (much like a patient information sheet containing demographic data and billing information). The completed form then can be inserted into the child's file for the doctor to review quickly before beginning the vision examination (similar to the way one might review pretesting results). If any areas on the form are marked yes, the doctor can investigate them further. If the doctor's findings (such as uncorrected refractive error) from his or her primary care vision examination do not appear to account for the items marked on the checklist, it is best to refer the child to a colleague for further diagnostic testing.

In addition to the case history supplement sheet, the doctor should take the standard case history that he or she would ordinarily take on any adult patient. With only a few key additions, this history can be easily adapted for a school-aged child (Box 9.10). In addition to the usual pertinent medical history (such as diabetes, thyroid problems), the following conditions should be specifically inquired about because of their association with learning difficulties: lead poisoning, chronic ear infections, and any chronic childhood illnesses, especially asthma and allergies. As always, medications the patient is taking should be identified. Table 9.1 contains medications commonly used for children that may be of special concern; the most common adverse reactions of these medications that either affect visual efficiency (such as convergence, accommodation) or attention (such as decreased mental alertness, drowsiness) are listed. A general query as to any unusual or significant events that occurred at birth is usually sufficient to identify common risk factors such as trauma or hypoxia at birth. Determining whether the child was carried to term and his or her birthweight will determine whether the child falls in the general category of low birthweight, with a risk for later visual processing, language, and motor deficits. A general inquiry as to whether there were any delays in the development of motor or language skills is usually sufficient to identify developmental milestone delays that might be associated with subsequent academic difficulties. A question about school performance and whether the child is performing at his or her potential will usually disclose whether the parents or school personnel believe that academic difficulties are present.

In most cases, this general line of questioning will uncover potentially significant information relating to learning-related vision problems and possible deficits in visual efficiency or visual information processing skills. If this scaled-down version of the case history uncovers such information,

---

Box 9.10 Additional Case History Questions for a School-Aged Child

- Has your child ever had lead poisoning, frequent ear infections, any significant accidents or trauma, or any chronic childhood illnesses?
- Does he or she have asthma or allergies?
- Was there anything unusual or significant at birth?
- Was the child carried to term and what was his or her birthweight?
- Were there any delays in the development of motor (such as walking or fine-motor) or language (when first talked, understanding the child's speech) skills?
- How is the child's school performance?
- Are you happy with the child's school performance?
- Is the teacher happy with the child's school performance?

the doctor then needs to decide only whether the patient should be rescheduled for further testing to be done by himself or herself or instead referred to a colleague well versed in this area.

SUMMARY

The case history provides the framework within which to view the child and provides clues for the generation of hypotheses. It is the doctor's initial opportunity to formulate clinical impressions and to establish a preliminary estimate of the nature and severity of the child's problem and then to generate an evaluation strategy. Because the case history is an integral part of the evaluation process, it should not be neglected. Although a comprehensive case history will generate the most complete and the most accurate data, the screening history presented should identify the majority of children who need optometric referral. A directed and thorough evaluation will be more likely to result in an accurate diagnosis, treatment program, and prognosis.

In addition to directing the examination, the case history information related to the child's visual, developmental, medical, behavioral, and educational histories is vital if the doctor is to have a complete understanding of the child and his or her school difficulties. With the knowledge obtained from a well-taken case history, the optometrist can better determine the significance of any visual problems identified from the visual assessment and then can develop a working alliance with the child and his or her parents.

CHAPTER REVIEW

1. List and discuss the key case history areas that should be investigated when a child is suspected of having a learning-related vision problem.
2. Discuss the common psychostimulant medications used for children with attention deficit disorder or hyperactive behavior. Describe the clinical and behavioral effects, as well as possible side effects of these medications.
3. List and discuss significant prenatal and intranatal risk factors.
4. Discuss the areas of previous assessment and treatment that one should investigate?
5. Discuss the aspects of a child's developmental history that one should investigate and why.

ACKNOWLEDGMENTS

We wish to thank Sue Mirman, O.D., for her help with various (too numerous to list) aspects of this project but especially for collecting, typing, verifying, formatting (and reformatting) the references—a tedious job well done! In addition, we wish to thank Sandra Engram for her cheerful but dogged pursuit of references through the interlibrary loan system,

Michelle Marciniak, O.D., for her library work and copying services (on and off campus), and Eric Borsting, O.D., for his helpful comments on an early version of the manuscript.

REFERENCES

1. Cutler P: The principal parts: data collection, data processing, problem lists. In Cutler P, editor: *Problem solving in clinical medicine: from data to diagnosis*, Baltimore, 1979, Williams & Wilkins.
2. Coulehan JL, Block MR: *The medical interview: a primer for students of the art*, Philadelphia, 1987, FA Davis, pp 38-54.
3. Korsch BM, Negrete VF: Doctor-patient communication, *Sci Am* 227:66-74, 1972.
4. Parmelee AH: Early intervention for preterm infants. In Brown CC, editor: *Infants at risk: assessment and intervention*, Pediatric Round Table Series 5, Skillman, NJ, 1981, Johnson & Johnson.
5. Gottfried AW: Intellectual consequences of perinatal anoxia, *Psychol Bull* 80:231-242, 1973.
6. Parmelee AH, Sigman M, Kopp CB, Haber A: Diagnosis of the infant at high risk for mental, motor, and sensory handicaps. In Tjossem TD, editor: *Intervention strategies for high risk infants and young children*, Baltimore, 1976, University Park Press.
7. Bee HL, Barnard KE, Eyres SJ, et al: Prediction of IQ and language skill from perinatal status, child performance, family characteristics, and mother-infant interaction, *Child Dev* 53:1134-1156, 1982.
8. Field TM, Dempsey JR, Shuman HH: Developmental follow-up of pre- and postterm infants. In Friedman SL, Sigman M, editors: *Preterm birth and psychological development*, New York, 1981, Academic Press.
9. Siegel LS: Reproductive, perinatal, and environmental factors as predictors of the cognitive and language development of preterm and full-term infants, *Child Dev* 53:963-973, 1982.
10. Cohen SE, Parmelee AH, Beckwith L, Sigman M: Cognitive development in preterm infants: birth to 8 years, *J Dev Behav Pediatr* 102-110, 1986.
11. Aylward GP, Gustafson N, Verhulst SJ, Colliver JA: Consistency in the diagnosis of cognitive, motor, and neurologic function over the first three years, *J Pediatr Psychol* 12:77-98, 1987.
12. Sameroff AJ, Chandler MJ: Reproductive risk and the continuum of caretaking casualty. In Horowitz FD, Hetherington ME, Scarr-Salapatek S, Sieger GM, editors: *Review of child development research*, vol 4. Chicago, 1975, University of Chicago Press.
13. Werner EE, Smith RS: *Vulnerable but invincible*, New York, 1982, McGraw-Hill, pp 24-35.
14. Thurman SK, Widerstrom AH: *Infants and young children with special needs: a developmental and ecological approach*, ed 2, Baltimore, 1990, Paul H Brookes Publishing, pp 13-27.
15. Sever JL: Perinatal infections and damage to the central nervous system. In Lewis M, editor: *Learning disabilities and prenatal risk*, Urbana, Ill, 1986, University of Illinois Press.
16. Simopoulos AP: Nutrition in relation to learning disabilities. In Lewis M, editor: *Learning disabilities and prenatal risk*, Urbana, Ill, 1986, University of Illinois Press.
17. Penrose LS: Some recent trends in human genetics, *Caryologia* 6(suppl):521-530, 1954, cited in Simopoulos AP: Nutrition in relation to learning disabilities. In Lewis M, editor: *Learning disabilities and prenatal risk*, Urbana, Ill, 1986, University of Illinois Press.
18. Van Dyke DC, Fox AA: Fetal drug exposure and its possible implications for learning in the preschool and school-age population, *J Learn Disabil* 23:160-163, 1990.
19. Burkett G, Yasin S, Palow D: Peri-

natal implications of cocaine exposure, *J Reprod Med* 35:35-42, 1990.

20. MacGregor SN, Keith LG, Chasnoff IJ, et al: Cocaine use during pregnancy: adverse perinatal outcome, *Am J Obstet Gynecol* 157:686-690, 1987.

21. Bandstra ES, Burkett G: Maternal-fetal and neonatal effects of in utero cocaine exposure, *Semin Perinatol* 15:288-301, 1991.

22. Spohr HL, Steinhausen HC: Follow-up studies of children with fetal alcohol syndrome, *Neuropediatrics* 18:13-17, 1987.

23. Gold S, Sherry L: Hyperactivity, learning disabilities, and alcohol, *J Learn Disabil* 17:3-6, 1984.

24. Barr HM, Darby BL, Streissguth AP, Sampson PD: Prenatal exposure to alcohol, caffeine, tobacco, and aspirin: effects on fine and gross motor performance in 4-year-old children, *Dev Psychol* 26:339-348, 1990.

25. Janowsky JS, Nass R: Early language development in infants with cortical and subcortical perinatal brain injury, *J Dev Behav Pediatr* 8:3-7, 1987.

26. Robertson CMT, Finer NN: Educational readiness of survivors of neonatal encephalopathy associated with birth asphyxia at term, *J Dev Behav Pediatr* 9:298-306, 1988.

27. Cohen SE: Low birthweight. In Brown CC, editor: *Childhood learning disabilities and prenatal risk*, Pediatric Round Table Series 9, Skillman, NJ, 1983, Johnson & Johnson.

28. Siegel LS: Reproductive, perinatal, and environmental variables as predictors of development of preterm (<1501 grams) and fullterm children at 5 years, *Semin Perinatol* 6:274-279, 1982.

29. Harvey D, Prince J, Bunton J, Parkinson C, Campbell S: Abilities of children who were small-for-gestational-age babies, *Pediatrics* 69:296-300, 1982.

30. Caputo DV, Goldstein KM, Taub HB: The development of prematurely born children through middle childhood. In Field T,

Sostek A, Goldberg S, Shuman HH, editors: *Infants born at risk*, Jamaica, NY, 1979, Spectrum Publications.

31. Klein NK, Hack M, Breslau N: Children who were very low birth weight: development and academic achievement at nine years of age, *J Dev Behav Pediatr* 10:32-37, 1989.

32. Hunt JV, Cooper BAB, Tooley WH: Very low birth weight infants at 8 and 11 years of age: role of neonatal illness and family status, *Pediatrics* 82:596-603, 1988.

33. Hunt JV, Tooley WH, Harvin D: Learning disabilities in children with birth weights ≤1500 grams, *Semin Perinatol* 6:280-287, 1982.

34. Behrman RE, editor: Infectious diseases. Chapter 12 in *Nelson textbook of pediatrics*, ed 14, Philadelphia, 1992, WB Saunders.

35. Bellinger D, Sloman J, Leviton A, et al: Low-level lead exposure and children's cognitive function in the preschool years, *Pediatrics* 87:593-873, 1991.

36. Needleman HL, Gunnoe C, Leviton A, et al: Deficits in psychologic and classroom performance of children with elevated dentine lead levels, *N Engl J Med* 300:689-695, 1979.

37. Bellinger D, Needleman HL, Bromfield R, Mintz M: A followup study of the academic attainment and classroom behavior of children with elevated dentine lead levels, *Biol Trace Elem Res* 6:207-223, 1984.

38. Needleman HL, Schell A, Bellinger D, Leviton A, Allred EN: The long-term effects of exposure to low doses of lead in childhood, an 11-year follow-up report, *N Engl J Med* 322:83-88, 1990.

39. Zinkus PW, Gottlieb MI, Schapiro M: Developmental and psychoeducational sequelae of chronic otitis media, *Am J Dis Child* 132:1100-1104, 1978.

40. Zinkus PW, Gottlieb MI: Patterns of perceptual and academic deficits related to early chronic otitis media, *Pediatrics* 66:246-253, 1980.

41. Bennett FC, Ruuska SH, Sherman R: Middle ear function in learning-

disabled children, *Pediatrics* 66: 254-260, 1980.

42. Adesman AR, Altshuler LA, Lipkin PH, Walco GA: Otitis media in children with learning disabilities and in children with attention deficit disorder with hyperactivity, *Pediatrics* 85:442-446, 1990.
43. Cravioto J, DeLicardie ER: Nutrition, mental development, and learning. In Falkner F, Tanner JM, editors: *Human growth.* 3: *Neurobiology and nutrition*, New York, 1979, Plenum Press.
44. Galler JR, Ramsey F, Solimano G, Lowell WE, Mason E: The influence of early malutrition on subsequent behavioral development. I. Degree of impairment in intellectual performance, *J Am Acad Child Psychol* 22:8-15, 1983.
45. Galler JR, Ramsey F, Solimano G, Lowell WE: The influence of early malnutrition on subsequent behavioral development. II. Classroom behavior, *J Am Acad Child Psychol* 22:16-22, 1983.
46. Galler JR, Ramsey F, Solimano G: The influence of early malnutrition on subsequent behavioral development. III. Learning disabilities as a sequel to malnutrition, *Pediatr Res* 18:309-313, 1984.
47. American Academy of Pediatrics Commitee on Nutrition: Megavitamin therapy for childhood psychoses and learning disabilities, *Pediatrics* 58:910-912, 1976.
48. Greenwood CT, Richardson DP: Nutrition during adolescence, *Wld Rev Nutr Diet* 33:1-41, 1979.
49. Benton D, Roberts G: Effect of vitamin and mineral supplementation on intelligence of a sample of schoolchildren, *Lancet* 1(8578): 140-143, 1988.
50. Schoenthaler SJ, Amos SP, Eysenck HJ, Peritz E, Yudkin J: Controlled trial of vitamin-mineral supplementation: effects on intelligence and performance, *Person Individ Diff* 12:351-362, 1991.
51. Eliason MJ: Neurofibromatosis: implications for learning and behavior, *J Dev Behav Pediatr* 7:175-179, 1986.

52. Eldridge R, Denckla MB, Bien E, et al: Neurofibromatosis type 1 (Recklinghausen's disease), *Am J Dis Child* 143:833-837, 1989.
53. Varnhagen CK, Lewin S, Das JP, et al: Neurofibromatosis and psychological processes, *J Dev Behav Pediatr* 9:257-265, 1988.
54. Fogarty K, Volonino V, Caul J, et al: Acute leukemia: learning disabilities following CNS irradiation, *Clin Pediatr* 27:524-528, 1988.
55. Ch'ien LT, Aur RJA, Stagner S, et al: Long-term neurological implications of somnolence syndrome in children with acute lymphocytic leukemia, *Ann Neurol* 8:273-277, 1980.
56. Waisbren SE, Norman TR, Schnell RR, Levy HL: Speech and language deficits in early-treated children with galactosemia, *J Pediatr* 102: 75-77, 1983.
57. Melnick CR, Michals KK, Matalon R: Linguistic development of children with phenylketonuria and normal intelligence, *J Pediatr* 98: 269-272, 1981.
58. Ewing-Cobbs L, Miner ME, Fletcher JM, Levin HS: Intellectual, motor, and language sequelae following closed head injury in infants and preschoolers, *J Pediatr Psychol* 14:531-547, 1989.
59. Gortmaker SL, Sappenfield W: Chronic childhood disorders: prevalence and impact, *Pediatr Clin North Am* 31:3-18, 1984.
60. Newacheck PW, Budetti PP, Halfon N: Trends in activity-limiting chronic conditions among children, *Am J Public Health* 76:178-184, 1986.
61. Newacheck PW, Taylor WR: Childhood chronic illness: prevalence, severity, and impact, *Am J Public Health* 82:364-371, 1992.
62. Taylor WR, Newacheck PW: Impact of childhood asthma on health, *Pediatrics* 90:657-662, 1992.
63. Hendeles L, Weinberger M: Drugs in perspective, *Pharmacotherapy* 3:2-44, 1983.
64. Furukawa CT, DuHamel TR, Weimer L, et al: Cognitive and behavioral findings in children taking

theophylline, *J Allergy Clin Immunol* 81:83-88, 1988.

65. Kasenberg DF, Bloom L: Potential neuropsychological side effects of theophylline in asthmatic children, *Pediatr Asthma Allergy Immunol* 1:165-173, 1987.

66. Rachelefsky GS, Wo J, Adelson J, Mickey MR, et al: Behavior abnormalities and poor school performance due to oral theophylline use, *Pediatrics* 78:1133-1138, 1986.

67. McLoughlin J, Nall M, Isaacs B, et al: The relationship of allergies and allergy treatment to school performance and student behavior, *Ann Allergy* 51:506-510, 1983.

68. Furukawa CT, Shapiro GG, DuHamel T, et al: Learning and behavioral problems associated with theophylline therapy [Letter], *Lancet* 1:621, 1984.

69. Springer C, Goldenberg B, Ben Dov I, Godfrey S: Clinical, physiologic, and psychologic comparison of treatment by cromolyn or theophylline in childhood asthma, *J Allergy Clin Immunol* 76:64-69, 1985.

70. Creer TL, Gustafson KE: Psychological problems associated with drug therapy in childhood asthma, *J Pediatr* 115:850-855, 1989.

71. Weinberger M, Lindgren S, Bender B, Lerner JA, Szefler S: Effects of theophylline on learning and behavior: reason for concern or concern without reason? *J Pediatr* 111:471-474, 1987.

72. Schlieper A, Alcock D, Beaudry P, Feldman W, Leikin L: Effect of therapeutic plasma concentrations of theophylline on behavior, cognitive processing, and affect in children with asthma, *J Pediatr* 118:449-455, 1991.

73. Feldman BR, Carroll D: *The complete book of children's allergies,* New York, 1986, Times Books.

74. Tannock R, Schachar RJ, Carr RP, Logan GD: Dose-response effects of methylphenidate on academic performance and overt behavior in hyperactive children, *Pediatrics* 84:648-657, 1989.

75. Shaywitz SE, Shaywitz BA: Attention deficit disorder: current perspectives. In Kavanagh JF, Truss TJ Jr, editors: *Learning disabilities: proceedings of the national conference,* Parkton, Md, 1988, York Press.

76. Swanson JM, Cantwell D, Lerner M, McBurnett K, Hanna G: Effects of stimulant medication on learning in children with ADHD, *J Learn Disabil* 24:219-230, 255, 1991.

77. Levine MD, Brooks R, Shonkoff JP: Medical therapies and interventions. Chapter 8 in *A pediatric approach to learning disorders,* New York, 1980, John Wiley & Sons.

78. Fraunfelder FT: *Drug-induced ocular side effects and drug interactions,* ed 3, Philadelphia, 1989, Lea & Febiger.

79. Lesher GA: *A quick reference to the top prescription drugs,* ed 2, Chicago, 1992, Illinois College of Optometry.

80. Hoffman MS: Early indications of learning problems, *Acad Ther* 7:23-35, 1971.

81. Lyle JG: Certain antenatal, perinatal, and developmental variables and reading retardation in middle-class boys, *Child Dev* 41:481-491, 1970.

82. Silva PA, McGee R, Williams S: The predictive significance of slow walking and slow talking: a report from the Dunedin multidisciplinary child development study, *Br J Disord Commun* 17:133-139, 1982.

83. Shapiro BK, Palmer FB, Antell S, et al: Precursors of reading delay: neurodevelopmental milestones, *Pediatrics* 85:416-420, 1990.

84. Brown FR: Neurodevelopmental evaluation (the physician's diagnostic role in learning disabilities). In Brown FR, Aylward EH, editors: *Diagnosis and management of learning disabilities: an interdisciplinary approach,* Boston, 1987, Little, Brown.

85. Levine MD, Brooks R, Shonkoff JP: The assessment process: systematic formulation. Chapter 5 in *A pediatric approach to learning disorders,* New York, 1980, John Wiley & Sons.

86. Aram DM, Ekelman BL, Nation JE: Preschoolers with language disorders: 10 years later, *J Speech Hearing Disord* 27:232-244, 1984.

87. Shapiro BK, Palmer FB, Wachtel RC, Capute AJ: Issues in the early identification of specific learning disability, *J Dev Behav Pediatr* 5:15-20, 1983.

88. McDonald MA, Sigman M, Ungerer JA: Intelligence and behavior problems in 5-year-olds in relation to representational abilities in the second year of life, *J Dev Behav Pediatr* 10:86-91, 1989.

89. Wolfson RJ, Aghamohamadi AM, Berman SE: Disorders of hearing. In Gabel S, Erickson MT, editors: *Child development and developmental disabilities*, Boston, 1980, Little, Brown.

90. Bishop DVM, Edmundson A: Language-impaired 4-year-olds: distinguishing transient from persistent impairment, *J Speech Hear Disord* 52:156-173, 1987.

91. Armstrong BL, Lewis JA, Cusick BD: Speech-language, occupational therapy, and physical therapy evaluation. In Brown FR, Aylward EH: *Diagnosis and management of learning disabilities: an interdisciplinary approach*, Boston, 1987, Little, Brown.

92. Ferholt JDL: *Clinical assessment of children: a comprehensive approach to primary pediatric care*, Philadelphia, 1980, JB Lippincott, pp 60-61.

93. Behrman RE, editor: The nervous system. Chapter 20 in *Nelson textbook of pediatrics*, ed 14, Philadelphia, 1992, WB Saunders.

94. Evans BJW, Drasdo N: Tinted lenses and related therapies for learning disabilities—a review, *Ophthalmic Physiol Opt* 11:206-217, 1991.

95. Solan HA, Richman J: Irlen lenses: a critical appraisal, *J Am Optom Assoc* 61:789-796, 1990.

96. Delacato C: *The treatment and prevention of reading problems (the neurological approach)*, Springfield, Ill, 1959, Charles C Thomas.

97. Pihl RO, Drake H, Vrana F: Hair analysis in learning and behavior problems. In Brown AC, Crounse RG, editors: *Hair, trace elements, and human illness*, New York, 1980, Praeger.

98. Cott A: *Dr. Cott's help for your learning disabled child, the orthomolecular treatment*, New York, 1985, Times Books.

99. Oliver JM, Cole NH, Hollingsworth H: Learning disabilities as functions of familial learning problems and developmental problems, *Except Child* 57:427-440, 1991.

100. Moser HW: Genetic aspects of learning disabilities. In Lewis M, editor: *Learning disabilities and prenatal risk*, Urbana, Ill, 1986, University of Illinois Press.

101. Pennington BF, Gilger JW, Pauls D, et al: Evidence for major gene transmission of developmental dyslexia, *JAMA* 266:1527-1534, 1991.

102. Omenn GS, Weber BA: Dyslexia: search for phenotypic and genetic heterogeneity, *Am J Med Genet* 1:333-342, 1978.

103. Finucci JM, Childs B: Dyslexia: family studies. In Ludlow C, Cooper G, editors: *Genetic aspects of speech and language disorders*, New York, 1983, Academic Press.

104. Griffin JR: Genetics of dyseidetic dyslexia, *Optom Vis Sci* 69:148-151, 1992.

CHAPTER 10

Optometric Assessment of Visual Efficiency Problems

MICHAEL W. ROUSE

KEY TERMS

visual acuity
refractive anomalies
ocular health
color vision
visual efficiency
oculomotor
saccades

accommodation
vergence
sensory fusion
amplitude
facility
accuracy
screening methods

The model of vision outlined in Chapter 8 separated the visual system into three board components: (1) visual acuity, which is largely dependent on eye health, refractive status, and the normal development of the visual system; (2) visual efficiency, which is composed of oculomotor, accommodative, vergence, and sensory fusion abilities; and (3) visual information processing. In this chapter I concentrate on developing a method for evaluating the first two components, whereas Chapter 11 provides a method for evaluating the patient's visual information processing ability.

The evaluation of the patient's visual efficiency represents an attempt to determine how clearly, efficiently, and comfortably a person's vision will be as he or she performs his or her daily tasks at school, work, or play. Ritty et al.[1] have recently identified that visual acuity, contrast-resolving abilities, accommodation and convergence abilities, and oculomotor abilites make up the primary, immediate physiological demands placed on the visual system by classroom ergonomics. Seventy-five percent of the academically related task time in the classroom is spent on reading and writing at the near distance and on tasks that require alternate near-distance and near viewing. An inadequate visual efficiency system may lead to specific signs and symptoms of visual fatigue. As the visual system becomes fatigued, the psychological system also becomes fatigued, affecting motivation and attention. Frequently patients may compensate for deficiencies by avoiding tasks that require efficient use of the two eyes. Therefore, in addition to the collection of data, behavioral signs and symptoms are critical components in the comprehensive evaluation of visual efficiency. Observations by the teacher or parent, such as seeing the student using his finger as a pointer, or rubbing his eyes after short periods of reading, may signal a potential vision problem though the patient may not report any specific subjective symptoms. The correlation of entering signs and symptoms with the diagnostic data is the doctor's primary problem-solving task.

Chapter 9 outlines the method for taking the case history on patients presenting with potential visually related learning disorders. Based on the information gained in the initial interview the doctor will have developed a list of hypotheses regarding the possible vision problems that may account fully or partially for the entering chief complaint and accompanying signs and symptoms. In this chapter I will concentrate on the diagnostic strategy for evaluating those hypotheses related to vision problems in the general area of visual efficiency skills. Secondly, I will emphasize the importance of conducting a comprehensive investigation that probes the integrity of specific visual functions within each of the systems outlined in the box, regardless of the patient's entering complaint.

I will focus on the diagnostic strategy, the methods that can be used to assess the visual functions in each area, normative data or criteria for determining if the results are normal or abnormal, the associated signs and symptoms, and finally the clinical characteristics of common diagnostic syndromes.

VISUAL ACUITY ASSESSMENT

Since we are concentrating on the school-aged child, the clinician can take a standard approach to assessing visual acuity. This will probably involve

---

Diagnostic Strategy

Visual acuities
- Refractive status
- Ocular health

Visual efficiency skills
- Oculomotor
- Accommodation
- Vergence
- Sensory fusion

Snellen visual acuities at distance and a reduced Snellen or point type for near visual acuity. For kindergartners and preschool children the doctor may have to vary the testing methods by using Tumbling E's, Broken Wheel Cards, HOTV chart or cards, or Lighthouse Cards in some cases. The reader is referred to Fern and Manny[2] and Rouse and Ryan[3] for a more detailed review of various visual acuity methods. The doctor will have to be careful in cases where reversals are reported in the case history. The child may miscall letters when conducting Snellen VA or have difficulty with the directionality concepts necessary in using Tumbling E targets. In addition, some patients with saccadic eye movement deficiencies may make omission and transposition errors during visual acuity testing.

REFRACTIVE ASSESSMENT

As pointed out in Chapter 6 there is an inverse relationship between the presence of myopia and school performance or more specifically reading. Generally, myopic patients are the good readers, whereas patients with hyperopia are more often found to be below average readers. In addition, hyperopes are much more likely to lag in the development of visual perceptual skills.[4,5] School screenings do a reasonably good job of identifying myopic children, whereas hyperopic children, except for cases of very high hyperopia (>4.00 D), will typically pass school vision screenings. As a result a large number of hyperopic children will go undetected until significant symptoms or poor school performance prompts a referral to a vision care practitioner.

When the clinician is evaluating a child or adult with a history of poor school performance, the doctor needs to be especially careful to rule out hyperopia, astigmatism, and anisometropia as contributing factors. These refractive conditions, especially hyperopia, can cause many signs and symptoms. Notice that the signs and symptoms listed in Table 10.1 are similar to those listed later for accommodative and vergence problems. The reason is that the signs and symptoms are not necessarily attributable solely to the refractive condition, but more often the result of the effect of refractive conditions on the accommodative-convergence interaction.

The doctor will want to conduct standard clinical testing including keratometry, retinoscopy, and subjective refraction. For details on conducting the refractive assessment of children see Rouse and Ryan.[3] Cycloplegic refraction is recommended in cases of suspected latent hyperopia or anisometropia. Additional hyperopia is often not suspected until additional conditions are found on subsequent testing of accommodation (such as high negative relative accommodation) and vergence (such as convergence excess). The suggested protocol for routine office cycloplegia is 1% cyclopentolate, 1 drop per eye or one spray application per eye,[6] refracting the patient in approximately 30 to 40 minutes. The amount of hyperopia uncovered by cycloplegia is not necessarily the amount you will prescribe but will serve as an important base-line value for making refrac-

TABLE 10.1   Signs and symptoms of refractive conditions

Condition	Sign or symptom
Hyperopia	• Complains of blurry vision at near (rarely at far) • Reports frontal headaches after near work • Avoids near tasks • Has red eyes • Rubs eyes during or after short periods of visual activity • Fatigues easily, reports ocular discomfort • Has poor comprehension • Inability to sustain reading • Concentration problems—daydreams
Myopia	• Has trouble seeing chalkboard • Squints • Holds book too close • Moves closer to see distant objects
Astigmatism	• Has difficulty seeing clearly at far and near • Has red eyes • Reports spatial distortions in size, shape, or inclination of objects • Frowns or squints • Blinks excessively at desk tasks • Reports nausea or motion sickness
Anisometropia	• Typically no symptoms if large anisometropia • For small imbalances, symptoms are similar to vergence symptoms

tive correction decisions once the visual efficient evaluation is complete. The dilated view of the fundus will also be important for assuring that ocular health is normal.

Any myopia over −0.50 should be considered significant and the need for correction should be reviewed based on the entering complaints and the needs of the patient. Often myopia is not corrected in early elementary school children until the magnitude is 1.00 D or greater because any detrimental effects can be compensated for by preferred placement in the classroom, such as sitting closer to the chalkboard. Any astigmatism greater than 1.00 D should be considered significant. Any anisometropia over 0.75 D should be considered significant because of the potential amblyogenic effect and the possibility of disrupting normal accommodative and binocular function. For hyperopia, any amount of hyperopia may be significant, depending on the status of the accommodative and vergence systems. Low hyperopia (+0.25 to +1.00 D) should not cause symptoms unless a primary binocular or accommodative dysfunction is present. In this case, even a low amount of hyperopia may exacerbate these conditions. Moderate hyperopia (+1.25 to +2.00 D) may or may not cause symptoms, but if the patient has borderline accommodative and vergence systems, this amount of hyperopia frequently exacerbates these conditions, causing symptoms. High hyperopia (+2.00 or greater D) in most cases causes significant accommodative-vergence problems, producing significant signs and symptoms, or leading to avoidance of near visual tasks.

OCULAR HEALTH ASSESSMENT

Although it is rare that an ocular pathological condition is a contributing factor to learning difficulties, the doctor evaluating patients presenting with learning problems should maintain the same diligence in regard to assessing ocular health as he or she would with any other primary care patient. The doctor should conduct a thorough ocular health assessment, including an evaluation of the anterior segment, pupillary function, clarity of the media, and posterior segment. Standard clinical testing of the anterior segment using biomicroscopy must be completed to rule out common childhood conditions, such as blepharitis, that may be responsible or contribute to entering signs or symptoms, such as red and irritated eyes. Pupillary function testing should be conducted as part of the standard neurological investigation of the patency of the visual system. The doctor will also want to carefully evaluate the media and fundus for any conditions that may need treatment or referral. Scheiman et al.[7] found that approximately 2% of 2025 consecutive cases (6 months to 18 years of age) required referral or follow-up care for posterior segment disorders. Tonometry should be attempt on all children over 5 years of age as well as a minimum-confrontation visual-fields screening.

One area that is often overlooked is the evaluation of the color vision system. One of the main reasons for testing color vision is to identify congenital problems at an early age. A color deficiency can cause problems in school, especially where extensive color coding is used in the classroom.[8] Color vision anomalies normally affect 6% to 8% of boys and only about 0.5% of girls. Evidence now exists to indicate that color deficient children's self-concepts are often affected. Several studies have reported that children suffered from problems such as anxiety, shame, embarrassment, confusion, frustration, and ridicule by peers.[9-12] Espinda[12] found that teachers reporting on children with difficulty acquiring color-discrimination skills often believed that these problems were suggestive of intellectual inadequacy. Espinda[12] also found a higher incidence of color vision failure among educationally handicapped boys (13%) than a normal control group (5%). Litton found similar results.[13] The conclusions from these studies indicate that color vision deficiencies should be considered as a possible factor contributing to learning disability. Identifying the type of color deficiency and its severity, and then communicating that information to the parents, teacher, and other school officials can help avoid mislabeling the child as learning disabled or wrongly accusing the child of laziness or carelessness. The Ishihara Color Test is the most common test used to screen red-green color vision defects. The reader is referred to Haegerstrom-Portnoy[14] for a more detailed discussion on screening and diagnostic testing methods.

VISUAL EFFICIENCY EVALUATION

There has been an enormous amount of research that has looked at the relationship of visual efficiency parameters and school performance. Dr. Garzia in Chapter 6 as well as many other authors have reviewed this body of literature and found a significant correlation between deficient binocular function and reading performance. Probably more important is the well-established relationship between both accommodative and vergence conditions and associated signs and symptoms. These signs and symptoms may not delay the learning-to-read process but may contribute to making the process of reading significantly more difficult. The strategy we will take is to look comprehensively at the patient's oculomotor, accommodative, accommodative-vergence, and sensory fusion skills to evaluate whether there are conditions present that account entirely or in part for the specific signs and symptoms (including reports of task avoidance) identified in the case history.

One of the doctor's major responsibilities is to assess the clinical data and make a judgment about whether the findings or groups of findings are within normal limits. There have been several case analysis systems (such as graphical analysis, Optometric Extension Program (OEP) analysis, and fixation-disparity analysis) as well as clinical criteria proposed to help the doctor make these decisions. In addition, there has been an enormous amount of research directed toward developing normative data for each of the clinical measurements of visual efficiency. Since some clinical measurements are not considered in classical case analysis systems, such as accommodative facility, the clinician will out of necessity need to refer to normative data. Normative data analysis employs the mean and standard deviation of clinical measures on a large number of subjects to describe the distribution of a particular clinical finding in the general population. Some suggestions have been made regarding the extent one should use for the standard deviation from the mean to determine the "normal" range of findings. This value has ranged from 0.5 standard deviation, in an attempt to avoid false-negative results, to 2.0 standard deviation in an attempt to avoid false-positive results. There has been a general trend in the literature to report the mean ±1 standard deviation. The doctor needs to be cautious about how normative data are used in clinical decision making. The clinician should use normative information as a method to identify clinical data that are more extreme than those typically found in the general population but not necessary abnormal. When these "extreme" clinical data are correlated with poor performance or associated clinical signs and symptoms, the findings can be considered abnormal. For example, accommodative facility rates below 1 standard deviation have been found to be associated with symptoms of blurred vision and asthenopia at near range; therefore clinical findings in this range have a higher probability of being abnormal.

Oculomotor system

The classroom task demands outlined by Ritty et al.[1] require that the student's oculomotor system be functioning in a coordinated and efficient manner and perform rapid, accurate saccadic eye movements during reading and smooth, accurate pursuit and tracking eye movements as the teacher moves through a variety of teaching routines. Therefore the primary objective when one is evaluating the oculomotor system is to evaluate the quality of fixation maintenance and pursuit and saccadic eye movements. *Fixation maintenance* represents the ability to maintain steady, accurate fixation of the macula (1° in diameter) on a stationary target;[15] whereas *pursuit eye movements* represents the ability to maintain fixation on a moving target, requiring a smooth coordination of the neuromuscular control mechanism.[15] Finally, *saccadic eye movements* represents the ability to change fixation quickly and accurately from one target to the next, as in the act of reading.[15] The optometric evaluation determines the quality of these skills and the ability to sustain them over time. Symptoms associated with deficient quality of oculomotor control are listed in the box. These types of symptoms are very common among children who are having learning problems.

The methods used to evaluate these skills range from gross observation, to quantitative rating of observation,[16-18] to indirect measures of eye movements,[19-21] and finally to sophisticated infrared eye-monitoring systems that directly measure eye movements.[22,23] Unfortunately, reasonably priced infrared eye-monitoring systems are currently unavailable for clinical use. The Eye Trac, which had been the clinical standard for evaluating eye-movement skills, is no longer available. If the doctor has an Eye Trac or is able to acquire one, he or she should consult Griffin[24] for the clinical protocol for evaluating eye-movement skills. The Ober 2: Visagraph system* has recently become available as a method for direct eye-movement recording.

*Dr. Paul Harris, 16 Greenmeadow Drive, #103, Timonium, MD 21093.

Symptoms Associated with Oculomotor System Deficiencies

Moves head excessively when reading
Frequently loses place when reading or copying
Omits words when reading or copying
Skips lines when reading
Uses finger or marker to maintain place
Lacks comprehension when reading
Rereads lines unknowingly

The practitioner will in the majority of cases have to rely on a combination of clinical observation and simple indirect measures of eye movement. Clinical observation can be improved by use of a rating system. The Southern California College of Optometry (SCCO) rating system is a quick and convenient testing and rating method for fixation maintenance, pursuits, and saccades.[17] There are other more-detailed rating systems that the doctor may want to consider.[16,18]

The SCCO rating system is outlined in the box, and the testing is conducted as follows. To evaluate fixation maintenance the practitioner should have the patient observe a small accommodative target (20/60 to 20/80) in primary gaze for approximately 10 seconds. I suggest two 10-second observation periods be used before rating the patient's performance. For pursuit testing a single target should be used and moved in a smooth manner (rate about 2 sec/20 cm) horizontally, diagonally, and then vertically. The patient is instructed to track the target as accurately as possible. Any head movements that are not controlled after instructions should be considered inadequate performance. For evaluation of saccadic eye movements, two targets are held about 40 cm in front of the patient, separated by not more than 15 cm. The patient is required to fixate one and then the other target upon command. The doctor should evaluate not only the accuracy, but also the latency involved in initiating each saccadic eye movement. Between 5 and 10 practice cycles should be conducted before rating the patient's performance. Any head movements that are not controlled after instructions should be considered inadequate performance.

Southern California College of Optometry (SCCO) 4+ System for Evaluating Oculomotor

Fixation maintenance—test binocularly; if deficient, test monocularly

4+   smooth and accurate
3+   one fixation loss
2+   two fixation losses
1+   more than two fixation losses

Pursuit ability—test binocularly; if deficient, test monocularly

4+   smooth and accurate
3+   one fixation loss
2+   two fixation losses
1+   more than two fixation losses or any uncontrolled head movement

Saccadic ability—test binocularly; if deficient, test monocularly

4+   smooth and accurate
3+   some slight undershooting
2+   gross undershooting or overshooting or increased latency*
1+   inability to do task or any uncontrolled head movement

---

*Normal latency of initiating a saccade is 120 to 180 msec.

Most practitioners will have to rely on a rating-assisted observation method. For a more quantitative method of evaluating saccadic eye movements that simulate reading, rapid number naming (or visual-verbal) tests have been developed. This type of test has a good correlation with results that are produced on an infrared eye-monitoring system.[25] The Pierce Saccadic Test was the original design, which was later modified by King and Devick to produce a test that evaluated smaller saccadic eye movements. The King-Devick Saccade Test was then extensively normalized in a study by the New York State Optometric Association (NYSOA) and is now available as the NYSOA K-D Saccadic Test.[26] This test is a three-part norm-referenced test in which a child is asked to vocalize as rapidly as possible a series of 40 numbers horizontally arranged on each test. The faster a patient completes the task, presumably the more efficient and accurate is the oculomotor performance. Unfortunately the introduction of a visual-verbal match can add a whole host of interfering factors that can affect the scoring of the test. Factors such as vigilance (sustained visual attention), number recognition and retrieval, and visual-verbal integration time are a few of the associated factors that influence these tests. A more significant factor resulting in poor performance is the patient's number-naming automaticity.[27] The child's poor performance on the K-D test may be caused by the child's slow number-naming automaticity rather than a true oculomotor dysfunction. In addition, both the Pierce and K-D saccade tests have been found to have poor test-retest reliability.[28,29]

To address the problems of automaticity and poor reliability and the continuing need for a practical, inexpensive, yet quantitative method of evaluating saccadic eye movements, the Development Eye Movement (DEM) was developed.[21] The DEM has two subtests (Figure 10.1). The first subtest consists of two cards Test A and Test B. Each card has 40 numbers arranged in a vertical column, which eliminates the requirement for horizontal eye movements. This subtest is dominated by automatic visual-verbal number-naming skills (automaticity). The second subtest introduces the demand for horizontal eye movements by presenting 80 numbers in a horizontal array of 16 rows of 5 numbers each. The doctor administers the first subtest and records the time for Test Cards A and B. The doctor administers the second subtest and records the number of errors (omissions, additions, transpositions, substitutions) and the time in seconds. A correct total time is calculated by use of the number of errors. The doctor then divides the horizontal time by the vertical time to arrive at a ratio score. The ratio score represents a method for directly comparing the vertical (automaticity) and horizontal (automaticity plus oculomotor control) test performance levels. This ratio procedure allows for parceling out the effect of automaticity on the oculomotor performance. The doctor then refers to age or grade level normative tables for the child's percentile rank performance for the three results. Although the authors do not give any specific recommendations for using the child's percentile rank, we use above the 50th percentile as normal, between the 50th and 16th percentile as suspect, and below the 16th percentile as significant. More important than the individual percentile rankings is the four patterns of test results that are typically found (see the box). Although there are some concerns about the reliability of the DEM,[30] at the present time it is the best indirect method of evaluating saccadic eye movements.

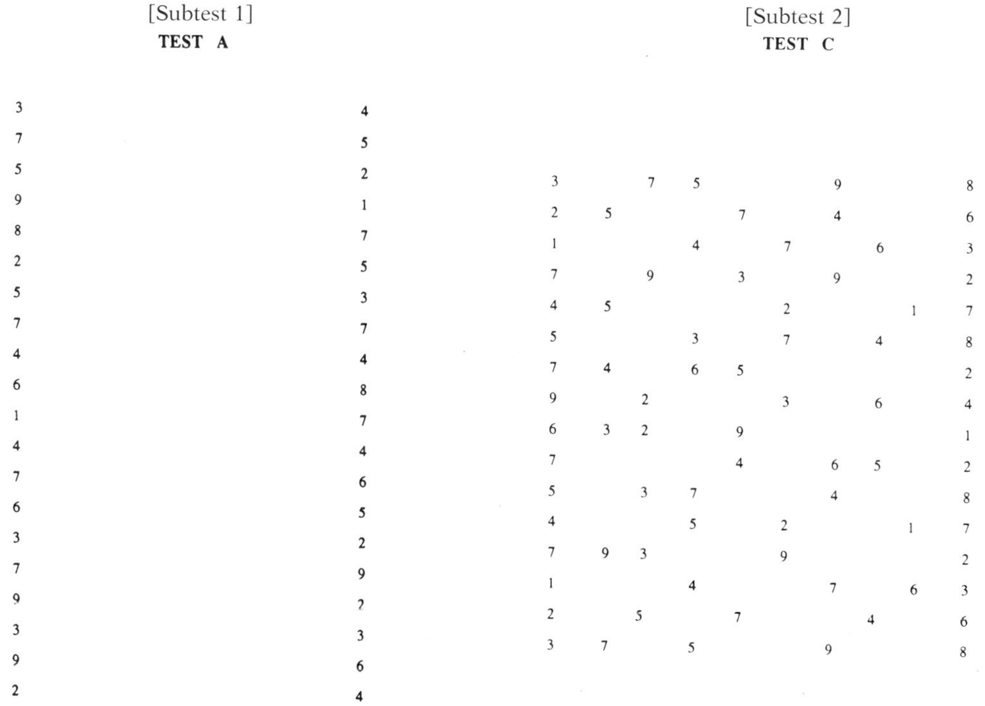

[Subtest 1]
TEST A

[Subtest 2]
TEST C

Test A (two columns):

3	4
7	5
5	2
9	1
8	7
2	5
5	3
7	7
4	4
6	8
1	7
4	4
7	6
6	5
3	2
7	9
9	7
3	3
9	6
2	4

Test C (horizontal array):

```
3       7 5       9       8
2 5         7   4       6
1       4   7     6     3
7       9 3     9       2
4 5       3   7   4     8
5       3 7     4       8
7 4     6 5         2
9   2       3 6       4
6 3 2     9             1
7       4     6 5       2
5       3 7     4       8
4         5   2     1 7
7 9 3       9           2
1       4     7   6     3
2       5   7       4   6
3 7       5       9       8
```

FIGURE 10.1 The Developmental Eye Movement (DEM) test is composed of two subtests. Subtest 1 is composed of test cards A (shown) and B (not shown). Subtest 2 is a single test card with 80 numbers in a horizontal array of 16 rows of 5 numbers each.

Four Clinical Patterns seen on the Developmental Eye Movement Test

Type I is characterized by normal performance on all subtests.

Type II is characterized by an abnormally increased horizontal time in the presence of relatively normal performance on the vertical subtest. The ratio is higher than expected. This pattern is characteristic of an oculomotor dysfunction.

Type III is characterized by abnormally increased horizontal and vertical times but a normal ratio score. This pattern is characteristic of a patient with a basic difficulty in number-naming automaticity.

Type IV is a combination of types II and III, where both subtest times are abnormally increased and the ratio score is also abnormal. This pattern is characteristic of both automaticity and oculomotor deficiencies.

Accommodative system

The ergonomic task demands of the classroom require a broad range of accommodative amplitude, flexibility, accuracy, and normal accommodative-vergence function. In particular, the average eye-to-desk distance of 30 cm (3.00 D accommodative demand) and the observation that students must be able to sustain this ergonomic demand for as long as 30 to 40 minutes at a time put school children at a very real risk for visual fatigue or avoidance behaviors.[1]

A thorough examination of accommodative function involves the monocular evaluation of amplitude and facility, and the binocular evaluation of amplitude, facility, accuracy (lag), and relative accommodation. The monocular test probes pure accommodative efficiency, whereas the binocular tests probe the adaptability and mutual interaction with the vergence system. Two additional characteristics are indirectly assessed during the accommodative evaluation, sustaining ability (capacity to maintain an appropriate response over an extended period of time), and consistency (ability to respond in a predictable fashion over a variety of stimulus conditions and demand levels). The importance of a comprehensive evaluation, rather than characterizing accommodative function based on a single measurement, has been emphasized repeated.[17,31,32] Symptoms commonly associated with an accommodative dysfunction are listed in the box.

Accommodative response characteristics have been reported by a number of investigators[33-35] to approximate adult abilities by 3 to 4 months of age. But the routine clinical assessment of accommodative function is usually not attempted before 4 to 5 years of age and the majority of children cannot be reliably tested by traditional subjective clinical methods until 6 to 7 years of age.

By 4 to 5 years, the subjective testing of *accommodative amplitude* on a large percentage of children can be accomplished by either Donder's Push-up Method[36] or the Minus Lens Method.[37] Donder's method involves moving a finely detailed target toward the spectacle plane until the target first becomes blurred. A slight modification, which we have found helpful

---

Symptoms Associated with Accommodative System Deficiencies

Reports blurry vision at near
Reports blurry vision at distance after near work
Reports eye fatigue after short periods of reading or writing
Holds book too closely (inside Harmon's distance) (see p. 284 for discussion)
Has difficulty sustaining near tasks
Rubs eyes excessively
Has red eyes
Avoids near visual tasks

when testing young children, involves first pushing the target up to the point of first blur. Then the target is pushed up to a point of "blur-out"; the target is changed and slowly receded until the child can first identify the new target. This point is recorded as the accommodative amplitude. Duane[38] established normative data for children 10 years of age and older, and Wold[39] later presented data for 6- to 10-year-olds. Based on Duane's data, Hofstetter[40] developed formulas predicting the range of accommodative amplitude expected at different ages. The minimum formula [D = 15 − 0.25(age)] has been used extensively as a clinical guideline. For example, the minimum amplitude expected for a 10-year-old would be about 12.5 D. Accommodative amplitudes falling below this guideline have been associated with symptoms.[41] The binocular accommodative amplitude is about 1 to 2 D greater than the monocular amplitude because of the added accommodation produced from the convergence-accommodation–to–convergence (CA/C) ratio. Sheard[37] pointed out a number of problems with Donder's Push-up Method, such as an increase in the visual angle of the approaching target, and suggested that the Minus Lens Method would provide a more accurate measure. Wold[39] and later Woodruff[42] have provided normative data for children 3 to 11 years of age. Abnormal findings would be less than 8 D for 3- to 9-year-olds and less than 9 D for 10- to 11-year-olds. The Minus Lens Method values are consistently lower than the Push-up Method, stressing the point of referring to appropriate normative data.

The reliable evaluation of *accommodative facility* starts at approximately 7 years of age. The standard clinical technique and initial normative data were established by Zellers et al.[43] A ±2.00 D accommodative demand is typically used with a 20/30 test target at 40 cm. Zellers et al. used the Van Orden attachment for the Keystone Correct-Eyescope to control the stability of the flipper mechanism and test distance, but a hand-held flipper is considered adequate (Figure 10.2). A Modified Bernell Acuity Suppression Slide (VO/9) has been used as the target because it can be used to monitor suppression under binocular conditions and can be back illuminated to improve contrast. The patient is asked to view the reduced Snellen letters 6/9 (20/30) on line 5 and say "now" when the letters on that line are clear and single and to report any letters missing from lines 4 and 6 during the binocular testing. Zellers et al.[43] established normative data for the age group 20 to 30 of about 11 cycles per minute (cpm) (±5) monocularly and about 8 cpm (±5) binocularly. While investigating the relationship between symptoms and accommodative facility rates, Hennessey et al.[44] found very similar monocular and binocular rates on a group of subjects (*n* = 60) between 8 and 14 years of age. Scheiman et al.[45] used a slightly different testing method and instructional set (the patient had to read three numbers accurately) on a large group of elementary school-aged children between 6 and 12 years of age. They reported much lower rates (Table 10.2). Similar to the problems experienced in oculomotor testing,

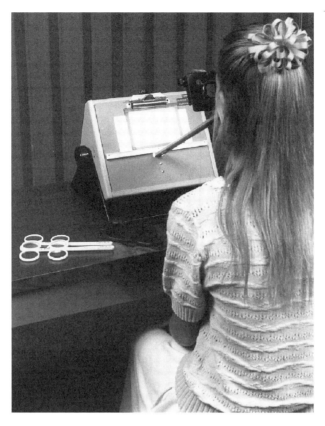

FIGURE 10.2 Example of a method for accommodative facility testing using Keystone Correct-Eyescope with Bernell Acuity Suppression Slide (VO/9) as the target. Simple hand-held flippers (on the left) can be used as an alternative method.

TABLE 10.2 Normative clinical data for accommodative facility

	Ages (years)	Monocular facility (cycles per minute)	Binocular facility (cycles per minute)
Zellers et al.*	18-30	11.6 (±5.0)	7.7 (±5.0)
Hennessey et al.†	8-14	11.8 (±6.0)	7.8 (±8.0)
Scheiman et al.‡	6	5.5 (±2.5)	3.0 (±2.5)
	7	6.5 (±2.0)	3.0 (±2.5)
	8-12	7.0 (±2.5)	5.0 (±2.5)

*Zellers JA et al: *J Am Optom Assoc* 55:31-37, 1984.
†Hennessey D et al: *Am J Optom Physiol Opt* 61:177-183, 1984.
‡Scheiman M et al: *Am J Optom Physiol Opt* 65:127-134, 1988.

the patient's number-naming automaticity may have had a significant effect on Scheiman et al.'s results. The Zeller et al. method values are consistently higher than the Scheiman et al. method, stressing the point of following a particular method and referring to appropriate normative data. We are inclined to use Zeller et al.'s normative data for all ages up to 35.

Normative information is of more value when links to signs and symptoms can be established. A strong link has been found between Zeller's normative values and the prevalence of symptoms,[44,46] especially where the patient's rate falls 1 standard deviation below the mean. Reliability studies indicate that the doctor may be confident of accommodative facility findings when the patient's rate is greater than the mean or when it is 1 standard deviation below the mean. However, patients with rates in the suspect range (between the mean and 1 standard deviation) often show improvement because of a practice effect and subsequently pass on the next retest. A mistaken diagnosis of accommodative disorder may therefore be made if only a single test is made, particularly if the patient score is within the suspect range. One can avoid misdiagnosis by repeating the test or extending it for an additional minute or two for suspect patients. Patients with rates above the mean are considered normal; those remaining 1 standard deviation below the mean are considered truly to have accommodative infacility.[47-49] We would also like to caution practitioners regarding the use of computerized methods for assessing accommodative facility. A recent comparison of the standard clinical method described previously and the Computer Orthoptics Diagnostic Program indicated that the computer method may not be a valid method for diagnosing accommodative facility deficiencies.[50]

For children of all ages, but especially younger children, dynamic retinoscopy provides one of the few practical objective methods to assess accommodative function. The monocular estimate method (MEM) has been shown to be a valid and reliable[51] measure of *accommodative accuracy* (lag or response). MEM controls the sources of retinoscopy error (such as scoping off axis) better than other methods of dynamic retinoscopy.[52] MEM retinoscopy is performed under normal reading conditions, including habitual refractive correction and working distance, target demand, illumination, and patient's posture (Figure 10.3). One performs the technique by having the patient read words or call out pictures that are arranged around a central hole in a card that is attached to the examiner's retinoscope. An estimate of the magnitude of the motion is made, and lenses are then interposed monocularly until the lag of accommodation is neutralized. The lenses are interposed only briefly, so that there is only minimal interference with the habitual accommodative response. The normal range of accommodative lag expected for 5- to 12-year-olds is plano to +0.75 D.[32,53] If the lag value is greater than +0.75 D, efforts should be made to rule out (latent) hyperopia, any ocular or systemic pathological condition, accommodative-convergence imbalances, subnormal accommodation, or medication-induced effects. If the lag values are minus, spasm of accommodation or accommodative-convergence imbalances should be ruled out as the cause. MEM retinoscopy results often provide useful objective information that influences prescribing decisions.[54,55]

The subjective evaluation of accommodative lag, using the cross-

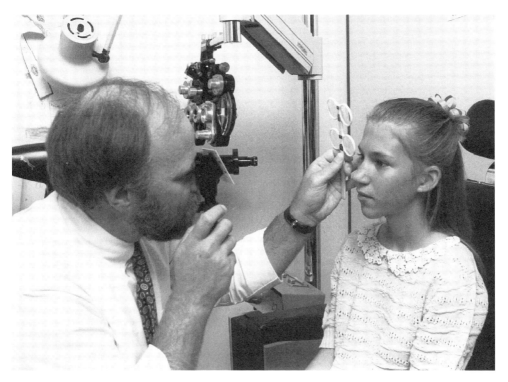

FIGURE 10.3 Monocular Estimated Method (MEM) retinoscopy is performed under normal reading conditions, including habitual refractive correction and working distance, target demand, illumination, and patient's posture.

cylinder method, is difficult before 6 to 7 years of age. In addition, there is some concern about the procedure's validity on prepresbyopes.[56] I prefer to use dynamic retinoscopy (MEM), regardless of the child's age, to evaluate accommodative lag.

The testing of *relative accommodation* involves increasing or decreasing the binocular accommodative stimulus while the vergence stimulus remains constant. This is exactly opposite to what occurs in the measurement of relative vergence. When performing tests of relative accommodation, the patient views a 20/20 to 20/30 target. The clinician introduces either minus (to stimulate positive relative accommodation, PRA) or plus (to stimulate negative relative accommodation, NRA) spherical lenses in 0.25 D steps binocularly until the patient notices first sustained blur. The clinician should not only evaluate the quantity of the response, but also the quality of the response; that is, How much effort was the response; Was the patient easily able to clear up to 2.00 D or did the patient labor over each 0.25 D change in stimulus? The patient will maintain clarity as long as there is sufficient relative vergence present. For example, as minus is added, there is an increase in convergence associated with the accommodative-convergence–to–accommodation (AC/A) ratio. There is an immediate compensatory stimulus to regain a fused and a stable binocular percept. As the patient reaches the limits of their negative relative vergence (NRV), he or she will cease to accommodate to the increased minus and the target will appear to blur. The reverse happens when the NRA is conducted, the target remains clear until the patient exhausts his or her positive relative vergence (PRV). Morgan reported a mean PRA of -2.37 (± 1.12) D and an NRA of $+2.00$ (± 0.50) D.[57,58] These normative findings have been relatively consistent across many studies of both adults and children (see Jackson and Goss[59] for a review).

A summary of normative data and clinical guidelines for accommodation are summarized in Table 10.3. Sustaining ability and consistency are indirectly assessed during the previous evaluation. One can assess the sustaining ability by noting the quality of the patient's performance on accommodative amplitude, facility, and PRA measurements. One evaluates consistency by looking at the intertest consistency and specifically intertest consistency with vergence measurements. For example, a low binocular accommodative facility rate with problems primarily on the minus lens side should correlate with a low first sustained blur on the NRV measurement and possibly a low PRA.

Vergence system

The ergonomic task demands of the classroom require a significant amount of time to be spent on reading and writing at the near distance, requiring a broad range of vergence skills, amplitude, flexibility, accuracy, and normal accommodative-vergence function as well. As mentioned previously, the average eye-to-desk distance of 30 cm and the observation that students must be able to sustain this ergonomic demand for as long as 30 to 40 minutes at a time[1] puts school children at a very real risk for visual fatigue or avoidance behaviors, especially if the vergence system is inefficient.

When evaluating the vergence system, the doctor can take an approach similar to that used in evaluating the accommodative system by measuring amplitude, facility, accuracy, and relative vergence (adaptability). Similarly sustaining ability and consistency can be indirectly assessed during

TABLE 10.3   Summary of normative clinical data or guidelines for assessing accommodative system measurements

Amplitude	15-0.25 (age)
Lag	0.33 (± 0.35) D
Facility	
Monocular	11.0 (± 5) cpm
Binocular	8.0 (± 5) cpm
Relative	
PRA	-2.37 (± 1.25)
NRA	$+2.00$ (± 0.50)

cpm, Cycles per minute; *NRA,* negative relative accommodation; *PRA,* positive relative accommodation.

the evaluation. The symptoms that are commonly associated with vergence anomalies are listed in the box.

The maximum amplitude of the vergence system can be assessed by measurment of the *near point of convergence* (NPC). The clinician should select a detailed target (20/20 to 20/30). The NPC is started at a point where the patient has single vision (typically 40 cm), and then the target is slowly advanced toward the patient until the patient reports double vision or the doctor detects that the patient has lost bifixation. Keep in mind that since convergence, like accommodation, is spatially nonlinear the clinician must move the target inward progressively more slowly to maintain a constant rate of stimulation.[60] Next the clinician should slowly move the target away from the patient until the objective and subjective recovery of bifixation are measured. Gallaway et al.[61] found the mean break on the NPC to be 2.5 (±2.5) cm from the bridge of the nose and the mean recovery to be 4.5 (±3.0) cm. To evaluate the patient's ability to sustain the initial NPC, the clinician can repeat the NPC measurement, such as 5 times. The patient's ability should remain reasonably consistent. The doctor may find that the NPC improves with repeated measurement, an indication that there is probably no gross convergence problem if normal measurements are finally found. On the other hand, the patient may show a gradual reduction in the NPC with repeated measurement, an indication that there are problems sustaining gross convergence.

The clinician will want to carefully rule out the presence of strabismus at far and near with the unilateral cover test (UCT). If strabismus is suspected, there are several additional tests that can be used to confirm the diagnosis. If strabismus is found, the doctor will want to identify carefully the characteristics of the deviation, including the direction, frequency, magnitude, laterality (eye preference), variability, and cosmesis. The reader should refer to Caloroso and Rouse[62] or Von Noorden[63] for a more in-depth review.

For the remainder of this discussion I will assume that the patient is heterophoric or if strabismic that the frequency of the deviation is relatively low. After the UCT, the alternate cover test (ACT) with prism neutralization (loose prism or prism bar) provides an objective quantitative method for determining the magnitude of any detected deviation. The cli-

---

Symptoms Associated with Vergence System Deficiencies

Reports asthenopia with reading or writing
Reports frontal headaches associated with visual tasks
Intermittently reports double vision
Squints, closes, or covers one eye during visual tasks
Reports that letters, words, or both appear to float or move around on the page
Has abnormal posture when doing near visual tasks.

nician should assess the deviation not only at the standard test distance of 40 cm, but also at the patient's actual ideal working distance. One can estimate this distance by measuring the distance from the middle knuckle of the second finger to the center of the elbow, often referred to as the "Harmon distance."[64] For patients with either a high or low AC/A ratio the magnitude of the deviation can change dramatically from the standard 40 cm test distance to, for example, the typical 20 cm working distance of an 8-year-old. In most cases of school-aged children the clinician will also measure the heterophoria as part of routine phorometry. Normative data on heterophoria at far and near are listed in Table 10.4. The normative data on the near and far phoria have been relatively consistent across many studies evaluating both children and adults.[59]

The determination of the patient's AC/A ratio is important for understanding and classifying the vergence condition, as well as designing an effective treatment plan. The AC/A ratio can be measured by either the gradient or calculated methods. The gradient method is preferred over the calculated method, since proximal vergence may contaminate the latter. This accounts for the fact that the calculated AC/A ratio usually has a higher value than the gradient AC/A ratio. One conducts the gradient technique by taking the near phoria first with the distance prescription and then by repeating the phoria measurement through an additional -1.00 D lens. The use of minus lenses is preferred because accommodation is stimulated only within the linear region of the accommodative stimulus-

TABLE 10.4   Normative clinical data for phorometry vergence system measurements

6 METERS	
Phoria	1XP ($\pm 2\triangle$)
Positive vergence	
Blur	9 ($\pm 4\triangle$)
Break	19 ($\pm 8\triangle$)
Recovery	10 ($\pm 4\triangle$)
Negative vergence	
Break	7 ($\pm 3\triangle$)
Recovery	4 ($\pm 2\triangle$)
40 CENTIMETERS	
Phoria	3XP ($\pm 5\triangle$)
Positive vergence	
Blur	17 ($\pm 5\triangle$)
Break	21 ($\pm 6\triangle$)
Recovery	11 ($\pm 7\triangle$)
Negative vergence	
Blur	13 ($\pm 4\triangle$)
Break	24 ($\pm 4\triangle$)
Recovery	13 ($\pm 5\triangle$)

XP, Exophoria.

response function.[60] For example, if the near phoria with the distance prescription was 2EP and then 10EP with −1.00 D, the stimulus AC/A = 8/1. One determines the calculated AC/A by taking the phoria measurement at two different distances (6 m and 40 cm) through the distance prescription. The phoria measurements are used in the following formula to arrive at the stimulus AC/A:

$$AC/A = pd + m \text{ (Near phoria} - \text{Far phoria)}$$

where the *pd* is patient's distance interpupillary distance (cm), *m* is near fixation distance (m), and esophoria has a positive value and exophoria a negative value. For example, a patient with a pd of 50 mm, near testing done at 30 cm and a near phoria of 10 exophoria and a distance phoria of ortho would have a calculated AC/A = 5.0 +0.30(−12−[−2]) = 2/1. An AC/A ratio of 6/1 has been considered a "normal" AC/A. However, a small amount of physiological exophoria at near is normal, and so it is reasonable to consider a normal range of AC/A to be 4/1 to 6/1. An AC/A less than this range would be considered a low AC/A, whereas values greater than this range would be considered high AC/A.

More important than the actual measurement of the magnitude of the heterophoria is the patient's ability to compensate comfortably for this demand on the fusional vergence system. Traditionally the method chosen to resolve this problem is to compare the patient's heterophoria and the relative fusional vergence ranges. The testing is conducted by having the patient view a 20/20 to 20/30 sized letter or number target at 40 cm. The clinician slowly increases base-out prism power symmetrically between the two eyes (typically by Risley prism) until the patient reports the first sustained blur. The first sustained blur is the result of the following process: the increasing base-out vergence demand increases the vergence-accommodative response through the CA/C ratio. The patient must use negative relative accommodation so that the target remains clear. At some point the relative accommodation is insufficient to compensate for the increasing vergence-accommodation and the target becomes blurred. The prism power continues to be increased until the base-out vergence demand becomes too great for the fusional vergence system to maintain single vision, and the patient reports diplopia. The base-out vergence demand is then reduced until the patient initiates a fusional movement. The scenario is similar for base-in vergence ranges, except that vergence accommodation is decreasing and the patient uses positive relative accommodation to maintain clarity of the target.

Several clinical criteria have evolved from graphical analysis to assist the clinician in quickly assessing whether a vergence disorder exists. The most common are Pervical's[65] and Sheard's[66] criterion. Pervical's criterion suggests that the demand line should fall within the middle third of the range of relative convergence (blur points) for the patient to be comfortable. To determine whether Percival's criterion has been met, the base-in and base-out blur limits are added to determine the total width of the zone of clear, single binocular vision, and this width is divided by thrcc. The middle third of this range was proposed to be the zone of comfort. If either the base-in or base-out blur is less than the width of the comfort zone, Pervical's criterion has not been met. For example, for a base-out blur of 16△ and a base-in blur of 5△, the total width of the zone of comfort would be 7△. Since the base-in blur is less than 7△, Pervical's criterion has not been met. Sheedy and Saladin[67,68] found that Pervical's criterion was not helpful in identifying symptomatic exophoric patients but that a modified criterion was valuable for identifying symptomatic esophoric patients. They suggested using the *break*, rather than the *blur* to improve the criterion's predictive ability. A simple way to remember this modified criterion is that the positive break should not be more than twice the negative break.

Sheard's criterion suggests that to maintain comfort the relative fusional vergence (the blur point) should be twice as great as the fusion demand (phoria). For example, if the patient had 10XP (exophoria) at near and a base-out to blur of 16△, the patient would fail Sheard's criterion. Sheedy and Saladin[67,68] found that Sheard's criterion is a powerful diagnostic aid for identifying symptomatic exophoric patients. In addition, Daziel[69] reported that improving the base-out to blur with vision therapy to a level that satisfied Sheard's criterion was effective in relieving asthenopia.

If a patient has a low phoria, he may easily pass either of the previous criteria, but still have a relatively narrow zone of clear and single binocular vision. In addition to applying the previous criterion, the doctor should also make sure that both the patient's positive and negative vergence abilities are within the normative data outlined in Table 10.4. If the patient's abilities are poorer than these normative values, the patient may have a fusional vergence dysfunction, even though the patient has no significant heterophoria.

As an alternative to comparing heterophoria and compensating vergence or as a supplemental test of vergence adaptation, the generation of a *forced vergence fixation disparity* (FVFD) *curve* is recommended.[70,71] Children under 8 years of age may have difficulty with the concepts involved in completing this testing. Using either the Disparometer (Figure 10.4) or the Wesson Fixation Disparity Card at 40 cm, the clinician increases in counterbalance order base-in (BI) and base-out (BO) vergence, usually in steps of 3△. The clinician plots the fixation disparity (FD) in minutes of arc at each measurement point to generate a forced-vergence FD curve (Figure 10.5). The clinician then evaluates the curve type, slope of the curve ±3△ around ortho, the amount of FD in minutes of arc at ortho, and the associated phoria or the amount of prism necessary to reduce fixation disparity to zero. The advantage of FVFD curves are that they permit

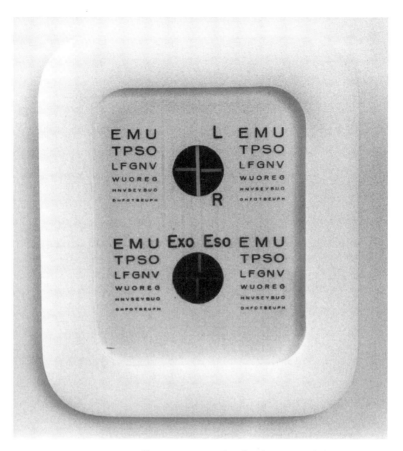

FIGURE 10.4 Disparometer allows testing for both vertical (target on top) and horizontal fixation disparity (target on bottom).

the evaluation of vergence adaptation under normal binocular conditions, rather than dissociated conditions of phoria-vergence analysis.

The type and shape of the curve helps assess whether the patient adapts to either convergent and divergent stimuli more efficiently or if the binocular system is equally adept at handling both. A steep slope (>45 degrees), suggestive of less than efficient vergence adaptation, has been associated with symptoms.[67,68] The magnitude of the FD in minutes of arc has been shown often to be a normal error signal,[72] but symptoms have been associated with exofixation disparity greater than 10 minutes of arc or the presence of any esodisparity.[67,68] Increasing amounts of fixation disparity have also been associated with increased stereothresholds. The associated phoria or the amount of prism necessary to reduce fixation disparity to zero has been shown to have limited value in allowing one to predict whether the patient will be symptomatic.[67,68] See Despotidis and Petito[73] for an in-depth review of the methods and evaluation of forced-vergence curves.

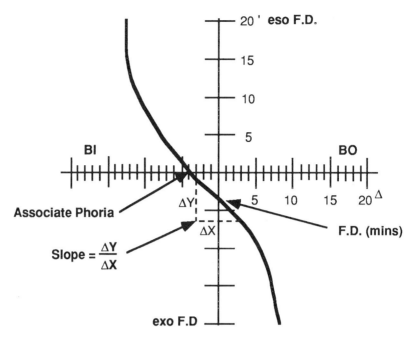

FIGURE 10.5 Forced vergence fixation disparity curve showing changes in the size and direction of fixation disparity as vergence demand is increased by BI and BO prism.

Vergence facility represents a dynamic test in which the vergence system's response to relatively large changes in vergence disparity are assessed over time. It has been suggested that the large disparity stimulus may "stress" an abnormal vergence system more than the slow incremental changes in relative vergence testing, and therefore may have greater diagnostic capabilities.[74] There have been some suggestions regarding the actual prism powers to be used in vergence facility testing (see Griffin[24]). We have found the 8BO/8BI prism flipper test to be a valuable clinical probe. The assumption for using 8BO/8BI is that these powers parallel the vergence response necessary on the ±2.00 D accommodative facility test for a patient with a 60 mm pd and a normal AC/A of 4 = 1. A −2.00 D lens change with the target at ortho vergence demand requires the patient to use about 8 BI to maintain single binocular vision. Conversely, a +2.00D lens change requires about 8BO to maintain single binocular vision.

The objective is not to stress the vergence system unduly but to probe the system's response characteristics, such as the latency (time to respond) and gain (speed to reach maximum response). There have been several studies that have established 8BO/8BI test normative data for third and sixth graders as well as adults[75-77] (see Table 10.5). There appears in these studies to be a developmental trend in the number of cycles per minute completed that is consistent with other studies using different flipper powers.[78] The relationship between vergence facility rate and symptoms has yet to be established[79] though reading-disabled children have been found

TABLE 10.5 Normative clinical data for vergence facility

Age range	n	Mean (SD) (cycles per minute)
Third graders (8-9)*	73	5.1 (2.6)
Sixth graders (11-12)*	293	6.6 (4.0)
Young adults (20-30)†	50	8.1 (4.3)

*Stuckle L, Rouse MW: *Norms for dynamic vergences,* Student Research Project 1979, and Mitchell R, Stanich R, Rouse MW: *Norms for dynamic vergences,* Student Research Project 1980, MB Ketchum Library, Southern California College of Optometry, Fullerton, Calif.
†Moser JE, Atkinson WF, Rouse MW: *Vergence facility in a young adult population,* Student Research Project 1980, MB Ketchum Library, Southern California College of Optometry, Fullerton, Calif.

be significantly slower on vergence facility tasks.[80] You may want to consult other sources for normative data for other flipper powers.[78]

Sensory system

An evaluation of the sensory system allows the clinician to gauge the quality of binocular vision. It has been suggested that patients may have particular symptoms, such as reporting the loss of absence of stereopsis, associated with a sensory system deficiency. This type of symptom is relatively rare, especially for school-aged children. It is more common to find sensory system deficiencies, in nonstrabismic patients, associated with accommodative and vergence system disorders. Therefore the *signs and symptoms* are the same as we have presented for accommodative and vergence disorders (see the boxes, pp. 277 and 283). In some cases a suppression (a sensory adaptation) will actually protect the patient from the consequences of these disorders; therefore identifying the presence of suppression is critical for understanding the possible discrepancy between what appears to be a significant binocular problem and a relatively symptom-free patient.

One can assess the components of the *sensory system* by checking *second-degree fusion* and *stereopsis.* One can assess second-degree fusion by using tests such as the Red Lens Test (RLT) or the Worth Dot Test (WDT). The RLT uses a red lens over typically the right eye, and the WDT uses a red filter over one eye and a green filter over the other to monitor suppression. The patient is typically asked to report what is seen as he or she fixates a penlight or transilluminator at 30 to 40 cm and 3 to 6 m. The test can be done under a variety of lighting conditions, bright to dim. The dim light conditions reduces the contours to fusion and probes the "strength" of fusional vergence. A fused response on the RLT would be reported as one single pink light, whereas the patient would report four dots, 2 green, 1 red, and 1 dot a mixture of red and green—or either red or green depending on which eye is dominant—on the WDT. A response of either 1 red and 1 white (RLT) or 5 dots (WDT) would indicate diplopia. In this case sensory fusion is absent and fusional vergence is inadequate to compensate for vergence demand. A response of 1 light either red or white (RLT) or 2 red dots or 3 green dots (WDT) would indicate suppression. The doctor should determine the eye being suppressed and the frequency of the suppression (intermittent to constant). Typically heterophoric patients give a stable second-degree fusion response on the RLT or WDT. Suppression is seldom reported on these tests unless the vergence disorder is severe. To detect central suppression the doctor may want to use tests that more closely approximate normal seeing, such as the Pola-mirror Test at near or portions of the Vectographic slide at distance. We have found it more helpful to closely monitor for suppression on all binocular accommodative and vergence tests, such as binocular accommodative and vergence facility. Suppression is much more likely when the demand on the accommodative-vergence relationship is increased.

Stereopsis testing should be conducted on each patient. The preferred method is random-dot tests or lateral-disparity tests where the monocular cues to depth are controlled by random-dot backgrounds, as in the Randot Test. The true random-dot portion is helpful when one is attempting to confirm if the patient is bifixating, as in cases of suspected small-angle esotropia, whereas the lateral disparity thresholding portions of tests provide an index of the quality of binocular sensory fusion. Generally patients should be able to reach the 20 to 40 second of arc thresholds on most commercial tests, since the normal visual system can typically resolve disparity down to 10 seconds of arc or less. If the patient is unable to reach normal clinical threshold values, the doctor should rule out reduced contrast caused by uncorrected refractive error or large accommodative lag, poorly compensated heterophoria resulting in increased fixation disparity (minutes of arc) or strabismus, anisophoria, aniseikonia, suppression, or amblyopia.

CLINICAL DIAGNOSTIC SYNDROMES

Once the doctor has completed a comprehensive systems evaluation he or she should have a list of objective problems and associated signs and symptoms. It is helpful both for diagnostic and billing reasons to arrange the data that have a tendency to vary together into groups or diagnostic syndromes.[57,58,81,82] It is not necessary that the patient have every finding listed, but there should be a sufficient number of findings present to constitute the syndrome. The clinician may need to use one or more of the data analysis methods described previously to analyze data and arrive at specific diagnoses listed under the board areas of oculomotor, accommodative, and vergence dysfunctions.

Oculomotor dysfunction may involve one or more of the following diagnoses:
1. *Fixation maintenance* (FM) *deficiency:* poor quality of FM noted on observation.

2. *Saccadic eye movement deficiency:* poor quality of saccadic eye movement noted on observation or indirectly assessed on DEM.

3. *Pursuit eye movement deficiency:* poor quality of smooth eye movement noted on observation.

Accommodative dysfunction may involve one or more of the following diagnoses:

1. *Accommodative insufficiency:* reduced amplitude, reduced PRA, difficulty on minus lens of accommodative facility, increased lag of accommodation.

2. *Accommodative infacility:* reduced monocular or binocular facility.

3. *Accommodative excess:* lead of accommodation (minus on MEM), difficulty on plus lens of accommodative facility, reduced NRA.

Duane's classification[83] sets the framework for the vergence syndromes we will be describing. Unfortunately, Duane's system uses only the difference of the phoria at far and near to classify the patient. Since no single-testing findings, such as phoria, is sufficient for classifying vergence disorders, we have used information from the literature and our clinical experience to list the findings in each diagnostic syndrome that have a tendency to vary together.

Vergence dysfunction typically involves one of the following diagnoses:

1. *Fusional vergence dysfunction.* Low phoria with reduced positive or negative relative and fusional vergence ranges, reduced vergence facility, reduced binocular accommodative facility (plus or minus, or both, may be difficult), reduced positive relative accommodation (PRA) and negative relative accommodation (NRA).

2. *Convergence insufficiency.* Low AC/A, higher exophoria at near, receded near point of convergence (NPC), reduced positive relative and fusional vergence ranges, reduced vergence facility (base-out more difficult), reduced binocular accommodative facility (plus lens more difficult), reduced NRA, possibly decreased second-degree fusion at near and increased stereoacuity.

3. *Basic exophoria.* Normal AC/A, approximately same magnitude of exophoria at far and near, receded NPC, reduced positive relative and fusional vergence ranges at far and near, reduced vergence facility, reduced binocular accommodative facility, reduced NRA, possibly decreased second-degree fusion at near and far and increased stereoacuity.

4. *Divergence excess.* High AC/A, higher exophoria at far than near, reduced positive relative and fusional vergence ranges at far, possibly decreased second-degree fusion at far.

5. *Convergence excess.* High AC/A, higher esophoria at near than far, reduced negative relative and fusional vergence ranges at near, reduced vergence facility (base-in, more difficult), reduced binocular

accommodative facility (minus lens more difficult), reduced PRA, possibly decreased second-degree fusion at near, and increased stereoacuity.

6. *Basic esophoria.* Normal AC/A, approximately same magnitude of esophoria at far and near, reduced negative relative and fusional vergence ranges at near and far, reduced vergence facility (base-in more difficult), reduced binocular accommodative facility (minus lens more difficult), reduced PRA, possibly decreased second-degree fusion at near and increased stereoacuity.

7. *Divergence insufficiency.* Low AC/A, higher esophoria at far than near, reduced negative fusional vergence at far, possibly decreased second-degree fusion at far.

VISUAL EFFICIENCY SCREENING FOR DETECTION AND REFERRAL

The comprehensive visual efficiency evaluation discussed in this chapter is just that—comprehensive. It is an in-depth review of a clinical strategy for evaluating visual acuity, refractive status, ocular health, oculomotor, and accommodative and vergence function and correlating the findings with entering signs and symptoms of patients presenting with suspected learning-related vision problems. Therefore this inclusive evaluation may be somewhat time consuming. This time is well spent for the doctor who plans on completely managing the identified visual efficiency disorders.

Most doctors in a primary care setting do not have either the time or the inclination to conduct the previously discussed comprehensive evaluation of visual efficiency. In an effort to provide the best vision care, however, the doctor will want to, first, use the supplemental case history screening checklist discussed in Chapter 9 and discuss further any signs and symptoms that were marked positive; second, conduct a routine primary care evaluation of visual acuity, refractive status, and ocular health; and, third, screen for potential visual efficiency problems. A suggested method for screening is outlined in the box. This limited battery of tests should detect the majority of visual efficiency problems encountered by the clinician. These procedures should take only 15 to 20 minutes to complete and will provide enough information to help in making initial prescribing and referral decisions. If the doctor's findings (such as uncorrected refractive error) from his or her primary care vision examination do not appear to account for the items marked on the checklist, the doctor will want to refer the patient to a colleague for more comprehensive diagnostic testing. If it appears that the findings from the primary-care examination might account for the signs and symptoms noted in the history, the doctor should refer to Chapter 15 for treatment methods.

SUMMARY

This chapter has concentrated on developing a comprehensive diagnostic strategy for evaluating the visual efficiency skills of patients presenting

---

Screening for Visual Efficiency Disorders

Oculomotor system

- Confrontation testing of saccades (4+ rating system)

Accommodative system

- Monocular accommodative amplitudes (push-up method)
- Binocular accommodative facility (±2.00 flipper)
- NRA and PRA (phorometry)
- Monocular estimate method (MEM) retinoscopy

Vergence system

- Near point of convergence
- Unilateral cover test/alternate cover test (UCT/ACT)
- Heterophoria at near (phorometry)
- Compensating vergence (phorometry)

Sensory system

- Stereopsis

---

with learning-related vision problems. We have focused on the methods that can be used to assess visual function within each system, normative data or criteria for determining if the results are normal or abnormal, the associated signs and symptoms, and finally the clinical characteristics of common diagnostic syndromes. Associating the entering signs and symptoms with the diagnostic findings will help the doctor determine the influence of visual efficiency problems on the patient's academic performance and the subsequent effect if the vision problems are resolved. In addition, I have suggested a strategy for screening the most important of these visual efficiency skills within the primary vision care setting, so that the doctor can make intelligent decisions about prescribing treatment and making referrals.

CHAPTER REVIEW

1. Visual efficiency is composed of what four systems?
2. Describe the symptoms typically associated with a oculomotor dysfunction.
3. A comprehensive evaluation of the accommodative system would involve testing which accommodative characteristics?
4. Contrast the use of clinical criteria, such as Pervical's and Sheard's, with the use of clinical norms for evaluating whether a vergence problem exists.
5. Describe the primary care strategy for evaluating visual efficiency that was presented in this chapter.

REFERENCES

1. Ritty MJ, Solan HA, Cool SJ: Visual and sensory-motor functioning in the classroom: a preliminary report of ergonomic demands, *J Am Optom Assoc* 64:238-244, 1993.
2. Fern K, Manny RE: Visual acuity of the preschool child: a review, *Am J Optom Physiol Opt* 63:319-345, 1986.
3. Rouse MW, Ryan JB: The examination and clinical management of children. In Rosenbloom AA, Morgan MW, editors: *Principles and practice of pediatric optometry*, Philadelphia, 1990, Lippincott.
4. Rosner J, Gruber J: Differences in the perceptual skills development of young myopes and hyperopes, *Am J Optom Physiol Opt* 62:501-504, 1985.
5. Rosner J, Rosner J: Some observations of the relationship between the visual perceptual skills development of young hyperopes and age of first lens correction, *Clin Exp Optom* 69:166-168, 1986.
6. Ismail E, Rouse MW, DeLand PN: A comparison of drop instillation and spray application of 1% cyclopentolate hydrochloride [abstract], *Optom Vis Sci* 70(suppl):101, 1992.
7. Scheiman M, Gallaway M, Coulter R, et al: Prevalence of vision and ocular disease conditions in a clinical pediatric population [abstract], *Optom Vis Sci* 69(suppl):108, 1992.
8. Zaba JN: Color deficiency, optometry and education, *J Am Optom Assoc* 45:94-95, 1974.
9. Thompson MA: Color vision screening in Price George County, *Sight Sav Rev* 32:216-217, 1962.
10. Thuline HC: Color-vision defects in American school children, *JAMA* 188:514-518, 1964.
11. Waddington M: Color blindness in young children, *Educ Res* 7:234-236, 1965.
12. Espinda SD: Color vision deficiency: a learning disability? *J Learn Disabil* 6:163-166, 1973.
13. Litton FW: Color vision deficiency in LD children, *Acad Ther* 14:437-441, 1979.
14. Haegerstrom-Portnoy G: In Rosenbloom AA, Morgan MW, editors: *Principles and practice of pediatric optometry*, Philadelphia, 1990, Lippincott, pp 449-466.
15. Gay AJ: *Eye movement disorders*, St Louis, 1974, Mosby.
16. Marcus SE: A syndrome of visual constrictions in the learning disabled child, *J Am Optom Assoc* 45:746-749, 1974.
17. Hoffman LG, Rouse MW: Referral recommendations for binocular function and/or developmental perceptual deficiencies, *J Am Optom Assoc* 51:119-126, 1980.
18. Maples WC, Ficklin T: Test retest reliability of the King-Devick saccade and the NSUCO ocularmotor tests, *J Behav Optom* 3(3):209-214, 1991.
19. Pierce J: Pierce Saccade Test, Bloomington, Ind, 1972, Cook Inc.
20. King AT, Devick S: *The proposed King-Devick test and its relation to the Pierce Saccade Test and reading levels*, Senior Research Project 1976, Carl F. Shepard Memorial Library, Illinois College of Optometry, Chicago, Ill.
21. Garzia RP, Richman JE, Nicholson SB, Gaines CS: A new visual-verbal saccade test: the Developmental Eye Movement test (DEM), *J Am Optom Assoc* 61:124-135, 1990.
22. Young LR, Sheena D: Survey of eye movement recording methods, *Behav Res Methods Instr* 7:397-429, 1975.
23. Winter J: Clinical oculography, *J Am Optom Assoc* 45:1308-1313, 1974.
24. Griffin JR: *Binocular anomalies: procedures for vision therapy*, ed 2, Chicago, 1982, Professional Press.
25. Gilbert LC: *Functional motor efficiency of the eyes and its relationship to reading*, Berkeley, Calif, 1953, University of California Press.
26. Liberman S, Cohen AH, Rubin J: NYSOA K-D test, *J Am Optom Assoc* 54:631-637, 1983.
27. Richman JE, Walker AJ, Garzia RP: The impact of automatic digit naming ability on a clinical test of eye movement functioning, *J Am Optom Assoc* 54:617-622, 1983.
28. Oride MKH, Marutani JK, Rouse MW, Deland PN: Reliability study of

the Pierce and King-Devick Saccade tests, *Am J Optom Physiol Opt* 63:419-424, 1986.

29. Maples WC, Atchley J, Ficklin T: Northeastern State University College of Optometry's oculomotor norms, *J Behav Optom* 3(6):143-150, 1992.

30. Nestor EM, Parot CJ, Rouse MW: *A re-evaluation on the reliability of the developmental eye movement test,* Student Research Project 1991, MB Ketchum Library, Southern California College of Optometry, Fullerton, Calif.

31. Wick B, Hall P: Relation among accommodative facility, lag, and amplitude in elementary school children, *Am J Optom Physiol Opt* 64:593-598, 1987.

32. Jackson TW, Goss DA: Variation and correlation of clinical tests of accommodative function in a sample of school-age children, *J Am Optom Assoc* 62:857-866, 1991.

33. Haynes HM, White BL, Held R: Visual accommodation in human infants, *Science* 148:528-530, 1965.

34. Banks MS: The development of visual accommodation during early infancy, *Child Dev* 51:646-666, 1980.

35. Brookman KE: Ocular accommodation in human infants, *Am J Optom Physiol Opt* 60:91-99, 1983.

36. Duane A: An attempt to determine the normal range of accommodation at various ages, *Trans Am Ophthalmol Soc* 11:634-641, 1908.

37. Sheard C: *Dynamic ocular tests: the Sheard volume,* Philadelphia, 1957, Chilton Co, pp 93-94.

38. Duane A: Studies in monocular and binocular accommodation with their clinical applications, *Am J Ophthalmol* 5:865-877, 1922.

39. Wold RM: The spectacle amplitude of accommodation of children aged six to ten, *Am J Optom Arch Am Acad Optom* 44:642-664, 1967.

40. Hofstetter HW: Useful age-amplitude formula, *Optom World* 38:42-45, 1950.

41. Daum KM: Accommodative dysfunction, *Doc Ophthalmol* 55:177-198, 1983.

42. Woodruff ME: Ocular accommodation in children aged 3 to 11 years, *Can J Optom* 49:141-145, 1987.

43. Zellers JA, Alpert TL, Rouse MW: A review of the literature and a normative study of accommodative facility, *J Am Optom Assoc* 55:31-37, 1984.

44. Hennessey D, Iosue RA, Rouse MW: Relation of symptoms to accommodative infacility in school-aged children, *Am J Optom Physiol Opt* 61:177-183, 1984.

45. Scheiman M, Herzberg H, Frantz K, Margolies M: Normative study of accommodative facility in elementary schoolchildren, *Am J Optom Physiol Opt* 65:127-134, 1988.

46. Levine S, Ciuffreda KJ, Selenow A, Flax N: Clinical assessment of accommodative facility in symptomatic and asymptomatic individuals, *J Am Optom Assoc* 56:286-290, 1985.

47. McKenzie KM, Kerr SR, Rouse MW, De Land PN: Study of accommodative facility testing reliability, *Am J Optom Physiol Opt* 64(3):186-194, 1987.

48. Rouse MW, DeLand PN, Chous R, Determan TF: Monocular accommodative facility testing reliability, *Optom Vis Sci* 66(2):72-77, 1989.

49. Rouse MW, Mozayani S, Smith JP, De Land PN: Binocular accommodative facility testing reliability, *Optom Vis Sci* 69:314-319, 1992.

50. Rouse MW, De Land PN, Freestone GM, Weiner BA: A comparative study of computer based and standard clinical accommodative facility testing methods, *Optom Vis Sci* 68:88-95, 1991.

51. Rouse MW, London R, Allen DC: An evaluation of the monocular estimate method of dynamic retinoscopy, *Am J Optom Physiol Opt* 59:234-239, 1982.

52. Haynes HM: Clinical observations with dynamic retinoscopy, *Optom Weekly* 51:2243-2246, 2306-2309, 1960.

53. Rouse MW, Hutter RF, Shiftlett R: A normative study of the accommodative lag in elementary school children, *Am J Optom Physiol Opt* 61:693-697, 1984.

54. Hutter RF, Rouse MW: Visually re-

lated headache in a preschooler, *Am J Optom Physiol Opt* 61:711-713, 1984.

55. Rouse MW, Polte L: Accommodative involvement with Adie's pupil, *Am J Optom Physiol Opt* 61:54-55, 1984.

56. Goodson RA, Afanador AJ: The accommodative response to the near point crossed cylinder test, *Optom Weekly,* pp 1138-1140, Dec 5, 1974.

57. Morgan MW: Analysis of clinical data, *Am J Optom Arch Am Acad Optom* 21:477-491, 1944.

58. Morgan MW: The clinical aspects of accommodation and convergence, *Am J Optom Arch Am Acad Optom* 21:301-313, 1944.

59. Jackson TW, Goss DA: Variation and correlation of standard clinical phoropter tests of phorias, vergence ranges, and relative accommodation in a sample of school-age children, *J Am Optom Assoc* 62:540-547, 1991.

60. Ciuffreda KJ: Components of clinical near vergence testing, *J Behav Optom* 3(1):3-13, 1992.

61. Gallaway M, Scheiman M, Frantz KA, et al: The significance of assessing nearpoint of convergence using different stimuli [abstract], *Optom Vis Sci* 68(suppl):93, 1991.

62. Caloroso EE, Rouse MW: *Clinical management of strabismus,* Boston, 1993, Butterworth-Heinemann.

63. von Noorden GK: *Binocular vision and ocular motility,* ed 4, St. Louis, 1990, Mosby.

64. Birnbaum MH: *Optometric management of nearpoint vision disorders,* Boston, 1993, Butterworth-Heinemann.

65. Percival AS: *The prescribing of spectacles,* ed 3, New York, 1928, William Wood & Co.

66. Sheard C: Zones of ocular comfort, *Am J Optom Arch Am Acad Optom* 7:9-25, 1930.

67. Sheedy JE, Saladin JJ: Association of symptoms with measures of oculomotor deficiencies, *Am J Optom Physiol Opt* 55:670-676, 1978.

68. Sheedy JE, Saladin JJ: Phoria, vergence, and fixation disparity in oculomotor problems, *Am J Optom Physiol Opt* 54:474-478, 1977.

69. Dalziel CC: Effect of vision training on patients who fail Sheard's criterion, *Am J Optom Physiol Opt* 58:21-23, 1981.

70. Sheedy JE: Actual measurement of fixation disparity and its use in diagnosis and treatment, *J Am Optom Assoc* 51:1079-1084, 1980.

71. Wick B, London R: Analysis of binocular visual function using tests made under binocular conditions, *Am J Optom Physiol Opt* 64(4):227-240, 1987.

72. Schor CM: Fixation disparity: a steady state error of disparity induced vergence, *Am J Optom Physiol Opt* 57(9):618-631, 1980.

73. Despotidis N, Petito GT: Fixation disparity: clinical implications and utilization, *J Am Optom Assoc* 62:923-933, 1991.

74. Grisham JD: The dynamics of fusional vergence eye movements in binocular dysfunction, *Am J Optom Physiol Opt* 57:645-655, 1980.

75. Stuckle L, Rouse MW: *Norms for dynamic vergences,* Student Research Project 1979, MB Ketchum Library, Southern California College of Optometry, Fullerton, Calif.

76. Mitchell R, Stanich R, Rouse MW: *Norms for dynamic vergences,* Student Research Project 1980, MB Ketchum Library, Southern California College of Optometry, Fullerton, Calif.

77. Moser JE, Atkinson WF, Rouse MW: Vergence facility in a young adult population. Student Research Project 1980, MB Ketchum Library, Southern California College of Optometry, Fullerton, Calif.

78. Buzzelli AR: Vergence facility: developmental trends in a school age population, *Am J Optom Physiol Opt* 63:351-355, 1986.

79. Delgadillo HM, Griffin JR: Vergence facility and associated symptoms: a comparison of two prism flipper tests, *J Behav Optom* 3(4):91-94, 1992.

80. Buzzelli AR: Stereopsis, accommodative and vergence facility: do they relate to dyslexia? *Optom Vis Sci* 68:842-846, 1991.

81. Flom MC: The use of the accommodative convergence relationship in

prescribing orthoptics, *Penn Optom* 14(3):3-18, 1954.

82. Schapero M: The characteristics of ten basic visual training problems, *Am J Optom Arch Am Acad Optom* 32:333-342, 1955.

83. Duane A: A new classification of the motor anomalies of the eye based upon physiological principles, together with their symptoms, diagnosis and treatment, *Ann Ophthalmol Otol* 5:969-1008, 1896.

CHAPTER **11**

Visual Information Processing: Assessment and Diagnosis

MITCHELL M. SCHEIMAN
MICHAEL GALLAWAY

KEY TERMS

visual information processing
visual-spatial skills
visual-analysis skills
visual-motor skills
auditory-visual integration skills
directionality
laterality
cognitive style

Z scores
scaled scores
standard scores
visual discrimination
visual figure ground
visual closure
visual memory
visualization

The objectives of this chapter are to provide an organized approach to the evaluation of visual information processing disorders and to demonstrate that the process of assessing visual information processing skills and reaching a diagnosis is comparable in many ways to that used for visual efficiency skills and other aspects of optometric care. Our goal is to present an assessment approach that requires the identical clinical reasoning and problem-solving skills as necessary for other aspects of optometric care.

When one is assessing visual efficiency skills, the following rules apply:

- To reach a diagnosis, the optometrist performs a standard battery of tests to elicit information about each important function. In Chapter 10, for example, we described the assessment of accommodation and included evaluation of amplitude, facility, and accuracy (lag).
- A classification of accommodative, binocular vision, and oculomotor

problems is recognized and several diagnostic categories are present for each area. For example, in Chapter 10 we reviewed the classification of accommodative, binocular vision, and oculomotor disorders. Within each broad area, such as accommodative anomalies , a subclassification of disorders is recognized (accommodative insufficiency, excess, and in-facility).

*   Each diagnostic entity has its own identifiable characteristics, signs, and symptoms.
*   Once a diagnosis is reached there are established and organized treatment methods to manage each diagnostic entity.

These rules also apply to the clinical assessment of visual information processing skills. In this chapter we present a test battery that has been designed to allow the clinician to elicit information about each diagnostic category. In addition, we introduce a classification of visual information processing disorders, including characteristics, signs, and symptoms for each. Finally we describe how to use the information gathered from the evaluation to reach a diagnosis.

It is important to understand that these disorders may not exist in isolation. In most cases patients present with a combination of visual information processing disorders, just as it is common for patients to have accommodative anomalies associated with binocular vision disorders. In addition, a large percentage of children with visual information processing problems also present with visual efficiency disorders. Diagnostic testing, however, is designed to try and isolate the various diagnostic entities described later in this chapter. This approach not only facilitates and organizes the diagnostic process, but also helps the clinician develop recommendations and treatment strategies.

VISUAL INFORMATION PROCESSING EVALUATION: PRELIMINARY \CONSIDERATIONS

The assessment battery includes tests to evaluate several diagnostic categories including visual-spatial, visual-analysis, visual-motor, and auditory-visual integration skills (Table 11.1). These diagnostic categories and their subclassification are described in detail later in this chapter. This text will not serve as a manual from which you can administer the various tests. Rather it is designed to provide background information and establish a model that can be applied clinically. It is therefore essential to have all the recommended tests accessible while you are reading this chapter. Although we will discuss each test in some detail and give a sample illustration for each, we will also extensively refer to the original manuals. As we discuss a particular test, have the test, test manual, and scoring instructions available. At the end of this chapter we have listed the companies that produce each of the tests in our battery.

The evaluation and classification system that we present is primarily

TABLE 11.1   Visual information processing test battery

Diagnostic category	Subclassification	Test
VISUAL-SPATIAL SKILLS		
	Bilateral integration	Standing Angels in the Snow
	Laterality	Piaget Test of Right/Left Concepts
	Directionality	Gardner Reversal Frequency: Recognition Subtest *Execution Subtest
VISUAL-ANALYSIS SKILLS		
	Visual discrimination	TVPS: Visual Discrimination
	Visual closure	TVPS: Visual Closure
	Visual form constancy	TVPS: Visual Form Constancy
	Visual figure ground	TVPS: Visual Figure Ground
	Visual-spatial relations	TVPS: Visual Spatial Relations
	Visual memory	TVPS: Visual Memory TVPS: Visual Sequential Memory
VISUAL-MOTOR INTEGRATION SKILLS		
	Visual-motor integration	Developmental Test of Visual-Motor Integration
	Fine-motor skills	Grooved Pegboard Wold Sentence Copy Test
AUDITORY-VISUAL INTEGRATION SKILLS		
	Auditory-visual integration	Auditory-Visual Integration Test

*Indicates auxiliary test.

based on the work of Richman,[1] Hoffman,[2] and Solan and Groffman.[3] It is important to understand, however, that visual information processing or visual-perceptual-motor anomalies can be assessed and subclassified in different ways. Through the years, in fact, a variety of testing and classification schemes have been recommended.[1-6] These different approaches are dependent on the underlying philosophy and model of the author.

Suchoff's[4] model of visual spatial development is representative of a very popular approach that is predicated on the concept that the development of visual perceptual skills is closely related to a child's motor development. This model is based heavily on the work of Gesell,[7] Kephart,[8] Getman,[9] and Piaget.[10] A key underlying concept in motor-based models, like that proposed by Suchoff, is that the primary purpose of vision in the human organism is the "organization and manipulation of space."[4] Suchoff classifies visual spatial development into three areas:

invariant The zero point or reference point from which vision functions in the organization and manipulation of space.

bilaterality The motoric and cognitive awareness of oneself as a two-sided being and the knowledge of the difference between the two sides.

spatial organization and manipulation The child's ability to relate to various spatial phenomena.

A very important idea in motor-based approaches, such as Suchoff's, is that as a child grows older, performance in certain task situations is characterized by more visual performance and less motor performance.[4] This concept has been referred to as the "visual-motor hierarchy." According to Weinstein,[11] in infancy there is little dependence on vision and much on motor activity. As a child develops, this relationship constantly changes and by 7 to 8 years of age the major dependence is on vision with relatively little on motor activity. The child moves through four stages—motor, motor-visual, visual-motor, and finally visual.

Although motor-based approaches like that just described have been very popular for optometric clinicians, we have found that teaching clinicians to understand and utilize this system can be difficult. Many of the evaluation tools used in these models are based very heavily on the clinician's ability to make sophisticated observations. In addition, the specific tests are primarily nonstandardized and unnormed. Although these factors do not negate the validity of this approach, they do limit its usefulness.

The approach we present is based on the work of Richman,[1] Hoffman,[2] and Solan and Groffman[3] and makes extensive use of standardized, objective tests. Standardized, objective testing has several important characteristics:

- Subjective judgments by the clinician are minimized (though not excluded).
- Testing is performed in a uniform way, and theoretically every trained observer should achieve the same result.
- Scoring follows specific rules, and performance is compared to normative data.

Using standardized testing we can more confidently know what we are measuring and we are better able to communicate our results to other professionals. For the less experienced clinician or for students learning to evaluate visual information processing for the first time, these characteristics are highly desirable. Although experienced clinicians can sometimes make meaningful decisions about visual information processing simply by watching the child in an unstructured task, less experienced clinicians are unable to do so. There is evidence that even an experienced clinician's subjective and intuitive judgments may not always be reliable or valid.[3] Solan and Groffman state that "there will always be some persons whose quality of judgment enables them to make more accurate estimates than others. Unfortunately, there are also persons who tend to utilize intuitive judgments based on inadequate data and whose conclusions are not accurate."[3] The use of standardized, objective testing eliminates this problem.

A significant difference between this system and the motor-based systems described above is that our approach is directed at identifying and treating specific visual information processing deficits. Concepts such as the importance of motor development and the visual motor hierarchy are retained in our model, though they are deemphasized.

The value of the approach and classification we present is that it follows the basic problem-oriented approach commonly practiced by today's optometrist. The same clinical reasoning skills that clinicians are accustomed to using in all other aspects of optometric care can be applied to visual information processing disorders. This makes the approach easier to learn and more readily accepted. The reliance on standardized testing deemphasizes the importance of observation and allows practitioners to communicate more effectively about their results and experiences with patients.

Case history

The case history helps direct the evaluation of the child with learning problems. As discussed in Chapter 9, children with visual information processing disorders present with a characteristic case history. Specific signs and symptoms also indicate problems in certain aspects of visual information processing. It is important to try and approach the visual information processing evaluation as we approach any other clinical problem. Based on the case history we should develop a list of clinical hypotheses and proceed to administer tests to confirm or deny these hypotheses.

The box lists the various diagnostic categories along with their characteristic signs and symptoms. If a patient presented with a chief complaint of difficulty with handwriting and copying skills, for example, the most likely clinical hypothesis would be a visual motor integration problem, as indicated in the box. A problem with reversals and learning left and right would indicate a clinical hypothesis of a visual spatial problem. Although a knowledge of the symptoms and signs of the various diagnostic categories may allow you to predict the results of the evaluation, we still recommend evaluation of all four areas discussed below.

Administration of tests

We have divided the test battery into two categories:

1. A core battery that should be administered to every patient.
2. Auxiliary tests that can be used when necessary. There may be occasions when the results of the core battery are equivocal. In such cases, additional tests can be selected from the auxiliary tests we have included to help in refining the diagnosis.

Symptoms and Signs of Visual Information Processing Disorders

Visual-spatial dysfunction

- Poor athletic performance
- Difficulty with rhythmic activities
- Lack of coordination and balance
- Clumsy; falls and bumps into things often
- Tendency to work with one side of the body while the other side doesn't participate
- Difficulty learning left and right
- Reverses letters and numbers when writing or copying
- Writes from right to left

Visual-analysis dysfunction

- Has trouble learning the alphabet, recognizing words, and learning basic mathematical concepts of size, magnitude, and position
- Confuses likenesses and minor differences
- Mistakes words with similar beginnings
- Difficulty recognizing the same word repeated on a page
- Difficulty recognizing letters or simple forms
- Difficulty distinguishing the main idea from insignificant details
- Overgeneralizes when classifying objects
- Has trouble writing and remembering letters and numbers

Visual-motor dysfunction

- Difficulty copying from the board
- Sloppy drawing or writing skills
- Poor spacing and inability to stay on lines
- Erases excessively
- Can respond orally but not produce answers in writing
- Difficulty completing written assignments in allotted period of time
- Seems to know the material but does poorly on tests
- Difficulty writing numbers in columns for mathematical problems

Auditory-visual integration dysfunction

- Poor spelling ability
- Difficulty learning to read phonetically
- Difficulty relating symbols to their relevant sounds

Table 11.1 illustrates those tests that are part of the core battery and those that are considered auxiliary tests.

When assessing visual information processing skills using standardized tests, it is important to follow some rules applying to these tests.

Instructional sets

The strength of standardized tests is that the procedures, instrumentation, and scoring have all been specified so that similar conditions can be duplicated at different times and places.[12] Therefore it is critical that the specific instructions and procedures be followed exactly as outlined in the instruction manual for each test. When these tests are being learned, we recommend that clinicians actually *read* the instructional sets found in the test manuals until the exact wording is memorized. Slight variations from the precise instructional sets are permissible as long as the intended meaning is not altered. This will sometimes be necessary when a child does not understand the instructions. In general, however, it is important to use the same instructional set each time you administer the test.

Observation of performance

Although the final result or quantitative score is important, it is equally vital to observe the way the child achieves a particular result. This information can add considerably to our understanding of the child's ability and is also important when planning a treatment program. As each test is administered, the clinician should carefully make observations about the child's performance. Behavior that a child exhibits during a particular test may provide additional information about the degree of difficulty he may be having or compensatory strategies being used to complete the task. Table 11.2 lists some of the observations that are important.

Some of the more critical areas include observations about attention and cognitive style. These issues are discussed in detail in Chapter 3. The child's attentional ability can greatly influence the results in many ways during the visual information processing evaluation. First, the child must be able to listen attentively to the instructional set. If the child cannot do so, he may fail to completely understand what is expected of him. Inability to attend and concentrate for adequate periods of time may also interfere with the child's overall performance on any test. For example, during the evaluation of visual memory does the child attend for the full 5 seconds on the stimulus? If not, poor results on the visual memory test may actually be caused by deficient attention rather than inadequate visual memory skills. Thus poor attentional skills may lead to test results that underestimate a child's visual information processing ability.

The child's cognitive style is another important issue about which clinicians should make careful observations. Cognitive style is the individual's characteristic approach to processing information. During the visual information processing evaluation it is important to observe whether the child has a reflective or impulsive style. Reflective children work slowly and produce few errors, whereas impulsive children work quickly and make more errors. During the testing process we try to assess whether the child's cognitive style is affecting his performance. For example, a child may score well on an untimed test but take an excessive amount of time. This is characteristic of a reflective style. Consideration of only the test result would tend to overestimate this child's visual information processing ability.

Issues such as attention and cognitive style must be considered in the design of the vision therapy program. The importance of these factors is covered in depth in Chapter 16.

TABLE 11.2 Important behavioral observations during the visual information processing evaluation

Category	Behavior
Performance style and overall approach to task	Short attention span Impulsive Reflective Gives up easily Perseveration Performs slowly Hesitant to give answers
Visual-spatial skills	Nondominant hand not used for support Switches hands during testing Motor overflow Rotates body Does not cross midline
Visual-analysis skills	Distractible Short attention span Difficulty with concentration Fear of failure Hyperactive Hypoactive Subvocalization Traces or touches figures Difficulty understanding directions Withdrawn
Visual-motor integration skills	Hand used to hold pencil Poor organization Excessive erasures Segmentation Does not recognize mistakes Cannot correct mistakes on second trial Inadequate pencil grip Excessive finger tension Motor overflow Rotates paper, constantly moves paper Rotates body Close working distance Poor posture when writing Nonwriting hand may not be involved in task
Auditory-visual integration skills	Needs to have directions repeated Taps out code with own finger Subvocalizes

Scoring and understanding test results

Just as important as using the precise instructional sets recommended for each test is applying the recommended scoring criteria. The specific rules described in each test's scoring manual must be applied consistently to eliminate the observer as a source of bias. A good example of this is the extensive scoring criteria for the Developmental Test of Visual Motor Inte-

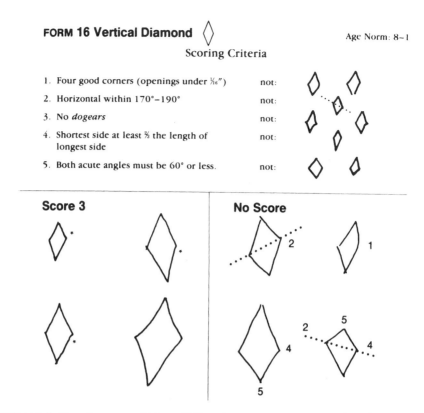

FIGURE 11.1 Developmental Test of Visual Motor Integration. (Modern Curriculum Press.)

gration (DTVMI). Figure 11-1 is an example of the scoring criteria used for one of the 24 forms of this test.

The raw scores that are generated from each test provide little valuable information about the child's level of performance. Clinically we want to determine if the child's performance is adequate or is better or worse than other children at his age. It is only after the raw score is compared to some standard that it becomes meaningful. When a raw score is converted to a score that facilitates comparison, it is called a "derived score." As a general rule, raw scores can be converted into three basic types of derived scores; standard scores, percentile ranks, and perceptual age equivalents.

Z scores, scaled scores, and standard scores. A Z (or z) score is used to express the distance of an individual's raw score from the mean. Typically a Z score of zero would indicate that the child's performance was equivalent to the mean for his age. The standard deviation for Z scores is 1. The higher the Z score the greater the deviation from the mean. A positive Z score indicates above–age level performance, and a negative Z score below–age level performance.

Many tests used by psychologists, educators, and optometrists use scaled scores to report results. Perhaps the most well-known test using scaled scores is the Wechsler Intelligence Test for Children–Revised

(WISC-R). This IQ test is described in detail in Chapter 12. A scaled score of 10 indicates that the child's performance is probably average for his age and is equivalent to the mean for children of that age. A standard deviation of 3 is used with scaled scores. Thus, if a child has a scaled score of 4 on a particular test, his score is 2 standard deviations below the mean. Scaled scores are useful when a test has several homogeneous subtests and allow the clinician to compare strengths and weaknesses across many areas. Scaled scores can be used in this manner with the Test of Visual Perceptual Skills (TVPS) described later in this chapter.

Another derived score that is similar to scaled scores is called a "standard score." Generally the standard score is assigned a mean of 100 with a standard deviation of 15. A standard score of 120 on the Developmental Test of Visual Motor Integration (DTVMI) described later in this chapter, indicates that the child scored more than 1 standard deviation above the mean for his age level.

Percentile ranks. Raw scores can also be converted to percentile scores. In most manuals, tables are available showing the percentile rank for each scaled or standard score. Table 4 in the *DTVMI Manual* and Table 18 in the *TVPS Manual* are examples of tables that can be used to convert raw scores and scaled scores to percentile ranks. Clinicians can also readily convert scaled and standard scores to percentile ranks even if such tables are not provided. This conversion is based on the fact that a scaled score of 10 represents the mean or the 50th percentile for the child. One standard deviation above the mean is the 85th percentile, and 1 standard deviation below the mean is the 15th percentile. The standard deviation with scaled scores is 3. Therefore a scaled score of 7 would represent a percentile rank of 16th percentile, and a scaled score of 13 would represent a percentile rank of 84th percentile. Table 11.3 can be used to convert scaled scores and two scores to percentile ranks.

With standard scores, the concept described above also applies. The only difference is that a standard score of 100 is equivalent to the 50th percentile and the standard deviation is 15. Thus a standard score of 115 is 1 standard deviation above the mean and is equivalent to the 85th percentile, whereas a standard score of 85 is 1 standard deviation below the mean and represents a percentile rank of 15th percentile.

Perceptual age equivalents. Raw scores can also be converted to a perceptual age equivalent. An age-equivalent score represents the raw score that is statistically characteristic of a particular age in the normative sample for a given task.[12] Age equivalents can be useful because they allow the clinician to compare quickly the child's chronological age to his age-equivalent score. Although age-equivalent scores can be very easily understood by parents, they are considered to be less precise than standard or scaled scores as statistical measures. Age equivalents are subject to the nonlinear characteristics of a child's development. This means that certain skills may develop more rapidly at one age level than at another. Use

TABLE 11.3 Conversion table for different derived scores

Scaled scores	Z scores	Percentile score
1	−3.00	0.1
2	−2.70	0.4
3	−2.25	1
4	−2.00	2
5	−1.60	5
6	−1.35	9
7	−1.00	16
8	−0.65	25
9	−0.35	37
10	0.00	50
11	0.35	63
12	0.65	75
13	1.00	84
14	1.35	91
15	1.60	95
16	2.00	98
17	2.25	99
18	2.70	99.6
19	3.00	99.9

of age equivalents alone may lead to overestimation or underestimation of a child's performance.[12]

Generally parents will not understand Z scores, scaled scores, or standard scores, and it will be necessary for you to convert these derived scores into either percentile ranks or age-equivalent scores. Parents certainly will understand the significance of age equivalents, and they are often familiar with percentile ranks. They have experienced the use of percentile ranks from the pediatrician who will talk of the child's height and weight in percentiles. Most children today also receive achievement tests each year in school, and a popular method of reporting the results of these tests is with percentile ranks.

Table 11.3 summarizes the relationship between the different derived scores just described and can be used to convert the various scores you obtain from testing into percentile ranks.

In the battery of tests we present in this chapter we use either percentile ranks or age equivalents as the method of reporting test results.

To facilitate recording the results of the evaluation, we recommend using the Visual Information Processing Evaluation Profile form, which can be found in Appendix F.

VISUAL INFORMATION PROCESSING EVALUATION: COMPREHENSIVE TEST BATTERY

The test battery described below is designed to assess four broad areas of visual information processing. These areas include visual-spatial, visual-analysis, visual-motor and auditory-visual integration skills. After a short description of each category we provide a general description of the recommended test for that category.

Visual-spatial skills

These skills allow the individual to develop normal internal and external spatial concepts and are used to interact with and organize the environment. They allow the individual to make judgments about location of objects in visual space in reference to other objects and to the individual's own body. Visual-spatial skills develop from an awareness within the individual's body of concepts such as left and right, up and down, and front and back.

Visual-spatial skills are important for the development of good motor coordination, balance, and directional senses. Component skills include bilateral integration, laterality, and directionality.

Bilateral integration

Bilateral integration is the ability to be aware of and use both sides of the body separately and simultaneously.

Laterality

Laterality is the ability to be internally aware of and identify right and left on oneself.

Directionality

Directionality is the ability of the individual to interpret right and left directions in three separate components of external space.

EVALUATION OF BILATERAL INTEGRATION

Standing Angels in the Snow

APPROPRIATE AGES: 3-8

Purpose, description of test, and scoring. This test evaluates the child's bilateral integration skills. The examiner should be seated with the child standing directly in front of the examiner. The examiner's legs should be separated so that the child is standing midway between them. There should be about 1 foot between the examiner's right foot and the child's left foot and the same for the other foot (Figure 11.2).

The examiner then proceeds to ask the child to make a very specific series of arm and leg movements. The movements range from very simple to complex. It is important for the examiner not only to observe if the correct movements are made, but also to watch for motor overflow, inappropriate movement, and other indications of performance breakdowns.

Since this test is not commercially available, we provide the specific instructional set that should be used.

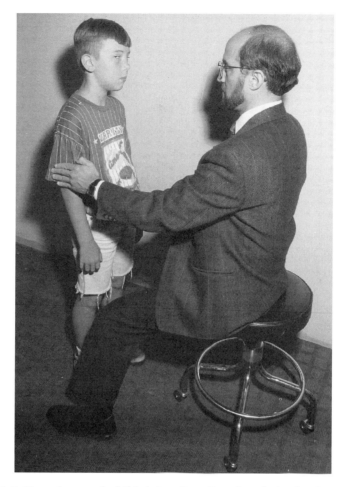

FIGURE 11.2 Examiner and child doing Standing Angels in the Snow.

Say to the child:

"We are going to play a game of touch and go. If I touch your arm, move only that arm to shoulder level (touch the child's arm and help him move it to shoulder level). If I touch your leg, slide it out until it just touches my foot (touch his leg and show him how to slide his leg to yours). If I touch more than one thing, you must move both things at the same time. Remember to move only the things that I touch. Do you understand?"

After each movement, instruct the child to move the leg, arm, or both back to the starting position.

Monolateral movements

1. Touch the right arm.
2. Touch the left arm.
3. Touch the right leg.
4. Touch the left leg.

TABLE 11.4   Scoring criteria for Standing Angels in the Snow

Child's performance	Age level
Movements are not related to body parts touched	3-year level
Homologous movements are performed, but monolateral are difficult	4-year level
Homologous, monolateral, and ipsilateral movements are performed but motor overflow is present	5-year level
Only contralateral movements produce overflow or performance breakdown	6-year level
Competent contralateral movement accompanied by minimal motor overflow and frequent segmentation (limbs touched are not moved simultaneously)	7-year level
Child succeeds in all movements without motor overflow	8-year level

Homologous movements

 5. Touch both arms.

Ipsilateral movement

 6. Touch both the right leg and right arm.
 7. Touch both the left leg and left arm.

Contralateral movement

 8. Touch the right arm and left leg.
 9. Touch the left arm and right leg.

Scoring. Use the criteria listed in Table 11.4 to score the results of Standing Angels in the Snow.

Important behavioral observations
• Does the child have to look at the limb to be moved?
• Were there abortive movements to get started?
• Does the child hesitate at the beginning of the movements?
• Are the movements hesitant and jerky?
• Is there motor overflow to limbs other than those touched?
• Do the instructions have to be repeated?
• If an error occurs, can correction be made after one repetition?

EVALUATION OF LATERALITY

Piaget Test of Left-Right Concepts
APPROPRIATE AGES: 5-11

Purpose, description of test, and scoring. This test evaluates the child's ability to differentiate right from left on his own body (laterality), on another person, and on the location of objects in space (directionality). The examiner asks the child a series of questions designed to probe his knowledge of right and left.

Since this test is not commercially available, we provide the specific instructional set that should be used.

Instructional set. During the entire test the child should be seated beside the examiner, except for section B and D where the examiner and the subject stand facing each other.

Section A (subject's body parts). Ask the child the following questions and record the responses as correct or incorrect.

    a. Show me your right hand.
    b. Show me your left leg.
    c. Touch your left ear.
    d. Show me your left hand.
    e. Show me your right leg.
    f. Point to your right eye.

Section B (examiner's body parts—Sit opposite the child)

    a. Show me my left hand.
    b. Point to my right ear.
    c. Show me my left leg.
    d. Show me my right hand.
    e. Point to my left ear.
    f. Show me my right leg.

Section C (Place a coin on the table to the left of a pencil in relation to the child)

    a. Is the pencil to the right or to the left of the coin?
    b. Is the coin to the right or to the left of the pencil?

NOW HAVE THE CHILD WALK AROUND TO THE OPPOSITE SIDE OF THE TABLE:

    c. Is the pencil to the right or to the left of the coin?
    d. Is the coin to the right or to the left of the pencil?

Section D (Sit opposite the child with a coin in your right hand and a watch or bracelet on your left arm):

    a. Do you see this coin. Do I have it in my right hand or my left hand?
    b. Is this bracelet on my right arm or my left arm?

Section E (Place three objects a pencil to the left, a key in the middle, and a coin to the right in relation to the child):

    a. Is the pencil to the left or to the right of the key?
    b. Is the pencil to the left or to the right of the penny?
    c. Is the key to the left or to the right of the penny?
    d. Is the key to the left or to the right of the pencil?
    e. Is the penny to the left or to the right of the pencil?
    f. Is the penny to the left or to the right of the key?

Scoring and interpretation. The child must answer all questions correctly in each section to pass that section. Refer to Table 11.5 to obtain an age equivalent (percentile scores are not available for this test).

EVALUATION OF DIRECTIONALITY
Gardner Reversal Frequency Test: Recognition Subtest

The Gardner Reversal Frequency consists of three subtests that probe different aspects of directionality. We have selected two of the three tests for inclusion in our test battery.

APPROPRIATE AGES: 5-15

Purpose, description of test, and scoring. This test evaluates the existence, nature, and frequency of occurrence of receptive letter and number reversals (reversals that the child can recognize). In this test the child is asked to mark off those letters and numbers that are written backwards or reversed (Figure 11.3). When this test is administered, it is important to seat the child so that he cannot observe books and other written material that may provide information about letter and number orientation.

Once seated properly the child is asked to carefully work through the six lines of the test worksheet and cross out the numbers or letters that appear backward. The test is untimed, and the child is allowed to erase. Nevertheless, it is important for the examiner to observe and take into consideration the amount of time it takes and the ease with which the child complete this task. For example, if one 7-year-old completes the test in 2 minutes with 5 errors and a second child completes the test in 8 minutes with 5 errors, there is certainly a qualitative difference in performance that must be noted.

The test is scored by counting the total number of errors. Two types of errors can occur, errors of omission and errors of commission. Errors of omission refer to mistakes in which the child fails to cross out a letter or number that is printed backwards. Errors of commission refer to errors in which the child crosses out a letter or number that is actually correct. The total of the two type of errors is the raw score, which can then be converted to a percentile score by using the tables supplied in the test manual.

TABLE 11.5 Scoring criteria for the Piaget Test of Left-Right Concepts

Age	Items passed by 75% of age level
5	A
6	A
7	A C
8	A B C D
9	A B C D
10	A B C D
11	A B C D E

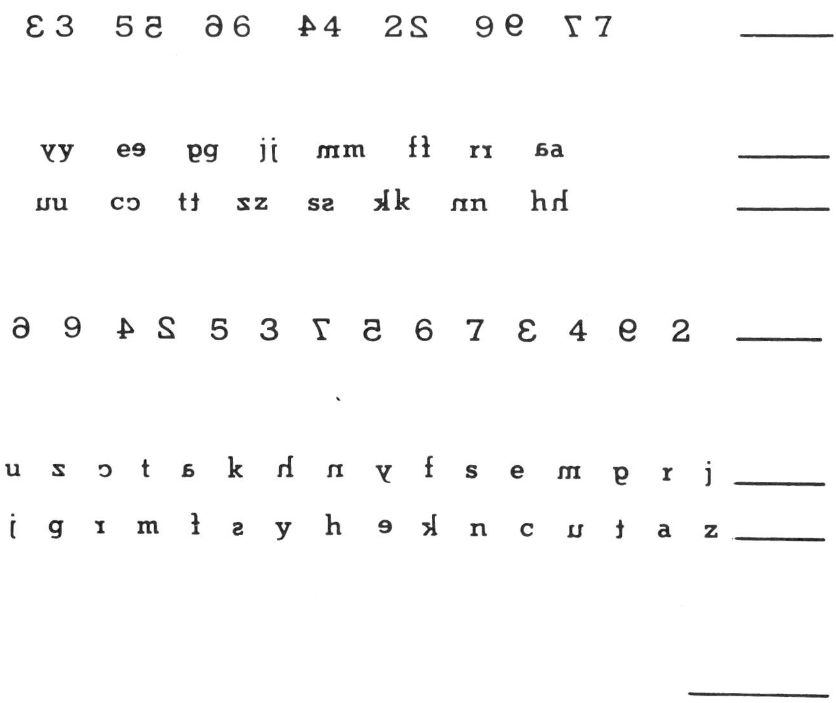

Ɛ3 5Ƨ ə6 ⱵꝐ 2Ƨ 9ə ⱵꞀ _____

ʏy eə ꮐg jį ɱm ƒꞁ ᴙɪ ꜱa _____
ɥɦ ᴎu cɔ ꞁꞁ sʐ sᴙ ʞk ᴎn ɦꞁ _____

ə 9 Ɱ Ƨ 5 3 Ꞁ ᴙ 6 7 Ɛ Ⱶ ə 2 _____

u ɔ ᴐ ꞇ ꜱ ʞ ꓔ ᴎ ʏ ʄ ꜱ ə ɱ Ꝓ ᴙ j _____
į g ᴙ m Ⱶ ꜱ y h ə ʞ n c ᴎ ꞇ ꜱ z ____

_____

FIGURE 11.3 Gardner Reversal Frequency Test—Recognition Subtest.

Important behavioral observations. In addition to obtaining a raw score, which should then be converted to a percentile score, it is important to make the following observations:

- Look for motor reinforcement such as the child tracing the letter or number in the air or attempting to write the letter or number.
- Some children will compare their responses in rows 4 to 6 to those in rows 1 to 3.
- Does the child become impulsive and careless as the test progresses?

Gardner Reversal Frequency Test: Execution Subtest

APPROPRIATE AGES: 5-15

Purpose and description and scoring. This test evaluates the existence, nature, and frequency of occurrence of expressive letter and number reversals (reversals that the child actually makes during a writing task). In this test the child is asked to write letters and numbers as they are dictated. As with the recognition subtest it is important to seat the child so that he cannot observe books and other written material that may provide information about letter and number orientation. Give the child a pencil with an eraser, place the test sheet in front of him, and ask him to print the numbers and letters you dictate. These numbers and letters are dictated one by one, and there is no time limit to this test. The letters must be reproduced as lower-case letters.

The numbers that are used include the numbers 2 5 6 3 9 4 7. After the child writes these numbers on the recording sheet the following letters are dictated one by one: h c q f j b k s r d y p t z g a e.

As with the recognition subtest it is important to remember that although the test is untimed the amount of time and ease with which the child can perform this task may indicate qualitative differences in performance that are important in diagnosis and treatment.

The test is scored by adding the number of errors. For this test there are two type of errors, reversals and unknowns. Unknowns refer to letters or numbers that the child cannot remember and therefore cannot write. Reversals refer to errors in which the child writes the letter or number in question but reverses it. If the number of total errors is greater than 16, the performance cannot be scored. If the score is less than 16, score the two types of errors separately, and the test manual provides tables that allow you to convert raw scores to percentile scores. There are separate tables for boys and for girls.

Important behavioral observations. In addition to obtaining a raw score, which should then be converted to a percentile score, it is important to make the following observations:

- Note which hand is used for writing.
- Notice if the child uses his nondominant hand to support the paper.
- Look for motor overflow.
- Does the child rotate the paper or his body?
- Is the working distance appropriate?
- Observe his pencil grip.
- Does the child make excessive erasures?
- Is the child impulsive?

Visual-analysis skills

These skills contribute to the individual's ability to analyze and discriminate visually presented information, to determine the whole without seeing all the parts, to identify more important features and ignore extraneous detail, and to use visual imagery to recall past visual information. It includes the ability of the child to be aware of the distinctive features of visual forms including shape, size, color, and orientation. Early in life a child uses visual analysis to recognize familiar faces, toys, or objects in the house. As the child approaches preschool age, he begins using visual analysis skills to analyze and comprehend more abstract shapes such as the visual symbols we use to represent sounds and quantities. Thus visual analysis skills represent one of the basic foundational skills that enable a child to learn to recognize letters and numbers and eventually whole words. These skills are also important for the development of mathematical concepts.

Clinically we subclassify visual spatial dysfunction into four categories including visual discrimination, visual figure ground, visual closure, and visual memory and visualization.

Visual discrimination is the ability of the child to be aware of the distinctive features of forms, including shape, orientation, size, and color.

Visual figure ground is the ability of the child to attend to a specific feature or form while maintaining an awareness of the relationship of this form to the background information.

Visual closure is the ability of the child to be aware of clues in the visual stimulus that allow him to determine the final percept without the necessity of having all the details present. In reading for example, visual closure allows us to perceive an entire word accurately when we may have seen only part of the word.

Visual memory and visualization is the ability of the child to recognize and recall visually presented information. Spelling requires recall of visual information, just as word recognition does in reading when we try to match the word on the page with an image that is stored in the brain. Visualization, or the ability to mentally manipulate a visual image, is important in reading comprehension and math.

EVALUATION OF VISUAL DISCRIMINATION

Test of Visual Perceptual Skills: discrimination, form constancy, and spatial relationships

APPROPRIATE AGES: 4-13

Purpose, description of test, and scoring. These three subtests evaluate the ability of the child to be aware of the distinctive features of forms including shape, orientation, and size. The three subtests are identical in their construction and administration and scoring.

Each test is made up of 16 different plates with stimuli that become more complex. Figures 11.4 to 11.6 are illustrations of one of the early

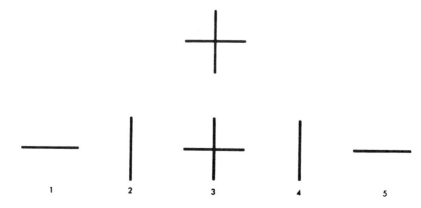

FIGURE 11.4 Test of Visual Perceptual Skills: Discrimination Subtest.

stimuli used in each of these tests. Introduce each test by telling the child that he may not be able to answer all the items correctly and that the pictures become more and more difficult. The child is asked to look at the picture on top and to find the exact form from among the forms below.

If the child correctly determines the answer to plate A, continue with the rest of the items until the child misses 4 out of 5 consecutive items. If the child cannot determine the answer to plate A, point out and explain the correct response and then proceed once the child seems to understand. It is important to prompt the child to try even if he or she is unsure.

To score the test, compute the raw score by adding up the number of correct responses. Using the TVPS scoring manual convert the raw score to a scaled score and then use Table 11.3 to convert the scaled score to a percentile rank.

When these tests are being performed, it is also important to observe the child's performance carefully and to look for the observations listed in Table 11.2.

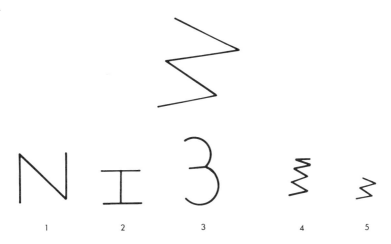

FIGURE 11.5 Test of Visual Perceptual Skills: Form Constancy Subtest.

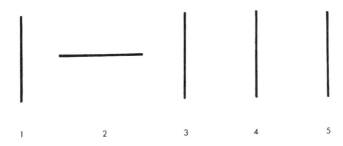

FIGURE 11.6 Test of Visual Perceptual Skills: Spatial Relationships Subtest.

EVALUATION OF VISUAL CLOSURE

Test of Visual Perceptual Skills: Closure

APPROPRIATE AGES: 4-13

Purpose and description and scoring. This subtest evaluates the ability of the child to be aware of clues in the visual stimulus that allow him to determine the final percept without the necessity of having all the details present The test is made up of 16 different plates with stimuli that become more complex. Figure 11.7 is an illustration of one of the early stimuli used in this test. The child is asked to look at the picture on top and to find the one that would look like the top form if the lines were connected or completed.

If the child correctly determines the answer to plate A, continue with the rest of the items until the child misses 3 out of 4 consecutive items. If the child cannot determine the answer to plate A, point out and explain the correct response and then proceed once the child seems to understand. Prompt the child to try even if he or she is unsure.

This subtest of the TVPS is scored as described above for other subtests of the TVPS. When this test is being performed, it is also important to

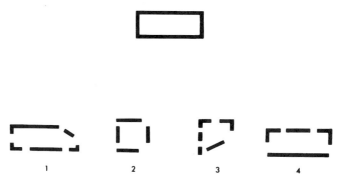

FIGURE 11.7 Test of Visual Perceptual Skills: Closure Subtest.

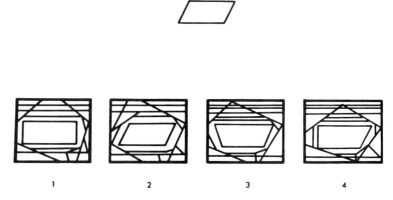

FIGURE 11.8 Test of Visual Perceptual Skills: Figure Ground Subtest.

observe the child's performance carefully and to look for the observations listed in Table 11.2.

EVALUATION OF VISUAL FIGURE GROUND

Test of Visual Perceptual Skills: Figure Ground

APPROPRIATE AGES: 4-13

Purpose and description and scoring. This subtest evaluates the ability of the child to attend to a specific feature or form while maintaining an awareness of the relationship of this form to the background information. The test is made up of 16 different plates with stimuli that become more complex. Figure 11.8 is an illustration of one of the early stimuli used in this test. The child is asked to look at the picture on top and to find the exact form from among the forms below.

If the child correctly determines the answer to plate A, continue with the rest of the items until the child misses 3 out of 4 consecutive items. If the child cannot determine the answer to plate A, point out and explain the correct response and then proceed once the child seems to understand. Prompt the child to try even if he or she is unsure.

This subtest of the TVPS is scored as described above for other subtests of the TVPS. When this test is being performed, it is also important to observe the child's performance carefully and to look for the observations listed in Table 11.2.

EVALUATING VISUAL MEMORY AND VISUALIZATION

Test of Visual Perceptual Skills: Visual Memory

APPROPRIATE AGES: 4-13

Purpose and description and scoring. This subtest evaluates the ability of the child to recognize and recall visually presented information. The test is made up of 16 different plates with stimuli that become more complex. Figure 11.9 is an illustration of one of the early stimuli used in this test. The child is asked to look at an isolated picture for 5 seconds. After

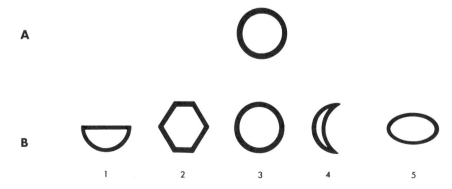

FIGURE 11.9 Test of Visual Perceptual Skills: Visual Memory Subtest. **A,** Isolated figure. **B,** That figure among five choices.

the stimulus is removed, he or she is asked to select the one that looks the same from among 5 choices.

If the child correctly determines the answer to plate A, continue with the rest of the items until the child misses 4 out of 5 consecutive items. If the child cannot determine the answer to plate A, point out and explain the correct response and then proceed once the child seems to understand. Prompt the child to try even if he or she is unsure.

This subtest of the TVPS is scored as described above for other subtests of the TVPS. When this test is being performed, it is also important to observe the child's performance carefully and to look for the observations listed in Table 11.2.

Test of Visual Perceptual Skills: Visual Sequential Memory

APPROPRIATE AGES: 4-13

Purpose and description and scoring. This subtest evaluates the ability of the child to recognize and recall visually presented information when sequence is important, as in spelling.

The test is made up of 16 different plates with stimuli that become more complex. Figure 11.10 is an illustration of one of the early stimuli used in this test. The child is asked to look at a series of pictures for 5 seconds. After the stimulus is removed, he or she is asked to select the one that has the same sequence from among 5 choices.

If the child correctly determines the answer to plate A, continue with the rest of the items until the child misses 4 out of 5 consecutive items. If the child cannot determine the answer to plate A, point out and explain the correct response and then proceed once the child seems to understand. Prompt the child to try even if he or she is unsure.

The time allowed for the child to view each plate varies depending on the number of forms in the sequence.

- 2 to 3 forms in sequence: 5 seconds
- 3 to 5 forms in sequence: 9 seconds
- 4 to 7 forms in sequence: 12 seconds
- 5 to 9 forms in sequence: 14 seconds

This subtest of the TVPS is scored as described above for other subtests of the TVPS. When this test is being performed, it is also important to

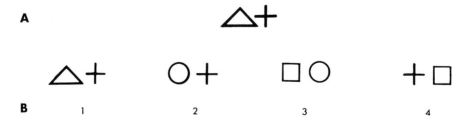

FIGURE 11.10 Test of Visual Perceptual Skills: Visual Sequential Memory. **A,** Isolated figure. **B,** That figure among four choices.

observe the child's performance carefully and to look for the observations listed in Table 11.2.

Visual-motor integration skills

These skills are related to the individual's ability to integrate visual information processing skills with fine-motor movement. Another term for visual-motor integration is eye-hand coordination. A very concrete example of a task requiring eye-hand coordination is catching a ball. A child must make many visual judgments about the ball including speed and direction and then translate the visual judgments into appropriate motor responses of his hand and body. If the visual-motor integration is accurate, the child will catch the ball.

A more abstract and higher level example of visual-motor integration is handwriting. As a child begins to write a letter, there is no external stimulus that guides his hand. Rather, he must use his "mind's eye" to guide his hand in the desired direction and pattern. As the written product emerges, the child must continuously use visual analysis skills to judge whether the shape or size of the letter is appropriate. He must also use fine-motor skills to manipulate the pencil. If he can accurately integrate (or combine) his visual analysis skills and his fine motor skill, the desired letter will be successfully completed. Thus visual-motor skills are a necessary prerequisite for learning good handwriting and keyboard skills as well as throwing and catching a ball.

The two subskills in this category are fine-motor coordination and visual-motor integration

Visual-motor integration skills are related to the individual's ability to integrate visual information processing skills with fine-motor movement.

Fine-motor skills are the ability to manipulate small objects or a pencil or pen.

EVALUATING VISUAL-MOTOR INTEGRATION
Developmental Test of Visual Motor Integration (Beery)

APPROPRIATE AGES: 3-15

Purpose, description of test, and scoring. This test evaluates the child's ability to integrate visual information processing and fine-motor skills by assessment of his ability to accurately copy a visual stimulus. The child is presented with pictures of increasing complexity and is asked to reproduce the pictures as accurately as possible. Figure 11.11 is a sample of some of the forms used in this test.

When this test is administered, the following issues are important:

- Keep the test booklet and the child's body centered with the desk and the booklet throughout the testing.
- Do not let the child trace the picture.
- Avoid calling the form by any descriptive name, such as a "diamond."

- Record your observations inconspicuously.
- Erasures or second tries are not allowed.

To score the test, use the very detailed scoring criteria that are included in the scoring manual. Testing should be discontinued after 3 consecutive incorrect responses. Each test form has a value from 1 to 4 depending on its complexity. Follow the scoring manual to determine the appropriate score for each correct form. The raw score is the total of all correct forms, and this score can be converted to a percentile score using Table 4 in the VMI manual.

Important behavioral observations

- Is the working distance close?
- Observe the pencil grip.
- Does the child use excessive finger tension?
- Is there motor overflow, tongue, head?
- Does the child rotate the body or paper?
- Which hand is used to hold the pencil?
- Does the child recognize mistakes?
- Can the child correct mistakes on second trial?
- Is the nonwriting hand involved in the task?

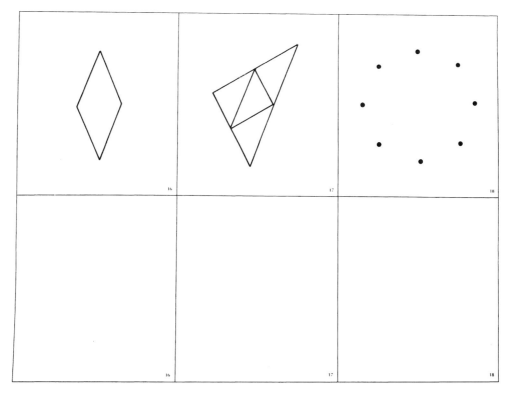

FIGURE 11.11 Developmental Test of Visual Motor Integration (Beery). (Modern Curriculum Press.)

Wold Sentence Copy Test

Purpose, description of test, and scoring. This test evaluates the child's fine-motor and visual-motor integration skills. The Wold Sentence Copy Test is a timed test used to determine a child's speed and accuracy in copying a sentence from the top to the bottom of a page (Figure 11.12). The test is comparable to a common school task of copying from a book to a notebook and provides the clinician with a sample of the child's handwriting skill.

To administer this test, place the test sheet in front of the child and tell the child to copy the sentence on the blank lines on the bottom of the test sheet. Tell the child to go as fast as he or she can but to be as neat as possible.

Important points

1. The child can be told to use either printing or cursive, whichever is preferred.

Four men and a jolly boy came out of

the black and pink house quickly to see

the bright violet sun, but the sun was

hidden behind a cloud

_____

_____

_____

_____

_____

_____

_____

Name _____ Age _____ Time_____

FIGURE 11.12 Wold Sentence Copy Test.

2. Start timing when the child begins.
3. Note where the child is at 1 minute.
4. The test can be discontinued at the 1-minute point or the child can be allowed to finish the sentence.
5. Do not allow the test to continue past 3 minutes or if the child is obviously frustrated by the task.

To score this test, count the total number of letters copied in 1 minute. Convert this raw score into a grade equivalent using Table 11.6.

Important behavioral observations
- Is the working distance close?
- Observe the pencil grip.
- Does the child lose his place excessively?
- Does the child use subvocalization?
- Is there motor overflow, tongue, head?
- Are there excessive erasures?
- Does the child rotate the body or paper?
- Note how many letters are copied after each fixation. Does the child look at each letter and copy it, or can he copy a word or several words after one fixation?
- Note the spacing of the letters and words. Is spacing consistent? Do the letters stay on the lines?
- Check for omissions or substitutions of words and letters. Are the letters and words in the proper order? Are any letters reversed?
- Note the formation of the letters. Are the lower-case and capital letters appropriately sized relative to each other?

EVALUATING FINE-MOTOR SKILLS

Grooved Pegboard Test

APPROPRIATE AGES: KINDERGARTEN TO FIFTH GRADE

Purpose, description of test, and scoring. This test evaluates the child's fine-motor skills. Other skills that are indirectly evaluated are visual attention, concentration, and directionality. The test requires the child to place pegs in a pegboard as quickly as possible (Figure 11.13). Before ad-

TABLE 11.6   Scoring criteria for the Wold Sentence Copy Test

Grade level	Letters per minute
1	20-25
2	30
3	40
4	50
5	60
6	67
7	75
8	80

Conversion from raw score to grade equivalent

ministration of the test, establish hand dominance by asking the child to demonstrate how he brushes his teeth, hammers a nail, cuts with a scissors, writes with a pencil, and throws a ball. The examiner tries to establish which hand is used for these activities. The dominant hand is the one that is used for the majority of the tasks.

Once the dominant hand is determined, tell the patient to place the pegs in the holes by matching the groove of the peg to the groove of the hole. Let the child try the first row to demonstrate that he or she understands the task. Once he or she understands the task, ask the child to place all the pegs in the holes as quickly as possible.

The raw score is the time in seconds required to complete the task. Use Table 11.7 to convert the raw score to percentiles.

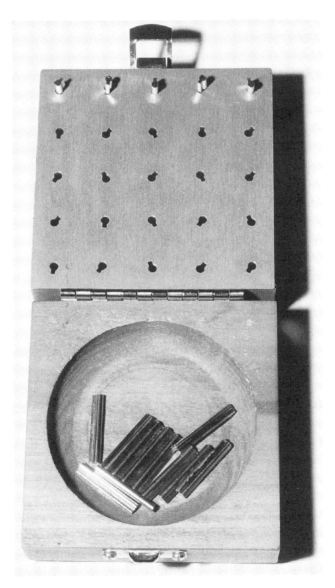

FIGURE 11.13 Grooved Pegboard Test.

Important behavioral observations
- Observe the dexterity with which the child picks up the pegs.
- Does he pick up all the pegs with one hand or does he use both hands?
- Does he cross the midline?
- Does he transfer the peg to the other hand and than insert the peg?
- Does the child orient the peg in his fingers and align the groove before inserting or does he try to force the peg into the holes?
- While inserting pegs, does the child demonstrate a tactile approach or a more visual approach?

Auditory-visual integration skills

These skills allow the child to equate a temporally distributed auditory stimulus to a spatially distributed visual stimulus. At least two important skills may contribute to inadequacy or problems in this area. The first is the ability to remember and identify the sequence and spacing of sounds. The second is the ability to integrate the auditory and visual modalities.

EVALUATING AUDITORY-VISUAL SKILLS
Auditory-Visual Integration Test
APPROPRIATE AGES: 6-15

Purpose, description of test, and scoring. This test evaluates the child's ability to equate a temporally distributed auditory stimulus to a spatially distributed visual stimulus. In other words, can a child match an auditory and a visual representation of the same stimulus? Reading is dependent on the child's ability to match a visual stimulus (letter) to an auditory stimulus (the sound the letter represents). There are at least two important skills that are being probed with this test. The first skill being evaluated is the ability to identify and remember the sequence and spacing of sounds. The second skill being assessed is the ability to integrate the auditory and the visual modalities.

TABLE 11.7 Scoring Criteria for the Grooved Pegboard Test

Percentile	Raw score (seconds)			
	Kindergarten	Grade 1	Grade 2	Grades 4 and 5
95	83	64	62	52
90	86	69	65	55
80	90	73	67	58
75	93	74	68	58
70	96	76	69	60
60	100	80	72	63
50	110	83	75	65
40	119	86	80	67
30	123	90	84	69
25	128	92	85	70
20	133	95	87	72
10	143	100	96	76
5	153	122	100	78

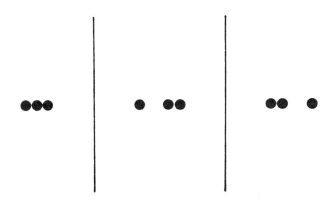

FIGURE 11.14 Auditory-Visual Integration Test. Demonstration Card A.

The test begins with three demonstration cards, A, B, and C. The examiner shows card A (Figure 11.14) to the child and asks the child to listen to the sound as he taps out the three patterns on the card. These patterns include two close dots, two dots separated farther apart, and three dots close together.

Once the child understands this concept the examiner asks the child to look at card B and, after listening to a pattern being tapped out, to identify the correct pattern.

Finally the examiner taps out a pattern, and the child has to listen and then identify the pattern tapped out on card C.

When this test is being administered, it is important that the hand used to tap out the patterns be hidden from the child's view. The first 10 cards are used for children up to and through 10 years of age, whereas 20 cards are used for children 11 to 15 years of age.

To score the test, determine the raw score by adding the number of correct responses. Convert the raw score to percentiles using Table 11.8.

Important behavioral observations
- Observe the child's response. Is it reflective, impulsive, random?
- Observe the child's strategy. Did he count the taps, verbalize?
- Were there any reversals?

ANALYSIS AND DIAGNOSIS

Diagnosis is based on a careful analysis of the case history, the actual test results, observation of the child's performance, and a review of all previous reports and testing.

Case history

The case history is used to learn about the main concerns of the parent and child. As we have stressed throughout this book, it is critical to establish as specifically as possible what type of learning or school problems the child is experiencing. In Chapter 5 Dr. Flax discussed the importance of defining the nature of the learning problem. For example, the chief complaint may be a "reading problem." Is this reading problem a failure to

TABLE 11.8   Scoring criteria for Auditory-Visual Integration Test

Grade and age	Kindergarten (5 to 6)	Grade 1 (6 to 7)	Grade 2 (7 to 8)	Grades 4 and 5 (9 to 11)
Percentile	Raw score			
95	8	10	10	20
90	8	9	—	20
80	7	9	—	19
75	—	—	—	—
70	6	8	—	18
60	—	7	9	18
50	5	7	—	17
40	—	6	8	16
30	4	6	—	15
25	—	—	—	—
20	—	5	7	14
10	3	5	6	12
5	—	4	5	11
Mean	**5.1**	**6.8**	**8.2**	**16.6**
Standard deviation	**1.7**	**1.9**	**1.6**	**3.1**

learn to read, or is it an inability to read lengthy assignments at a more sophisticated level? Is it a failure to recall previously encountered words, or is it an inability to utilize phonetic analysis to decode an unfamiliar word? This is the type of information that we must acquire through the case history. Chapters 5 to 7 and 9 review these issues in great detail, and an understanding of this information creates a solid foundation for diagnosis and analysis of the results of the visual information processing evaluation.

Each of the four major categories of visual information processing disorders, visual-spatial dysfunction, visual-analysis dysfunction, visual-motor dysfunction, and auditory-visual integration dysfunction, have characteristic signs and symptoms that can be elicited from the case history.

Children who have difficulty with visual-spatial skills may not know their right from their left, exhibit excessive reversals of letters and numbers when writing, be clumsy or accident prone, or have difficulty riding a bike or throwing a ball.

Problems in visual-analysis skills may cause difficulty learning to recognize letters and numbers consistently, identifying words when reading (sight-word recognition), or spelling properly.

Children with visual-motor integration difficulties often have difficulty with handwriting, copying from the board, and organizing written material on the page. Handwriting may be slow or sloppy, with inconsistent spacing and sizing of letters. Words or letters may be omitted during copying. Sometimes a child will be able verbally to spell a word correctly but misspell it when writing the word.

Children with auditory-visual integration dysfunction will present with many representative signs and symptoms such as difficulty sounding out words when reading, poor spelling ability, and difficulty relating symbols to their relevant sounds

The box on p. 303 has a more complete list of the characteristic signs and symptoms associated with each type of visual information processing disorder.

Analysis of Visual Information Processing Test results

Norms, expected findings, means, and standard deviations have all been established for the tests we reviewed in this chapter. Significant deviation from the expected findings indicate problems in that particular area. It is important to understand, therefore, how we define a significant deviation from expected findings.

When standardized, objective testing is used, a significant deviation is generally defined as performance greater than 1 standard deviation from the mean, or a significant deviation from the individual's overall level of function.[3] We have recommended conversion of all raw scores to percentile ranks when possible (only age equivalents are available for the Standing Angels in the Snow, the Piaget Test of Left-Right Concepts, and the Wold Sentence Copy Test). Table 11.3 indicates that a score below the 15th percentile is greater than 1 standard deviation below the mean and a score above the 85th percentile is greater than 1 standard deviation above the mean. Thus the general rule is that we consider a score to be significantly low if the patient scores below the 15th percentile on any given test. There are some exceptions, however, to this general rule.

1. Scores between the 15th percentile and the 50th percentile are considered suspicious findings and may be clinically significant when compared to the child's overall level of functioning.

It is certainly possible for a child to have a series of suspicious test scores all falling below the 50th percentile yet not have any score below the 15th percentile. In such a situation, clinical interpretation depends on analysis of the specific learning problem and the child's overall cognitive and intellectual functioning. For example, if previous testing indicates that the child has an above-average IQ (above the 50th percentile), a large number of suspicious scores between the 15th percentile and the 50th percentile become clinically significant. On the other hand, if previous testing revealed a below-average IQ (below the 50th percentile), a large number of suspicious scores between the 15th percentile and the 50th percentile simply indicate that the child is performing at an expected level.

2. Scores at or above the 50th percentile are generally considered normal but may be clinically significant when compared to the child's overall level of functioning.

If previous testing indicates that the child is very bright and has scored, for example, at the 95th percentile on IQ testing, scores that fall significantly below that level may be considered abnormal relative to the child's overall capability. Thus scores falling at the 50th percentile for such a child may be indicative of a visual information processing disorder for this child.

When interpreting the results of visual motor integration tests such as the Developmental Test of Visual Motor Integration, one must consider three possible reasons for inadequate performance.

The child may have difficulty copying the design because he has a visual analysis dysfunction. If the child cannot adequately analyze the stimulus, he will be unable to make an accurate reproduction.

The poor performance may have been secondary to a fine-motor problem. Thus, even if the child is able to analyze the stimulus adequately and has normal visual-motor integration skills, if his fine-motor coordination is poor, the reproduction may be inaccurate. One can rule out this issue by administering the Grooved Pegboard Test. Adequate performance on this test indicates normal fine-motor skills.

Finally, a child may perform poorly on visual-motor integration testing even if fine-motor coordination and visual-analysis skills are adequate. If testing indicates normal functioning in both of these areas the deficiency is in the area of visual-motor integration.

Analysis of behavioral observations

It is not enough to just look at a child's test scores to arrive at a diagnosis. Behavioral observations refer to behaviors that the child exhibits during testing that can be directly observed by the clinician. These behaviors provide us with clues about how the child arrives at his answer or response. Certain behavioral observations can indicate that the child is using an inappropriate or inefficient strategy. They may also be suggestive of the level of effort and energy that a child needs to exert to perform a task. This information can be used to predict when a child's performance is likely to break down as the task increases in complexity or duration.

The following are some of the key behavioral signs and symptoms for each visual information processing category.

Visual-spatial skills. On the Standing Angels in the Snow test, the behavioral observation called "motor overflow" refers to the child's inability to limit his movement to only the parts of his body that he is instructed to move. For example, when asked to move his right arm, the child with motor overflow may move both arms or even a foot on the same side. This indicates a possible difficulty with bilateral integration and, when combined with the child's actual score, will help us predict how the child would perform with activities in which both sides of the body must perform a different function.

Visual-analysis skills. A common behavioral observation seen when one is evaluating visual-analysis skills is a child's tracing over the test figure with his finger before responding. This type of response indicates that the child needs tactile or kinesthetic reinforcement to aid visual judgment. This may make learning letters and numbers slower and less consistent because a child is expected to use primarily a visual approach to these tasks by the time he is in first grade.

Visual-motor integration skills. There are several important and interesting behaviors to observe during visual-motor integration testing. A poor pencil grip or excessive finger tension can be a sign of poor fine-motor skills. Such behaviors can quickly fatigue a child and result in sloppy or slow performance when copying from the board or writing. A child who rotates his body when copying a shape on the Developmental Test of Visual Motor Integration or who moves his whole arm instead of just his hand and wrist is exhibiting motor overflow. A child with a very close working distance is likely to display inefficient performance on a prolonged visual-motor integration task.

These behaviors can contribute to a diagnosis of a visual-motor integration deficit when analyzed along with depressed scores. Such observations can also support a diagnosis of a subtle disorder when test scores are in the borderline range.

Review of previous testing

In addition to the information that you acquire orally from the parent and patient during the case history, the tests, and behavioral observations, it is important to review previous educational and psychological testing. Much of the detail that parents will not remember or understand can be found in these reports. Chapter 12 reviews the educational and psychological evaluation in detail. Reading this chapter should enable you to understand and interpret educational and psychological reports. Reviewing these reports is often a critical part of the process of defining the nature of the learning problem.

Based on the history and review of previous testing the clinician will generally be able to establish one or more clinical hypotheses. The evaluation of visual information processing skills is designed to confirm or deny these clinical hypotheses and lead to a diagnosis. It is very important to understand that for the test results to have any real meaning they must be related to the case history and the child's specific problems. Test results from the visual information processing evaluation can generally be interpreted in several ways when reviewed in isolation. For example, a child scoring between the 15th percentile and the 25th percentile on all tests may have a visual information processing problem. Alternatively, the child may be performing adequately based on his overall intellectual potential. The only way for the clinician to make this distinction is to review previous psychological and educational testing. If previous psychoeducational testing reveals that the child has a low-average IQ (between the 15th percentile and 50th percentile), performance on the visual information processing evaluation in the same percentile range is merely consistent with the child's overall potential and may not indicate a problem.

The important underlying concept is that the significance of the actual test results can be established only in relationship to the case history and after the nature of the child's learning problem is defined. This concept is true in the diagnostic process for visual information processing disorders or for any other visual, ocular, or medical disorder.

CASE STUDY

When the results of the evaluation are being analyzed, it is important to be as specific as possible about the diagnosis. For example, the test results listed below were found with a 7-year, 6-month-old boy in the second grade. The case history revealed that he was having great difficulty with tasks involving copying from the board or from a book to his desk. When asked questions and allowed to respond orally, his performance improved. However, when asked to respond in writing, his performance was considerably poorer. He also tended to reverse letters and numbers more frequently than his classmates did. Previous psychoeducational testing revealed an IQ of 118 (this is greater than 1 standard deviation above the norm).

The results of his visual information processing examination are illustrated below.

VISUAL SPATIAL SKILLS	Test	Score
Bilateral integration	Standing Angels in the Snow	7-year level
Laterality	Piaget Test of Left-Right Concepts	7-year level
Directionality	Gardner Reversal Frequency Test:	
	Recognition Subtest	5th percentile
	Execution Subtest	15th percentile
VISUAL-ANALYSIS SKILLS		
Visual discrimination	TVPS: Visual Discrimination	63th percentile
Visual closure	TVPS: Visual Closure	50th percentile
Visual form constancy	TVPS: Visual Form Constancy	63th percentile
Visual figure ground	TVPS: Visual Figure Ground	63th percentile
Visual spatial relations	TVPS: Visual Spatial Relations	37th percentile
Visual memory	TVPS: Visual Memory	63th percentile
	TVPS: Visual Sequential Memory	75th percentile
VISUAL-MOTOR INTEGRATION		
Visual-motor integration	Developmental Test of Visual Motor Integration	25th percentile
Fine-motor skills	Grooved Pegboard	50th percentile
	Wold Sentence Copy Test	First grade
AUDITORY-VISUAL INTEGRATION SKILLS		
Auditory-visual integration	Auditory-Visual Integration Test	84th percentile

If we apply the general rule that any score below the 15th percentile is suggestive of an area of weakness, these results indicates difficulty in the broad categories of visual-spatial skills and visual-motor integration skills. It is important to be more specific, however. Within these two broad areas some subskills were normal whereas others were abnormal. In the area of visual-spatial skills, bilateral integration and laterality were at age level or at the 50th percentile. Directionality skills, however, were below the 15th percentile as evaluated with both the recognition and execution subtests of the Gardner Reversal Frequency Test.

Visual-motor integration testing revealed significant weaknesses in visual-motor integration, whereas fine-motor skills were normal.

Applying only the general rule that scores below the 15th percentile are significant would yield a diagnosis of directionality problems only. However, it is important in this case and all others to also consider the child's overall level of functioning. For this child, previous IQ testing revealed that he has above-average intelligence. Clinically, this indicates that borderline or suspicious scores may be significant for this child. Specifically the 37th percentile score in visual-spatial relations and the 25th percentile score in visual-motor integration should be considered significantly low for this child

The diagnosis in this case would be visual information processing dysfunction with specific weaknesses in:

- directionality
- visual-spatial relations
- visual-motor integration

A vision therapy program would then be developed to treat the specific areas of deficiency.

PRIMARY CARE SCREENING BATTERY FOR DETECTION AND REFERRAL

The comprehensive visual information processing evaluation described above will enable a practitioner to evaluate these skills, reach a specific diagnosis, and plan a treatment program for the patient. For clinicians choosing to become involved with learning-related vision problems in a more limited way, a screening battery can be utilized.

If the objective is simply detection of a visual information processing disorder, we suggest using only the Gardner Reversal Frequency Test (Recognition Subtest) and the Developmental Test of Visual Motor Integration. Like all screening approaches, some children with problems may be missed. However, in our experience most problems will be detected when this approach is used. If a problem is detected, the clinician should refer the child to an optometrist with more expertise in this area to provide a comprehensive evaluation, diagnosis, and treatment.

SUMMARY

We have presented an organized approach to the evaluation of visual information processing disorders and demonstrated that the process of assessing visual information processing skills and reaching a diagnosis is comparable in many ways to that used for visual efficiency skills and other aspects of optometric care.

In this chapter we have also introduced a classification of visual information processing disorders, including characteristics, signs, and symptoms for each. The test battery presented allows the clinician to elicit information about each diagnostic category. An important objective of this evaluation system is that it is designed to assess systematically the strengths and weaknesses of the child's visual information processing leading to an appropriate therapy program to deal with each deficient area.

CHAPTER REVIEW

1. Describe the similarities between the diagnosis of visual efficiency and visual information processing disorders.
2. What are the advantages of using standardized testing for the evaluation of visual information processing disorders?
3. Name three different derived scores and describe the advantages and disadvantages of each.
4. What is considered to be an average percentile? At what percentile score do we believe that a clinical problem is present?
5. How do we relate the results of the visual information processing evaluation to tests results from IQ testing?
6. Describe the various reasons why a child would possibly have difficulty copying a shape from the Developmental Test of Visual Motor Integration?
7. What are the key behavioral observations clinicians should be aware of for visual-spatial, visual-analysis, and visual-motor integration testing?
8. Practice the administration and scoring of each core test and auxiliary test in our visual information processing evaluation on a child. After the administration determine the raw score and then convert the raw score to a percentile score.

SOURCES OF VISUAL INFORMATION PROCESSING EVALUATION TESTS

1. Creative Therapeutics
   155 County Rd
   Cresskill, NJ 07626
   (800)-544-6162

   Gardner Reversal Frequency Test

2. Psychological and
   Educational Publications,
   1477 Rollins Rd
   Burlingame, CA 94010
   (800)-523-5775

   Test of Visual Perceptual Skills (TVPS)

3. Vision Extension
2912 South Daimler Street,
Suite 100
Santa Ana, CA 92705-5811
(714)-250-0846

Developmental Test Of Visual Motor
 Integration
Wold Sentence Copy test

4. Lafayette Instruments Co., Inc
P.O. Box 5729
Sagamore Parkway
Lafayette, IN 47903
(800)-428-7545

Grooved Pegboard

5. Bernell Corp.
750 Lincolnway E.
P.O. Box 4637
South Bend, IN 46634
(800)-348-225

Auditory-Visual Integration Test

REFERENCES

1. Richman J: *Visual Development Profile*, Philadelphia, 1972, Pennsylvania College of Optometry.
2. Hoffman LG: *An optometric learning disabilities evaluation*, Part I, 78-81, February 1979; Part II, 77-82, March 1979; Part III, 70-77, April 1979.
3. Solan HA, Groffman S: Understanding and treating developmental and perceptual motor disabilities. In Solan HA, editor: *The treatment and management of children with learning disabilities*, Springfield, Ill, 1982, Charles C Thomas.
4. Suchoff IB: *Visual spatial development in the child: an optometric theoretical and clinical approach*, New York, 1981, State University of New York.
5. Roach EG, Kephart NC: *The Purdue perceptual motor survey*, Columbus, Ohio, 1966, Charles E. Merrill.
6. Rosner J, Richman V: *The identification of children with perceptual motor dysfunction*, Pittsburgh, Penn, 1968, Division of Mental Health Services, Pittsburgh Public Schools.
7. Gesell A, Bullis GE: *Vision: its development in infant and child*, New York, 1949, Paul Hober, Inc.
8. Kephart NC: *The slow learner in the classroom*, Columbus, Ohio, 1960, Charles E. Merrill.
9. Getman GN: *Techniques and diagnostic criteria for the optometric care of children's vision*, Duncan, Okla, 1960, Optometric Extension Program Foundation, Inc.
10. Piaget J, Inhelder B: *The child's conception of space*, New York, 1967, The Norton Library.
11. Weinstein M: A rational of vision and visual behavior, *J Am Optom Assoc* 38(12):1029-1033, 1967.
12. Solan HA, Suchoff IB: *Test and measurements for behavioral optometrists*, Santa Ana, Calif, 1991, Optometric Extension Program.
13. Gardner RA: *The objective diagnosis of minimal brain dysfunction*, Cresskill, NJ, 1979, Creative Therapeutics.

CHAPTER 12

Psychoeducational Evaluation

PENNI BLASKEY
RICHARD SELZNICK

KEY TERMS

psychoeducational testing	Wechsler Intelligence Scale–III
attention-deficit hyperactivity disorder (ADHD)	(WISC-III)
	expressive language
learning disability	receptive language
cognitive functioning	memory testing
academic achievement	attention and concentration
emotional functioning	decoding
intelligence quotient (IQ)	projective testing

Parents frequently bring their child to an optometrist wanting to know whether their child's academic difficulties might be related in some way to an underlying vision problem. At times, the school or a private psychologist has already done psychoeducational testing, and the parents present the report as one piece of information for the optometrist to integrate into his or her findings. At other times the child has received no testing, and the optometrist is the first professional consulted about the academic difficulties. The optometrist must be familiar with the process of psychoeducational testing to answer the parents' questions, to know when to refer for further testing, to explain what the family should expect from testing if none has been done, and to be part of the decision-making process regarding when to intervene if a vision problem is suspected of contributing to the learning problem. In addition, not all psychological reports are written in language that a "nonpsychologist" would be able to understand. Thus, at times, the parent may be unclear about what the psychologist has said and written and is seeking help from the optometrist in interpreting the findings stated in the report. This is particularly true when the psychologist has indicated to the parent that the child has visual perceptual problems.

The objectives of this chapter are to review the basic components of the psychoeducational evaluation and to discuss the important issues, testing instruments and relevance of each component. An understanding of this information is essential for management of learning-related vision problems.

Psychoeducational evaluations are usually performed by a certified school psychologist, a psychologist who has specialized in school-related issues. In some states the entire evaluation is divided into two components, with the psychologist doing the cognitive and emotional testing and a learning specialist doing the educational and academic testing. Based on the results of this basic evaluation the psychologist may refer the child for more extensive testing in a particular area. Examples of areas that might require additional testing are speech and language, more extensive visual perceptual testing, and neurological and medical evaluations to rule out attention-deficit hyperactivity disorder. The psychologist must integrate all the information from other professionals and help the parents and teacher implement appropriate methods that will allow the child to function successfully.

A child is usually referred for psychoeducational testing because of academic or behavioral problems at school and at home. The parents and teachers want to know what is causing the problem or problems and how to ameliorate them. As discussed in other chapters of this book, it is clear that learning and behavior problems can be caused by a myriad of factors. The psychologist must explore each possible contributing factor listed in the box to assure that areas are not missed.

For example, even the best reading remediation plan will not be effective if the child is very hyperactive and cannot sit still long enough to concentrate. If, in addition, he is depressed because of repeated school failures and negative interaction with his parents, the reading program and possible stimulant medication for the hyperactivity might also not be enough. The self-esteem issues and depression must also be addressed. The evaluation process can be viewed as a puzzle, with each piece needing to be put into place to help achieve the finished product.

Often parents will start the process of determining why their child is having academic problems with the optometrist. No information will be available, other than possible school reports such as report cards and parent observations. The optometrist may carry out his testing and find that a problem exists, either in the visual efficiency area or visual-perceptual area. However, to begin treatment based only on the results of the vision evaluation is inadvisable. Rather, a psychoeducational evaluation should be recommended to determine the child's level of functioning in other areas. Without this additional information, many potential problems (see box) may be overlooked.

Contributory Factors to Learning Problems

Neurological processing problems

Visual processing
Auditory processing
Linguistic comprehension and expression

Memory

Attention and concentration problems

Physiological problems

Vision problems
Hearing problems
Allergies
Coordination, gross/fine-motor problems
Other medical problems
Nutrition

Emotional disturbance

Anxiety disorders
Depression
Conduct disorders

Interpersonal factors

Parent-child relationships
Marital discord
Peer relationships

Educational issues

Readiness for instruction
Match between teaching style and student's learning needs
Classroom environment

Environmental issues

Poverty
Chaotic home circumstances
Access to adequate education
Emotional trauma, such as abuse

A common example is a case in which visual-perceptual testing reveals significant deficits. One potential explanation for poor performance on visual-perceptual testing is overall cognitive problems. For example, a child with an IQ of 68 is by definition mentally retarded and would generally have difficulty with visual-perceptual testing. Another example is when a visual efficiency problem is found in a child with a learning disability. The optometrist may hypothesize that the visual efficiency problem is the basis of the sixth grader's reading problems. However, the child's decoding and language skills may be poorly developed, and these need to be addressed along with the visual efficiency problem. In another example, a significant visual efficiency problem may be contributing to the child's difficulty concentrating on reading. The child may also be in a chaotic family situation with many personal problems. Correcting the visual efficiency problem may not alleviate the concentration problem entirely, leaving the optometrist wondering why the child is still having difficulty when reading.

It is therefore important for the optometrist to recommend psychoeducational testing either through the school or from a private psychologist who specializes in learning problems. Only then will the optometrist know whether to intervene at all and at what point in the total remediation plan will intervention have the most chance of success.

BASIC COMPONENTS OF PSYCHOEDUCATIONAL TESTING

A standard psychoeducational evaluation consists of four major components. The first component is a comprehensive history gathered through parent and child interviews and the use of questionnaires. It is important to understand that the actual testing process is an artificial situation in which the child may not display typical behavior. The additional information received from the history and questionnaire therefore is useful in developing an accurate understanding of the child's performance in other settings. Also, because the parents and teachers are important members of the treatment team, their perspectives are essential.

Once the appropriate history has been gathered and rapport established, the formal testing process begins. A comprehensive psychoeducational evaluation probes four broad areas, including history, cognitive functioning, academic achievement, and emotional functioning. The box on the next page lists the different areas evaluated for each category.

Each area is relevant to the overall functioning of a child and will be reviewed in greater detail. In most states, to be classified as learning disabled (Chapter 4) and to receive special education services, a discrepancy must exist between a child's aptitude, or intellectual level, and actual level of academic achievement.[1] Thus both intellectual level and academic achievement must be assessed thoroughly to make that determination. Furthermore, for the academic underachievement to be considered a learning disability, the academic problems must not be attributable primarily to emotional disturbance, vision, hearing problems, or environmental deprivation. Such difficulties, however, may exist along with the learning disability. As a result, from the perspective of qualification for services, these areas also must be understood thoroughly.

Another important reason for evaluating cognitive functioning, academic achievement, and emotional functioning is related to development of appropriate remediation methods. As mentioned previously, all areas of functioning are interrelated and must be considered for treatment methods to be effective.

Four Components of a Psychological Evaluation

History

Cognitive functioning

IQ level
Language skills
Attention and concentration
Memory
Visual-perceptual skills
Auditory-perceptual skills
Cognitive style
Processing speed

Academic achievement

Reading—decoding and comprehension
Mathematics
Spelling
Writing—handwriting, paragraph composition, thematic maturity, grammar,
   punctuation

Emotional functioning

Self-concept
Frustration tolerance and coping mechanisms
Relationships with significant others
Reality testing
Diagnostic classifications for emotional disturbance

A comprehensive psychoeducational evaluation that includes the four areas described above generally takes approximately 5 to 8 hours to perform. Testing is often completed in two or three sessions, depending on the age and attention span of the child being tested.

DETAILED DESCRIPTION OF THE PSYCHOEDUCATIONAL EVALUATION
History

The process of gathering a comprehensive history is crucial to the understanding of the problem or problems for formulating a diagnosis and developing intervention methods. Frequently parents are asked to complete comprehensive history questionnaires[2] and behavior rating scales (such as Child Behavior Checklist,[3] Connor's Parent Rating Scale–Revised,[4] Home Situations Questionnaire[5]) before meeting with the psychologist. Teachers are also generally asked to provide their input in the same manner (such as Child Behavior Checklist–Teacher Report Form,[6] Connor's Teacher Rating Scale–Revised[7]). These checklists come with age norms for the various behaviors under consideration, providing a guideline for age-appropriate behaviors.

The Connors and Achenbach Parent forms were completed for case 1

Sample Questions to Gather Information about the Child

Pregnancy and birth

Were there complications during pregnancy?
To what extent were medications, drugs, alcohol, cigarettes used?
Was the pregnancy full term?
What was the length of labor, and what type of delivery?
Were there any complications during delivery?
What was the Apgar score?

Infancy and preschool period

How would you describe your infant in regard to temperament, sleeping patterns, feeding, etc.?
At what ages were developmental milestones attained, particularly for speech, walking, toilet training?
Did any stressful events occur in the family during this period?

Medical history

Describe your child's current health.
Have there been any accidents, major illnesses, hospitalizations?
Are there sleep, bowel, or bladder problems?
What medications is the child currently taking?

Peer relationships/socialization/interests

Approximately how many friends does your child have?
Are friends of same age, younger, older?
To what extent is your child sought out by other children?
What activities does your child enjoy?
What things does your child do well?
What activities does your child dislike?
What things does your child have trouble doing?
What chores and responsibilities does your child have?

(Appendix B). It can be noted that impulsivity was a problem noted by the parents on the Connors form, and attention and thought problems were seen as concerns on the Achenbach form.

The actual interview with the parents is a vehicle for establishing rapport with them. It begins the process of working cooperatively and allows the psychologist to gain perspective about the learning problems. It is also an opportunity to search for contributing factors and to decide what tests should be administered during the testing process. Information must be gathered about three general areas. These include information about the child, school history, and the family. The three boxes on pp. 341 to 343 list sample questions that are generally asked in these three areas.

Structured interview forms are available to assist in gathering a thorough history, such as the ADHD Clinic and Parent Interview.[8]

The history obtained by the psychologist is generally summarized in the Background Information section of the written report (in Appendix B).

Sample Questions to Gather School History

Preschool

At what age did your child start preschool?
Were there any difficulties reported in terms of peer interactions, speech and language skills, task participation, activity level?

Elementary school

What type of academic problems is your child having?
What type of behavior problems is your child having?
At what point did you become aware your child was having problems?
Has your child repeated a grade?
What types of interventions have occurred to deal with the above problems?
What remedial services (such as tutoring, speech therapy) have been provided and what has been the effect?
What have recent report cards and standardized tests shown?
What have your child's peer relationships been like?

High school

Same questions as above.
Are there different levels in your child's school, and what level classes is your child taking?
How has your child adjusted to class cycling (such as dealing with different teachers' styles, organization for classes, getting to classes on time)?
How much homework does your child do nightly?
In what extracurricular activities is your child involved?

The optometrist can utilize this information as the basis for obtaining his or her own history, probing those areas related to the referral question. It is particularly important for the optometrist searching for a connection between vision and learning to understand the age of onset of academic problems and how they became manifest. For example, the child with an onset of reading difficulty in first grade is very different from the child who had no reading problems until fifth grade and then began doing very poorly.

Cognitive testing

Cognitive testing includes assessment of various abilities, including language, memory, auditory and visual perceptual skills, visual-motor abilities, attention and concentration, and cognitive style. One gathers this information by administering an intelligence test as well as supplemental tests. An intelligence test provides an IQ (intelligence quotient) as well as information about the various aspects of cognitive functioning mentioned above. It is beyond the scope of this chapter to discuss the controversy over the possible cultural bias of IQ tests. The interested reader can consult Sattler[9] and Kaufman[10] for a discussion on this topic. IQ tests do provide valuable information about learning style and current levels of

Sample Questions to Gather Family History Information

Family history

Is there a history of learning problems in your (mother or father's) family or with your other children? Describe.

Is there a history of hyperactivity in your (mother's or father's) family or with your other children? Describe.

What significant medical problems exist in your (mother's or father's) family or with your other children? Describe.

Marital relationship

How long have you been married? Have there been previous marriages? Describe.

What factors in your marital relationship might be affecting your child?

If divorced situation:

How long have you been divorced?

What are the custody and visitation arrangements?

How has your child adjusted to the divorce?

What is the current relationship like between you and your ex-spouse?

Stressful life events

What events in your life would you consider to have been particularly stressful?

How might these events have affected your child?

Parent-child interactions

Who is the primary disciplinarian for your child?

To which parent do you feel your child is closer to?

What type of things do you do as a family?

How do you feel you get along with your child?

functioning, and when administered by an experienced, sensitive clinician and interpreted cautiously as one part of an overall evaluation, they can be useful in understanding the child's strengths and weaknesses.

Intellectual functioning is generally classified in the following way: The IQ scores have a mean of 100 and a standard deviation of 15. About two thirds of all people obtain an IQ score within 1 standard deviation of the mean (between 85 and 115). Ninety-five percent of all people obtain a score between 70 and 130, which is two standard deviations from the mean.[11] Children are compared to other children the same age. The intelligence classification system illustrated in Table 12.1 is commonly used.

An IQ score of 115, for example, falls in the high-average range of functioning, whereas a score of 88, is in the low-average range of intelligence. It is important to remember that the IQ score itself provides only one piece of information. A critical analysis of the various subtests of the IQ test is necessary to obtain a more accurate perception of the person's functioning and learning style.

There are two major IQ tests that are predominantly used by psychologists; the Wechsler Scales[11] (Wechsler Intelligence Scale for Children

TABLE 12.1   IQ classification system

IQ	Classification
130 and above	Very superior
120-129	Superior
110-119	High average
90-109	Average
80-89	Low average
70-79	Borderline
69 and below	Mentally deficient

TABLE 12.2   Weschler Intelligence Scale for Children–III (WISC-III)

Verbal Scale Subtests	Performance Scale Subtests
Information	Picture Completion
Similarities	Picture Arrangement
Arithmetic	Block Design
Vocabulary	Object Assembly
Comprehension	Coding
Digit Span (optional)	Mazes (optional)
	Symbol Search (optional)

[WISC-III], Wechsler PreSchool and Primary Scale of Intelligence [WPPSI-R], and the Wechsler Adult Scale of Intelligence [WAIS-R]) and the Stanford Binet Scale of Intelligence: Fourth Edition.[12] Both tests provide an overall IQ score, various IQ or standard age scores for different scales, and subtest scores for each individual subtest within the scales.

Wechsler Scales. The Wechsler Scales are three separate tests, distinguished by the age range they cover. The WISC-III, which is administered to children from 6 through 16 years of age, is the test that optometrists are most likely to encounter in a report. It is divided into two scales, the Verbal and Performance Scales. Three IQ scores are obtained from this test, the Verbal IQ, the Performance IQ, and the Full Scale IQ, which is a combination of the Verbal and Performance IQs. Furthermore, factor scores that will be discussed later are also given. One is able to compare a child's functioning on verbally related subtests with nonverbal, or more visual-spatial, tasks, by comparing the Verbal IQ with the Performance IQ. Obviously, such a comparison would be quite relevant for an optometrist, who may be exploring the role of vision in learning. A description of each subtest allows the optometrist to understand the various abilities being measured and the relevance to optometric testing.

Verbal Scale. The Verbal Scale consists of five mandatory and one optional subtests (Table 12.2).

Information measures a child's general fund of information. Long-term memory skills and acquired school learning are important contributing factors for adequate performance on this subtest. Questions vary in difficulty level, with questions ranging from the most basic, such as, "How many wings does a bird have?" to more difficult questions, such as, "Who wrote Tom Sawyer?"

The *Similarities* subtest measures verbal abstract reasoning and verbal conceptualization, through determining similarities among items or concepts. Examples of the type of questions asked include, "How are a pencil and a pen alike?" and "In what ways are an hour and a week alike?" This subtest relies more on general knowledge and is less related to the effects of schooling.

The *Arithmetic* subtest is a part of the verbal scale because the questions are asked orally and the child must respond orally. However, it has been found to be related more to attention and concentration abilities and numerical reasoning than to general verbal abilities. On this subtest, children are asked word problems, and they must solve them mentally, that is, without the use of paper and pencil. Psychologists believe that this requires a great deal of attention and concentration. Examples include, "Jane had three pieces of candy and Joe gave her four more. How many pieces did she have all together?" "If two buttons cost 15 cents, what will be the cost of a dozen buttons?" This is the only verbal subtest that is timed. For this subtest the child must determine the correct answer within a certain time limit (such as 30 seconds) to receive credit for the response.

The *Vocabulary* subtest measures a person's word knowledge and general language skills. A child is required to define words of varying complexity, such as "car" or "constitution." School-related learning is a factor in a person's ability to perform adequately on this test because a child must have been exposed to a variety of experiences to be able to define particular words.

Comprehension is a subtest measuring social reasoning and common-sense judgment. General knowledge, rather than school-related information, is tapped on this subtest. Questions often require a child to think through solutions to problems or interpret information in novel ways. Examples of the types of questions include, "What should you do if you see someone forget his book when he leaves a restaurant?" "What are the advantages of keeping money in the bank?"

The final subtest, which is optional, and is not used when one is computing the Verbal IQ is *Digit Span*. This subtest requires a child to repeat increasing strings of numbers both forwards and backwards. Psychologists believe that attention and concentration, to a greater extent than general verbal abilities, are needed to perform adequately on this subtest. In addition, it is generally believed that this subtest measures short-term auditory memory and perhaps visualization as well, depending on the manner in which the child attempts to accomplish this task.

In summary, the Verbal Scale is composed of a series of subtests in which the child listens to questions and must respond orally. Performance on some subtests is related to the adequacy of the educational process to which the child has been exposed, whereas for other subtests performance is dependent on adequate attention and concentration, or on reasoning abilities. All subtests, however, provide assessment of oral skills to some degree.

Performance Scale. The primary distinction between the Verbal and Performance Scales is that in the Performance Scale the child must deal with visual information or concrete objects and does not need to respond orally. Although on one subtest oral responses are requested, if the child can explain only by pointing, the answer is accepted as correct. It is important to understand that all directions are given orally, and so the Performance Scale is not a totally language-free measure of ability. Another difference between the Performance Scale and Verbal Scale is that all subtests are timed on the Performance Scale. Thus a child is given bonus points for timely completion of the tasks but may not receive any credit for a correct response if given after the time limit expires. Finally, the performance subtests provide valuable information on the person's independent, problem-solving strategies and capabilities.

The Performance Scale consists of five mandatory and two optional subtests (see Table 12.2).

Picture Completion requires that a child look at a picture and indicate, either by an oral response or by pointing, what is missing from the picture. Thus this task requires the person to distinguish essential from non-essential differences as well as attend to visual details. Adequate visual memory is required for skilled task performance. For example, in Figure 12.1, in a picture of a filing cabinet, a drawer handle is missing, which is the essential missing element.

A child would have to know that each filing cabinet drawer should have a handle and see that one is missing and find that missing part within the given time limit (that is, 20 seconds).

The *Picture Arrangement* (Figure 12.2) Subtest requires that the child rearrange a series of pictures in the proper sequence to tell a logical story.

Again, the child must pay attention to visual details. In addition, he must understand cause-and-effect relationships, as well as have some understanding of social situations. Although no oral responses are required, many children use oral mediation to perform this task by telling the stories either in their heads mentally or aloud. These first two subtests require a minimum of visual-motor integration. The remainder of the subtests require higher level visual-motor integration skills and spatial-reasoning abilities.

The *Block Design* Subtest (Figure 12.3) involves the use of red and white cubes that are used to reproduce designs on cards.

This subtest requires visual perception and the ability to apply logical reasoning to abstract visual relationships. Inductive and deductive reasoning are also involved in completing this task. The faster the designs are reproduced, the more points a child receives for successful completion.

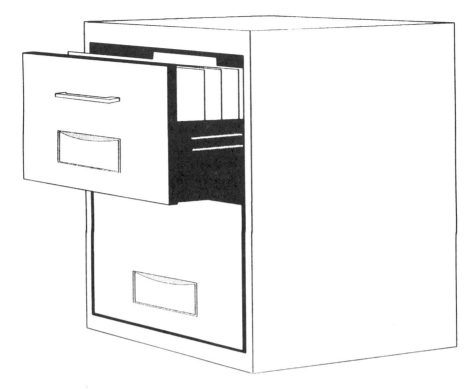

FIGURE 12.1 A simulation of the Picture Completion Subtest of the WISC-III. The child looks at a picture and indicates, either by a oral response or by pointing, what is missing from the picture.

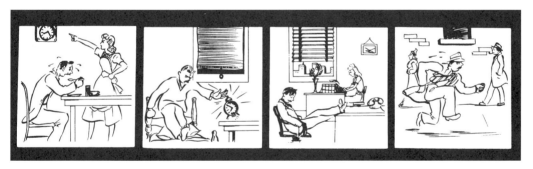

FIGURE 12.2 Simulation of the Picture Arrangement Subtest of the WISC-III. The child rearranges a series of pictures in the proper sequence to tell a logical story.

Assembling puzzles from individual pieces is required on the *Object Assembly* Subtest. This task measures a child's flexibility, ability to perceive part-whole relationships, and visual retention. An example (Figure 12.4) of one of the five puzzles on this subtest is that of a cow, which is displayed before the child in separate components, and the child is asked to assemble the puzzle quickly.

On the first two puzzles, the child is told what the puzzle is to be, but on the last three, the child must make that determination on his or her

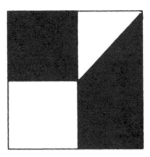

FIGURE 12.3 Simulation of the Block Design Subtest of the WISC-II. The child must use red and white cubes to reproduce designs on cards.

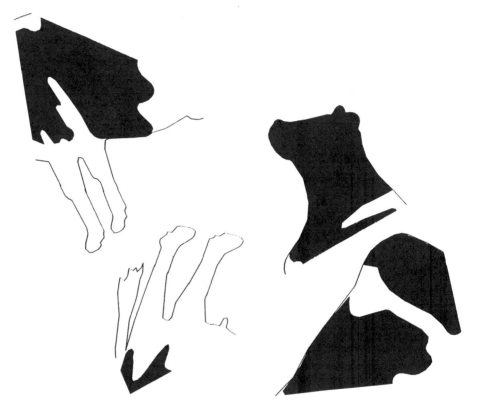

FIGURE 12.4 Simulation of the Object Assembly Subtest of the WISC-III. The child is asked to quickly assemble the puzzle.

own. It is on this task that much can be learned about the person's ability to employ trial-and-error and problem-solving skills.

The *Coding* Subtest is a paper-and-pencil task requiring the child to quickly pair a number with a symbol (Figure 12.5). Visual memory, attention and concentration, psychomotor speed, accurate eye movements, visual tracking, and coordination are all component skills required for adequate task performance.

The first optional subtest, *Mazes* (Figure 12.6), is not computed in the

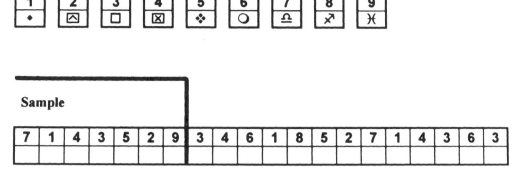

FIGURE 12.5 Simulation of the Coding Subtest of the WISC-III. This a paper-and-pencil task requiring the child to quickly pair a number with a symbol.

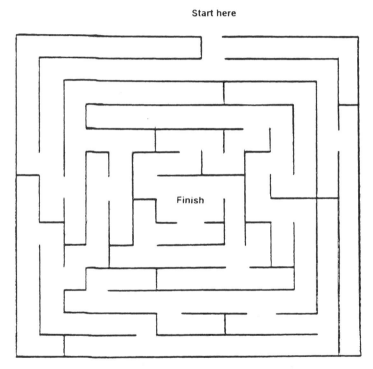

FIGURE 12.6 Simulation of the Mazes Subtest of the WISC-III. On this paper and pencil task, the child must find the way from the center of the maze to the outside without going through any lines.

Performance IQ score. On this paper-and-pencil task, the child must find the way from the outside of the maze to the center without going through any lines. Planning and forethought, flexibility, and fine-motor coordination are necessary on this subtest.

The second optional subtest (Figure 12.7) (also not computed in the Performance IQ score) is Symbol Search. This subtest is new to the Wechsler scales. It measures processing speed. The student is required to dis-

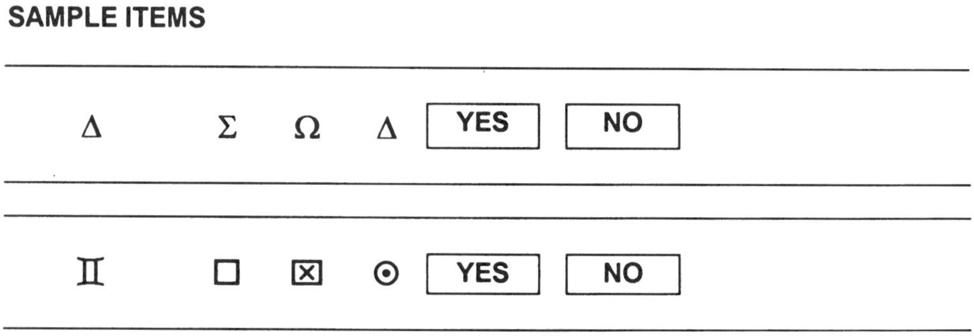

SAMPLE ITEMS

Δ	Σ	Ω	Δ	YES	NO

Ⅱ	□	☒	⊙	YES	NO

FIGURE 12.7 Simulation of the Symbol Search Subtest of the WISC-III. The child is required to discriminate among various symbols to determine whether there is an exact match.

criminate among various symbols to determine whether there is an exact match. Efficient visual scanning is needed for successful completion of this task.

The WISC-III is an instrument that can provide the optometrist with valuable information. First, by looking at the Full-Scale IQ, one can determine whether a child would be expected to achieve at an average rate in comparison to other children the same age or might be expected to achieve at a faster or slower pace.

In case 1 (Appendix B), the boy's Full-Scale IQ of 90 is in the beginning of the average range of intelligence. The child in case 2 has a Full-Scale IQ in the superior range. Thus one would expect inherent differences in the rate at which these two boys would be expected to achieve.

Next, by comparing Verbal and Performance IQs, the optometrist can determine whether verbal and nonverbal abilities are fairly consistent, or whether one area is weaker than the other. This is one important issue to consider when determining whether vision therapy for visual processing skills is indicated. Intervention should occur when visual processing abilities are significantly weaker than verbal abilities.

In making such a decision the clinician should determine if test results from the visual-perceptual evaluation are consistent with the WISC-III scores. If visual-perceptual test results are below average and both Verbal and Performance IQs are at similar below-average levels, the visual-perceptual skills would not necessarily be considered a significant area of weakness. Rather, the poor visual-perceptual abilities would be consistent with overall abilities. A situation in which visual-perceptual test results are below average and the Performance IQ is significantly below the Verbal IQ (a difference of 12 to 15 points is considered a significant difference) is indicative of relatively weak processing skills. In such cases the visual-perceptual disorder probably represents a significant problem area for the child. Case 1 (Appendix B) represents such a situation in which the Verbal IQ is significantly higher than the Performance IQ.

Similarly, if visual-perceptual test results were average for the child's age, but Verbal IQ was in the superior to very superior range and significantly above the Performance IQ, this would again indicate an area of significant weakness for the child (despite average test results on the perceptual evaluation).

Finally, one might be confronted with the situation in which the child has scored below average on perceptual testing, but when he looks at the WISC-III results, the Performance IQ is significantly higher than the Verbal IQ. In such a situation, one might question whether perceptual therapy would be the most appropriate intervention. It might be more important to work on improving weak language skills. Such a decision should be based on more information, specifically the presenting problem and the hypothesized contributing factors to that problem.

It is apparent, therefore, that it is necessary for the optometrist to have complete information from a psychoeducational evaluation when trying to determine the significance of visual efficiency or visual-perceptual problems. Case 2 (Appendix B) represents a boy who has a visual efficiency problem as well as a significant difference between Verbal and Performance IQ, with the Performance IQ being significantly higher than the Verbal IQ.

The final way in which the WISC-III may be important to the optometrist is in analyzing the individual subtests on the WISC-III. Subtest scaled scores range from 1 to 19, with a score of 10 being the mean. Scaled scores between 7 and 13 are within 1 standard deviation from the mean. Scaled scores from 14 to 16 are within 2 standard deviations above the mean, whereas scaled scores from 4 to 6 are within 2 standard deviations below the mean. Thus one not only can compare how the child is performing in comparison to other children of the same age, but also can look for strengths and weaknesses within the individual child's profile.

WISC-III factors. The WISC-III subtests have been factor analyzed[10] and have been found to measure several dimensions of cognitive ability. The four factors include verbal comprehension, perceptual organization, freedom from distractibility, and processing speed (see box on next page). Such factors go beyond the verbal and performance IQ and aid in determining specific areas of strength and weakness.

By looking at these factors and comparing them with results from visual testing, one can obtain a clearer picture of the child's problems. Several examples will demonstrate how such an analysis can be helpful.

If everything on the WISC-III is high, except for the two subtests that constitute the freedom-from-distractibility factor, one can hypothesize that there is an attention and concentration or memory problem. This is the situation for case 2 (Appendix B), where the mean on the Arithmetic and Digit Span Subtest is 6.5 whereas the mean for the other verbal subtests is 13.

The relevance for the optometrist would be twofold: first, poor perfor-

---

WISC-III Factors

Verbal comprehension factor

Information
Similarities
Vocabulary
Comprehension

Perceptual organization factor

Picture completion
Picture arrangement
Block design
Object assembly
Mazes

Freedom from distractibility

Arithmetic
Digit span

Processing speed

Coding
Symbol search

---

mance on some subtests of the perceptual evaluation can be questioned as being related to attentional deficits rather than perceptual weaknesses, and, second, such findings would alert the optometrist to the possibility of potential refractive, oculomotor, and accommodative/convergence problems if poor reading comprehension were also a factor.

If Coding and Symbol Search had shown weaknesses, the possibility of ocular motility problems should be considered as causing the poor performance. Likewise, difficulty processing visual information efficiently must also be assessed.

If a child performed poorly on Coding and Mazes in comparison to the other performance tests, fine-motor coordination and other paper-and-pencil tasks, such as the Beery Test of Visual Motor Integration, as well as a handwriting sample should be examined.

If Picture Completion and Picture Arrangement were weaknesses, one would search for indications of lack of attention to visual detail on visual tests. In contrast, if Picture Completion and Picture Arrangement were strengths in comparison to the other performance subtests because they require the least fine-motor abilities, it would be hypothesized that visual organization skills were well developed whereas visual-motor integration problems were evident. Such is also the situation with case 2, where the mean of 16.5 for Picture Completion and Picture Arrangement is significantly discrepant from the mean of 13 for the tests that require visual motor integration. Alternatively, with case 1, the two subtests that require an equal degree of visual motor skills are widely discrepant (Block Design 9, Object Assembly 4). One must therefore search for another explanation. One alternative is that Block Design involves imitating, whereas Object Assembly requires seeing the parts forming a complete whole. One would need to look to other test data for confirmation of this hypothesis. (For example, this boy also did very poorly on the Visual Closure Subtest of the Woodcock Johnson Test of Cognitive Ability.[13])

It is useful to determine how a child responds to concrete or meaningful stimuli versus abstract stimuli if one compares those Performance subtests that use abstract stimuli (Block Design, Coding) with those that use meaningful stimuli (Picture Completion, Picture Arrangement, and Object Assembly). Again, this comparison could lead to interpretation of perceptual tests along similar lines.

Another way of looking at these same Performance subtests relates to imitation in comparison to problem solving. Both Block Design and Coding require children to imitate or reproduce models, in a way similar to that of other tests such as the Beery,[14] Bender,[15] and Benton Visual Retention tests.[16] Problem-solving tasks, however, require more input from the person being tested in terms of organizing and carrying out the task. The lack of planning and organization might be the overriding problem in poor task performance, rather than the visual processing required.

The spatial subtests, specifically Picture Completion, Block Design, and Object Assembly, tend to be among the least dependent on specific cultural and educational opportunities[10] and can shed important information for children who may come from culturally or educationally deprived environments.

Stanford Binet. The Stanford Binet, fourth edition, is similar in organization to the WISC-III, in that an overall test composite score is obtained, derived from subtests that are clustered into various scales. The major differences between the two tests is that the Stanford Binet has separate scales for quantitative reasoning and short-term memory, in addition to verbal reasoning and abstract/visual reasoning (thus four scales to determine the test composite score as opposed to two on the WISC-III). There is a total of 15 subtests though all subtests are not usually administered to each student. Rather, the psychologist selects appropriate subtests based on the age of the examinee. The other major difference is that for the subtests the mean score is 50 with a standard deviation of 3. The four overall clusters, however, have a mean of 100 and a standard deviation of 15, similar to those of the WISC-III.

These subtests on the Stanford Binet are the basis for exploring cognitive functioning in the various areas mentioned, such as language, visual perceptual functioning, memory, attention and concentration, and cognitive style.

Because the WISC-III is used by psychologists more frequently than the Stanford Binet, it is much more likely that optometrists will be presented with the former measure of intelligence as part of test batteries than the latter.

Language assessment

When one is evaluating language, it is important to consider expressive language skills, which involves communicating one's own ideas through speaking, and receptive skills, which is ability to understand what is spoken. Expressive language can be further delineated into speaking one's own thoughts extemporaneously, which is considered spontaneous, versus demand language, which consists in speaking in response to questions and requires specific answers. Formalized testing as well as informal observation can provide information about these skills. The psychologist will generally make a referral to a speech and language therapist for more extensive testing and remediation when significant problems are uncovered in the language area.

Receptive language. Two popular tests for the assessment of receptive language are the Token Test for Children[17] and the Peabody Picture Vocabulary Test (PPVT).[18]

The *Token Test* uses large and small multicolored circles and squares that are arranged in front of the child. The child then follows examiner directions by manipulating the blocks in various ways. For example, the child might be asked to "Point to the small red circle," or "Put the green square between the yellow square and red square." The child is asked to act on increasingly complex linguistic directions. The task measures receptive language because the child demonstrates an understanding of what is being said to him or her.

On the *Peabody Picture Vocabulary Test* (PPVT), the child is shown a page with the pictures of four objects or concepts on it, and the child must point to the picture associated with a particular word spoken by the examiner. Again, this test measures the understanding of language because it does not require an oral response. Children with receptive language problems may have difficulty understanding spoken instructions or information given aloud. This may be especially true if the speaker talks quickly or there is background noise.

Expressive language functioning. Expressive language problems may be seen in the child who says, "I have really good ideas and know what I want to say, but it doesn't come out right, or it's too much trouble to try to say what I mean." They may have word-retrieval problems, difficulty finding or recalling the right words in a timely fashion. Two tests to measure expressive language include the *Boston Naming Test*,[19] where a child must name a picture, and the *Rapid Automatized Naming Test* (RAN),[20] where the child quickly names numbers, letters, colors, and commonly used objects as quickly as possible. The child in case 2 (Appendix B) received an age-equivalent score of 9-0 on the Boston Naming Test. Given that his IQ is in the superior range and he is 11 years of age, this area was a significant weakness for him.

It is important for the optometrist to understand the pervasive nature of language problems. Such problems can affect not only academic functioning, but social functioning as well. Adequate language skills are important for making and keeping friends. If a child does not understand what is being said, it may lead to embarrassment and withdrawal. Similarly, a child may withdraw rather than attempt to explain what he or she means in a particular situation. Young children with language problems may have more frequent temper outbursts because of the frustration of not being understood or being able to express their needs or thoughts. The alert optometrist can pick up either receptive or expressive language problems during the routine eye examination. For example, when asking the child to follow certain instructions, it may be clear that the child does not understand what is being asked. Certain position words, such as *next to, on top of,* may be misunderstood. Or, when gathering history information, the child may be unable to answer questions clearly, or may appear to search for appropriate descriptive words. This information can then be shared with the parent as part of the overall picture of the child's performance. In addition, when doing perceptual testing, if there is a known or suspected language processing problem, the clinician must be certain that the child understands the task requirements, particularly if there are complex instructions, or the test results might be invalid.

Memory testing

Memory is important in almost all aspects of daily life, ranging from such diverse activities as tying a shoe, doing multiplication tables, and finding one's way home from school. When one is evaluating memory, it is important to look at both the process involved in remembering information, as well as the various types of memory.

Process of remembering information. There are several components to remembering that generally occur naturally without thought. However, each of these components can be the source of a memory problem.

attention and concentration To remember information, a person must first focus on the information to be remembered.
storage The information must be either used immediately or stored in the brain for future use.
retrieval If the information has been stored, it must be found, when needed.
active working memory Ideas must be kept together while one is working on them.

A child might have difficulties with any or all of these aspects of memory.

To further complicate matters, the sensory modality used to receive and remember information also might influence the child's effective memory skills. Visual memory involves gathering and remembering information through sight, whereas auditory memory involves obtaining information through hearing. Motor, or kinesthetic, memory involves gathering information through the motor system, and is important for effective performance of physical tasks such as riding a bicycle or writing.

Types of memory

sequential memory Information remembered in a certain order or sequence.
short-term memory Information that needs to be remembered for a brief period of time (such as just long enough for dialing a telephone number).
long-term memory Information retained over a long period of time.
procedural memory Remembering how to do something, such as the steps in doing a particular chemistry experiment.
episodic memory Memory for things or events that happened in one's life.
factual memory Memory for knowledge, such as baseball statistics for a particular team.
automatic memory Something that was once learned but has been used so much it has become automatic, such as driving a car, writing in cursive writing.

Although listed as such, these memory categories cannot be seen as discrete. They overlap and interrelate in many ways. For example, in doing a chemistry experiment, along with procedural memory one would have to have stored and then retrieved various pieces of information, such as the types of equipment needed (such as a Bunsen burner) and how the equipment was operated. Also sequential memory would be important so that the experiment could be carried out in the right order. The various sense modalities would come into play if the student was picturing the way the teacher demonstrated the project, remembering the directions the teacher gave to the class, using the motor modality to carry out the experiment, and remembering how a similar experiment was handled previously. Factual, long-term memory would also be utilized, since the student would be expected to be familiar with the periodic table of the elements and know which chemicals might react together in a specific way.

Clearly, memory testing is not easy to accomplish, and no one test will give us all the answers. It is important to utilize history and behavioral observations as well as specific tests to obtain as complete a picture as possible about memory.

The WISC-III gives some information about memory skills (see Table 12.3. Within the Verbal Scale, several subtests are dependent on acquired learning and involve long-term memory skills. These include the Information and Vocabulary subtests. In addition, the Arithmetic subtest probes short-term auditory memory, as well as active working memory, or being able to hold onto and manipulate discrete bits of information. The Digit Span subtest is a measure of short-term auditory sequential memory. The Digits Backwards portion of the WISC-III also tends to measure visual sequential memory and visualization, as many people try to make a mental image of the numbers to manipulate them and say them backwards. One can determine the strategy the child uses by asking appropriate questions.

Several of the Performance Scale subtests also include a memory component. On the Picture Completion subtest, in order to determine the essential missing element, one must use long-term visual memory to get an image of the complete picture. To perform well on the Coding subtest a symbol must be associated with a number. Although the code is always available to the child, the more the task can be done without referring to it, the faster the task can be accomplished and the higher the score can be. Thus short-term visual memory is involved. Automatic memory for directionality also plays a role because some of the symbols are just mirror images of each other. On the Object Assembly subtest, if the child has a visual image of the actual object stored in memory (such as the image of a cow or a bicycle), it will be easier to put the puzzle pieces together to make that image. Thus the WISC-III is very useful for the assessment of memory skills.

Other memory tests. See Table 12.3.

The *Stanford-Binet* has a short-term memory scale that measures both visual and auditory memory. There are four memory subtests, requiring the child to repeat numbers or sentences, reproduce a pattern of beads, or remember a series of objects. The *Woodcock Johnson Tests of Cognitive Ability* have several subtests that comprise either the short-term memory or long-term retrieval components. Repetition of sentences, words, and numbers (in a reversed order) are measured as part of the short-term memory component. The ability to associate a picture with a name, or a symbol with a word, is required in the long-term retrieval component.

The child in case 2 (Appendix B) did well on one memory test of the Woodcock Johnson (Memory for Sentences), performed at an average rate on two others (Memory for Words, Numbers Reversed), and had great difficulty on the Memory for Names subtest, which combined visual and auditory information. The patient in case 2 also did well when recalling sentences or words but had great difficulty with names and listening to a story and answering questions about what he heard.

The *Detroit Tests of Learning Aptitude II*[21] also assesses memory skills as one component of the overall battery. These tests allow one to attempt to tap the various component aspects of memory as well as the various types of memory listed above.

The *Denman Neuropsychology Memory Scale*[22] is a test for children 10 years of age through adult that specifically concentrates on memory functioning. It measures immediate recall as well as retention after a period of time (such as 45 minutes). The patient in case 2 (Appendix B) was also given the Denman, where he had greatest difficulty remembering the facts of a paragraph-length story. Thus he can remember small bits of written verbal information (sentences and words), but longer, more complex verbal material is problematic.

The *Rey Auditory Verbal Learning Test*[23] assesses the person's ability to learn a list of 15 words over five trials. Thus a learning curve can be established. The child in case 1 (Appendix B) was given this test, and as can be seen, he was initially able to recall 4 of 14 words and after five learning trials recalled 8, which is indicative of a problem in this area.

The *Wide Range Assessment of Memory and Learning* (WRAML)[24] is a comprehensive memory battery normed for students 5 through 17 years of age. There are three major divisions within the test. The first differentiates between "memory and learning." Each memory subtest measures a specific amount of information with immediate recall, whereas each learning subtest involves the acquisition of new information over repeated trials. The second division differentiates between verbal and visual information, progressing from rote memory demands with minimally meaningful materials to memory demands with increasingly meaningful material.[24] Finally, the length of time between task administration and recall is assessed. Although all subtests evaluate short-term recall, several subtests also allow for a delayed recall. This allows for the assessment of forgetting over time. There are three verbal, three visual, and three learning subtests. (See Table 12.3).

Relevance to optometric care. Optometrists often assess visual memory and visual sequential memory as part of a perceptual evaluation. It is important to determine whether memory skills are weak across modalities or are specific to the visual modality. Such an understanding is valuable when one is determining whether to remediate visual memory weaknesses, to use compensatory strategies, or to use a combination of both. It is also helpful for the optometrist to know that a child with memory problems often requires repeated exposure to information before it can be easily recalled. Thus vision therapy for visual efficiency or visual information processing problems might be expected to take longer than normal.

Attention, concentration, and impulse control

The ability to control attention and to concentrate is an important variable related to academic success. It is therefore necessary to assess this area as part of a comprehensive psychoeducational evaluation. Children with severe difficulties are said to have attention deficit hyperactivity disorder (ADHD) (Chapter 4). At present, it is believed that the root of this difficulty lies in the child's tendency to gravitate off task to whatever else is more immediately reinforcing.[8] Thus poor self-regulation and motivation to do tasks that may be boring lead a child to difficulty with sustained attention.

Behavioral rating scales (Achenbach, Connors), informal observations during testing, and formal tests believed to measure attention and concentration are used to measure these skills. A problem associated with the assessment of all skills is that it is often easier for a child to attend during formal one-on-one testing than in a classroom situation. There are fewer distractions, less noise, and an examiner to motivate and encourage the child during formal testing. Some children will do well in the testing situation but through parental report will have great difficulty in school. For these reasons it is important to utilize the behavior rating scales completed

TABLE 12.3 Commonly used tests with memory components

Test	Memory subtests	Measure
WISC-III	Arithmetic	Auditory sequential Active working memory
	Digit Span	Auditory sequential
	Picture Completion	Long-term visual
	Coding	Short-term visual
Stanford-Binet	Bead Memory	Visual sequential
	Memory for Sentences	Short-term auditory
	Memory for Digits	Short-term auditory sequential
	Memory for Objects	Short-term visual
Woodcock-Johnson Tests of Cognitive Ability	Memory for Sentences	Short-term auditory
	Memory for Words	Short-term auditory
	Numbers Reversed	Auditory sequential
	Memory for Names	Visual/auditory long-term—immediate, delayed
Detroit Tests of Learning Aptitude	Sentence Imitation	Syntax, auditory
	Oral Directions	Auditory/visual
	Word Sequences	Auditory
	Object Sequences	Visual sequential, concrete
	Letter Sequences	Visual sequential, symbolic
Denman Neuropsychology Memory Scale	Story Recall, Immediate, Delayed	Auditory linguistic
	Paired Associates Learning Immediate, Delayed	Auditory
	Recall Complex Figure	Visual motor
Rey Auditory Verbal Learning Test		Auditory
Wide Range Assessment of Memory and Learning	Picture Memory	Visual
	Design Memory	Visual motor
	Verbal Learning	Auditory learning
	Story Memory	Auditory linguistic
	Finger Windows	Visual sequential
	Sentence Memory	Auditory
	Sound Symbol	Visual auditory association
	Visual Learning	Visual learning
	Number/Letter Recall	Auditory

by the parents and teacher. Other children will demonstrate such weaknesses even under the ideal circumstances of the formal testing situation. Please refer to case 1 (Appendix B) where the child scored at the 99th percentile for attention problems, based on the parents' observations.

Vigilance, or continuous-performance, tests and direct, systematic behavioral observations of ADHD symptoms in the home, school, or test situation are the best measures of ADHD.[8] Although the WISC-III Freedom from Distractibility Factor has also been used to assess ADHD, Barkley's research has found that this factor was unable to distinguish children with ADHD from learning-disabled children and normal children.

There are both computerized instruments as well as paper and pencil versions of Continuous Performance Tests. The Gordon Diagnostic System[25] is one such computerized version. The child observes a screen while individual letters or numbers are quickly projected onto it. The child responds when a certain stimulus appears. This test measures both sustained attention and impulse control.

Cancellation tests, such as the Cancellation of Rapidly Recurring Target Figures,[26] require the child to scan a series of symbols in rows on paper and cross out the target stimulus with a pencil. Although the test measures visual discrimination and eye-movement skills, it is also a measure of vigilance and the ability to sustain attention.

The Matching Familiar Figures Test[27] is often used to measure impulsivity, a common attribute of children with ADHD. The child must find an exact match to a sample picture from an array of six similar pictures. Both accuracy and the degree of reflection are assessed in the way the child accomplishes the task. The child in case 1 (Appendix B) was both impulsive and inaccurate in his performance on this task. This is consistent with the parents' report of impulsivity on the Connors Parent Rating Scale.

An additional way to measure attention and concentration is through the use of the Restricted Academic Situation.[8] A child is asked to complete math problems at his or her independent level on his or her own. The examiner observes from a two-way mirror the amount of time the child is off task. The number of problems completed and the number correct are also computed. As can be seen in case 1 (Appendix B), the child completed 12 of 100 problems in 15 minutes, with 8 of the 12 (66%) correct. In addition, he was off task 46% of the time. Thus this child appears to have a significant problem with sustained attention.

Achievement testing

Overview. Educational testing has an important place in a complete psychoeducational evaluation. At a very basic level such testing is designed to answer the following questions:

What skills does the child possess?
At what point does the child start to need help with the material?
What causes the child to be overwhelmed and frustrated?
What does the information indicate about specific remedial goals?
Is the child making adequate progress?
Is the classroom work and homework in concert with current skill and ability level?
Are expectations (that is, parents', teachers', student's) appropriate?

Assessment process

Achievement testing is a process that varies from clinician to clinician. Examiners develop their own battery of tests and approaches. The following description of the educational assessment process represents a typical approach to achievement testing for those who are attempting to answer the questions indicated above.

Reading assessment. The first stage of the assessment involves an evaluation of the child's ability to recognize words and apply word-analysis methods. If the child has significant difficulty in these areas, there are many implications about how this could affect his functioning overall. Adequate word recognition is the foundation of reading skill and for a vast number of learning disabled children, their learning problems are directly a result of their deficiencies with word recognition and decoding.

Many different tests exist to assess this area. The actual test chosen is not nearly so crucial as the methodology of obtaining information. The Boder Test of Reading-Spelling Patterns[28] differentiates the child's ability to respond automatically and immediately to word patterns (immediate-sight vocabulary) from his performance when he is provided with an unlimited amount of time to determine (decode) an unfamiliar word. As a supplement to the Boder, a list of nonsense words from the Woodcock Reading Mastery Tests[29] can be presented to further assess the child's ability to apply word analysis and phonological principles. The nonsense words (such as *roo, dud's, cigbet, gouch*) help to identify specific skill deficits that should be targeted in remediation. For example, if the child responded "goach" to *gouch,* it is reasonable to assume that he is having specific difficulty with the *ou* vowel combination. Similarly, if the child gives a one-syllable response to *cigbet,* we would be looking to see whether there is a consistent pattern of difficulty with syllabication principles.

Letter and word reversals are also assessed during this portion of the evaluation. This area is particularly relevant to the optometrist, since children are often referred because they are reversing letters or words. The most typical letter reversals involve the letters that have the same configuration (p/g, p/q, b/d). However, other letter confusions are also seen (f/r, h/n). Similarly, the common word reversals are those words that have like configurations (was/saw, no/on). It is important to remember that reversals are expected and considered a normal part of acquiring early reading skills. Beyond 7 years of age, however, the frequency of reversals should greatly diminish. Persistence of a significant number of reversals beyond this age is suggestive of probable learning disabilities. The Gardner Test of Letter Reversals is another test often used with the ones mentioned in this section.

The child in case 1 has severe deficiencies in the areas of word recognition and word analysis. The youngster has a very limited understanding of sound-to-symbol relationships and tends to guess at words based on their configuration and initial consonant. For example, when he was exposed to the word *boat,* the response was *but,* and for the word *ride* the stated word was *red.* A very different picture emerged with the child in case 2. This youngster had superior abilities to apply word-analysis methods and recognize words.

After analysis of the child's word recognition and decoding methods using isolated words and nonsense-word patterns, it is beneficial to assess how the child handles word reading demands while reading in context from representative text material. This is typically accomplished through an assessment instrument known as the Informal Reading Inventory (IRI).[30] In contrast to the typical standardized reading tests given in the schools, the IRI provides a wealth of qualitative information about how the reader manages text. The examiner listens attentively to the person reading and transcribes exactly what the reader does with the text.

The following example is a sample of the responses of the child in case 1. The italicized words show where the reader requested help from the examiner because he could not apply any strategy to figure out the word. Words written above the text are the actual substitution errors that were made by the reader.

will   to show

One day *when* Mary was *at school* the

kibs

kittens ran away.

From this sample one can well understand how laborious and frustrating the reading process is to this youngster. The qualitative assessment of oral reading provides a vivid sense of what the child is capable of doing and what causes frustration. The information from the IRI and the word recognition tests mentioned above offer much in terms of establishing instructional goals for future remediation.

Another aspect of the IRI assessment is the evaluation of the child's ability to derive meaning from the text. Since reading is a complex process involving symbol recognition and understanding, an exploration of the child's comprehension of the material is crucial. It is important to understand that simply because the child can read text fluently, without error, does not mean that his understanding of the material is adequate. There are many "word callers" whose critical thinking skills and ability to respond appropriately to text material is very limited. Again the format of the IRI goes well beyond the multiple-choice format of group standardized achievement testing.

In the IRI assessment, the examiner asks a range of questions that tap the person's understanding. These include his ability to recall important facts stated in the selection, to think and respond inferentially when asked questions that are not directly stated in the text, to draw conclusions, and to respond to the vocabulary demands of the text. Listening to and recording the responses provides a real sense of readers' approaches. Do they actively seek information as they read? Are they just looking to "get through the material" without taking the time to reflect? Can they organize information in a logical and sequential manner? Do they respond differently to fiction versus nonfiction material. These and other such questions can be addressed in an IRI assessment.

Both of the cases in Appendix B provide very different pictures of the comprehension area. In case 1 (Appendix B), the comprehension of the material is impaired by the degree of word-recognition problems interfering in the text material. In case 2 (Appendix B) difficulty with reading comprehension is not grounded in problems with the mechanics of reading, since most of the words that he read were done so flawlessly and effortlessly. However, the child's language-based weaknesses overlap with the thinking skills involved in reading comprehension. Thus recognizing cause-effect relationships, organizing details, formulating inferences, and drawing conclusions is difficult for this child, based on the weaknesses that were observed on the verbal section of the WISC-III.

As rich as the IRI is in its diagnostic information that is yielded, there are other reading tests given in the evaluation. By definition the IRI is an informal test, which means that there is no normalizing group used or statistical information on validity and reliability. Therefore giving a standardized or formal test complements the findings from the IRI. Further, a youngster may do poorly with one format and more effectively with another.

The Woodcock Reading Mastery Test[29] is an example of a reading test that utilizes a totally different format and means of assessing reading from that of the IRI. In this format the youngster is asked to read a small paragraph and supply a word that is missing from the paragraph. Such a format allows for comparison to a normalizing group, which is typically not a part of informal testing.

The Wechsler Individual Achievement Test (WIAT)[30] is a relatively recent addition to the standardized test market. It covers all the major academic areas (reading recognition and comprehension, written language, and mathematics). An interesting feature of the WIAT is that the norming group was the same population used for the WISC-III normalizing, which may allow for more reliable intertest comparisons.

Assessing spelling, arithmetic, and written expression. Other important components of achievement testing include assessing the basic skill areas of spelling, written expression, and arithmetic.

Spelling. In the spelling area several standardized and informal measures are available. A popular standardized assessment tool is the Wide Range Achievement Test.[31] This test simply asks the person to spell in a traditional spelling-test format, with words increasing in difficulty as the test proceeds. Most spelling tests follow this format.

Spelling errors, when interpreted diagnostically, may provide important clues as to how the youngster understands phonological information. The following are typical questions that are asked of a clinical spelling evaluation:

Does the person understand the regular patterns present in words?
Does he have particular difficulty with less regular patterns? Is he hearing the subtle differences between the various sound frequencies?
Does he spell in an overly phonetic manner?
Does he understand principles of syllabication?

The spelling sample of a 12-year-old learning-disabled youngster reproduced below, with the errors spelled exactly as written by the student, provides valuable information about how this youngster understands basic sound-to-symbol, phonological relationships:

Spelling word	Child's response
make	mack
him	hemes
shout	sout
cook	cuk
must	maust
correct	corat
circle	colce

Written expression. Once a spelling sample is obtained the student is asked to produce a paragraph for a sample of his written expression. This has been a difficult area to standardize, but there is a growing number of standardized measures of writing on the market. The WIAT has a standardized writing subtest. Most clinicians, however, assess writing informally by asking the person to organize a written paragraph about something that is relevant to the student.

The writing sample reproduced below is written in its exact form by the student in case 1:

> *The reson school stinch is, the teacher are awails on my Back aBolt evering i do and say. The teacherno ever thing I do, every thing wrong and wright every stupit move I make and every other thing.*

Another, less dramatic sample from a student with writing problems is reproduced below:

> *My expectations for this year are to greatly improve my grades, have better study habits. Make myself more determined in my work. Improve from my former years in school. Never skip a night of homework.*

Clearly, suggestions for remediation emerge from these writing samples. Clinicians typically assess the sample as a whole. Does it state a unified theme? Is the theme coherent? From there, questions about sentence structure, fragments, run-ons, and so on are considered. The samples above have significant sentence structure problems. The problems aid the clinician in formulating specific goals for future remediation.

Arithmetic. A similar approach to analyzing a student's product is used when one is assessing arithmetic skills. Again, of greater importance than the actual grade-equivalent score is the process by which the youngster approaches mathematics. An astute clinician observes the child's approach and organization to determine where it is that the process breaks down and what he is capable of doing independently.

The Key-Math Diagnostic Test[32] is the most widely used instrument for an in-depth assessment of different aspects of mathematics. For a quick screening the Wide Range Achievement Test–Revised has an arithmetic calculations test. The WIAT has a calculations and mathematics reasoning section.

Importance of the educational assessment for the optometrist. It is important for the optometrist to understand that there is a tremendous range of possible approaches to achievement testing, from fairly superficial approaches to those that are much more qualitative assessments of process and approach. This does not imply that superficial approaches are necessarily poor ones. The important issue is the purpose of the evaluation, which helps to determine the level of assessment that is necessary. There are many occasions where quick screenings in the major areas are totally appropriate. Thus, greater and more in-depth testing is not always the most prudent course. Clinicians are often guilty of unnecessary overtesting. Good practice will take into consideration the referral question, as well as the existing documentation and history before one decides about the level of assessment.

When one is reading the educational assessment section of a psychoeducational report the most important consideration for the optometrist will be the type of reading or learning problem being described. This may have implications as to how much involvement the optometrist will have in the treatment. First, it is imperative that the optometrist determine where the problem falls on a continuum from mild to moderate to severe. The degree of the problem dictates the levels of treatment. Second, categorizing the reading problem as one that is primarily based on decoding or one that involves higher level thinking skills, as in comprehension, will also help guide the optometrist. The major issue is about who should be involved in the treatment and what type of treatment is most effective. This is not always apparent, especially when there are multiple layers of problems and deficiencies.

Emotional and personality functioning

Just as other aspects of a person's functioning, such as cognitive deficiencies, perceptual abilities, memory skills, and visual disorders, can interfere with progress in learning, so too can emotional issues interfere and exacerbate learning problems. For example, reading is a developmental task that cannot be obtained until a youngster is ready. This includes an assumption that the central nervous system is mature enough to handle the complex demands of the act of reading. To some youngsters, taking that next developmental step is intimidating and frightening, and emotional issues may surface. Reading may be perceived to be an act that only "the big people do," and this little person may not feel equipped to tackle such an adult activity.

In the assessment of emotional and personality functioning there is a myriad of issues that need to be considered. These issues are related to the child's level of age, development, and experiential background.

How is a person tested and what are the major issues that are considered? The nature of the referral and the time constraints placed upon the testing determine the extent and depth of testing. Reports received from schools frequently make reference to fairly brief screenings done in the emotional and personality areas. This is a function of the massive case loads that await the school psychologist. They simply do not have the time to give more extensive evaluations.

Typical psychoeducational assessments evaluate emotional state and personality on a continuum from objective measures that ask the person directly how he feels about a certain issue, to much more indirect or projective methods of gaining information. In the more direct method the person is asked a range of questions in what is called a "clinical interview." Insight from this interview can be gained about the person's feelings about himself, key people in his life, school, and so on. It is very important for the clinician to try to understand the youngster's self-perceptions because most people with learning problems feel bad about themselves. Determining whether the person has pervasive negative feelings or is negative about a specific area (such as home, school friends) has different implications for treatment and prognosis.

For example, compare the following two responses to this question: What do you not like about yourself? The first youngster said, "There's not much I don't like. I just get down about my grades." Contrast this statement with another child who said, " It's hard to say what I don't like. There are so many things; I just hate myself." Obviously, the pervasive sense of negativity that is suggested by the statement of the second youngster will likely be a significant obstacle to overcome if progress in the academic arena is to take place.

Also important in the clinical interview is the child's view of the family. Family problems weigh heavily on children. Often, the children are the "lightning rods" for marital discord. In fact, many families who are unable to admit they have a problem use a psychoeducational evaluation as a means of broaching sensitive subjects that otherwise would remain unstated. Discussing the family with the child and observing him in the family context and listening to the family's view of the different relations provide important insights in the assessment process.

Other ways of gaining insight into a person's emotional life include the more projective methods. The concept of projective testing is that a person's responses to tests reflect personal associations which are "projected" onto the material. These are often believed to represent less conscious thoughts. Sentence completions tests ask that a person complete a sentence stem with the first thing that comes to mind, such as "All my life I. . . . Other methods include projective drawings, in which drawings are used to interpret major themes and issues that are relevant to the individual. Figure 12.8 was drawn by the youngster in case 1.

The size of the drawing and the helpless looking arms indicate that this youngster feels fairly insecure and uncertain about himself. Stories told to picture cards and responses to unstructured stimuli such as in the Rorschach Inkblot test[33] provide "deeper" insight into the person's personality and emotional makeup. The story below from the Thematic Apperception Test was told about a picture of a boy looking down at a violin sitting

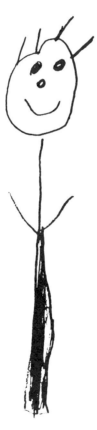

FIGURE 12.8 A drawing of a child used by psychologists to study themes and issues that are important to the individual.

on his desk. Typically, this picture provides insight into a person's feelings about achievement, motivation, and goal orientation.

> *He's looking at the violin and he's wondering whether he should practice or not. His mother's forcing him to even though he hates it. (Examiner asks how the story ends?) He breaks the violin and sneaks out to play.*

The student's "projective" story reveals the sense of frustration and anger being experienced and implies his own internal lack of motivation.

Importance of the emotional and personality assessment for the optometrist. When optometrists consider the emotional and personality section of the report the same basic concepts that were discussed in the achievement section apply. How severe are the emotional problems? What can an optometrist expect from the youngster? Will he be very difficult to manage? Is the child overly withdrawn? Is there too much anger and tension in the family system to expect consistent follow-up?

Understanding a child's emotional experience is very difficult. Children are not forthcoming about their feelings, and much needs to be done by way of inference. It is crucial to understand, though, that negative feelings, such as anger, depression, and anxiety can deplete a child and leave him with little energy for sustained academic tasks. Many children who are considered to be learning disabled may well be masking emotions that interfere with schooling. To the extent that professionals can understand these, it is well worth the time and effort involved.

SUMMARY

It has been a theme of this chapter that a more successful outcome will be obtained when the various professionals involved in treating children with learning problems work together. The more thorough the understanding of the varied elements composing the child's problems, the more effective is the remedial plan that can be developed and carried out. The educator will be most effective in addressing learning problems when vision, hearing, medical, neurological, emotional, and behavioral concerns have been discovered and corrected, or addressed to the extent possible.

Communication is the key to accomplishing the above results. However, to avoid a problem like the blind men touching the elephant in various places and then describing completely different perceptions, the optometrist, psychologist, and educator must have an understanding of the others' roles. When a referral is made to an optometrist, it is hoped that any barriers to learning within the vision sphere will be corrected. Thus, if glasses or vision therapy are needed to allow more sustained reading ability and concentration and better visual information processing skills, the optometrist plays a key role. The optometrist will need to explain the nature of the vision problem and how it would be expected to interfere with learning, unless successfully remediated. It is easier for other professionals to understand the need for glasses than the need for vision therapy.

Having access to research regarding the effects of accommodative, binocular, ocular motility, and visual information processing disorders on learning is often helpful. The different effects of various vision problems at different times in the child's educational career must also be explained to other professionals. For example, if a parent has been told that the child has had a long-standing binocular vision problem, why did it not cause problems for the child until he entered junior high school? Why would an accommodative problem be related to difficulty copying from the blackboard? The more the optometrist is able to associate the visual requirements related to adequate task performance that a child faces on a daily basis, the greater is the cooperation of the educator or other professionals who will be able to see concrete results from the therapy.

The two cases described in Appendix B required optometric intervention in completely different ways. Neither boy had received a thorough eye examination before the psychological evaluation. In case 1, a 7-year-old who was struggling to develop beginning reading skills and who had a family history of dyslexia, significant visual information processing problems were noted from the psychological evaluation. In addition, speech and language, and audiological evaluations also noted areas of concern. The optometrist could be a valuable member of the treatment team regarding ways to help this child. First, visual acuity problems need to be ruled out. Second, the child had greatest problems with visual closure and letter reversals, areas that could be addressed in vision therapy and could have a positive influence on the child's being able to begin to develop a sight vocabulary and influence on other aspects of word-learning methods.

In case 2 it was observed during the psychological evaluation that the boy seemed more tired and less able to concentrate during reading tasks. Despite this, his reading comprehension skills were above average. It was also noted that he had great difficulty on the Gardner Reversal Frequency Test, though reversals were not noted in his reading or writing. An optometric evaluation was requested to determine whether a visual efficiency problem might exist. The visual examination did indeed indicate that a visual efficiency problem was present and bifocal glasses were prescribed (see Appendix B).

Because emotional problems were paramount, family and individual psychotherapy was the primary intervention needed. Continued language therapy was also indicated, particularly regarding appropriate language for interpersonal communication. However, the prescription of glasses clearly had a beneficial effect and allowed all aspects of the boy's situation to be addressed. This case again points to the importance of the optometrist in evaluating learning problems. Yet, if the boy had been seen initially by the optometrist and glasses prescribed, without a more thorough psychoeducational evaluation recommended, the glasses alone would not be effective in helping this boy be a happy, successful person.

The psychologists and educators must learn to include an optometrist as a key member of the assessment and remediation team. The optometrist must learn to treat vision problems in the context of the whole child and not in isolation. When this occurs consistently, the student will receive the greatest benefits.

CHAPTER REVIEW

1. What four areas are assessed in a psychoeducational evaluation?
2. Why is it important to gather information from many professionals when performing a psychoeducational evaluation?
3. Why must the optometrist have a clear understanding about the onset of reading problems? What differences would be hypothesized between a reading problem beginning in the first grade or the fifth grade?
4. What comparisons between Verbal IQ and Performance IQ scores are important for the optometrist to make?
5. What are some indications for a possible language problem that an optometrist could quickly become aware of during a routine eye examination?
6. What is a possible effect of a child's significant visual and auditory memory problems on vision therapy outcomes?
7. How should an optometrist respond to letter-reversal questions that are raised by parents?
8. How might emotional factors influence a child's learning development?

REFERENCES

1. Silver LB, editor: *The assessment of learning disabilities: preschool through adulthood*, Boston, 1989, College Hill Publication.
2. Gardner R: *Psychotherapeutic techniques of Richard Gardner*, Cresskill, NJ, 1986, Creative Therapeutics.
3. Achenbach TM, Edelbrock, C: *Manual for the Child Behavior Checklist and Revised Child Behavior Profile*, Burlington, 1983, University of Vermont, Department of Psychiatry.
4. Goyette CH, Connors CK, Ulrich RF: Normative data on Revised Connors Parent Rating Scale, *J Abnorm Child Psychol* 6:221-236, 1978.
5. Barkley RA: *Defiant children: a clinician's manual for parent training*, New York, 1987, Guilford Press.
6. Edelbrock CS, Achenbach TA: The teacher version of the Child Behavior Profile: boys aged 6-11, *J Consult Clin Psychol* 52:207-217, 1984.
7. Goyette CH, Connors KS, Ulrich RF: Normative data for Revised Connors Teacher Rating Scales, *J Abnorm Child Psychol* 6:221-236, 1978.
8. Barkely RA: *Attention deficit hyperactivity disorder: a handbook for diagnosis and treatment*, New York, 1990, Guilford Press.
9. Sattler JM: *Assessment of children's intelligence*, Philadelphia, 1974, WB Saunders.
10. Kaufman AS: *Intelligent testing with the WISC-R*, New York, 1979, Wiley.
11. Wechsler D: *Manual for the WISC-III*, New York, 1990, Psychological Corp.
12. Thorndike RL, Hagen EP, Sattler, JS: *Stanford-Binet Intelligence Scale: Fourth Edition*, Riverside, Calif, 1986, Riverside Publishing Co.
13. Woodcock RW, Johnson MB: *Woodcock-Johnson Tests of Cognitive Ability*, Allen, Texas, 1989, DLM Teaching Resources.
14. Beery KE, Buktenica RA: *The Beery-Buktenica Developmental Test of Vi-*

sual Motor Integration, Chicago, 1967, Follett Publishing Co.

15. Bender L: *Bender Motor Gestalt Test,* Odessa, Fla, 1938, Psychological Assessment Resources.

16. Benton AL: *The Revised Visual Retention Test,* New York, 1955, Psychological Corporation.

17. DiSimoni F: *Token Test for Children,* Allen, Texas, 1978, DLM Teaching Resources.

18. Dunn LM, Dunn LM: *Peabody Picture Vocabulary Test–Revised,* Circle Pines, Minn, 1981, American Guidance Service.

19. *Boston Naming Test,* Philadelphia, 1983, Lea & Febiger.

20. Denkla M, Rudel R: Rapid automatized naming of pictured objects, colors, letters, and numbers by normal children, *Cortex* 10:186-202, 1974.

21. Hammill DD: *Detroit Tests of Learning Aptitude–2,* Austin, Texas, 1985, Pro-Ed.

22. Denman SB: *Denman Neuropsychology Memory Scale,* Charleston, SC, 1984, Sidney Denman.

23. Rey A: *Rey Auditory Verbal Learning Test. L'Examen clinique en psychologie,* Paris, 1958, Presses Universitaires de France.

24. Sheslow D, Adams W: *Wide Range Assessment of Memory and Learning (WRAML),* Wilmington, Del, 1990, Jastak Assessment Systems.

25. Gordon M: *The Gordon Diagnostic System,* DeWitt, NY, 1983, Gordon Systems.

26. Rudel RG: Rapid silent response to repeated target symbols by dyslexic and nondyslexic children, *Brain Lang* 6:52-62, 1978.

27. Kagan J: *Matching Familiar Figures Test,* Cambridge, Mass, 1964, Harvard University.

28. Boder EA, Jarrico SJ: *The Boder Test of Reading-Spelling Patterns,* New York, 1982, Grune & Stratton.

29. Woodcock RW: *Woodcock Reading Masters Tests–Revised,* Circle Pines, Minn, 1987, American Guidance Service.

30. *Wechsler Individual Achievement Test,* New York, 1992, Psychological Corporation.

31. Jastak S, Wilkinson G: *Wide Range Achievement Test–Revised,* Odessa, Fla, 1984, Psychological Assessment Resources.

32. Connolly AJ: *Key Math–Revised,* Circle Pines, Minn, 1988, American Guidance Service.

33. Rorschach H: *Rorschach Psychodiagnostic Test Plates,* Odessa, Fla, 1921, Psychological Assessment Resources.

CHAPTER **13**

Case Presentation

MITCHELL M. SCHEIMAN
MICHAEL W. ROUSE

KEY TERMS

communication
treatment goals

case presentation sequence
written correspondence

Successful case presentation and communication for visual efficiency and visual information processing disorders depends on several factors including the clinician's ability to:

- Communicate the nature and extent of the vision problem
- Communicate the relationship between the vision problems and the entering complaints, signs, and symptoms
- Communicate the nature of the proposed treatment and expected outcomes
- Communicate with other professionals orally and in writing about the diagnosis, proposed treatment, and expected outcomes

DETERMINATION OF TREATMENT GOALS

During the case presentation it is important for the clinician to establish the patient's goals and his or her own treatment goals. These two sets of objectives should match. If they do not, the possibility of patient dissatisfaction increases. If the patient and the clinician have different goals, it would be possible for the doctor to believe that the patient has been "cured," whereas the patient may believe that there has been no improvement.

For the patient presenting with a visual efficiency problem without learning problems, the chief concern of the patient is overcoming symptoms. The goal of the practitioner is to improve certain visual functions in some measurable way. The criterion that practitioners use to define functional correction of these cases therefore involves some combination of decrease in symptoms and improvement in measured visual functions. After treatment the patient should feel that his or her original symptoms have been eliminated or significantly improved. In addition, accommodative and binocular test findings should fall within normal parameters. In this type of case the objectives of the clinician and the patient are compatible. After treatment, if the clinician is satisfied and has achieved his objectives, the patient will also be content.

For patients with visual efficiency and visual information processing disorders along with learning problems this issue is more complex. These patients may present with asthenopia, blurred vision, diplopia, reversals, sloppy handwriting, or other school-related problems. If so, their goal will be to eliminate these symptoms and improve learning performance. Alternatively they may present with complaints or concerns about school performance without visual symptoms. In such cases, the patient's goal will be to improve learning and school performance. In both instances there is a critical difference between this patient and one with a visual efficiency problem without learning-related issues. These patients may expect more from us than just feeling better. They are looking for a solution to their learning problems.

Although there are certainly some instances in which treatment of a visual efficiency or a visual information processing problem will directly influence some aspect of learning, this is not always the case. It is so critical that the clinician emphasize that although the treatment of the visual problems is designed to eliminate symptoms and improve visual function it may not lead to direct improvement in school performance. In Chapters 5 and 6, Drs. Flax and Garzia discussed the various situations in which you would expect direct improvement and those for which you would not. In this chapter we present several "model" case presentations that clinicians can use as a basis for developing their own clinical presentations for these complicated situations.

CASE PRESENTATION

The clinician's ability to communicate his thoughts about diagnosis and treatment to the patient is critical to the success of any treatment plan. In all cases of learning-related vision problems, this presentation will require more time and effort than more routine vision care.

Most people have little or no knowledge of these vision problems and have not had any personal experience with them. It is therefore necessary to educate the patient or parents about the nature of these conditions. It is best to speak to both parents at the case conference. If this is not possible, then after the parents receive your report, the parent that was unable to attend the conference should be encouraged to call with any questions.

Case Presentation Sequence

Review the chief complaint and symptoms.
Explain the vision disorder found and the relationship between the chief complaint and symptoms.
Explain the treatment plan and prognosis for improvement of the vision problem and elimination of associated symptoms.
Explain the time and financial commitment.
Open questions and discussion.

We try to organize the case presentation into several phases. Each phase of the presentation has a specific objective. The phases are listed in the box.

Sample case presentation for visual efficiency problem related to learning requiring vision therapy

The following is an example of a presentation to the parents of a 12-year-old child, seventh grader, with a convergence insufficiency. He was brought in for an examination because of concern about his school performance. Specifically, Jimmy had been experiencing difficulty keeping up with his reading assignments. He had always been an outstanding student and achieved good grades with limited effort. This year he changed schools and several teachers regularly assigned large amounts of reading. Jimmy found that after reading for 10 to 15 minutes he began to feel uncomfortable and had difficulty concentrating on reading. As a result his performance was considerably poorer than in previous years.

Phase one: Review the chief complaint and symptoms. Beginning the presentation with a review of why the patient was brought in to see you is an important starting point and allows you to build a relationship between the visual complaints and the diagnostic findings.

> I am going to begin by first reviewing the various problems and complaints that Jimmy has been reporting. As you remember, he has been complaining of eyestrain, blurred vision and words moving on the page after reading for about 10 to 15 minutes. In previous years in school Jimmy did very well, but as we discussed, he really did not have to read for extended periods of time. You mentioned that currently two of his teachers are assigning large amounts of reading. Because of Jimmy's inability to complete and concentrate on these reading assignments his marks have been much poorer. You brought Jimmy to see me to learn if there might be a vision problem that could explain his school performance problems.
>
> You mentioned that he has never had a full vision examination, although he has always passed his school screening. In fact, he passed his school eye test just two months ago.
>
> Does that seem like a reasonable summary of why you brought Jimmy to see me?

Give the parents an opportunity to add any additional information or to agree that the key elements of the problem have been reviewed.

Phase two: Explain the nature of the vision problem.

I want to spend a little more time than usual reviewing my findings because Jimmy has a type of vision problem with which many people are not familiar. Most people are aware of vision problems, such as nearsightedness or farsightedness, that effect our ability to see clearly. You know that we treat these conditions using eyeglasses. In Jimmy's case he sees clearly. In fact, he has perfect 20/20 eyesight in both eyes, his eyes are healthy and he is neither nearsighted nor farsighted.

However, I want to stress that good vision is more than being able to see 20/20. It is possible to have excellent vision in each eye and still have a significant vision problem. For example, focusing, eye teaming and tracking problems can all be present even though a person has 20/20 vision. People who have problems like these often see clearly but have uncomfortable vision, eyestrain, headaches, double vision, and similar symptoms when reading. This is the reason why a school vision screening which tests only for 20/20 vision will often fail to detect significant vision problems. That is exactly what has happened to Jimmy.

In Jimmy's case he has an eye teaming problem. I am sure that you have seen children with severe eye teaming problems in which an eye actually turns in or out. Jimmy does not have a severe problem like this. However, when he reads or does any close work, his eyes have a very strong tendency to drift out, and his ability to compensate for this is inadequate.

We encourage the parent or parents to be present during the examination so that we can demonstrate deficient findings such as the near point of convergence, fusional vergence, and accommodative facility. If the parent or parents were not present at the examination, this is a good opportunity to demonstrate these problems.

If his eyes actually turn out, he would experience double vision. Therefore, whenever he reads he has to use excessive effort to prevent his eyes from drifting out. This constant need to use excessive effort can lead to the types of symptoms described by Jimmy. Patients with eye teaming problems complain of a variety of problems including eyestrain, headaches, blurred vision, double vision, sleepiness, difficulty concentrating on reading material, loss of comprehension over time, a pulling sensation around the eyes, and movement of the print.

I believe that the school problems that he is experiencing this year may be due to this eye teaming problem. We know that Jimmy is very bright and has succeeded in previous years. The only significant difference this year is the increase in reading that has been expected. His inability to concentrate and read comfortably is obviously interfering. It seems reasonable that if we can successfully treat this problem so that he is completely comfortable his reading and school performance may improve. Do you have questions about Jimmy's vision problem?

Stop at this point to give the parents or patient an opportunity to ask any questions about the nature of the problem, how it may cause symptoms, and how it may be related to learning. It is a good idea to ask the parent to summarize what he or she believes the problem may be after hearing your presentation.

Phase three: Explain the proposed treatment plan.

> I have been stressing that Jimmy's vision problem is different from the usual vision problems that are treated with eyeglasses. Jimmy does not have an optical problem such as nearsightedness or farsightedness. As a result, standard optical treatment using eyeglasses alone would not be successful. Rather, I am recommending that we treat Jimmy using an approach called "vision therapy."
>
> Vision therapy is a treatment approach involving a series of office visits in which we use a variety of instruments and procedures to teach Jimmy how to overcome this eye teaming problem. I know you have heard of children receiving therapy or tutoring for speech, reading, or math. You know that with an effective therapist or tutor these skills can be improved.
>
> The good news is that vision therapy has also been shown to work very well and will almost always lead to improved eye teaming skills. In fact, we are successful in about 9 out of 10 patients. The key to success is motivation and a commitment to attending the therapy sessions and performing the recommended home therapy techniques. Treatment for the type of vision problem that Jimmy has generally requires about 3 months of vision therapy. We will need to see Jimmy two times each week and each visit will last 45 minutes. We will also ask Jimmy to do 10 to 15 minutes of home vision therapy for 5 days per week. I will give you a packet of information about vision therapy as you leave today.
>
> Once vision therapy is complete, we ask all our patients to work on their own at home with several procedures. For example, for the first 3 months after the completion of vision therapy we ask the patient to work 3 times a week, 5 minutes each time. We reevaluate the patient at this time, and if everything seems fine, we ask the patient to work once a week for 5 minutes for the next 6 months. If at this 6-month reevaluation the patient is still comfortable and the vision findings are normal, we ask the patient to check his eyes once a month using one very simple procedure.
>
> As Jimmy begins to overcome his eye teaming problem we expect that he will be able to read comfortably for considerably longer periods of time. If this occurs we should see improvement in his school performance.
>
> Do you have any questions about my recommendations?

Stop and give the parents an opportunity to question you about vision therapy. If you are not sure if the patient understands, it is useful to ask the parent to summarize the treatment plan.

Phase four: Discuss the time and financial commitment. If vision therapy has been recommended, it is particularly important for the optometrists to spend time discussing the time and financial commitment that will be necessary.

> The treatment approach that I am recommending is going to require both a time and financial commitment on your part. To successfully treat Jimmy's eye teaming problem we will need to work with him for about 3

months. As a general rule we need to see the child twice a week over this period of time, and each visit lasts 45 minutes. In addition, he will be asked to work at home on various home vision therapy techniques for about 15 minutes, five times per week. Vision therapy visits are scheduled late afternoons and early evenings.

The fee for each therapy visit is $50. In many cases medical insurance covers about 80% of the cost of vision therapy. My staff will be happy to assist you in finding out whether your insurance company will cover Jimmy's therapy.

One important idea to keep in mind when discussing this with your insurance company is that the treatment we have recommended is not considered vision care. Rather, Jimmy has a medical condition, and we have recommended medical treatment called "vision therapy," or "orthoptics." This distinction is important because most medical insurance will cover only one vision examination once a year or every 2 years, and some do not cover routine vision care at all. Vision therapy, however, is not routine vision care, and for insurance purposes is considered a form of medical treatment. It is very important that you use the correct terminology when you communicate with your insurance company. In my correspondence to you I will include a letter with a full explanation of the diagnosis and treatment plan that you can forward to your insurance company for a predetermination of benefits (Appendix G).

It might take several weeks for your company to respond. If they do not give a positive response, make sure you get any denial of benefits in writing and send it to us. If we know the basis for the denial we can sometimes reverse the company's decision to deny benefits.

Do you have any questions about scheduling, the cost of vision therapy, or the insurance?"

Phase five: Open questions and discussion. This last phase is designed to allow the parents one more opportunity to ask you questions about any issues discussed in the case presentation. It is also your opportunity to summarize the presentation and determine if the parents would like you to send a report to the school or other professionals.

At this time we tell the parents that we will send a report summarizing the evaluation, diagnosis, and recommended treatment. If vision therapy has been recommended we also send a letter of predetermination to the insurance company.

Sample explanation of proposed treatment using prism

Regardless of the diagnosis and treatment, we follow the case presentation sequence described in Table 13-1 for all learning-related vision disorders. If added lenses in a bifocal format or prism are recommended, the explanation of the proposed treatment and prognosis for improvement will require additional time. Most people have no personal experience with the use of prism, and bifocals are almost universally associated with vision problems of middle age and older people. It is necessary therefore to educate the parents about the use of these treatment options. The presentation is significantly shorter and less complex when vision therapy is not necessary. However, even if the only treatment necessary is a single vision prescription for reading, time should be spent in each of the five phases outlined above.

Phases one and two. Reviewing symptoms and reasons for the visit, explanation of the vision disorder, and relating the vision disorder to learning are similar to the previous sample explanation.

Phase three: proposed treatment and prognosis for improvement

I have been stressing that Billy's vision problem is different from the usual vision problems that are treated with traditional eyeglasses. Billy does not have an optical problem such as nearsightedness or farsightedness. As a result, standard optical treatment alone with regular eyeglasses would not be successful. Rather, I am recommending that we treat Jimmy using eyeglasses that contain a special lens called "prism."

Prism is used when a person has a particular type of eye teaming problem. As we discussed earlier, Billy has a problem in which his eyes have a strong tendency to drift in. To control this tendency he has to use excessive amounts of effort. A prism is a special type of lens that decreases the amount of effort that a person must use to control an eye teaming problem. The glasses will not look very different from regular glasses, though if you look closely you will see that one edge will be thicker then the other. It is important for you to realize that although prism will help Billy when he wears the glasses the underlying problem will still be present. Prism does not correct the eye teaming problem. Rather, it will allow Billy to function more comfortably despite the eye teaming problem.

Sample explanation of proposed treatment using a bifocal

Phases one and two. Reviewing symptoms and reasons for the visit, explanation of the vision disorder, and relating the vision disorder to learning are similar to the previous sample explanation.

Phase three: proposed treatment and prognosis for improvement

I have been stressing that Paul's vision problem is different from the usual vision problems that are treated with traditional eyeglasses. Paul does not have an optical problem such as nearsightedness or farsightedness. As a result, standard optical treatment alone would not be successful. Rather, I am recommending that we treat Paul using glasses with a special lens called "bifocals."

We often prescribe bifocals for people that have focusing or eye teaming problems. Bifocals are used when the power of the lens necessary for reading is different from the power of the lens needed for looking at a distance. Bifocals are useful for focusing problems because they decrease the amount of focusing effort the patient must use. They are also helpful for some eye teaming problems. In Paul's case, for example, his eyes have a tendency to drift in, and his ability to compensate is inadequate. He must therefore use effort to control the eye teaming problem. The bifocals I am prescribing will reduce the amount of effort that Paul must use. It is important for you to realize that although the bifocal lens will help Paul while he wears the glasses the underlying problem will still be present. Bifocals do not correct the eye teaming problem. Rather, they will allow Paul to function more comfortably despite the eye teaming problem.

Sample case presentation for visual information processing problems requiring vision therapy

The following is an example of a presentation to the parents of a 8-year-old child (second grade) with a visual information processing problem. He was brought in for an examination because of concern about his school performance. Specifically, Steven had been experiencing difficulty since kindergarten. He was still reversing letters and numbers and transposing words. Steven was having difficulty getting information down in writing. He seemed very bright because he had strong language skills, but any task in school that involved getting information down on paper was very frustrating for him. Copying his homework assignments from the chalkboard was particularly difficult. He was retained in first grade because his teachers felt he was immature. Despite repeating first grade, he continued to struggle. He had recently been tested by the school psychologist who had referred him for a visual information processing evaluation because of a 25-point difference between his verbal and performance IQ's on the WISC-R (verbal higher than performance).

Phase one: Review the symptoms and reasons for the visit. Beginning the presentation with a review of why the patient was brought in to see you is an important starting point and allows you to build a relationship between the visual complaints and the diagnostic findings.

> I am going to begin by first reviewing the various problems that you are concerned about. As you mentioned earlier, Steven had been experiencing difficulty since kindergarten. He reverses letters and numbers and transposes words. He is frustrated by any task in school that involves getting information down on paper. Copying his homework assignments from the chalkboard is particularly difficult. He was retained in first grade because his teachers felt he was immature. Despite repeating first grade, he continues to struggle. His recent test by the school psychologist showed a 25-point difference between his verbal and performance IQ's on the WISC-R (verbal higher than performance). Although he is in second grade and was retained once, he is reading at only a first-grade level.
>
> You mentioned that he has never had a full vision examination, though he has always passed his school and pediatrician screenings.
>
> Does that seem like a reasonable summary of why you brought Steven to see me?

Give the parents an opportunity to add any additional information or to agree that the key elements of the problem have been reviewed.

Phase two: Explain the nature of the vision problem.

> I want to spend a little more time then usual reviewing my findings because Steven has a type of vision problem with which many people are

not familiar. Most people are aware of vision problems such as nearsightedness or farsightedness that affect our ability to see clearly. You know that we treat these conditions using eyeglasses. In Steven's case he sees clearly. In fact, he has perfect 20/20 vision in both eyes, his eyes are healthy, his eyes work together in a coordinated way, and he is neither nearsighted nor farsighted.

However, I want to stress that good vision is more than being able to see 20/20. It is possible to have excellent vision in each eye and still have a significant vision problem. For example, children may see clearly but have difficulty processing and analyzing the information coming in through their visual system.

In Steven's case he has problems in several areas of visual information processing that appear to explain some of the difficulties he has in school. Let's review the special testing that we completed today.

First I want to give you just a little background information about the way we interpret the tests we used. To make sense of the tests we just gave Steven we have to compare his performance to other children his age and at his grade level. The score we use is called a "percentile." I know that you are probably familiar with percentile scores because pediatricians and schools often use these scores. For instance, I am sure you have heard your pediatrician talk about Steven's height or weight in these terms. If the pediatrician tells you that Steven is in the 10th percentile in height you would know that he is short for his age. If he is in the 95th percentile he is tall for his age. When the school reports the results of achievement tests, they often use percentile scores. The 50th percentile is considered average. Below the 50th percentile is below average, though we generally do not become concerned about scores until they drop below the 30th percentile.

Do you understand this concept of percentile scores? Remember that this is different from a test in school. If Steven received a grade of 50 out of out of 100 points on a math test it would be a problem of course. But in the testing we are talking about a score of 50th percentile is considered normal.

For the next part of the case presentation we recommend that you have the child's actual test results along with samples of the various tests used. For example, we photocopy one or two items from each test and place them in a binder that we can use during the presentation.

With that background let's look at Steven's tests results.

Show the parents the results from the Gardner Reversal Frequency Recognition Subtest.

On this test we asked Steven to cross out the number or letter in each pair that is backwards. I think you can see that he had considerable difficulty with this task. He made a total of 22 errors, which is very poor for his age. In fact this places him below the 1st percentile. This test looks at his ability to differentiate left and right and apply this understanding to letters and numbers. This may be one reason why he continues to reverse and transpose letters, numbers, and words.

The other area in which he had great difficulty was a skill called "visual motor integration." This test is an example of how we test this area.

Show the parents the Visual Motor Integration Test forms along with the child's test results.

Look how Steven copied some of these shapes. On this test he scored at only the 10th percentile for children at his grade level. Again this means that if we tested 100 children in second grade, 90 of them would have performed better than Steven. This test tells us that Steven has difficulty analyzing and reproducing visual information. Children that have problems with visual motor integration often have difficulty with copying tasks, and writing and organizing information on a page. Again this test result seems to explain some of Steven's problems.

It is important to point out that in several other areas Steven performed very well. On this test that evaluates his ability to discriminate fine likeness and differences he scored at the 75th percentile and in visual memory at the 63rd percentile. His auditory processing skills were also above average.

To summarize, we found that Steven has problems in directionality, the ability to apply the concepts of left and right, and visual motor integration, the ability to reproduce visual information.

Do you have any questions at this point?

Stop at this point to give the parents or patient an opportunity to ask any questions about the nature of the problem, how it may cause symptoms, and how it may be related to learning. It is a good idea to ask the parent to summarize what he or she believes the problem is after hearing your presentation.

Phase three: Explain the proposed treatment plan.

I have been stressing that Steven's vision problem is different from the usual vision problems that are treated with eyeglasses. Steven does not have an optical problem such as nearsightedness or farsightedness. As a result, standard optical treatment using eyeglasses alone would not be successful. Rather, I am recommending that we treat Steven using an approach called "vision therapy."

Vision therapy is a treatment approach involving a series of office visits and home therapy in which we use a variety of instruments and procedures to improve Steven's visual information processing skills. I know you have heard of children receiving therapy or tutoring for speech, reading, or math. You know that with an effective therapist or tutor these skills can be improved.

The good news is that vision therapy has also been shown to work very well and will lead to improved visual information processing skills. The key to success is motivation and a commitment to attending the therapy sessions and performing the recommended home therapy techniques. Treatment for the type of vision problem that Steven has generally requires about 6 months of vision therapy. We will need to see Steven two times each week and each visit will last 45 minutes. I will give you a packet of information about vision therapy as you leave today.

It is very important for you to understand that we will be treating his visual processing problems. In most cases we are able to improve these skills quite effectively and decrease or eliminate the symptoms we have associated with these problems. However, it is important for you to understand that we will not be teaching writing, reading, or math. The vision therapy by itself is not expected to directly improve his reading or math skills. Rather, vision therapy is designed to improve the underlying skills necessary for Steven to learn reading and math. Thus vision therapy improves the child's readiness for the classroom environment. We therefore expect that when he finishes vision therapy he will be able to benefit more from his lessons at school. We strongly recommend that he continue his reading tutoring. We have found that after vision therapy children get more out of their reading or math tutoring.

Do you have any questions about my recommendations?

Stop and give the parents an opportunity to question you about vision therapy. If you are not sure if the patient understands, it is useful to ask the parent to summarize the treatment plan.

Phase four: Discuss the time and financial commitment. If vision therapy has been recommended, it is particularly important for the optometrists to spend time discussing the time and financial commitment that will be necessary. The explanation is identical to the one used for vision efficiency problems.

Phase five: Open questions and discussion. This last phase is designed to allow the parents one more opportunity to ask you questions about any issues discussed in the case presentation. It is also your opportunity to summarize the presentation and determine if the parents would like you to send a report to the school or other professionals.

At this time we tell the parents that we will send a report summarizing the evaluation, diagnosis, and recommended treatment. If vision therapy has been recommended we also send a letter of predetermination to the insurance company.

COMMUNICATING THROUGH WRITTEN CORRESPONDENCE

Because most people have little or no knowledge of visual efficiency, visual information processing disorders, and vision therapy, it is important to follow up your case presentation with a written report. We write a report after each evaluation summarizing the symptoms, diagnosis, and proposed treatment plan. From a public relations standpoint, if you are dealing with a child, it is also helpful to send a copy of this report to other professionals who have contact with the child. We often send reports to the teachers, reading specialists, school psychologists, and pediatricians. If you practice in a small to medium-sized community, after a short amount of time these professionals will soon understand that your practice is unique and may begin to refer patients to your office when they encounter children with similar problems. We have enclosed examples of this correspondence in Appendix G.

COMMUNICATING YOUR FINDINGS TO OTHER PROFESSIONALS

Communication with other professionals is important for two reasons. First, communication can help develop your reputation in the community. Sending reports allows you to let other professionals know that your practice is different and unique. Your reports will inform them that you practice full-scope optometric care including the use of vision therapy when appropriate.

Communication is also important because of some of the misconceptions that persist about vision therapy. Despite extensive scientific support of the efficacy of vision therapy for the conditions described in this text, some professionals persist in their opposition to vision therapy. Parents often rely on the judgment of these professionals when decisions about health issues are necessary.

It is therefore essential that you use handouts, reports, and copies of articles to provide as much educational information at the time of your presentation to the patient or parents to prepare them for the negative advice they may receive. We included sources for brochures and articles that can be provided to your patients in Appendix A.

SUMMARY

The case presentation is an important step in the management of learning-related vision problems. We have presented an organized sequence of steps to follow to make the case presentation as effective as possible along with examples of the most common types of presentations. Because of the complicated nature of learning-related vision problems, we have also emphasized the importance of good written communication to parents and other professionals. This written communication provides reinforcement for the concepts that you discuss during the case presentation.

CHAPTER REVIEW

1. Outline the importance of determination of treatment goals during the case presentation.
2. You are treating a child with a visual efficiency problem and the parent asks you what the effect of this treatment will be on the child's reading level. What would your response be?
3. Using the case presentation sequence described in this chapter, play the role of the doctor and make a case presentation to a friend for each of the following type cases:
   a. Visual efficiency problem related to school performance
   b. Visual information processing problem related to school performance

PART FOUR

TREATMENT

CHAPTER 14

Development of the Overall Management Plan

MICHAEL W. ROUSE
MITCHELL M. SCHEIMAN

KEY TERMS

general treatment strategy

problem-oriented therapy

master problem list

patient progress note

office vision therapy

home vision therapy

working level

visual attention

cognitive style

motivation

The clinical challenge of managing patients presenting with learning-related vision problems can range dramatically from patient to patient. Some patient problems are managed simply with a spectacle correction of their ametropia, whereas other patients appear to have an overwhelming number of problems to manage. The initial clinical challenge is to integrate all the information gathered in the evaluation phase: comprehensive case history, status of refraction, visual efficiency skills, visual information processing skills, and psychoeducational information, and to arrive at an accurate assessment of the relationship between the objective problems and the entering signs and symptoms. The subsequent challenge is to effectively communicate the diagnosis and its relationship to the entering complaints to the parents or patient. The final challenge is to design a therapy program that will resolve or improve the objective problems the patient is experiencing. The ultimate management goal is to resolve the vision problems and eliminate the associated signs and symptoms, which in many cases removes a significant obstacle to effective learning in the academic setting.

OVERALL MANAGEMENT STRATEGY

The management of learning-related vision problems is greatly simplified when the doctor has a overall management strategy. The objective of this chapter is to provide the doctor with the overall management strategy, present the concept of problem-oriented record keeping and therapy, and discuss the role of the doctor in the therapy process. We will also discuss the role of office and home therapy and some patient factors that need to be addressed in order to achieve successful results. The details of the management plan are developed in Chapters 15 and 16 and then illustrated with case examples in Chapter 18.

The overall treatment strategy is outlined in the box. The first step in the general treatment strategy is to correct any significant refractive anomalies. Specific recommendations and guidelines on amounts of refractive error that are significant and strategies for prescribing are provided in Chapter 15. The second step is to treat the visual efficiency deficiencies. Treatment strategies are outlined in Chapter 15 for the most common diagnostic syndromes. After the treatment of the refractive condition and visual efficiency problems, the doctor will want to reassess deficient visual information processing skills. Successful remediation of visual efficiency problems often results in improved visual information processing skills.[1,2] The last step for the doctor providing comprehensive vision care for patients with learning-related vision problems is to treat any remaining visual information processing deficiencies. Chapter 16 provides a comprehensive management model for treating visual-spatial, visual-analysis, and visual-motor deficiencies. The chapter provides specific goals and subgoals that need to be achieved along with example patient interactions. The tables in Chapter 16 provide a number of representative treatment techniques for each area, and Chapter 17 provides a core of therapy procedures. There are some exceptions to this general strategy, which are discussed in Chapters 15 and 16.

General Treatment Strategy

1. **Correct significant refractive anomalies**
   a. Consider added lens power to address accommodative and vergence anomalies.
   b. Consider added prism power to address vergence anomalies.
   c. Consider occlusion to address amblyopia or other sensory anomalies.
2. **Treat residual visual efficiency anomalies.**
   a. Improve monocular eye movement and accommodative skills.
   b. Improve smooth (or tonic) vergence skills.
   c. Improve jump (disparity) vergence skills.
   d. Improve accommodative-vergence integration skills.
   e. Improve binocular eye movement skills
   f. Develop automaticity of these skills.
3. **Treat residual visual information processing anomalies.**
   a. Develop visual spatial-skills: bilateral integration, laterality, and directionality.
   b. Develop visual analysis-skills: visual discrimination, visual figure ground, visual closure, visual memory, and visualization.
   c. Develop visual-motor skills: general eye-hand coordination, efficient visual-motor ergonomics, accurate and rapid visually guided fine-motor control, ability to plan visually guided motor actions in order to reproduce complex spatial patterns.
   d. Develop automaticity of these skills.

PROBLEM-ORIENTED THERAPY

An important issue in the management approach that we are presenting is the concept of problem-oriented therapy. The initial therapy plan is designed to treat only those visual skills that are found to be objective problems in the evaluation phase. For example, a patient may have normal monocular accommodative amplitudes, but an abnormally low monocular accommodative facility, or the patient is found to have normal laterality skills but has problems with directionality concepts. For these patients, therapy would be directed to treat those specific deficient visual skills, and valuable time would not be wasted on training prerequisite skills that were determined to be adequate. So the management plan will not be a "canned" or "global" approach that will be the same for every patient. On the contrary, the management plan will be carefully planned and sequenced for the individual patient's specific visual problems.

From the evaluation that was conducted in Chapters 9 to 11 the doctor will have generated a list of specific subjective and objective problems. Subjective problems are those signs and symptoms reported by the patient, parent, teacher, or others. Objective problems are those abnormal clinical findings found in the primary care and in visual efficiency and visual information processing evaluations. To assist the doctor in designing a management plan for these problems it is extremely helpful to adopt a problem-oriented clinical recording system.[3] The heart of this system is the master problem list (MPL), which lists all the significant signs and symptoms (subjective problems) and specific clinical (objective) problems (not a syndrome diagnosis but the specific findings that were considered abnormal; see Figure 14.1). The MPL serves as a practical and convenient index to the patient's file. Placing the MPL as the top page of the patient's file keeps the doctor constantly reminded of the patient's chief compliant, syndrome diagnosis (International Classification of Diseases–Clinical Modification, ICD-CM, codes), and subjective and objective problems. Each follow-up, progress, or therapy visit would then be recorded in SOAP (subjective, objective, assessment, and plan) format (Figure 14.2). The MPL would be updated when subjective or objective problems were improved or resolved or periodically reassessed during the therapy process.

PATIENT AND DOCTOR EXPECTATIONS

During the case presentation, discussed in Chapter 13, the clinician determined the patient's or parent's treatment goals. It is very important to reinforce the agreed-upon goals of the treatment program throughout the therapy. The doctor will want to review the objectives of each phase of the therapy program and review the progress of the case with the patient or parents on a regular basis. This constant reinforcement is critical for maintaining an interested and motivated patient and parent. To assess the direct influence of therapy on the subjective complaints the doctor will, in almost all cases, find it helpful to contact the patient's teacher. This con-

MASTER PROBLEM LIST

Patient_____*Jimmy T.*_____ DOB *2/2/84*   File # ____*10067*____

Chief Compliant: ___*Problems reading for any longer than 10-15 minutes, school*___
*performance has decreased significantly over past year*_____
Syndrome DX (code): __*CI (378.83), Accom Dysf (367.55), Oculomtr Dysf (378.90)*___

| Date | P# | Specific Problem | Patient Progress/Units |||||
			1: 3/27	2: 5/1	3: 11/6	4:	5:
2/20/93	SP1	fatique with reading	B	AB	AB		
2/20/93	SP2	frontal headache	B	AB	AB		
2/20/93	SP3	interm near blur	AB	AB	AB		
	SP4						
	SP5						
	SP6						
	SP7						
	SP8						
	SP9						
	SP10						
	SP11						
	SP12						
	SP13						
	SP14						
	SP15						
2/20/93	OP1	monoc saccades	B	AB	AB		
2/20/93	OP2	binoc saccades	B	AB	AB		
2/20/93	OP3	monoc accom ampl	AB	AB	AB		
2/20/93	OP4	binoc accom ampl	B	AB	AB		
2/20/93	OP5	monoc accom fac	AB	AB	AB		
2/20/93	OP6	binoc accom fac (+)	B	AB	AB		
2/20/93	OP7	NRA	B	AB	AB		
2/20/93	OP8	PRA	B	AB	AB		
2/20/93	OP9	receded NPC	AB	AB	AB		
2/20/93	OP10	12 XP'	11XP	9XP	10XP		
2/20/93	OP11	PFC'	B	AB	AB		
2/20/93	OP12	verg fac (BO)	NC	AB	AB		
2/20/93	OP13	12" exo FD	8"	2"	2"		
2/20/93	OP14	2º fusion	B	AB	AB		
	OP15						
	OP16						
	OP17						
	OP18						
	OP19						
	OP20						

Codes: AB=Abated, B=better, NC=No Change, W=worse, NT=Not Tested

FIGURE 14.1 Example of a Master Problem List used in cases of learning-related vision problems. *SP,* Subjective problems; *OP,* objective problems.

Patient Progress Note

Patient Jimmy T.   File # 10067   Visit #   2

(S) Subjective:
No change in SPs, did HVT daily for 20mins, some near dot on 3-Dot-Card, All other procedure goals were achieved.

(O) Objective:
OP9: Pencil Pushups, 8cm to break, 14 cm recovery, is aware of physiol diplopia and effort.

OP9: 3-Dot-Card, able to fuse all but near dots, gets physiol diplopia & color fusion, is aware of effort.

OP9: Brock String, able to achieve accurate bifixation and physiol diplopia up to 12cm, is aware of effort and suppression checks

OP11: Lifesaver Card, able to achieve first two rows by using pencil, has trouble getting target clear, not sure of where to look.

OP11: Vectograms (Clown), can achieve 8BO/4BI ranges, but having difficulty with SILO concept, kinesthetic feedback improved response.

OP5: ±1.50 MAF, worked on different effort of + & -, used some lens ordering to help initially, patient awareness, able to do ~8cpm this week.

OP3: Hart Chart accom pushups, appreciates effort, quick improvement to 10cm. understands facility procedure and appreciates different effort from far to near.

(A) Assessment:
Patient is making good progress on gross convergence (OP9) procedures, relative vergence is difficult (OP11), MAA & MAF improving (OP5).

(P) Plan: HVT:
OP9: PPU, 20 repetitions to break and recovery, goal 5 cm break 10cm recover.

OP9   3-dot-card, 20 repetitions, goal be able to get near dot and quickly move between the 3 dots.

OP3   Hart Chart accom pushups and facility, 10X pushups each eye, goal 8cm, facility 20cycles each eye, goal quick change concentrate on effort difference from far to near.

OP5   ±1.50 continue monocular practice ~5mins/day, concentrate on different effort for + & -, goal 12-15cpm.

FIGURE 14.2 Example of a vision therapy progress note.

tact also keeps the teacher informed of the therapy program's goals and progress.

ROLE OF THE DOCTOR IN THERAPY

We view vision therapy as an interactive process between the patient and the doctor. The role of the doctor is to act as a facilitator, helping the patient to learn a strategy or "process" to achieve an intended skill. To fulfill this role as a facilitator the doctor should keep in mind several educational principles[4] (see the box). The ultimate goal of the doctor is to teach the patient to "internalize" changes in the visual process, as opposed to simply teaching the patient to "do" the training technique or "obtain" the desired response.[5] To facilitate this process the doctor must first emphasize the "process" or "awareness" of how the technique is accomplished, rather than the technique itself. For example, the patient with poor visual memory cannot simply be told to remember visual items more efficiently. The patient works with a therapy technique to achieve a strategy defined by the doctor (for example, Form an image in your head). The therapy technique is viewed as a tool that is necessary to mediate the acquisition of new skills and strategies. Through an interactive process, the doctor helps the patient to achieve an appropriate strategy and subsequently to improve his or her performance. Therapy requires the doctor to interact with the patient by asking questions, providing feedback of the patient's responses, and helping the patient develop alternative strategies. The doctor should never tell the patient that an answer is incorrect; there are no incorrect or correct responses in therapy. There are, however, appropriate and inappropriate strategies that can be applied to achieve a specific skill or goal.

The second concept the doctor needs to emphasize to facilitate the internalization of changes in the visual process is that the changes the patient observes during the training procedures (such as blur, diplopia) in fact result from the patient's own level of visual function. The patient should come to recognize that the changes occur internally, not externally. The changes are not created by the lenses, prisms, instruments, or the therapist, but solely by the patient. Once the patient recognizes that the changes are internal, the likelihood of the patient creating these changes

---

Educational Principles that Facilitate Vision Therapy (Spivey 1970)

1. Learning is better accomplished in an active rather than a passive manner.
2. Learning is an individualized process that occurs at different rates and in different ways for different patients.
3. Learning is accomplished more easily when it is meaningful and relevant to the patient.
4. The goals and objectives of the task at hand should be realistic and achievable to avoid patient discouragement.
5. Learning is best accomplished when the patient is provided with feedback to allow the patient to monitor his or her own performance. The feedback should be positive and rewarding, not negative or punishing.
6. Learning is best facilitated in the presence of pleasant surroundings and good interpersonal relationships.

greatly improves. In addition, it gives the patient a sense of control and accomplishment.

Once the patient can adequately perform all the skills and demonstrate the methods necessary to achieve a particular procedure, the emphasis of therapy shifts to increasing the speed and accuracy of performance. The goal is automaticity, which is the ability to perform a visual task with minimal attention and effort.[6,7] The patient is expected to maintain visual performance even in the presence of concurrent motor and cognitive demands. In this phase of therapy the doctor demands that the patient responds more quickly, adds distractors, or overloads the patient with other sensory information. The box outlines five general procedures that can be used to increase either the cognitive or motor "loading" of a technique.

The contention that automaticity is important is based on the premise that most of the visual skills addressed in the therapy program are visual processes that should function without the patient's conscious awareness during cognitive activities. For example, accommodative accuracy and visual motor integration should be occurring automatically in the act of writing. Frequently, when a new skill is learned, a tremendous amount of energy is required for adequate performance. If the patient expends the majority of his or her cognitive resources on lower level skills, poor performance on the higher level cognitive act may result. In our experience, if therapy is stopped at this point, the newly learned visual skills tend not to transfer to everyday activities.

ROLE OF OFFICE AND HOME THERAPY

The therapy sequences outlined in this text are designed to include a combination of office vision therapy (OVT) and home vision therapy (HVT) procedures. OVT procedures are structured to teach the patient a "strat-

---

**Techniques for Increasing the Cognitive and Motor "Loading"
of a Therapy Procedure**

1. The patient performs visual efficiency procedure through *increased accommodative and vergence demands* (such as base-out therapy through a +2.00 flipper).
2. The patient performs the procedure with an *increased motor demand* (such as bouncing on a rebounder (small trampoline), standing on a balance board, and shifting weight in different directions).
3. The patient performs the procedure keeping pace to an *auditory rhythm demand* (by metronome).
4. The patient performs the procedure with an *increased cognitive demand* (such as a doctor engaging the patient in conversation; a patient solving a continuous arithmetic task such as, "How much is 7 + 3? plus 4? minus 6?" or doing a difficult backwards counting task, such as "Count backwards by threes from 121.").
5. The doctor combines two or more of the above demands.

egy" or "process" to achieve a specific therapy goal. Once the patient is aware of the "process", he or she will be sent home so that the newly acquired skill or techniques can be practiced. The amount of time spent in both the office and home may need to be modified based on the number of patient factors, such as developmental level and motivation, that we discuss later in the chapter. Additionally, the parents' schedules and ability to work with their own child may limit the effectiveness of home vision therapy and necessitate an increased number of office visits per week.

Office vision therapy

When HVT is possible and good results are anticipated, OVT can be prescribed on a once-per-week basis. However, for difficult patients or when HVT cannot be performed, a minimal schedule of two to three times per week of OVT is recommended. The average in-office training time is approximately 45 minutes, though variations between 30 and 60 minutes are common.

Each OVT session usually begins with a review of the patient's HVT. This review allows the doctor to monitor the level of compliance and progress on each of the procedures. To confirm the patient's and parent's verbal reports of compliance and progress, the doctor should ask the patient to demonstrate each HVT technique. In this way, the doctor can verify whether the training was performed correctly and whether the patient achieved the prescribed therapy goals for each technique. This is also a good time to monitor for any changes in the patient's subjective complaints.

Next, OVT is conducted. The emphasis is on developing a conscious awareness of the process and strategies to successfully accomplish the procedures. When programming OVT, it is helpful to keep the four levels of difficulty described by Betts[8] in mind (see the box). Initially it is important to give the patient a visual task that can be performed correctly and easily, referred to as the basic level. Therapy should begin on a level where success is guaranteed. For example, a patient with convergence insufficiency may have difficulty on binocular accommodative facility, though monocular facility is normal. Therefore monocular activities can be in-

---

Four Levels Of Difficulty (Betts 1946)

1. The *basic level*, on which the patient can perform smoothly and easily.
2. The *probable capacity level*, the maximum (or target) that the individual could be expected to master.
3. The *frustration level*, on which activity results in disordered behavior. This lies between level 1 and level 2.
4. The *working level*, which lies above the basic level and below the frustration level. Here learning is most effective.

cluded at the beginning of the office session, not only to further improve monocular facility, but also to reinforce the positive accomplishment of a task. New techniques should be kept within the patient's range of ability but requiring some challenge. The doctor will want to carefully select and set goals at the working level of the patient. This will help avoid the frustration level. If too many techniques are assigned at one time or the difficulty level approaches the capacity level too quickly or the patient does not experience a reasonable level of success, the patient may reach the frustration level, which often results in a loss of interest and motivation. Although the doctor will want to avoid too many techniques, a sufficient variety of techniques must be prescribed to maintain the patient's interest. Four to six therapy techniques per session usually satisfies this requirement. During therapy it will often be necessary to use behavior modification techniques to maintain the patient's interest and motivation (see discussion later in this chapter).

During the review of HVT and the conducting of OVT, the doctor will be assessing the patient's progress on each procedure and the changes in visual function that is being targeted by the procedure. Based on this assessment the doctor will determine the plan for HVT and the next OVT visit. The doctor may change or modify existing procedure goals, practice time or repetitions, or add new procedures. It is important to avoid assigning too many techniques at one time, otherwise the patient may be overwhelmed. The doctor needs to demonstrate carefully each change in procedure and each new procedure to the patient. It is the doctor's responsibility to ensure that the patient is capable of performing the assigned procedures at least at a minimal level before leaving the office. This is an excellent time to get parents involved because the doctor needs to make sure that the parent understands his or her role in the HVT process. Both verbal and written instructions should be given to the patient or parent. The written instruction should outline the procedure, goals, and practice time, as well as provide some system for the patient or parent to record daily compliance and progress (Figures 14.3 and 14.4). This is an excellent tool when reviewing and assessing HVT compliance at the next OVT.

The OVT session should be documented in SOAP format (see Figure 14.2 for a sample recording). The doctor should also plan a periodic reevaluation of the visual skills being treated to monitor the effectiveness of the therapy program. In addition, the doctor should monitor for changes in the patient's subjective complaints. Because some of the initial signs were probably reported by the teacher, the doctor will need to speak with the teacher periodically to assess changes in behavior that he or she has noticed. A reasonable schedule of reevaluation would be every fifth or sixth visit. The reevaluation should be conducted with the same methods or procedures that were used to make the original diagnosis. For example, the Risley prism method was used to test and make the initial diagnosis of

HOME THERAPY INSTRUCTION FORM

Patient's Name_____ File #_____ Date _____

Technique(s)	Practice Time Repetitions	Goals
1._____ _____ _____ _____ _____	_____	1._____ _____ 2._____ _____ 3._____ _____
2._____ _____ _____ _____ _____	_____	1._____ _____ 2._____ _____ 3._____ _____
3._____ _____ _____ _____ _____	_____	1._____ _____ 2._____ _____ 3._____ _____
4._____ _____ _____ _____ _____	_____	1._____ _____ 2._____ _____ 3._____ _____

FIGURE 14.3 Example of a Home Therapy Instruction Form.

reduced positive relative vergence. Although we might have trained this visual function with several different techniques, such as Vectograms and chiastoptic fusion cards, the reevaluation would be conducted by use of the Risley Prism Method. The MPL should then be updated after the reevaluation. Again the MPL provides an index to the current condition of the patient's subjective and objective problems.

HOME THERAPY PRACTICE RECORD

TECHNIQUE	MON	TUES	WED	THURS	FRI	SAT	SUN
1.							
2.							
3.							
4.							

Record under each day, for each technique your practice time and how well you did and any problems you experienced.

FIGURE 14.4 Example of a home therapy record form that can be used to monitor home vision therapy compliance. This form is usually printed on the back of the Home Therapy Instruction Form.

Home vision training

Home vision therapy, when properly programmed and complied with, can have a significant effect on the success of the overall vision training program. Because vision training attempts to establish conditioned reflexes, frequent repetition of the correct response is necessary before conscious effort is no longer needed, and a reflex response is achieved. The suggested HVT training time is usually 20 to 30 minutes of daily home therapy for 5 days during the week. As an adjunct to OVT, HVT provides the continuity that is absent in an active therapy program managed entirely in the office. We recommend that HVT be included as part of the total training process whenever possible because it (1) provides regular practicing periods necessary for correct responses to eventually become reflexive in nature, (2) enables the patient to make progress on his or her own, (3) results in a reduction in the number of office visits necessary, (4) prevents regression between office visits, and (5) maintains the patient's interest.[9]

Parental involvement is a critical requirement for successful HVT if the patient is a child. Optimum results will be achieved when the parent clearly understands his or her role as the home therapist. HVT failures are more often attributable to a parent's inability to deal with the family dynamics and stress created during active therapy than attributable to the inadequacies of the prescribed home training techniques.[10] Whoever, such as parent, grandparent, or older sibling, assists the child with HVT should be present and observe the in-office instruction of all HVT. This allows the doctor to instruct that person on how to correctly perform and provide the necessary feedback for each HVT procedure. That person should be informed of the subgoals and final goal of each procedure. Additionally, the parent observes the optometrist's behavior and interaction with the child and models these characteristics in the HVT. The parent's role as the home therapist is to understand the optometrist's goals, administer and monitor the HVT, give positive emotional support to the child, adapt the HVT schedule to meet any variations in the emotional and physical status of the child, and bring the child on time and for all OVT sessions.

PRELIMINARY THERAPY CONSIDERATIONS

Programming and selecting the appropriate vision therapy procedures for both OVT and HVT is influenced by several patient factors, which include the patient's age and developmental status, auditory abilities, cognitive development and style, cooperation, and motivation. Accounting for these factors will affect how well the patient responds to therapy, the treatment time, level of compliance, and the ultimate therapy outcome. For example, a patient who is asked to perform a procedure that is developmentally too difficult will be easily frustrated, resulting in lower levels of cooperation, motivation, and compliance.

Age and developmental level

The age of the patient will have a profound effect on the communication style, procedures selected, and level of performance expected. The younger patient is generally more challenging for the doctor. Patients of all ages learn most readily when performing a task that is both interesting and meaningful to them. Therefore, discovering each patient's interests allows a better selection of techniques and targets. Using a variety of training techniques, employing interesting and varying targets that are appropriate for the patient's age, introducing competitive games, and establishing a reward system can all be used to increase motivation, concentration, and compliance.

Young children (less than 7 years of age) require short periods (such as 5 to 10 minutes) of training with frequent changes in activity or targets. This requires adaptability and flexibility on the doctor's part. Vision training techniques that requires a high level of visual attention should be alternated with gamelike activities that demand less concentration on the child's part. Targets must be attractive and interesting; bright colors, moving objects, musical accompaniment, and flashing lights can help to hold the child's interest. Competitive games help stimulate a child's interest (especially if there is a reward for the winner!).

Communication and activities should be geared to the patient's age. Young children may listen to statements about "helping their eyes to work better" but perform best when they like the doctor and enjoy doing the therapy procedure. Older patients like to be taught the mechanics and physiological functioning of the visual system during the training session. They can be told about the specific subskills to be achieved and how they relate to subjective observations and progression toward binocular vision that is both comfortable and efficient. Unlike older patients, young patients often fail to understand the purpose of vision training and the potential importance of remediating their visual problem. They will need external rewards from the doctor and parents to maintain their interest and motivation.

In addition to the patient's chronological age, the doctor has to take into account the patient's developmental status. The patient's developmental level can be determined by a review of each deficient area in the visual information processing evaluation. For a patient operating at a developmental level of 7 years of age or less, therapy procedures should emphasize a multisensory approach. In a multisensory approach, additional sensory modalities, such as visual, auditory, kinesthetic, and tactile, are used in the presentation of materials to develop normal perception in another modality.[11] For patients with delays in visual information processing skills, kinesthetic or tactile reinforcement of the visual response is typically used in vision therapy procedures. For example, a patient may need to trace a square with his finger before drawing one. This parallel information creates a motor memory trace of the visual stimuli that is being processed through the visual channel.[12] Processing equivalent information in the two senses facilitates a visual motor match, which in turn expedites the achievement of the specific goal defined in the therapy program. Once the appropriate visual response is achieved, the nonvisual cues are gradually removed and the patient is encouraged to use only the visual information to achieve the desired goal. When reviewing the goals of therapy outlined in Chapter 16, you should take note that many of the initial phases of treatment use multisensory learning. When an older patient has difficulty achieving the desired goal using only the visual channel, the addition of multisensory input should be considered.

Auditory processing ability

Auditory processing skills can have a significant effect on the presentation of the therapy technique. The ability to attend to and process verbal instructions is an integral component of each therapeutic procedure. As an example, if the patient has poor auditory memory, he may not be able to process directions that contain multiple steps. Therefore verbal directions should be simplified and presented at the developmental level of the patient. In some cases the doctor may need to present procedures as a package of small sequential steps. In contrast, when auditory processing skills are above average, the therapist can use verbal mediation of the visual task to develop the weaker visual processing skills. The patient essentially talks through the vision therapy procedure while the doctor slowly begins to point out the visual clues that can be used to make the task easier to perform. This strategy is built on the theory that processing in a weaker sensory modality is facilitated when it is paired with a stronger one.[13]

Visual attention and cognitive style

When a patient performs a therapy procedure, three components of attention are necessary for effective processing: coming to attention, decision making, and sustaining attention.[14,15] Diagnostic measurement of all three components of attention are available,[14] though close observation of the patient during testing can yield a reasonable assessment of each component of attention that should be considered in designing therapy procedures. The doctor should constantly monitor these three aspects of attention and modify therapy techniques to account for the patient's attention style.

The first attention requirement is for the patient to correctly orient himself to the therapy task. This is referred to as coming to attention, or the patient's ability to focus his attention on the requirements of the task. This involves understanding the instructional set and identifying the salient features within the therapy procedure that are necessary for performing the task. For example, in an accommodative facility therapy procedure, the patient has to sit in an upright position, identify the letters to keep clear, and look through the appropriate lenses. The second attention requirement in a therapy procedure is for the patient to make a decision. Decision making refers to the cognitive style of the patient. This represents a continuum from the impulsive patient (a fast and inaccurate decision maker) to the reflective patient (a thoughtful problem solver). The patient that is an impulsive decision maker will answer quickly without looking at alternative answers or considering alternative strategies. These patients should be allowed to make mistakes, but the doctor should have the patient express his or her strategy for solving the problem rather than just pointing out the correct solution. The doctor should then help the patient generate a more appropriate problem-solving strategy. In contrast, the doctor should encourage the overly reflective patient to respond more rapidly without sacrificing accuracy. The third attention requirement is for the patient to be able to sustain performance over the duration of the procedure. Many patients with visual problems lack this ability. As coming to attention and decision-making abilities improve, there is a tendency for the patient to also increase his ability to sustain attention. The doctor can promote this process by gradually lengthening the amount of time spent on a therapy procedure.

When working with the visual style of a patient, it is unlikely that therapy will change him from one processing style to another. However, there is evidence that supports the premise that one can modify the patient's style, especially that of the impulsive decision maker.[16,17] As part of the vision therapy program, it is often necessary to modify the processing style to the extent that the patient can participate effectively in the program. For impulsive patients the doctor may want to consider one or more of the methods mentioned on pp. 105 to 107. These involve delaying the patient's response time, having the doctor model more reflective behavior, develop more efficient scanning techniques for the patient or what appears to be the most effective method—cognitive self-instructional training procedures. Clinically, we have observed this modification of visual style seen in the therapy room transfer to the classroom and other settings.

Patient motivation and cooperation

Motivation is a very important ingredient in a successful therapy program. It is hoped that each patient entering into a vision therapy program is cooperative and self-motivated. Unfortunately, patients with a history of learning problems often have poor motivation. In addition, experience has shown that the possibility of improvement in the distant future is not always sufficient to develop or sustain the motivation of a patient. The problem is even more pronounced with children, who are less likely to fully appreciate the long-term advantages of vision therapy. The use of behavior modification in vision therapy is critical for developing and sustaining the patient's motivation, especially for children.[18-21]

Behavior modification studies have shown that behavior is controlled by its own immediate effects. A behavior followed by a satisfying result will be repeated with increasing frequency, whereas a behavior resulting in a neutral or unpleasant effect will decrease in frequency of occurrence. The process in which a behavior is maintained or increased in frequency when it is followed by an effect is called "positive reinforcement." The hypothesis would then be that the doctor could motivate a patient to carry out even boring procedures regularly by rewarding the patient immediately upon starting the procedure. The doctor must take care to target the appropriate behavior for reinforcement. In the beginning of therapy, the doctor will want to reward the child for "looking carefully" and for "working hard," rather than the positive outcome of the therapy. The target behavior will change depending on the stage of therapy and objectives of the particular therapy procedure.[20]

The choice of the reinforcing stimulus to sustain behavior has to be made carefully. For each case, the doctor has to find the reinforcer that is appropriate to sustain the target behavior. The doctor can usually discover a good reinforcer by asking the patient or parent about his or her interests and hobbies. With children, the parents can usually supply a list of games, events, and physical objects of interests to the child. Simple reinforcers, such as verbal praise have been shown to be effective.[21] The reinforcer should be given only when the target behavior is carried out. It is often useful also to choose several possible reinforcers. If the same reinforcer is given too often and too freely, it can lose its ability to sustain behavior (satiation occurs). Feldman[20] reported on using behavior modification to develop prerequisite behaviors for visual therapy and to facilitate the acquisition of visual skills. This paper is required reading for anyone involved in vision therapy.

An important but often overlooked factor is providing the patient with a success-oriented environment. Many patients with learning problems have a long history of failure and often develop adaptive behaviors such as avoidance. The clinician will frequently encounter patients who are either hesitant to perform activities or perform the activity rapidly to provide an excuse for poor performance. Therefore office and home therapy encounters should be positive experiences for the patient. It is often necessary to have the patient perform activities, in the office and at home, that he is already able to do with reasonable success as noted previously under office vision therapy. A simple expression should always be kept in mind when one is working with these patients: "Nothing succeeds like success." This provides a positive environment for both the child and the parent and will promote better cooperation and motivation in the future.

SUMMARY

This preliminary discussion should have prepared the reader with a general treatment strategy, a model of problem-oriented therapy and record keeping, an appreciation of the important role of the doctor in therapy, the different roles that office and home therapy play, and important patient attributes that can influence the sequencing and selection of therapy techniques.

CHAPTER REVIEW

1. Describe the general treatment strategy when a patient presents with both visual efficiency and visual information processing problems.
2. Describe the concept of problem-oriented therapy and the components of problem-oriented record keeping.
3. What is the role of the doctor in the therapy process?
4. List the preliminary therapy considerations that influence the programming and selecting of appropriate vision therapy procedures.

REFERENCES

1. Weisz CL: Clinical therapy for accommodative responses: transfer effects upon performance, *J Am Optom Assoc* 50:209-215, 1980.
2. Hoffman LG: The effect of accommodative deficiencies on the developmental level of perceptual skills, *Am J Optom Physiol Optics* 59(3):254-262, 1982.
3. London R, Caloroso EE, Barresi BJ: Problem orientation in vision therapy, *Am J Optom Physiol Optics* 58:393-399, 1981.
4. Spivey BE: Some considerations in orthoptic education, *Am Orthopt J* 20:141-147, 1970.
5. Birnbaum MH: The role of the trainer in visual training, *J Am Optom Assoc* 48:1035-1039, 1977.
6. Peachey GT: Minimum attention model for understanding the development of efficient visual function, *J Behav Optom* 2:199-206, 1991.
7. Birnbaum MH: *Optometric management of nearpoint vision disorders*, Boston, 1993, Butterworth-Heinemann.
8. Betts EA: *Foundations of reading instruction*, Chicago, 1946, American Book, Chapt. 21.
9. Caloroso EE, Rouse MW: *Clinical management of strabismus*, Boston, 1993, Butterworth-Heinemann, pp 135-139.
10. Shivas GC: Parents and visual training, *Optom Weekly* 62:170-174, 1971.
11. Gearheart BR: *Learning disabilities educational strategies*, St Louis, 1977, Mosby, pp 91-92.
12. Hulme C: *Reading retardation and multi-sensory teaching*, London, 1981, Routledge, Kegan, & Paul.
13. Frostig M: Visual perception, integrative functions and academic learning, *J Learn Disabil* 2:30-33, 1969.
14. Borsting E: Measures of visual attention is children with and without visual efficiency problems, *J Behav Optom* 2:151-156, 1991.
15. Keogh BK, Margolis J: Learn to labor and to wait: attentional problems of children with learning disorders, *J Learn Disabil* 9:276-286, 1976.
16. Blackman S, Goldstein KM: Cognitive styles and learning disabilities, *J Learn Disabil* 2:105-115, 1982.
17. Brown RT, Alford N: Ameliorating, attentional deficits and concomitant academic deficiencies in learning disabled children through cognitive training, *J Learn Disabil* 17:20-26, 1984.
18. Groffman S: Operant conditioning and vision training, *Am J Optom Arch Am Acad Optom* 46:583-594, 1969.
19. Granger L, Letourneau J: Behavior modification techniques in vision training, *Optom Weekly* 68:423-427, 1977.
20. Feldman J: Behavior modification in vision training: facilitating prerequisite behaviors and visual skills, *J Am Optom Assoc* 52:329-340, 1981.
21. Punnett AF, Steinhauer GD: Relationship between reinforcement and eye movements during ocular motor training with learning disabled children, *J Learn Disabil* 17:16-19, 1984.

CHAPTER 15

Treatment of Visual Efficiency Problems

MITCHELL M. SCHEIMAN

KEY TERMS

refractive error
added lenses
prism
occlusion
vision therapy
Aperture Rule

Vectograms
Tranaglyphs
Eccentric Circles
Free Space Fusion Cards
Hart chart

This chapter is designed to provide the clinician with an organized, sequential treatment strategy for managing visual efficiency problems. The specific context is of the patient presenting with a visual efficiency problem related to a learning difficulty. A primary objective of the model we are presenting is to emphasize the significance of considering all treatment options for every accommodative, ocular motor, and binocular vision anomaly encountered.[1] There is a limited number of management options for any patient with these disorders. When managing such patients, one would best acquire the habit of always considering each option and then either using or rejecting that management for a particular patient. This approach will ensure that no management option has been ignored and should lead to more frequent and rapid success. For example, several of the treatment options discussed below (that is, occlusion, vision therapy for amblyopia) are rarely necessary when accommodative and nonstrabismic binocular vision problems are being managed. In heterophoria cases associated with anisometropia, however, occlusion and amblyopia treatment will often be necessary. Thus it is prudent to consider all treatment options for each case.

GENERAL TREATMENT SEQUENCES FOR VISUAL EFFICIENCY PROBLEMS

In the system we describe, the size of the accommodative-convergence–to–accommodation (AC/A) ratio (low, normal, and high) determines the specific treatment sequence. The direction of the distance phoria and the analysis of the other data determine certain particulars of treatment, such as whether base-out or base-in prism should be prescribed and the nature of the vision therapy recommended. The following is a list of the various treatment approaches that should be considered for all patients with visual efficiency problems:

> **Sequential management approach for visual efficiency problems**
> Optical correction of ametropia
> Added lens power
> Prism
> Occlusion
> Vision therapy

Optical correction of ametropia

The first consideration for all patients with accommodative, ocular motor, and nonstrabismic binocular anomalies is the optical correction of the patient's ametropia. Prescription of lenses to correct the refractive error is generally not thought of as management for accommodative and binocular problems because we so routinely prescribe lens corrections. However, such prescriptions are often essential in the management of these conditions, and so it is wise to think routinely of correction of ametropia as the first consideration.

Significant degrees of refractive error. As a general rule, it is advisable to first prescribe for any significant refractive error. There are several basic underlying assumptions that form the basis for the approach of first considering management of refractive error.

The presence of an uncorrected refractive error may:

- result in either underaccommodation or overaccommodation, leading to disorders of accommodative function.
- result in a high phoria and an unusual demand on either negative or positive fusional vergence.
- create an imbalance between the two eyes leading to sensory fusion disturbances.
- create decreased fusional ability because of blurred retinal images.

The strategy of first prescribing for significant refractive error is therefore based on the assumption that there may be a cause-and-effect relationship between refractive error and accommodative and binocular vision anomalies. There are some differences in refractive errors between patients with esodeviations and exodeviations. Esodeviations tend to be associated with greater amounts of hyperopia, whereas exodeviations tend to be associated with myopia. By prescribing for the refractive condition we are attempting to minimize a possible underlying etiological factor.

Table 15.1 lists criteria for significant refractive error. It is important to view these criteria as only guidelines. With any given patient a variety of factors must be considered. For example, the general guideline is that any degree of myopia over −0.50 should be considered significant. However, there are some instances in which we would not suggest prescribing for this level of myopia. For the early elementary school child we do not prescribe until the magnitude of the myopia is 1.00 D or greater because any detrimental effects can be compensated for by preferred placement in the classroom. With low degrees of myopia it is also important to rule out an underlying accommodative or convergence problem as a cause of the myopia. In the presence of accommodative-convergence problems with low degrees of myopia we recommend elimination of the underlying problems using vision therapy before prescribing for myopia.

Although our general guideline is that 1.50 D or greater is a significant degree of hyperopia, any amount of hyperopia may be significant, depending on the status of the accommodation and vergence systems. Even low degrees of hyperopia become significant in the presence of esophoria and accommodative disorders.

When one is deciding on a prescription for ametropia, it is therefore important to consider and understand that the correction influences the vergence posture of the eyes through the AC/A ratio. As a result, we generally recommend prescribing maximum plus for esodeviations and minimum plus for exodeviations. If a patient has a condition such as convergence excess and a degree of hyperopia that might be less than the level we describe as significant, we would still prescribe to assist in the management of the convergence excess. Optical correction may also have a negative effect on binocular vision. An example is an exophoric patient with uncorrected hyperopia of 2.00 D. With correction of the ametropia the magnitude of exophoria would be expected to increase, and he may experience asthenopia and diplopia. Another example is a patient with a small amount of esophoria and 4.00 D of uncorrected hyperopia. With correction this patient may become exotropic. Management of these patients is more complex and requires the use of additional steps described below.

TABLE 15.1 Guidelines for correction of refractive error in school-aged children

Type of refractive condition	Significant amount
Hyperopia	+1.50 D or greater
Myopia	−0.50 D or greater
Astigmatism	−1.00 D or greater
Anisometropia	0.75 D difference in either the sphere or the cylinder

If a significant refractive error is present, the patient is generally asked to wear the prescription for 4 to 6 weeks and another evaluation is performed for reassessment of the status of accommodative and binocular function. In some instances, the previously detected disorders will have resolved and no additional treatment will be necessary. If accommodative, oculomotor or binocular disorders still persist after the prescription glasses are worn, additional treatment alternatives must be considered.

Insignificant degrees of refractive error. There is far less agreement about the management of small amounts of refractive error. This would be defined as a refractive error less than the values listed in Table 15.1. An example would be a patient presenting with a history of eyestrain associated with reading and the refraction is:

OD: $+0.25 -0.50 \times 90$
OS: $+0.25 -0.50 \times 90$

The question a clinician must answer is whether such a refractive error could be a contributing factor to the patient's discomfort or school-related difficulties. This decision should be based on additional testing and analysis of accommodative and binocular data and the specific type of learning problem. There are two scenarios that generally could occur. First, the patient may also present with significant accommodative and binocular problems. Assume this patient also had a near point of convergence of 15 cm/30 cm, orthophoria at distance, 12 exophoria at near and reduced positive fusional vergence. In the presence of these additional data, the low refractive error is likely to be insignificant.

Another possible situation would be a patient with the low refractive error listed above and all accommodative and binocular testing within the expected values. In this case the clinician may be left with no other possible visual basis for the patient's discomfort and must make a decision about prescribing for the low refractive error. It is wise in such a situation to ask additional questions about the nature of the symptoms to clarify whether there truly appears to be a relationship between the use of the eyes and the discomfort. If based on this additional questioning there seems to be a relationship, prescription for the low refractive error may sometimes be helpful; especially if small astigmatism corrections axis 90 or oblique are present.

In our experience, however, there is often an accommodative, oculomotor, or binocular vision disorder present in addition to the low refractive error. It is very unusual to find a low refractive error in isolation that accounts for significant symptoms.

Added lens power (minus and plus)

The other primary use of lenses in the treatment of accommodative and binocular disorders is to alter the demand on either the accommodative or binocular systems. The important clinical data that are used to determine whether such an approach will be effective are listed in Table 15.2

TABLE 15.2   Consideration for prescribing added plus lenses

Test	Consider the use of added plus	Added plus not indicated
AC/A ratio	High	Low
Refractive error	Hyperopia	Myopia
Near phoria	Esophoria	Exophoria
NRA/PRA	Low PRA	Low NRA
Positive relative vergence	Normal to high	Low
MEM retinoscopy	High	Low
Amplitude of accommodation	Low	Normal
Accommodative facility testing	Fails minus	Fails plus

AC/A, Ratio of accommodative convergence to accommodation; *MEM,* Monocular Estimate Method; *NRA,* negative relative accommodation; *PRA,* positive relative accommodation.

TABLE 15.3   Consideration for prescribing added minus lenses

Test	Consider the use of added minus	Added minus not indicated
AC/A ratio	High	Low
Phoria	Exophoria	Esophoria
Negative relative vergence	Normal to high	Low
Amplitude of accommodation	Normal	Low
Accommodative facility testing	Fails plus	Fails minus

AC/A, Ratio of accommodative convergence to accommodation.

and 15.3. Table 15.2 lists the eight findings that should be considered when one is trying to determine whether added plus lenses should be prescribed, and Table 15.3 lists the findings that should be considered one is when trying to determine whether added minus lenses should be prescribed.

The primary test finding that helps determine the effectiveness of added lenses is the magnitude of the AC/A ratio. If the AC/A ratio is higher than expected (such as ³⁄₁ to ⁶⁄₁), the use of added lenses will generally be an effective approach. A high AC/A ratio indicates that a very large change in binocular alignment can be achieved with a small addition of lenses. A low AC/A ratio indicates that the use of lenses will have little desirable effect. When the AC/A ratio is in the normal range of ³⁄₁ to ⁶⁄₁, the other data in Tables 15.2 and 15.3 must be taken into consideration before one determines the potential value of prescribing added lenses. It is important to understand the effect that plus or minus lenses will have on all optometric findings. Tables 15.4 and 15.5 provide examples of these effects.

If one keeps in mind the effect that a prescription of additional plus or minus will have on all the different optometric tests it becomes easier to make decisions about appropriate treatment for any particular patient.

The most common example of the effectiveness of the use of lenses in the absence of refractive error is convergence excess. In such a case, the

TABLE 15.4   Example of the effect of plus lenses on test results

Given: AC/A ratio = 8/1; if a +1.00 add is prescribed, it would be expected
to lead to the following changes:

Test	Expected change with +1.00
Near phoria	About 8 pd less esophoria
NRA	Decrease of about 1.00 D
PRA	Increase of about 1.00 D
Positive relative vergence (near)	Decrease of about 8 pd
Negative relative vergence (near)	Increase of about 8 pd
MEM retinoscopy	Decrease in plus
Amplitude of accommodation	Increase of about 1.00 D
Accommodative facility testing	Better performance with −2.00

TABLE 15.5   Example of the effect of minus lenses on test results

Given: AC/A ratio = 8/1; if a −1.00 add is prescribed, it would be expected
to lead to the following changes:

Test	Expected change with −1.00
Near phoria	About 8 pd less exophoria
NRA	Increase of about 1.00 D
PRA	Decrease of about 1.00 D
Positive relative vergence (near)	Increase of about 8 pd
Negative relative vergence (near)	Decrease of about 8 pd
MEM retinoscopy	Increase in plus
Amplitude of accommodation	Decrease of about 1.00 D
Accommodative facility testing	Better performance with +2.00

patient will generally have no significant phoria at distance and a moderate-to-high degree of esophoria at near. Tests assessing negative fusional vergence will be decreased and the AC/A ratio is typically high. These findings indicate that one could achieve a significant change in the amount of esophoria at near simply by prescribing plus lenses for near. If the patient has 12 prism diopters (pd) of esophoria at near, for example, with base in at near of 4/6/2 and an AC/A ratio of 10/1, an add of +1.00 would be expected to have considerable beneficial effect. In this case the add would result in a near-point phoria of about 2 esophoria and the base-in-range measured through this add would be expected to increase as well. If, however, the clinical data are somewhat different and the patient has the moderate esophoria at near with a low AC/A ratio, the use of added lenses may not be sufficient to lead to a resolution of the patient's complaints.

The classic example of the ineffectiveness of the use of lenses in the absence of refractive error is convergence insufficiency. In such a case the distance phoria is insignificant while a moderate-to-large exophoria may be present at near along with a low AC/A ratio, a receded near point of convergence, and low positive fusional vergence. The use of lenses in this case to achieve a desirable change in the near phoria would not be expected to be helpful. For instance, one might consider the use of additional minus at near. If the patient has 12 exophoria at near with an AC/A ratio of 2/1 and base-out at near of 2/4/−2, the use of −1.00 or even −2.00 at near would have little effect on the exophoria or base-out relationship. Thus, because of the low AC/A, the use of lenses in this situation would not be an effective strategy.

The use of added plus or minus lenses is particularly helpful for the conditions listed in the box. Prescription guidelines for prescribing added plus lenses are based on the information in Table 15.2. This table lists all the findings from the optometric evaluation that contribute to the final decision about prescribing added plus. The important concept is that groups of data should be analyzed rather than a single isolated finding. Although all the datum points do not have to agree, there will generally be a trend suggestive of the amount of plus that should be prescribed.

When added plus lenses are prescribed, a bifocal prescription is almost always preferable. With children below about 10 years of age I recommend setting the segment height at about the lower pupil margin to ensure that the child reads through the segment. A flat top 28 mm segment works well with young children. In older children the segment height can be set at the lower lid margin.

Added minus lenses also should be considered in certain cases. Added minus lenses are generally used for intermittent exotropes. In such cases the lenses are used to reduce the angle of deviation using accommodative convergence to supplement fusional vergence. These lenses can be prescribed as training lenses to be used only during active vision therapy or for general wear. When minus lenses are used as a training device, large amounts of minus can be prescribed (such as greater than −2.00). To determine the prescription the clinician would find the least amount of minus that allows the patient to fuse. The power of the lenses would gradually be reduced as therapy progresses and the patient's ability to fuse improves.

Added minus lenses can also be prescribed for full-time wear. This

---

Conditions Responding Favorably to Added Lenses

Added plus lenses
Convergence excess
Basic esophoria
Accommodative insufficiency

Added minus lenses
High basic exophoria
Divergence excess

would be done to reduce the percentage of time that an intermittent exotropia occurs or to provide more comfortable fusion in high exophoria. When prescribed for this purpose smaller amounts of minus (such as 1.00 to 2.00 D) are used. In such cases the AC/A ratio is not the critical factor in determining the amount of minus to prescribe. The objective of the added minus is to create a stimulus to convergence. Once this is accomplished the patient is able to maintain fusion using fusional vergence. When added minus lenses are used to help in the early treatment of an intermittent exotropia, a bifocal prescription is generally used to avoid the need to use excessive accommodative effort at near.

Prism

The use of prism to treat binocular anomalies should be a consideration in all visual efficiency cases. Generally there are five situations in which the use of prism may be helpful. These include:

- horizontal relieving prism
- vertical relieving prism
- prism as an aid to begin vision therapy
- prism used when vision therapy is inappropriate or impractical
- prism used at the end of vision therapy

Horizontal relieving prism (horizontal prism used to decrease the demand on the fusional vergence system). If a large lateral heterophoria or an intermittent strabismus is present, it may be helpful to prescribe prism to decrease the demand on fusional vergence. Prism is most often effective in cases of high tonic vergence (esophoria at distance) along with a normal-to-low AC/A ratio. Prism can be prescribed as a temporary measure until a vision therapy program has been completed, or it can be prescribed as an attempt to eliminate the patient's symptoms without vision therapy. The approaches used most often to prescribe prism are fixation disparity analysis, Sheard's criterion, and Percival's criterion.[1]

Vertical relieving prism (prism to correct vertical heterophoria). London and Wick[2] have reported that correction of a vertical fixation disparity may have a beneficial effect on the horizontal deviation. They suggest that when a vertical and horizontal deviation are both present the clinician should first consider prism correction of the vertical component. Wick[3] does not believe that vertical prism needs to be prescribed in all cases, however. He suggests that vertical prism should be prescribed when it results in improved visual performance such as decreased suppression and increased fusion ranges. When management of a horizontal heterophoria is not proceeding well, it is worthwhile to recheck for a small vertical component that may have not been detected initially. As little as ½ pd of vertical prism may be beneficial for fusion.

The most accepted criterion for determining the amount of vertical prism to prescribe is the associated phoria measurement.[3,4] In vertical heterophoria, prescribe the prism that reduces the fixation disparity to zero. Another method that has been described is Sheard's criterion. Enough vertical prism is prescribed to establish a situation in which the vertical vergence is twice the vertical phoria. There is sufficient evidence in the literature, however, demonstrating that the use of the associated phoria is preferable to Sheard's criterion.[5]

Other uses of prism

Prism as an aid to begin vision therapy. With very high degrees of heterophoria or when an intermittent strabismus is present, prism is sometimes helpful in the initial phase of vision therapy. Prism is used in such a case to decrease the overall demand on the binocular system. For example, base-out prism would be used to reduce the demand on negative fusional vergence. This enables the clinician to more easily find a starting point for vision therapy. When prescribed for this purpose, prism glasses are generally used primarily during office or home therapy.

Prism used when vision therapy is inappropriate or impractical. Although vision therapy may be indicated for a particular patient, there are factors that may limit the prognosis for vision therapy. Such factors include cooperation, motivation, the age of the patient, scheduling issues and finances. If a child is too young to be able to communicate or cooperate, if an elderly patient is unable or unwilling to perform vision therapy, or if there is simply a lack of time or money for vision therapy, prism becomes an option that should be considered.

Prism used at the conclusion of vision therapy. If the patient's symptoms persist after the conclusion of a vision therapy program, prism should be considered. In such cases prism is prescribed as a relieving prism to reduce the demand of the fusional vergence system. Criteria for prescribing are identical to those described for horizontal and vertical relieving prism.

OCCLUSION

Occlusion is a commonly used treatment option in the management of strabismus and its associated conditions: amblyopia, eccentric fixation, suppression, and anomalous correspondence. There are also instances in which occlusion is necessary in the treatment of patients with heterophoria, and it must be included as part of the sequential considerations in the management of nonstrabismic binocular anomalies.

Occlusion is used when heterophoria is associated with anisometropic amblyopia. This topic is discussed in depth in other texts.[1,6] The length of occlusion is important in anisometropic amblyopia. There have been reports in the literature of strabismus caused by the use of full-time occlusion.[7] Full-time occlusion generally refers to the use of an occluder for 8 or more hours per day. I therefore recommend direct, total occlusion for 2 to 3 hours per day, with a maximum of 4 to 6 hours. There are exceptions to this rule, however. I suggest more aggressive occlusion in anisometropia of greater than 7 D and cases of high, unilateral myopia. In these cases minimal occlusion is not always effective, and longer periods of occlusion may be necessary. Even in such cases, it is prudent to begin with short amounts of occlusion. If acuity does not improve, the number of hours of occlusion can be increased gradually until a treatment effect occurs.

Another type of occlusion that should be considered in heterophoria is the use of regional occlusion of a lens. This is particularly useful when a strabismus is present at one distance or one direction of gaze, whereas a heterophoria exists at other distances or positions of gaze. An example is a patient with a 25 pd constant, right exotropia at distance and 5 pd exophoria at near. An appropriate treatment option would be occlusion of the upper portion of the lens of the right eye, with the lower portion of the lens clear. This setup permits reinforcement of binocularity at near, while preventing suppression and other adaptations at distance.

VISION TRAINING

A significant percentage of patients with binocular vision, oculomotor, and accommodative problems cannot be successfully treated with lenses or prisms alone. Of the 12 different accommodative, oculomotor, and binocular disorders (Table 15.6) only accommodative insufficiency, diver-

TABLE 15.6 Recommended treatment approach by diagnosis

Diagnosis	Primary recommended treatment approach	Secondary treatment recommendations
Oculomotor dysfunction	Vision therapy	Added plus
Accommodative insufficiency	Added plus	Vision therapy
Accommodative excess	Vision therapy	
Accommodative infacility	Vision therapy	
LOW AC/A CONDITIONS		
Convergence insufficiency	Vision therapy	Prism
Divergence insufficiency	Prism	Vision therapy
HIGH AC/A CONDITIONS		
Convergence excess	Added lenses	Vision therapy
Divergence excess	Vision therapy	Added lenses
NORMAL AC/A CONDITIONS		
Basic esophoria	Vision therapy and added lenses	Prism
Basic exophoria	Vision therapy	Added lenses prism
Fusional vergence dysfunction	Vision therapy	
VERTICAL DISORDERS		
Vertical phoria	Prism	Vision therapy

AC/A, Accommodative convergence to accommodation.

gence insufficiency, convergence excess, basic esophoria, and vertical heterophoria are readily treated with lenses or prism alone. Prism is generally most effective for divergence insufficiency. For the other conditions the use of lenses and prism would not be expected to be totally effective. The goal of a lens or prism prescription for many of these cases, however, is maximally to increase binocularity optically. This can then be reinforced with vision therapy management.

Vision therapy is the treatment of choice for convergence insufficiency, divergence excess, fusional vergence dysfunction, basic exophoria, accommodative excess, accommodative infacility, and ocular motor dysfunction.

Effectiveness of vision therapy

Vision therapy has been shown to be effective for accomplishing the following in accommodative, oculomotor and nonstrabismic binocular vision disorders.[8,9]

- increase amplitude of accommodation
- increase accommodative facility
- eliminate accommodative spasm
- increase fusional vergence amplitudes
- increase fusional vergence facility
- eliminate suppression
- improve stereopsis
- improve the accuracy of saccades and pursuits
- improve stability of fixation

The prognosis for all accommodative and nonstrabismic binocular vision problems is excellent, except for divergence insufficiency.[8-11] In recent years there have been several studies that have reviewed success rates for various types of accommodative and binocular disorders. These studies clearly demonstrate the efficacy of vision therapy for these conditions.

Studies investigating the clinical efficacy of vision therapy for accommodative dysfunction have shown success in approximately 9 of 10 cases. Daum,[12] in a retrospective study of 96 patients found partial or total relief of both objective and subjective difficulties in 96% of the subjects studied. Hoffman et al.[13] reported a vision-therapy success rate of 87.5% in a sample of 80 patients with accommodative problems.

Other studies, using objective assessment techniques, have investigated the actual physiological changes that occur because of vision therapy. Both Liu et al.[14] and Bobier and Sivak[15] found that the dynamics of the accommodative response were significantly changed after therapy. Liu et al. found that the latency of the accommodative response was decreased and the velocity of the response was increased. Bobier and Sivak were able to show a decrease in symptoms along with objective changes in accommodative dynamics.

Numerous investigators have shown that vision therapy for nonstrabismic binocular vision disorders leads to improved fusional vergence ranges. In both prospective[16] and retrospective studies[17] Daum showed that relatively short periods of vision therapy can provide long-lasting increases in fusional vergence. Other[18-21] studies have used both experimental and control groups to demonstrate the efficacy of binocular vision therapy. Duam[18] investigated the effectiveness of vision therapy for improving positive fusional vergence using a double-blind placebo-controlled experimental design. He found statistically significant changes in vergence in the experimental group with no changes in the control group. Vaegan[19] also found large and stable improvement in vergence ranges in his experimental group with no changes in the control group. Cooper et al.[20] studied patients with convergence insufficiency using a matched-subjects control group crossover design to reduce placebo effects. They found a significant reduction in asthenopia and a significant increase in fusional vergence after the treatment. During the control phase significant changes in symptoms and vergence were not found.

Clinical studies have also been performed to investigate the efficacy of treating oculomotor dysfunction. Wold et al.[22] reported on a sample of 100 patients who had completed a vision therapy program for a variety of problems including accommodation, binocular vision, pursuits, and saccades. Saccadic and pursuit function was determined using subjective clinical performance scales like those described in Chapter 10. Vision therapy consisted of three 1-hour visits per week. The number of visits ranged from 22 to 53. It is important to understand that these patients did not have only eye movement disorders; almost all patients had accommodative and binocular vision problems as well. Pretesting and posttesting revealed statistically significant changes in both saccadic and pursuit function.

In a more recent clinical study, Rounds et al.[23] used a Visagraph Eye-Movement Recording System to assess reading eye movements before and after vision therapy. This investigation is one of the few specifically to study eye movement therapy alone. They used 19 adults with reading problems and assigned 12 to the experimental group and 9 to a control group. The experimental group received 4 weeks (12 hours) of exclusively oculomotor skill-enhancement vision therapy. The therapy consisted of three 20-minute office sessions and six 20-minute home sessions per week for 4 weeks. The control group received no intervention of any kind. Although no statistically significant changes were found, the experimental group showed trends toward improving reading eye movement efficiency (less regressions and number of fixations and increased span of recognition) compared to the control group.

Young[24] also used an objective eye movement recording instrument (Eye Trac) to assess reading eye movements before and after therapy. She studied 13 school children who had failed a vision screening. They each had three 5-minute vision therapy sessions per day for 6 weeks. They received a total of 6 hours of eye movement vision therapy. Posttesting revealed significant decrease in number of fixations, an increase in reading speed, and a decrease in fixation duration.

Fujimoto et al.[25] investigated the potential for using vision therapy procedures prerecorded on videocassettes for eye movement vision therapy. They had three groups of subjects. The first group of 9 subjects received standard eye movement vision therapy. The second group received videocassette-based eye movement therapy, and the third group received no treatment. The results showed that both standard eye movement vision therapy and videocassette-based therapy were equally effective in improving saccadic ability.

Punnett and Steinhauer[26] studied two different approaches for eye movement therapy. They compared the effectiveness of vision therapy for eye movements using feedback versus no feedback. They used the Eye Trac to monitor eye movements and studied 9 subjects. They found that the use of verbal feedback and reinforcement during vision therapy led to better treatment results.

Indications for prescribing vision therapy

Although the success rates are excellent for all cases of binocular, oculomotor, and accommodative disorders, all patients with these problems may not be good candidates for vision therapy. Many factors must be taken into consideration before a recommendation is made for vision therapy (Chapter 14). These include:

- age and developmental level of the patient
- auditory processing ability
- visual attention and cognitive style
- patient motivation and cooperation

Management decisions are particularly complicated when dealing with children with learning disorders. It is not unusual for several other critical problems to be present in addition to the visual efficiency or visual information processing problems. Sometimes conditions may not be appropriate for vision therapy, and other alternatives may have to be suggested at least temporarily.

OVERVIEW OF VISION THERAPY FOR VISUAL EFFICIENCY PROBLEMS

Vision therapy for accommodation, eye movement, and nonstrabismic binocular vision problems has been covered in great detail in other texts.[1,27] Rather than reiteration of specific details about administering vision therapy for these conditions our objective is to provide a general overview about vision therapy for visual efficiency disorders, with emphasis on the issues that are important when performing vision therapy for learning-related visual efficiency problems.

If visual information processing problems are also present, the vision therapy program will need to incorporate procedures to treat both visual efficiency and visual information processing disorders. As we discussed in Chapter 14, the treatment sequence is generally to remediate visual efficiency problems first and then reevaluate visual information processing. At times, however, it is appropriate to work simultaneously on both areas.

It is important to understand that there are general principles and guidelines that apply to all vision therapy techniques and specific principles and guidelines for binocular vision, oculomotor, and accommodative techniques. Vision therapy is similar in many ways to other types of therapy that involve learning and education. For any learning situation there are specific guidelines to facilitate learning and success. Since vision therapy can be considered to be a form of learning and education, similar principles and guidelines must be used to achieve success (Chapter 14, box, see p. 392).

These issues are important for any vision therapy patient. When one is dealing with a child who has learning problems, these factors take on even greater significance.

VISION THERAPY FOR BINOCULAR VISION AND ACCOMMODATIVE DISORDERS

Vision therapy for binocular vision and accommodative disorders generally requires between 12 to 24 office visits if vision therapy is office based. If home vision therapy can be effectively administered, the total number of office visits can sometimes be reduced. The key concept is that a given amount of vision therapy is necessary. Whether it takes place in the office or at home is less important, as long as the therapy can be effectively administered at home. The total number of therapy sessions also depends on the age of the patient, motivation, severity of the learning disorder, and compliance.

As a general rule a vision therapy program for a visual efficiency problem, regardless of the specific diagnosis, can be divided into three general phases.[1]

Phase 1

This first phase of therapy is designed to accomplish the objectives listed under phase 1 in the upper box on the next page.

Since vision therapy requires communication and cooperation between the therapist and patient, it is important to develop a working relationship with the patient during the first few sessions. The establishment of such a relationship is vital to the success of vision therapy and must therefore be a specific objective of the early visits. Some of the key issues that may need to be discussed or clarified are the nature of the vision problem being treated, the reason vision therapy is necessary, and the goals of vision therapy. Although these issues generally have been discussed before the beginning of vision therapy, misconceptions and misunderstandings

Vision Therapy for Binocular and Accommodative Disorders

Phase 1 subgoals

- Develop a working relationship with the patient
- Develop an awareness of the various feedback mechanisms that will be used throughout therapy
- Develop voluntary convergence or divergence (diagnosis dependent)
- Normalize smooth fusional vergence amplitudes (diagnosis dependent)
- Normalize accommodative amplitude and ability to stimulate or relax accommodation (diagnosis dependent)

Phase 2 subgoals

- Normalize smooth fusional vergence amplitudes not addressed in phase 1
- Normalize fusional vergence facility (diagnosis dependent)
- Normalize fusional vergence in opposite direction

Phase 3 subgoals

- Develop ability to change from a convergence to a divergence demand
- Integrate vergence procedures with changes in accommodative demand
- Integrate vergence procedures with versions and saccades

Feedback Cues Used in Vision Therapy

1. Diplopia
2. Blur
3. Suppression
4. Luster
5. Kinesthetic awareness
6. SILO (small in, large out)
7. Float
8. Localization
9. Parallax

can occur because many people have little previous knowledge of vision therapy. A short amount of time spent reiterating previous discussions about these topics can be very valuable.

It is equally important in this first phase to make the patient aware of the various feedback mechanisms that will be used throughout therapy. If the patient develops a good understanding of the nine feedback cues listed in the lower box, therapy will progress more rapidly. These feedback cues are discussed in detail elsewhere.[1]

The first goal of the therapy itself is to teach the concept and feeling of converging or diverging and accommodating or relaxing accommodation depending on the specific diagnosis. The patient should be able to voluntarily converge and diverge to any distance from 2 inches to 20 feet. Once the patient can voluntarily initiate a controlled convergence and divergence movement the other goals of the vision therapy program become much easier to accomplish. Three commonly used procedures to accomplish this first objective are the Brock string, Bug-on-String, and the Red-Green Barrel Card.[1]

If a binocular vision problem is present, the patient will have either limited positive or negative fusional vergence findings. Therefore another objective of the first phase of vision therapy is to normalize fusional vergence amplitudes in the direction of the deficiency. The initial goal is to reestablish a normal vergence range for a smooth, or tonic, type of vergence demand. A smooth vergence demand is easier for the patient to accomplish in the early part of a vision therapy program. It is important, however, to move to the next phase involving jump vergence as soon as possible. This tends to shorten the course of therapy.

Another advantage of beginning with smooth vergence procedures is that in some cases the introduction of any vergence demand is enough to cause suppression or diplopia. Smooth vergence techniques provide a starting point for therapy with such patients. If the patient is unable to fuse any convergence demand, for example, the procedure can begin with a divergence demand. For example, a variable Tranaglyph can be set at 10 base-in and then gradually reduced to zero. This approach at least allows the patient to get started and to experience some success, and the change from 10 base-in to zero can be viewed as convergence therapy relative to the starting point. Speed is of little importance initially. Rather, we simply want the patient to be able to maintain fusion as the convergence demand is slowly increased.

Examples of instrumentation that can be used to accomplish these objectives are the Variable Tranaglyphs, Variable Vectograms, and the Variable Prismatic Stereoscope from Bernell (see list, p. 428). These three devices can be used to create a smooth, gradual increase in convergence or divergence demand.

When an accommodative problem is also present, another objective of the first phase of therapy is to normalize monocular accommodative amplitude and the ability to stimulate and relax accommodation. The emphasis in this early phase of accommodative therapy depends on the specific diagnosis. For accommodative insufficiency, phase one of therapy is designed to improve the ability to stimulate accommodation. For accommodative excess the initial emphasis is on relaxation of accommodation. Typical vision therapy techniques used in this phase of accommodative therapy include lens sorting, loose lens rock, and Hart Chart.

Phase 2

This second phase of therapy is designed to accomplish the objectives listed under phase 2 in the upper box on p. 418.

Once smooth vergence is normalized, phasic or jump vergence demand should be emphasized. Variable Tranaglyphs and Vectograms can still be used. However, the specific modifications to create a step vergence demand must be implemented. These include:

1. Changing fixation from the target to another point in space
2. Covering and uncovering one eye
3. Using a loose prism or flip prism
4. Flip lenses to create a step vergence change in vergence demand
5. Two different Tranaglyphs or Vectograms set up in a Dual Polachrome Illuminated Trainer
6. Polaroid or red/green flippers

Other valuable techniques at this stage are the nonvariable Tranaglyphs, the Aperture Rule, Keystone Eccentric Circles, Bernell Free Space Fusion Cards, Lifesaver Cards, and computerized fusional vergence activities (RC Instruments; see list, p. 428).

In contrast to phase 1, in which speed was not a factor, during this second phase of therapy the emphasis should be on the qualitative aspects (speed, accuracy) of fusion rather than quantitative (magnitude) aspects. It is important to increase the speed of the fusional vergence response and quality of the recovery of fusion.

A second objective of this phase of therapy is to begin working with the fusional vergence amplitude, which was not stressed during phase 1. For example, when one is treating a convergence insufficiency patient, the initial emphasis in phase 1 would be on positive fusional vergence. It is not unusual to find a reduction occurring in negative fusional vergence in these patients when the entire vision therapy program emphasizes only convergence techniques. Once the patient begins to demonstrate normal smooth positive fusional vergence it is important to also implement therapy with smooth negative vergence demand. The same techniques used in phase 1 to work with positive fusional vergence are repeated for negative fusional vergence.

Finally, during the end of this phase of therapy, incorporate fusional vergence facility techniques using the same procedures as listed above for jump vergence demand for the fusional vergence amplitude that was not stressed during phase 1. For the patient with convergence insufficiency this would involve working with negative fusional facility.

If an accommodative problem is also present, the speed of the monocular accommodative response should now be emphasized. In addition, it is important to continue working with using both plus and minus lenses. The objective is for the patient to be able to relax and stimulate accommodation as quickly as possible. The same techniques used during phase 1 can be repeated using plus and minus lenses with an emphasis on the speed of the accommodative response. We also begin working with *biocular* accommodative facility procedures such as Red Red Rock and *binocular* accommodative facility procedures such as bar readers and accommodative facility with targets such as Vectograms and Tranaglyphs.

In addition, we now incorporate divergence therapy in addition to convergence therapy and move toward binocular vision techniques that emphasize phasic vergence changes. By the end of this phase, the patient should be using the Aperture Rule (for both convergence and divergence) and the Computer Orthoptics Random Dot Program (RC Instruments, Cicero, Ind.) for both convergence and divergence therapy.

Phase 3

This third phase of therapy is designed to accomplish the objectives listed under phase 3 in the upper box on p. 418.

Until this point the patient has either worked separately with convergence techniques or divergence techniques. Now the objective is to develop the patient's ability to change from a convergence to a divergence demand and to integrate vergence procedures with versions. Several excellent procedures are available to help accomplish this objective. Vectograms with Polaroid flippers or Tranaglyphs with red/green flippers can be used. Each time the flippers are changed the demand switches from divergence to convergence. The transparent Keystone Eccentric Circles or transparent Bernell Free Space Fusion Cards are inexpensive, excellent methods for achieving this objective. The patient has already learned by this time to fuse these cards with a divergence or convergence demand separately. Now the patient is taught to switch from convergence and then back to divergence. As this skills improves, speed or the number of cycles per minute is emphasized.

During phase 3 the emphasis is also on integration of accommodation and binocular therapy. Phasic binocular techniques like the Aperture Rule, Eccentric Circles, Free Space Cards, and the step/jump vergence program of Computer Orthoptics are useful techniques. Binocular accommodative facility with flip lenses should be used with phasic binocular techniques listed above. It is also important to integrate accommodative and binocular therapy with saccades and versions. Moving the Eccentric Circles or Free Space Fusion Cards into different positions of gaze or using several sets of cards in various positions along with flip lenses is an excellent procedure to accomplish this goal. Other techniques such as the Brock String with rotation and Computer Orthoptics vergence with rotation are useful.

The final objective of therapy is to integrate vergence procedures with versions and saccades. Under normal seeing conditions patients are constantly trying to maintain accurate vergence while changing fixation from one location to another. It is therefore important to combine vergence therapy with versions and saccades. Techniques such as the Brock String with rotation and Eccentric Circles or Lifesaver Cards with rotation or lateral movements and saccades are techniques that can be used to accomplish this goal. The Computer Orthoptics program that combines horizontal vergence with rotation is also useful for this objective.

Since the objectives of vision therapy are to eliminate the patient's symptoms and normalize binocular and accommodative findings, a reevaluation should be performed every five or six visits and again at the end of therapy. During these evaluations the clinician should refer to the original complaints and determine if the patient is now comfortable. All tests of binocular and accommodative function should be repeated and compared to the initial findings as well as the expected findings.

When all vision therapy objectives have been reached and the vision therapy program is completed, we recommend the home vision therapy maintenance program outlined in the box. For the first 3 months after completion of vision therapy the patient works with the Eccentric Circles or Free Space Fusion Cards 3 times a week, 5 to 10 minutes each session. The patient is reevaluated after 3 months, and if all findings are still normal and the patient is comfortable, the amount of home therapy can be decreased. For the next 6 months the patient is asked to work with the same procedure 1 session each week for 5 to 10 minutes. Another reevaluation is scheduled in 6 months. If all findings are normal and the patient is still asymptomatic, I advise the patient to practice the Eccentric Circles or Free Space Fusion Cards the first day of each month to monitor his or her own visual systems. If these patients can still perform the task as expected, they need not do any therapy that month. If they feel that there has been some deterioration, they work with the technique until they reach the expected level of performance. We then advise the patients to return on an annual basis for routine vision care.

The boxes on pages 423 to 425 provide a sample detailed vision therapy program for convergence insufficiency, one of the more common visual efficiency problems encountered in clinical practice.

Vision Therapy Maintenance Program

1. Three months after completion of vision therapy work with the Eccentric Circles or Free Space Fusion Cards 3 times a week, 5 to 10 minutes each session.

   Reevaluation in 3 months

2. For the next 6 months the patient is asked to work with the same procedure 1 session each week for 5 to 10 minutes.

   Reevaluation in 6 months

3. Patients are to try the Eccentric Circles or Free Space Fusion Cards the first day of each month to monitor their visual systems. If they can still perform the task as expected, they need not do any therapy that month. If they believe that there has been some deterioration, they work with the technique until they reach the expected level of performance.

   Annual routine vision care

VISION THERAPY FOR OCULAR MOTOR DYSFUNCTION

A vision therapy program for ocular motor dysfunction generally requires between 12 to 24 in-office visits if vision therapy is office based. As we discussed above, if home vision therapy can be effectively administered, the total number of office visits can be reduced.

Phase 1

This first phase of therapy is designed to accomplish the objectives listed under phase 1 in the box on p. 426.

Sample Vision Therapy Program For Convergence Insufficiency

Phase 1

Sessions 1 and 2
In office
- Discuss nature of vision problem, goals of vision therapy, various feedback cues, importance of practice
- Brock String
- Lens sorting
- Loose lens rock (begin with plus if accommodative excess, with minus if accommodative insufficiency)
- Tranaglyph or Vectograms: convergence. Begin with a peripheral target like Tranaglyph 515 or the Quoit Vectogram
- Computer Orthoptics Random Dot Vergence Program: convergence
Home therapy
- Brock String
- Loose lens rock

Sessions 3 and 4
- In office
- Bug-on-string
- Loose lens rock
- Tranaglyph or Vectograms: convergence
    Use targets with more central demand (Clown, Bunny Tranaglyphs, Clown, Topper Vectograms)
- Computer Orthoptics Random Dot Vergence Program: convergence
Home therapy
- Brock String
- Loose lens rock

Sessions 5 to 8
In office
- Barrel Card
- Voluntary convergence
- Loose lens rock
- Tranaglyph or Vectograms: convergence
    Use even more detailed targets such as Tranaglyphs Sports slide and Faces targets and the Spirangle Vectogram
- Computer Orthoptics Random Dot Vergence Program: convergence
Home therapy
- Tranaglyph: convergence

Continued.

Sample Vision Therapy Program For Convergence Insufficiency—cont'd

Phase 2

Sessions 9 and 10
In office
• Tranaglyph or Vectograms with modifications to create jump vergence demand: convergence
• Non-Variable Tranaglyphs
• Tranaglyph 515 or the Quoit Vectogram: divergence
• Binocular accommodative therapy techniques: Use any of the binocular techniques listed above with +/− lenses
Home therapy
• Non-Variable Tranaglyphs

Sessions 11 and 12
In office
• Tranaglyph or Vectograms with modifications to create jump vergence demand: convergence
• Aperture Rule: convergence
• More central Tranaglyphs or the Vectograms: divergence
• Binocular accommodative therapy techniques: Use any of the binocular techniques listed above with +/− lenses
Home therapy
• Non-Variable Tranaglyphs with loose prism jumps

Sessions 13 to 16
In office
• Aperture Rule: convergence
• Eccentric Circles or Free Space Fusion Cards
• Computer Orthoptics Random Dot Vergence Program: both convergence and divergence
• Aperture Rule: divergence
• Tranaglyph or Vectograms with modifications to create jump vergence demand: divergence
• Binocular accommodative therapy techniques: Use any of the binocular techniques listed above with +/− lenses
Home therapy
• Eccentric Circles or Free Space Fusion Cards

Phase 3

Sessions 17 to 20
In office
• Tranaglyph or Vectograms with Polaroid or red/green flippers
• Eccentric Circles or Free Space Fusion Cards
• Computer Orthoptics Random Dot Vergence Program: step jump vergence
Home therapy
• Eccentric Circles or Free Space Fusion Cards: convergence

Sessions 21 and 22
In office
• Tranaglyph or Vectograms with Polaroid or red/green flippers
• Eccentric Circles or Free Space Fusion Cards
• Lifesaver cards
• Computer Orthoptics Random Dot Vergence Program: jump/jump vergence
Home therapy
• Eccentric Circles or Free Space Fusion Cards: divergence

Sessions 23 to 24
In office
• Tranaglyph or Vectograms with Polaroid or red/green flippers
• Eccentric Circles or Free Space Fusion Cards with rotation and versions
• Lifesaver cards with rotation and versions
• Computer Orthoptics Vergence Program with rotation
Home therapy
• Eccentric Circles or Free Space Fusion Cards: convergence/divergence

After a working relationship with the patient is established, the primary goal of this first phase of therapy is to improve large or gross saccadic ability and small excursion pursuit ability. It is important to note that the training progression is from large-to-small movements for saccades and small-to-large excursions for pursuits.[28,29]

One of the important changes in vision therapy equipment in recent years has been the introduction of the computer. Computers are ideally suited for creating the stimuli and variability necessary for vision therapy techniques. This is particularly true for eye movement training. There are several excellent programs for this purpose. The two primary systems available are the software from Opti-Mum (Learning Frontiers) and from Computer Orthoptics (RC Instruments; see list, p. 428). Both systems have many programs designed for saccadic or pursuit training. All these programs allow the practitioner to vary a wide range of parameters and accurately monitor progress. This ability to vary the stimuli in a controlled fashion allows us to begin therapy at a level at which the patient can succeed and gradually increase the demand. I highly recommend incorporation of computerized vision therapy equipment. During this first phase of therapy I recommend using monocular pursuits and saccades from the Opti-Mum system or pursuits and saccades from the Computer Orthoptics vision therapy software. Several comprehensive reviews are available in the literature with detailed information about these programs[30,31]

Other common procedures that can be used include wall fixations with afterimages for feedback, Hart Chart saccades, the pegboard rotator, and Groffman Tracings.

In almost all cases, an accommodative or convergence problem will be present in addition to the eye movement disorder. Therefore I have also included accommodative and binocular therapy procedures in the treatment plan. Even if accommodative and binocular function is normal, I still suggest incorporation of these techniques because adequate performance on accommodative and binocular therapy procedures is dependent on good fixation and attention.

Phase 2

This second phase of therapy is designed to accomplish the objectives listed under phase 2 in the box below.

During this second phase of therapy the objective is to develop more accurate saccades using finer, more detailed targets and more accurate pursuits using larger excursions. Commonly used saccadic techniques include Ann Arbor Letter Tracking and loose prism jumps (monocular). For pursuits continue working with the pegboard rotator and add flashlight pursuit techniques. I also suggest incorporating computer vision therapy techniques for both saccades and pursuits. Some of the programs I have found to be most helpful include saccades, pursuits, visual memory, visual search, visual scan, and tachistoscope from Computer Orthoptics and alphabet jumbles, monocular and bi-ocular visual pursuits and saccades and tachistoscope from Opti-Mum. It is also important to work monocularly until performance is equalized for fine saccadic and pursuit ability in the two eyes.

Goals during this second phase of therapy also include normalization

---

Vision Therapy for Oculomotor Dysfunction

Phase 1 objectives
- Develop more accurate gross saccades and fine pursuits
- Equalize gross saccadic and pursuit ability in the two eyes

Phase 2 objectives
- Develop more accurate fine saccades and large excursion pursuits
- Equalize fine saccadic and pursuit ability in the two eyes

Phase 3 objectives
- Integrate accurate saccades and pursuits with changes in vergence and accommodation

of both positive and negative fusional vergence amplitudes using both smooth or tonic vergence demand and jump or phasic vergence demand.

Phase 3

This third phase of therapy is designed to accomplish the objectives listed under phase 3 in the box on p. 426.

By this stage in therapy the patient should have developed excellent accommodative and fusional vergence amplitude and facility as well as normal fixational skills and monocular saccadic and pursuit ability. This last phase of therapy is primarily designed to integrate saccadic and pursuit eye movements with changes in accommodative and vergence demand. Thus during this stage the patient should be working binocularly during all procedures.

The use of two or more Brock Strings is a simple task that combines all the necessary elements desired at this point. The patient simply holds two or three strings at the bridge of his nose, rather than one. The origin of the Brock Strings can be placed to the patient's right, left, and directly in front. With two beads on each string, the patient has multiple targets in various positions of gaze. Instruct the patient to change fixation in a given pattern and use a metronome to provide an auditory stimulus to control the speed of change of fixation. To accomplish this task the patient must make accurate saccades and accommodate and converge accurately.

The Brock String can also be used to integrate pursuits with accommodation and convergence. Tie the end of the Brock String to a pencil. Have the patient hold one end of the string against the bridge of his nose while holding the other end (tied to the pencil) with his arm outstretched. Instruct the patient to move his arm slowly in a circular fashion while also changing fixation every 5 seconds from the far to the near bead. If a rotating pegboard device is available, one end of the Brock String can be attached to the rotator to accomplish the same effect.

Another common procedure is to use two or more Tranaglyphs, Vectograms, or Eccentric Circles. The patient is already familiar and has succeeded with all these procedures. The objective at this stage is to have the patient fixate from one target to another and quickly to achieve clear, single, binocular vision. Finally, the Eccentric Circles and Lifesaver cards can be hand held by the patient and rotated in a circular or any other pattern. This is another excellent method of integrating pursuits with changes in vergence and accommodative stimulus levels.

SUMMARY

The management sequence described above represents one approach that will lead to successful elimination of a patient's symptoms and normalization of optometric data. A primary objective of the model we have presented is an emphasis on considering all treatment options for every accommodative, oculomotor, and binocular vision anomaly encountered. When one is managing such patients, it is best to acquire the habit of always considering each option and then either using or rejecting that management for a particular patient. This approach will ensure that no management option has been ignored and should lead to more frequent and rapid success.

The number of sessions we recommended for vision therapy are approximations and will vary from one patient to another. An important variable is the use of home therapy techniques to supplement the activities used for in-office therapy. Home therapy can be useful with a highly motivated adult patient. It can also work when the patient is a motivated, compliant child with a parent that has the capability to function as the home therapist. In some cases, however, the parent may not interact well with the child in this role, and home therapy will not be helpful.

LIST OF MANUFACTURERS

Bernell Corporation
750 Lincolnway East
PO Box 4637
South Bend, IN 46634
(800) 348-2225

RC Instruments
1558 East Port Court
PO Box 197
Cicero, IN 46034
(800) 346-4925

Learning Frontiers
190 Admiral Cochran Drive, #180
Annapolis, MD 21401
(800) 331-6412

CHAPTER REVIEW

1. Describe a general treatment sequence for visual efficiency problems.
2. Why is it important to prescribe for significant refractive error first?
3. List and describe three situations in which the use of added lenses would be appropriate for visual efficiency problems.
4. List eight tests that can be used to decide if added plus is an appropriate treatment strategy.
5. Describe the effect that the addition of +1.00 would have on the following findings:
   • NRA
   • PRA
   • Base out at near
   • Base in at near
   • Accommodative facility testing
6. Describe five clinical situations in which prism would be helpful.
7. Describe a general vision therapy approach for binocular vision and accommodative disorders.

REFERENCES

1. Scheiman M, Wick B: *Clinical management of heterophoric, accommodative, and eye movement disorders,* Philadelphia, 1994, Lippincott.
2. London RF, Wick B: The effect of correction of vertical fixation dispar-ity on the horizontal forced vergence fixation disparity curve, *Am J Optom Physiol Optics* 64:653-656, 1987.
3. Wick B: Horizontal deviations. In Amos JF, editor: *Diagnosis and man-*

agement in vision care, Boston, 1987, Butterworth.

4. London R: Fixation disparity and heterophoria. In Barresi BJ, editor: *Ocular assessment: the manual of diagnosis for office practice*, Boston, 1984, Butterworth.

5. Sheard C: Zones of ocular comfort, *Am J Optom* 7:9-25, 1930.

6. Ciuffreda KJ, Levi D, Selenow A: *Amblyopia: basic and clinical aspects*, Boston, 1991, Butterworth-Heinemann.

7. Crewther DP, Crewther SG, Mitchell DE: The efficacy of brief periods of reverse occlusion in promoting recovery from the physiological effects of monocular deprivation in kittens, *Invest Ophthalmol Vis Sci* 21:357-362, 1981.

8. The efficacy of optometric vision therapy. The 1986/1987 AOA Future of Visual Development/Performance Task Force. *J Am Optom Assoc* 59:95-105, 1988.

9. Suchoff IB, Petito GT: The efficacy of visual therapy, *J Am Optom Assoc* 57:119-125, 1986.

10. Grisham JD: Visual therapy results for convergence insufficiency: a literature review, *Am J Optom Physiol Optics* 65:448-454, 1988.

11. Griffin JR: Efficacy of vision therapy for non-strabismic vergence anomalies, *Am J Optom Physiol Optics* 64:11-14, 1987.

12. Daum K: Accommodative insufficiency, *Am J Optom Physiol Optics*, 60:352-359, 1983.

13. Hoffman L, Cohen A, Feuer G: Effectiveness of non-strabismic optometric vision training in a private practice, *Am J Optom Arch Am Acad Optom* 50:813-816, 1973.

14. Liu JS, Lee M, Jang J, et al: Objective assessment of accommodative orthoptics: 1. Dynamic insufficiency, *Am J Optom Physiol Optics* 56:285-291, 1979.

15. Bobier WR, Sivak JG: Orthoptic treatment of subjects showing slow accommodative responses, *Am J Optom Physiol Optics* 60:678-687, 1983.

16. Daum K: The course and effect of visual training on the vergence system, *Am J Optom Physiol Optics* 59:223-227, 1982.

17. Daum K: Convergence insufficiency, *Am J Optom Physiol Optics* 61:16-22, 1984.

18. Daum K: Double blind placebo-controlled examination of timing effects in the training of positive vergences, *Am J Optom Physiol Optics* 63:807-812, 1986.

19. Vaegan JL: Convergence and divergence show longer and sustained improvement after short isometric exercise, *Am J Optom Physiol Optics* 56:23-33, 1979.

20. Cooper J, Selenow A, Ciuffreda KJ, et al: Reduction of asthenopia in patients with convergence insufficiency after fusional vergence training, *Am J Optom Physiol Optics* 60:982-989, 1983.

21. Daum K: A comparison of results of tonic and phasic training on the vergence system, *Am J Optom Physiol Optics* 60:769-775, 1983.

22. Wold RM, Pierce JR, Keddington J: Effectiveness of optometric vision therapy, *J Am Optom Assoc* 49:1047-1053, 1978.

23. Rounds BB, Manley CW, Norris RH: The effect of oculomotor training on reading efficiency, *J Am Optom Assoc* 62:92-99, 1991.

24. Young BS, Pollard T, Paynter S, Cox R: Effect of eye exercises in improving control of eye movements during reading, *J Optom Vis Dev* 13:4-7, 1982.

25. Fujimoto DH, Christensen EA, Griffin JR: An investigation in use of videocassette techniques for enhancement of saccadic movements, *J Am Optom Assoc* 56:304-308, 1985.

26. Punnett AF, Steinhauer GD: Relationship between reinforcement and eye movements during ocular motor training with learning disabled children, *J Learning Disabil* 17:16-19, 1984.

27. Griffin J: Binocular anomalies: procedures for vision therapy. ed 2, Chicago, 1982, Professional Press.

28. Griffin JR: Pursuit fixations: an overview of training procedures, *Optom Monthly* 67:35-38, 1976.

29. Griffin JR: Saccadic eye movements—recommended testing and training procedures, *Optom Monthly* 72:27-28, 1981.

30. Press LJ: Computers and Vision Therapy Programs, Optometric Extension Program, Curriculum II, series I, 1988, vol 60, no 1-12.

31. Maino DM: Applications in pediatrics, binocular vision and perception. In Maino JH, Maino DM, Davidson DW, editor: *Computer applications in optometry*, Boston, 1989, Butterworth.

CHAPTER 16

Management of Visual Information Processing Problems

MICHAEL W. ROUSE
ERIC BORSTING

KEY TERMS

overall therapy goals
therapy subgoals
therapy techniques
multisensory
visual-spatial dysfunction

automaticity
visual-analysis dysfunction
computerized techniques
visual-motor dysfunction
visual-motor ergonomics

Historically, optometry has been involved in providing vision care to patients with developmental vision problems for over 30 years. These therapy regimens were outlined in the 1950s and the 1960s and were based on two central theoretical constructs.[1-3] First, the development of visual-perceptual skills was intimately linked to the patient's motor development. In particular, vision was said to develop as the dominant sense that guides the motor system. Therefore, therapy activities requiring motor movement were emphasized, and it was assumed that training in the motor modality should cause improvement in visual-perceptual skills. Recent investigations of visual processing in infants and toddlers clearly indicates that visual development is not entirely linked to motor development.[4]

The second important concept intrinsic to these early theories was that improvement of visual skills would subsequently result in improved school performance. However, success in school is dependent on numerous factors such as intelligence, cultural factors, emotional stability, and motivation. Trying to equate the improvement of a single factor with a complex function such as school performance often results in unfulfilled expectations. For example, it would be unreasonable to expect that improvement of visual-motor integration would necessarily result in an improved ability to read. A more realistic expectation would be one that is more closely related to the visual skill's specific effects on performance. In the previous example, it would be reasonable to expect that an improvement in visual motor-integration would lead to an improvement in the patient's ability to copy written work more accurately. Therefore, optometric care should be directed at the identification and treatment of specific visual deficits, and the treatment expectations should be more closely tied to elimination or

431

reduction, as much as possible, of the signs and symptoms that are associated with those specific visual deficits.

The model of developmental vision care proposed by Getman[5] has influenced subsequent thinking about vision therapy, and we owe a great debt to his legacy. We have combined parts of these early models with current psychological and optometric research to devise a treatment model that is based on a visual information processing approach to vision.[6-9] Despite advances in our understanding of vision development and the effects of vision problems on learning, there is no adequate source to help the clinician design a vision therapy program for the learning-disabled patient who has developmental visual information processing (DVIP) dysfunction. This chapter helps to fill that void by providing the clinician with a systematic strategy for managing patients with specific deficits in DVIP skills.

EFFICACY OF DVIP THERAPY

When one is evaluating the efficacy of optometric vision therapy as a treatment tool for improving DVIP skills, it is important to address two separate issues. First, how effective is vision therapy at improving DVIP skills? For example, when a therapy program for visual-motor skills is provided, is it likely that this ability will improve? Second, if there are improvements in DVIP skills, is the child more available or responsive to educational instruction; that is, after remediation of specific visual deficits will the child respond more appropriately to academic intervention for specific educational deficits?

In addressing the first issue, most studies evaluating the effectiveness of visual therapy had involved use of a broad variety of training procedures in all three areas of visual information processing (visual spatial, visual analysis, and visual motor) at the same time. Academic performance was then reevaluated after the treatment. Several of these studies had found significant improvements in DVIP skills after therapy.[10,11] Studies that have concentrated on the treatment of isolated visual-perceptual skills have also supported the effectiveness of therapy for visual-spatial,[12,13] visual-analysis,[14,15] and visual-motor skills.[16] For example, Greenspan[13] administered a program of perceptual-motor therapy, which included therapy for bilaterality and body-image development, to a group of underachieving children and measured the frequency of reversal errors. The control group received only standard orthoptic therapy. The experimental group showed a statistically significant improvement in directionality and reduction in the total number of reversal errors after the perceptual therapy. These studies indicated that the level of performance of individual visual information processing skills can be enhanced through an optometric vision therapy program designed to address specific DVIP deficits.

Improving the ability of the child to benefit from academic instruction has been supported by similar research.[11,15,17-19] These studies have demonstrated statistically significant improvements in standardized tests of academic skills compared to a control group. For example, Seiderman[11] provided visual and perceptual therapy to 18 learning-disabled children who were matched with a control group. The experimental group showed an improvement on the Word Reading and Paragraph Meaning subtests of the Stanford Achievement Test.

These studies taken from an interdisciplinary group of researchers provide positive evidence that therapy for DVIP can be expected to improve specific skills and help the child benefit from academic instruction. In reviewing the literature that addresses therapy for perceptual skills, Solan and Ciner[20] cite several factors that are important for a successful therapy program. First, the patient should have a documented perceptual deficit that is associated with the reading or learning disorder. Broad-based therapy programs to improve readiness skills in normal patients may not be effective. Second, therapy programs should be individualized to address the specific deficits that the patient manifests. Therapy programs should address specific problem areas while·taking into account the patient's developmental level, auditory processing, and visual attention and cognitive style. Finally, therapy should complement and not replace reading and other educational instruction. The role of the optometrist in the managing of DVIP deficits is to improve visual-spatial, visual-analysis, and visual-motor skills in those patients who manifest these problems. This should enable the patient to participate more effectively in the classroom and benefit from other educational therapies.

GENERAL TREATMENT STRATEGY

Chapter 15 presented the initial phases of the management regimen, specifically correction of significant refractive anomalies and treatment of visual efficiency problems. Management of these problems is typically completed before therapy addresses the deficits in DVIP. It must be remembered that treatment of deficient visual efficiency skills has resulted in concurrent improvement in DVIP skills.[21,22] Therefore, reevaluation of deficient DVIP skills is essential before treatment is started.

There are exceptions to this general strategy. First, some DVIP dysfunctions, such as laterality and directionality, appear to have little relationship to deficient visual efficiency skills and are relatively unaffected by their improvement.[22] Consequently, therapy for these types of DVIP problems are often sequenced concurrently with the visual efficiency phase of treatment. Second, some children are not developmentally ready to understand the concepts underlying some visual efficiency therapy procedures.[23] The clinician may find that performing sophisticated accommodative and vergence procedures (such as chiastoptic fusion) is too difficult and frustrating for the patient. In these cases the doctor may need to start the DVIP therapy before or concurrently with the visual efficiency therapy. Finally, certain patients with a primary deficiency in DVIP skills may have only minor visual efficiency deficits. Delaying DVIP therapy until these minor deficits are resolved could result in poor compliance and adversely affect the treatment outcome.

The therapy program is designed to remediate deficits within three general systems in the following order: (1) visual spatial, (2) visual analysis, and (3) visual motor. The diagnostic evaluation reveals specific deficits within each general system, which then allows the clinician to design a problem-oriented treatment plan. The therapy plan is designed to treat only those component abilities that are deficient in each general system. For example, a patient may have difficulties only with directionality concepts within the general system of visual-spatial skills. For this patient, therapy would be directed toward treating those directionality skills, and valuable time would not be wasted on training prerequisite skills that were determined to be adequate.

DEFINING AND SEQUENCING THERAPY GOALS

Successful treatment of a dysfunctional system (such as visual spatial) depends on developing an understanding of the individual therapy goals and their appropriate sequencing. To assist the reader in defining and sequencing therapy goals, which may seem overwhelming at first, we are presenting the following model (see Figure 16.1 for a visual overview of this model). For each system there is an overall therapy goal that characterizes the patient's performance after successful completion of therapy. Each system is composed of a sequence of component abilities that have associated therapy goals. For example, in the visual-spatial system, bilateral integration, laterality, and directionality are considered component abilities. Achievement of these goals depends on the successful completion of a sequence of subgoals that are typically organized in a hierarchical manner. The subgoal is divided into either an individual skill or a sequence of underlying skills that must be successfully achieved. Skill development is so important that the majority of the doctor's office therapy time will be spent on developing patient strategies to treat deficient skills.

SELECTION OF THERAPY PROCEDURES

Our intention is not to provide the clinician with a "cookbook" list of techniques that will address deficits found in the diagnostic profile. Instead, we want the doctor to develop an understanding of the overall goals and subgoals that must be achieved in order to remediate visual processing deficits. In addition, to illustrate how to address each subgoal, example interactions are used. The example interactions typically use a single therapy technique for illustration. A more expanded list of techniques can be found in the accompanying tables. The tables provide an overview of the therapy goal and subgoals, as well as the expanded list of techniques. The techniques that are marked with an asterisk can be found in Chapter 17. Other techniques are identified by the source and can be acquired by reference to the resource list at the end of the chapter.

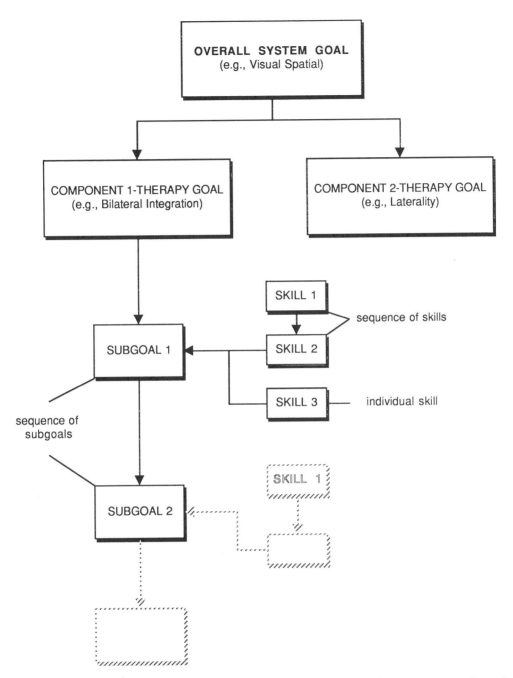

FIGURE 16.1 The flow chart illustrates the organization of component goals and subgoals within an overall system goal.

As the clinician becomes familiar with this area of treatment, he or she will find that many techniques and procedures can be used to address the same dysfunction. In fact there are several excellent compilations of techniques that are invaluable for the clinician.[24-29] In addition, there are several computer programs available for remediating DVIP deficits. The computer offers the unique advantage of arranging stimulus conditions that are difficult to set up in other ways. For example, alterations of time, distractor targets, and level of difficulties can be changed very quickly. Children are familiar with computers and in most cases enjoy working in this environment, which in turn can improve the motivation of the patient. However, it should be emphasized that the computer does not teach the child the process or strategy needed to succeed at a particular activity. The doctor still needs to interact with the patient and teach appropriate strategies. An exhaustive description of all the computer systems available is beyond the scope of this chapter, and you are referred to other sources for this information.[30,31]

We believe that once an understanding of specific goals and methods of teaching strategies are understood, the clinician will be able to apply the vast array of therapy techniques that have been compiled.

PRELIMINARY THERAPY CONSIDERATIONS

Programming and selecting the appropriate vision therapy procedures for both office and home vision therapy is influenced by several patient factors. These include the patient's age and developmental status, auditory abilities, cognitive development and style, cooperation, and motivation. Accounting for these factors will affect how well the patient responds to therapy, the treatment time, level of compliance, and ultimate therapy outcome. For example, a patient who is asked to perform a procedure that is developmentally too difficult will be easily frustrated, resulting in lower levels of cooperation, motivation, and compliance. Review Chapter 14 for a detailed discussion of these important patient factors.

TREATMENT OF VISUAL-SPATIAL DYSFUNCTION

The visual-spatial system is the first area treated in DVIP therapy. This system is made up of the following abilities or components: bilateral integration, laterality, and directionality. The overall goal of visual-spatial skills therapy is to develop the individual's internal and external spatial concepts that help organize the environment. The sequence of therapy outlined below starts at the most rudimentary level of training and proceeds to more complicated skills. Therapy programs outlined by McMonnies,[32] Kirshner,[24] and Lane[28] use similar techniques as the program outlined below. However, we have stressed a sequential set of subgoals that the patient needs to achieve to develop efficient visual-spatial ability. Information from the case history and diagnostic profile regarding the status of bilateral integration, laterality, and directionality skills provides the doctor with the starting point in the therapy sequence.

Goal 1: Develop bilateral integration

Bilateral integration is the ability of the individual to plan motor actions by performing isolated, simultaneous and sequential movements of the right and left sides of the body. Bilateral integration can be thought of as the patient's ability to control and plan movements of the gross motor system. Therapy for bilateral integration does not directly remediate a visual deficit but can be considered a prerequisite skill that will aid in the development of laterality and visually guided fine-motor skills. Having the patient develop a motor understanding of how the right and left sides of the body are different will aid in the development of laterality skills. Developing the ability to plan sequential gross-motor movements will aid in the development of visually guided fine-motor system planning skills. These are not absolute prerequisite skills (for example, a patient can perform laterality tasks with poor bilateral integration ability), but in our experience they serve to promote better performance in the visually based skills. Finally, patients who exhibit excessive nondirected motor activity, often referred to as motor overflow, can benefit from this type of therapy. Improvements in goal-directed motor behavior often parallel the effects seen when modifying visual styles[10] (see Chapter 14).

Before bilateral integration therapy is begun, it is important to determine if the patient has developed a dominant hand. Developmentally a dominant hand is typically established by 5 years of age.[33] The dominant hand serves as the primary tool for teaching laterality skills. If it is not obvious by observation that the patient has established a dominant hand, the doctor may need to administer a standardized test (such as a grooved pegboard; Solan[34]) to evaluate the motor proficiency of each hand. In those cases where a dominant side has not been established, the doctor should emphasize the performance differences between the two hands in the subsequent therapy procedures.

The overall goal of bilateral integration therapy is to develop motor planning ability by performing isolated, simultaneous and sequential movements of the right and left sides of the body. The box on p. 438 outlines the sequence of subgoals necessary to achieve the overall goal of adequate bilateral integration. The estimated treatment time is 2 to 4 in-office therapy sessions.

Bilateral integration: subgoal 1. The first subgoal is to develop a motor memory of the difference in performance between the right and left sides of the body. For example, in the procedure called "chalkboard squares"[28] the patient draws a line simultaneuosly with his and her right and left hands from edge to edge of two boxes drawn on the chalkboard (Figure 16.2). Typically the performance of one hand will be different from that of the other one. The doctor needs to ask the patient questions such as, "Which hand arrived at the edge of the box first?" or "Which hand drew smoother lines?" This will illustrate to the child that one hand performs differently from the other and will further develop the child's internal awareness of the differences between the two sides of the body. During therapy, the patient may improve the performance of the nondominant or the poorer performing hand. However, it is not the goal of therapy to equal-

Goals and Techniques for Developing Bilateral Integration

Therapy goal: Develop the patient's motor planning ability by performing isolated, simultaneous and sequential movements of the two sides of the body.

  Subgoal 1: Develop the patient's motor memory of the difference between the right and left sides of the body.

   Therapy techniques:
     Balance activities
     Ball bounce*
     Chalkboard squares*
     Gross eye-hand activities
       Bean bag toss

  Subgoal 2: Develop the patient's motor planning ability by performing isolated, simultaneous and sequential movements of the two sides of the body.

   Therapy techniques:
     Ball bounce*
     Chalkboard squares*
     Jumping jacks*
     Randolf shuffle*
     Slap tap*

*Techniques are detailed in Chapter 17.

ize the performance of the right and left sides. Rather, it is through the patient's exploration of the right and left sides of the body by altering the performance of each that helps develop a knowledge of laterality.[3] The estimated treatment time is 1 to 3 therapy sessions.

Bilateral integration: subgoal 2. The next subgoal is to develop the patient's motor planning ability by performing isolated, simultaneous and sequential movements of the two sides of the body. Isolated refers to the ability to isolate a single motor movement without overflow from other body parts. Simultaneous refers to either a coordinated movement of two or more body parts at the same time. A sequence of movements refers to a series of movement patterns. The first step in therapy is to develop simple motor planning of isolated motor movements. A representative technique is the Randolf shuffle.[35] The technique begins by having the patient extend either an individual arm or leg without overflow from other body parts (Figure 16.3, *A*). Initially the role of the doctor is to help the patient inhibit or activate simple motor-movement patterns. Frequently in the initial therapy steps the doctor may have to restrict certain body parts physically to help the patient inhibit excessive motor movements. These supports should be gradually removed as the patient is able to isolate motor movements more effectively. The patient should be able to achieve smooth performance within 2 to 3 weeks. If the patient's performance does not improve, referral to an occupational therapist should be considered.

The next phase in therapy is to proceed to more complicated motor activities that stress simultaneous movements and sequential movements

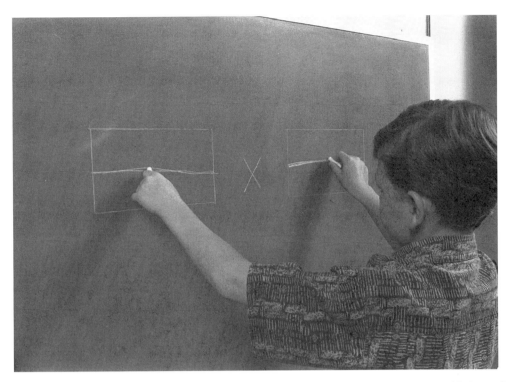

FIGURE 16.2 Chalkboard squares technique for addressing subgoal 1 of bilateral integration therapy. The patient simultaneously moves both hands from edge to edge of the boxes. The goal is to be aware of the performance difference of the two sides of the body.

of the right and left sides of the body. The Randolf shuffle can also be used for this phase of therapy. The technique begins with the patient moving both arms simultaneously and one leg in a coordinated five-step sequence (Figure 16.3, *B*). The next step has the patient isolate the movement of one arm and one leg on the ipsilateral side (Figure 16.3, *C*). Finally, the patient has to perform a contralateral movement that is similar to the previous phase but requires a more complex pattern of neurological inhibition and activation of body parts (Figure 16.3, *D*). Refer to Figure 17.3, *B* to *D*, for a complete illustration of the movement sequences for the three steps above. As the therapy proceeds to complex motor tasks, the doctor's role changes to helping the patient evaluate his or her own performance. If an incorrect sequence of motor movement is completed by the patient, the doctor should ask the patient to relate whether the sequence was correct or incorrect and to identify where in the sequence a mistake was made. Finally, the patient needs to tell the doctor what he will do to improve his or her own performance. These interactions between the doctor and the patient promote the development of an appropriate strategy for improving motor planning skills. The patient should be able to achieve smooth performance within 2 to 3 weeks. The skill will need to be reinforced regularly during

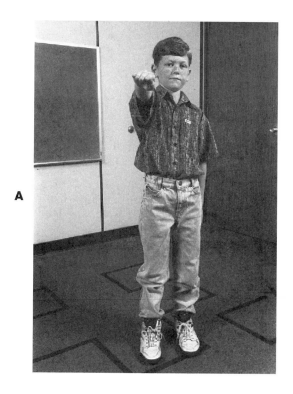

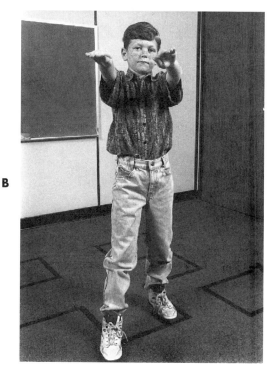

FIGURE 16.3 Randolf shuffle technique for addressing subgoal 2 of bilateral integration therapy. **A,** Isolated motor movement of right arm. **B,** Simultaneous motor movement of both arms and right leg.

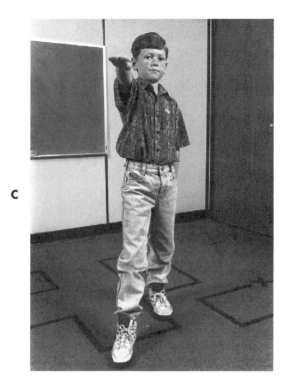

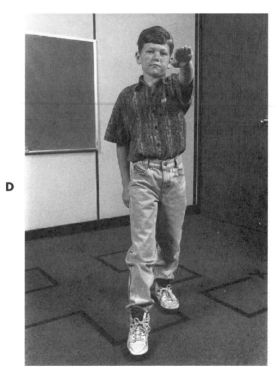

FIGURE 16.3, cont'd. C, Ipsilateral motor movement of right arm and right leg. **D,** Contralateral motor movement of left arm and right leg.

the early phases of laterality development. Other activities that are appropriate for this phase of therapy are listed in the box on p. 438.

Goal 2: Develop laterality

Laterality is the ability to be internally aware and to identify right and left on oneself. Therapy for bilateral integration establishes an internal, or motor, awareness of the difference between the right and left sides of the body. The overall goal of laterality therapy is to develop the patient's internal awareness of how the right side is different from the left side into concepts that the patient expresses orally. The box below outlines the sequence of subgoals necessary to achieve the overall goal of adequate laterality. The estimated treatment time is approximately 5 therapy sessions.

Laterality: subgoal 1. The first subgoal is to have the patient build upon the motor awareness developed in bilateral integration therapy by recalling a series of everyday tasks where he uses his dominant hand. For example, in a game of catch the patient needs to identify which hand to use in throwing a ball. Other examples include: "Which hand do you use for writing?" or "What hand do you use for holding your fork while eating?" If the patient has difficulty recalling which hand to use in throwing or writ-

---

Goals and Techniques for Developing Laterality

Therapy goal: Develop the patient's internal awareness of how the right side is different from the left side into concepts that the patient expresses orally.

Subgoal 1: Develop the patient's awareness of laterality by recalling a series of everyday activities where the patient uses the right and left hands.
Therapy techniques:
Laterality questions*

Subgoal 2: Develop the patient's ability to identify laterality of his or her own body parts.
Therapy techniques:
Children's games:
Mother May I
Simon Says*
Enhancing automaticity
Ball bounce
Jumping jacks
Randolf shuffle
Slap tap

Subgoal 3: Develop the patient's ability to use his or her own internal reference system (laterality) for making right and left judgments while moving through space.
Therapy techniques:
Directional mazes*
Floor map I*

*Techniques are detailed in Chapter 17.

ing, the doctor should let the patient actually throw a ball or write with either hand. This reinforces the patient's motor memory of the differences between the two sides. This initial step develops the underlying strategy that the patient will use when performing subsequent laterality procedures. Patients are usually able to grasp this concept in one or two therapy sessions, but the concept will need to be reinforced throughout the laterality therapy sequence.

Laterality: subgoal 2. The second subgoal is to have the patient identify laterality of his or her body parts. This will solidify the patient's internal reference system for judging right and left. For example, in the game Simon Says[35] the doctor asks the patient to touch or point to various body parts using right and left directions (for example, Touch your right ear). Initially the doctor should ask the patient how he or she reached the solution after each set of instructions. This helps rule out the possibility that the patient is simply guessing. When the patient is unsure of the response, the doctor should direct him or her to apply the strategy developed in subgoal 1 (for example, Recall what hand you use for writing). It is important not to use external markers (such as bracelets, rings, or watches) for making right and left judgments. An internal awareness of the opposition of right and left is a superior strategy to external markers because the patient is able to reach a higher level of automaticity, which facilitates transfer to other contexts. The patient is usually able to establish reasonably good performance in 1 or 2 therapy sessions but will need reinforcement of the underlying concept throughout the laterality therapy sequence.

Laterality: subgoal 3. The next subgoal is to have the patient use his internal reference system for making right and left judgments as he moves through space. The floor map I (Figure 16.4) shows an example of how this stage of laterality proceeds.[35] The patient identifies whether he will make a right or a left turn while trying to find his way through the map. At each turn the patient should describe the strategy used to make the right or left decision. When the patient reaches a point of indecision, the doctor should help him generate a strategy. In the above example, the doctor might ask the patient which hand he uses to throw a ball and then apply this previous strategy to the new learning situation. As therapy progresses, the patient should be able to verbalize a strategy to differentiate the right and left sides of the body: "I throw a ball with my right hand" or "I use my left hand for writing." The patient should be able to demonstrate smooth and consistent laterality on these tasks in 2 or 3 office visits.

Finally, the patient should be able to guide themselves through the map without having to think about the difference between right and left at each turn in the map. This and similar procedures that emphasize the speed of the response without sacrificing accuracy are designed to improve automaticity. Techniques for bilateral integration therapy can also be reintroduced at this point to work on the automaticity of laterality skills. The doctor should realize that the goal has changed from coordinating move-

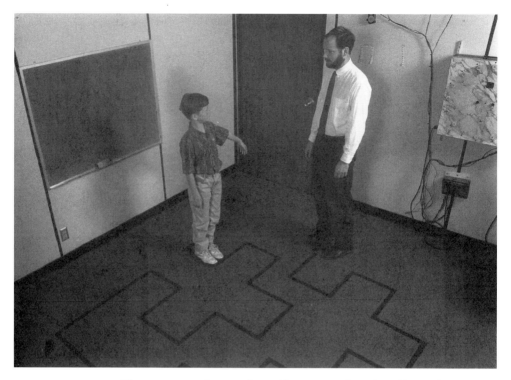

FIGURE 16.4 Floor map I technique for addressing subgoal 3 of laterality therapy. The patient identifies whether he will make a right or a left turn as he goes through the map.

ments of the two sides of the body to isolated movements of the right and left body parts. For example, on the first phase of Randolf shuffle the patient can perform two repetitions with left arm and then two repetitions with only the right arm. Here the patient is responding to verbal instructions about the right- and left-sided body parts with the motor system. The development of automaticity is the most challenging part of therapy and may require reinforcement over several therapy visits before the patient's responses are consistent at a high level of automaticity.

Goal 3: Develop directionality

Directionality is the ability to use directional concepts to organize external space. The patient needs to be aware of both his position in space as well as the relationship of objects to himself. The development of directionality involves three separate but interrelated concepts. First, the patient has to generate an awareness that his internal knowledge of laterality can be used to make right-left judgments of objects in space. Second, for animate objects (such as another person), which can turn by themselves in space, the patient needs to learn that right and left coordinates depend on the orientation that the object has chosen. In this case the patient cannot simply project his own internal right and left coordinate system to determine directionality. Instead, he needs to use perspective judg-

Goals and Techniques for Developing Directionality

Therapy Goal: Develop the ability to use directional concepts to organize external space.
  Subgoal 1: Develop an awareness that laterality skills taught previously can be used to make right and left judgments of objects in space.
    Therapy techniques:
      Directional "U" saccades (Lane[28])(9)
      Kirshner arrows I and II*
      Directional Triangles*
  Subgoal 2: Develop the patient's ability to identify right and left on another person while that person is engaged in a variety of activities.
    Therapy techniques:
      Directional mazes*
      Floor map II*
      Simon Says*
      Stickman
  Subgoal 3: Develop the patient's ability to apply directionality concepts to the spatial orientation of linguistic symbols
    Therapy techniques:
      b-d-p-q sorting (8)
      Letter find*
      Letter reversals*
      Recognition of reversals (8)

*Techniques are detailed in Chapter 17; numbers in parentheses refer to source list at end of chapter.

ments to interpret the possible right and left orientations that the object can assume (such as judging right and left on a person). Finally, directional concepts are used to determine the distinctive features of letters and numbers. These three distinct concepts of directionality are taught separately in therapy (see the box). The patient usually achieves the first subgoal relatively quickly, 1 or 2 therapy sessions, whereas consistent performance with the concept of perspective requires 1 or 2 additional therapy sessions. The final subgoal requires a significant amount of practice, and the underlying concepts will need to be reinforced over several therapy sessions.

Directionality: subgoal 1. The first subgoal of therapy is to have the patient generate an awareness that the laterality skills taught previously can be used to make right and left judgments of objects in space. In this phase, the patient is asked to make judgments of nonlinguistic symbols that have right and left orientation. The role of the doctor is to have the patient apply the strategies used in laterality therapy to make these directional judgments. Kirshner arrows[24] is a representative technique (Figure 16.5) that requires the patient to name the direction of a series of arrows that are drawn on a chalkboard or printed on paper and then describe how he arrived at that decision. The patient may say "This is my right hand

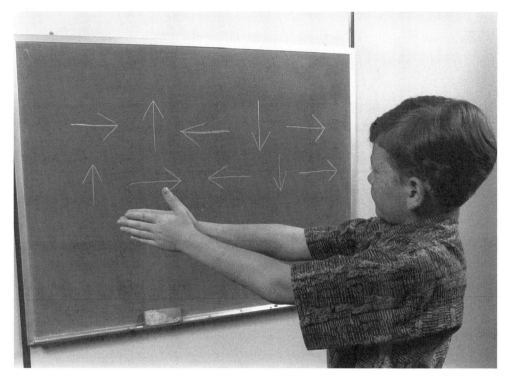

FIGURE 16.5 Kirshner arrows technique for addressing subgoal 1 of directionality therapy. Patient calls out or moves hands in the direction of the arrows.

and this is to the right" or "Right is this way." While making an explanation, the patient will typically use a motor gesture, moving his hand in the direction of the arrow, toward the right or left. Once accurate performance is achieved with minimum effort, a variety of procedures can be used to increase the automaticity of the response (see box on p. 393). For example, an auditory component can be added to the previous procedure by use of a metronome. The patient calls out the directions according to a specific pace, requiring the patient's right and left decision making to become more automatic in order to keep pace with the metronome. Another tactic is to have the patient move his or her hands in the direction of the arrow but to say the opposite direction. This step is very difficult and will probably not be performed smoothly by the young patient (less than 7 years of age) even with practice. These are examples of progressively overloading a therapy procedure to help create efficiency in the directionality response. Other activities that are appropriate for this stage of therapy are listed in the box on p. 445.

Directionality: subgoal 2. Direct projection of an individual's right and left coordinate system works especially well for interpreting verbal directions (for example, "Put your name in the top right hand corner") and linguistic symbols but will lead to erroneous answers when judging the rights and lefts of other people. This leads to the second subgoal where the patient develops an awareness that the right and left coordinates of animate objects depends on that object's orientation. The doctor needs to instruct the patient that if the object can turn by itself in space then right and left is not directly related to his or her own laterality. This requires interpretation of right and left directions from a different perspective. It should be remembered that developmentally this level of right and left knowledge is attained at approximately 8 years of age.[36,37] Therefore this stage of therapy is not emphasized for patients under 7 years of age. We have found that some 7 year olds can understand this concept, but they typically cannot achieve the stage of automaticity.

The therapy for subgoal 2 is directed at having the patient identify right and left directions on the doctor while the patient is engaged in a variety of activities. The doctor needs to help the patient understand how to alter the perspective of right and left by using concrete examples. Initially, it is helpful to hold the patient's dominant hand while the patient makes a 180-degree turn. This illustrates how a change in body position alters where right and left are in space. The next step is to identify right and left on the doctor using motor support. For example, the doctor directs the patient to turn himself to match the doctor's body orientation before making a judgment of right and left. Once the patient achieves accurate performance he should make the right or left decision first and then move his body to see if his decision was correct. Finally the patient needs to identify right and left on the doctor without using motor support. This phase is often difficult for children under 7 years of age.

Floor map II[35] is a representative therapy procedure that illustrates the above sequence (Figure 16.6). Instead of having the patient guide himself through the map, the patient guides the doctor through the floor map using right and left directions. It is important to have the patient use a fixed perspective from which to make the right and left decisions. Initially, the doctor can allow the patient to use his own knowledge of laterality to make the right and left judgments. For example, the patient would turn in the same direction as the doctor. If the patient can direct the doctor accurately using this strategy, he should then maintain a fixed position and only turn in the same direction as the doctor to confirm or check his decision. The goal is to have the patient direct the doctor using a fixed perspective, without having to rely consciously on his own laterality knowledge, and describe the strategy he is using to make his decision. Typical patient explanations include: "You are opposite of me, so you need to turn to the right" or "If I turn this way, then that is a right turn." The patient will often use illustrations, using his own laterality, to help verbalize the strategy. Alternative techniques for this phase of the therapy are listed in the box on p. 445. The patient is usually able to establish reasonably good performance in 2 or 3 therapy sessions but will

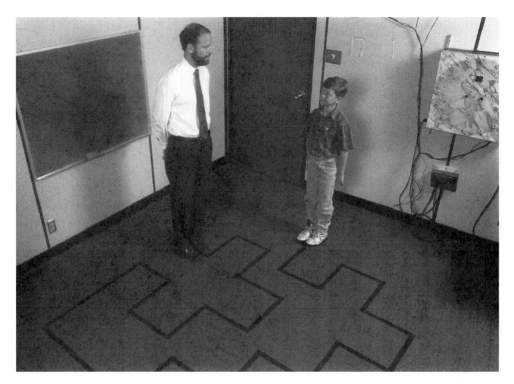

FIGURE 16.6 Floor map II technique for addressing subgoal 2 of directionality therapy. Patient identifies whether the doctor is to make a right or a left turn as the doctor goes through the map. The patient maintains a stationary position during the procedure.

need reinforcement of the underlying concept throughout the directionality therapy sequence.

Directionality: subgoal 3. The next subgoal for directionality therapy is to have the patient apply the concepts from subgoal 1 to the spatial orientation of linguistic symbols. In this stage the patient should be able to describe the distinctive features of those letters that are mirror images of each other. This is initially done with isolated letters, for example, a **b** is different from a **d** because the bump is on the right. The next step is to identify commonly reversed letters under increasing demands. Finding letters among other similar but reversed letters is a representative technique (Figure 16.7, *A*).[28,35] Once the patient understands the initial strategy, the therapy emphasizes the rapid identification of reversed letters. The next step would be to have the patient identify the reversed letter when it is part of simple words (Figure 16.7, *B*). Before this technique is attempted, it is important to have an idea of the patient's decoding level. The doctor should use only words that the patient knows eidetically (by sight). Dolch word lists are a good source of eidetic words if the doctor is interested in creating his or her own worksheets. If the patient does not know the word eidetically he or she may have difficulty determining whether there is a

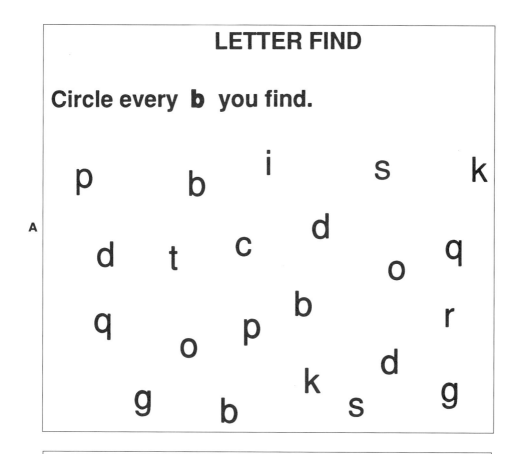

FIGURE 16.7 Letter finding technique for addressing subgoal 3 of directionality therapy. **A,** Letter finding requires the patient to circle the letters that match the target letter. **B,** Letter reversal requires the patient to circle all the backward letters that are within the words.

reversed letter within the word. The estimated treatment time is 2 to 4 therapy sessions. Periodic reinforcement may be necessary throughout the remainder of DVIP therapy.

The outcome of visual-spatial therapy is to provide the patient with a greater ability to understand and manipulate concepts that organize the external world. The patient not only gains a greater understanding of his own body's right and left, but also is able to project this understanding and interpret the directional characteristics of symbols. Additionally, the patient has developed the ability to use perspective to make spatial judgments. These skills will have some overlap with goals taught in the next section but in most instances will act as a foundation that will help the clinician remediate visual analysis dysfunctions.

TREATMENT OF VISUAL ANALYSIS DYSFUNCTION

The next phase of the therapy program addresses visual analysis skills. We recommend that treatment proceed in five sequential phases: (1) visual discrimination, (2) visual figure ground, (3) visual closure, (4) visual memory, and (5) visualization. This sequential approach is consistent with current notions in visual information processing such that different levels of organization have been found within the visual system.[9] Visual efficiency and visual-spatial skills therapy often has a positive affect on the first three phases of the visual analysis therapy sequence.[22] Before implementing therapy in this phase the doctor should reevaluate any deficient areas. Therapy for any remaining problem areas should start at the lowest level where a dysfunction exists. For example, if visual discrimination is adequate but figure ground was deficient, therapy should start with visual closure.

Goal 1: Develop visual discrimination

Visual discrimination is the ability to be aware of the distinctive features of forms, including size, shape, color, and orientation. These features are used to determine the similarities and differences between forms. This area includes the skills tested on both the visual discrimination and the spatial relationship sub-tests of the Test of Visual Perceptual Skills (TVPS). Most visual discrimination tasks that the patient will encounter will require the patient to make judgments of several visual parameters simultaneously (such as size and position). However, in therapy it is helpful initially to isolate each parameter before attempting to handle several judgments at once. The therapy sequence and representative therapy techniques are listed in the facing box. The estimated treatment time is 3 to 5 therapy sessions.

Visual discrimination: subgoal 1. The first subgoal requires the patient to be aware of similarities or differences between simple forms using multisensory (vision and tactile) input. The first step is to have the patient describe the distinctive features of individual forms. The use of parquetry

---

Goals and Techniques for Developing Visual Discrimination

Therapy goal: Develop the ability to be aware of the distinctive features of forms, including size, shape, color, and orientation.
  Subgoal 1: Develop the patient's awareness of similarities or differences among forms using multisensory input.
    Therapy techniques:
      Parquetry blocks*
      Winterhaven templates*
  Subgoal 2: Develop the patient's ability to use only visual clues to find similarities or differences of increasingly complex forms.
    Therapy techniques:
      Geoboard*
      Parquetry blocks*
      Perceptive (4)
      Sames/differences (7)
      Visual discrimination (10)

*Techniques are detailed in Chapter 17; numbers in parentheses refer to source list at end of chapter.

---

blocks[25] is a representative technique (Figure 16.8, *A*). For example, the patient traces the four sides of a square with his finger. The doctor then asks the patient to describe the characteristics of the square. Frequently, questions such as, "How many sides does this have?" "Are all the sides the same size?" or "How many corners does the figure have?" are necessary to elicit responses from the patient. The next step is to have the patient identify all the similar shapes when they are mixed in with a variety of other shapes (for example, Find all the squares in the box).

Once the patient consistently identifies the features of individual forms the doctor asks the patient to find similarities and differences between forms. For example, the patient describes the similarities and differences between a square and a triangle parquetry block. Again the doctor may have to prompt the patient to respond with specific questions such as, "Do the forms have the same number of sides?" The patient functioning at a lower developmental level will often need to use tactile support to help him explain the difference between forms (for example, They may trace the differences in the lengths of the individual sides between a square and a diamond). Additionally, certain features such as angles or oblique lines are difficult for children to explain without motor support. Most patients will understand these basic concepts in 1 or 2 therapy sessions.

Visual discrimination: subgoal 2. The next subgoal is to have the patient be aware of similarities and differences of increasingly complex forms relying primarily on visual clues. For example, the patient would physically build a parquetry block design directly on top of a simple design that the doctor constructed (Figure 16.8, *B*). It is helpful to have the patient pick out all the pieces he needs to build a parquetry block design

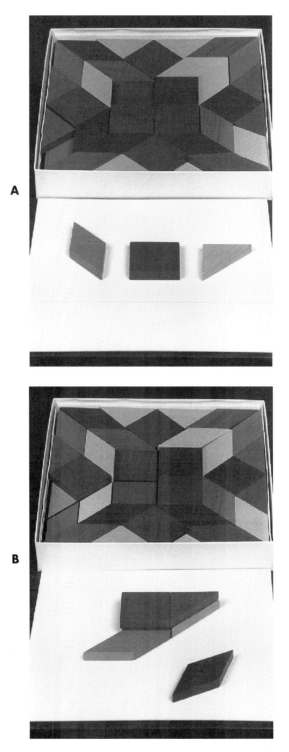

FIGURE 16.8 Parquetry blocks technique for addressing subgoals 1 and 2 of visual discrimination therapy. **A,** Subgoal 1 requires the patient to identify the similarities and differences of the three figures and then sort and match the figures. **B,** Patient builds a design on top of the doctor's design.

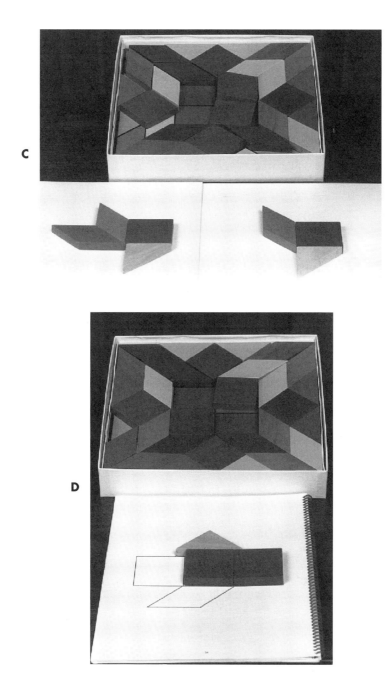

FIGURE 16.8, cont'd. C, Patient builds a design next to the doctor's design, **D**; patient builds design on the parquetry block workbook. **B** to **D** are techniques used in addressing subgoal 2 of visual discrimination therapy.

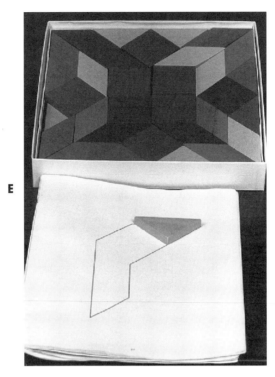

FIGURE 16.8, cont'd. E, Parquetry blocks technique for addressing subgoal 2 of visual closure. Patient is asked to identify what blocks are necessary to build the design on a pattern with no internal lines.

before attempting to construct it. This forces the patient to make both shape and color discriminations allowing the doctor to observe the accuracy of the patient's analysis. Next the patient would attempt to build an exact parquetry block design replicate alongside the parquetry block design the doctor built (Figure 16.8, *C*). Frequently the patient will be able to select the correct color and shape forms and build the correct design but ignores the proper orientation of the total design. For example, the patient may have the figure rotated to the left or right by 30 degrees. The doctor should ask the patient to identify the similarities and differences between the doctor's design and the one the patient built. If the patient is unable to identify subtle orientation differences, the doctor needs to physically pick up the patient's design of blocks and place it on top of the doctor's design. This serves as a concrete illustration of the difference between the two designs. The doctor then asks the patient to identify the differences between the two designs. Once accurate performance is achieved the doctor can present more complex figures, and the patient is required to make more subtle judgments of similarities and differences. Once the patient is able to build the designs on top and then alongside the block design created by the doctor, the patient can be asked to do a parallel task using parquetry block design workbooks (Figure 16.8, *D*). This is a more abstract task than building designs on or alongside the actual

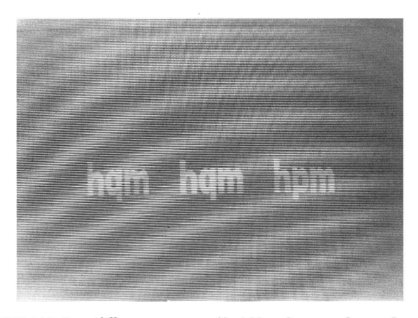

FIGURE 16.9 Same/differences program (Opti-Mum Computer System, Learning Frontiers, Inc., Hillsboro, Oreg.) for addressing subgoal 2 of visual discrimination therapy. Patient is asked to choose which of the targets is different.

parquetry blocks. The parquetry workbooks typically start with simple designs and progress to more complex designs. In addition, there are several other workbooks, which do not require parquetry blocks, that can used in developing visual discrimination skills at this stage in therapy (see the box on p. 451). The estimated treatment time to complete the sequence in subgoal 2 is 2 or 3 therapy sessions.

Once the patient can identify distinctive features of a design or form based only on visual clues, the automaticity of the response is stressed. A representative technique is the "Sames/Differences" program on the Opti-Mum Computer System. This program requires the patient to identify whether a target was the same or different when compared to other targets (Figure 16.9). For example, the patient would have to choose which one of the following targets is different: **hqm**, **hqm**, **hpm**. The program can be made progressively more difficult when more distractor targets are added or the amount of time the patient is given to respond is decreased.

Goal 2: Develop visual figure ground

Visual figure ground is the ability to attend to a specific feature or form while maintaining an awareness of the relationship of this form to the background information. This may be a prerequisite skill for performing several visual efficiency therapy procedures such as Michigan Tracking, Percon saccades, and Hart Chart saccades. In these therapy activities, the patient is asked to find a target stimulus that is "buried" in background information. Poor figure-ground ability may initially make these kinds of

Goals and Techniques for Developing Visual Figure Ground

Therapy goal: Develop the ability to attend to a specific feature or form while maintaining an awareness of the relationship of this form to the background information.

  Subgoal 1: Develop the patient's ability to separate the figure from the ground using a multisensory approach.

    Therapy techniques:

      Visual tracings (1)

      Parquetry blocks*

  Subgoal 2: Develop the patient's ability to conduct an organized or structured search pattern to find a particular figure.

    Therapy techniques:

      Alphabet jumbles (7)

      Find the word (1)

      Geoboard*

      Hart chart coordinates*

      Jumbled pictures*

      Michigan tracking (1)

      Perceptive (4)

      Visual figure ground (10)

      Visual scan (2)

      Visual search (2)

  Subgoal 3: Develop the speed of the patient's response without sacrificing the accuracy of the performance as distractors are added to the background.

    Therapy techniques:

      Visual tracings* (1)

      Jumbled pictures*

      Michigan tracking (1)

      Hart chart coordinates*

      Visual search (2)

      Visual scan (7)

      Alphabet jumbles (7)

      Find the word (1)

      Perceptive (4)

      Visual figure ground (10)

*Techniques are detailed in Chapter 17; numbers in parentheses refer to source list at end of chapter.

techniques more difficult and frustrating for the patient and in turn impede patient cooperation. In these cases the clinician should either alter the visual efficiency therapy to include procedures with minimal figure-ground requirements or remediate figure-ground skills before or concurrently with visual efficiency therapy. On the other hand we have seen minor figure-ground problems resolved after visual efficiency therapy without the need to specifically address the figure-ground problem. The therapy sequence and representative therapy techniques are listed in the box. The estimated treatment time is 3 to 5 therapy sessions.

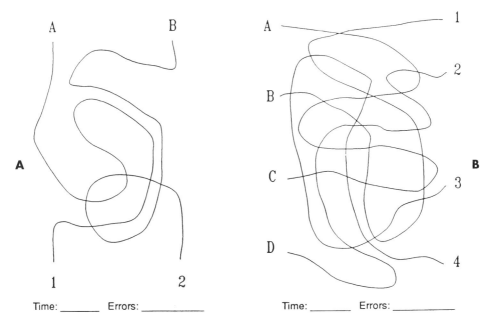

FIGURE 16.10 Visual tracings technique for addressing subgoals 1 and 3 of visual figure ground therapy. Patient is asked to trace a line from the beginning letter to the number at the end of the line. **A,** Simple figure ground task using only two lines. **B,** More complex figure ground task using four lines.

Visual figure ground: subgoal 1. The first subgoal is to separate the figure from the ground using a multisensory approach. For example, the patient can visually and motorically trace the figure simultaneously. A representative therapy procedure is visual tracing (Figure 16.10). In this procedure, the patient traces the line from point A to the number at the end of the line. Initially the patient uses a pencil for tracing the lines, and such tracing reinforces the visual cues of separating figure from ground. Later the patient is encouraged to scan the line visually from beginning to end. The doctor should foster the development of this strategy by asking the patient to describe how he knows that he should continue on the same line. In this initial phase where the patient is tracing the line, children typically have trouble expressing their strategy orally but will often be able to show the doctor by tracing the line through an intersection of lines with their finger or pencil. At this point in the therapy sequence the doctor should not be overly concerned with the patient's visually guided fine-motor accuracy. The estimated treatment time is 1 or 2 therapy sessions.

Visual figure ground: subgoal 2. The next subgoal is to have the patient use an organized or structured search pattern to find a particular figure. The patient needs to perform a systematic search strategy that he can explain to the doctor. Initially, it is helpful to have the patient perform a task and observe what type of strategy he uses. Patients with poor figure ground skill tend to be impulsive and demonstrate a random or disorganized search strategy resulting in many items being skipped or missed. The doctor should ask questions that direct the patient's attention to items that have been overlooked. Once the patient identifies missing items the doctor should encourage the patient to change his original strategy to search systematically through all the items again. This might involve having the patient take a left-to-right and top-to-bottom strategy.

Jumbled pictures[37] is a representative therapy procedure. The patient's task is to find the number of items in Figure 16.11, *B*, that are different from Figure 16.11, *A*. Initially, the doctor observes the patient's strategy and notes those items that were overlooked. The doctor should ask the patient to describe the patient's search plan and then identify the items that were overlooked. The doctor should ask the patient to reexamine the picture this time stressing an organized search strategy that starts with one item in Figure 16.11, *A*, and comparing that in Figure 16.11, *B*. For example, the doctor could ask the patient "Does the pot in this picture look the same as the one in the other picture?" Once the patient can identify individual differences it is helpful to have him verbalize his strategy by telling the doctor what items he is comparing. Eventually, the patient should be able to compare a group of figures to each other by remembering chunks of information in each glance. This last step is not intended to train visual memory but to encourage a more efficient visual search strategy. The estimated therapy time is 1 to 3 therapy sessions.

Visual figure ground: subgoal 3. The next subgoal of therapy is to increase the visual demand by adding distractors to the background and increasing the speed of the patient's response without sacrificing the accuracy of the performance. In this phase, we are progressively overloading the visual response with other sensory information and in turn establishing automaticity. Initially the doctor would add distractors to the background information and stress accurate performance. Once the responses are accurate then speed is stressed along with adding other sensory information. For example, the complexity of visual tracings can be increased to four or five lines, instead of two lines (Figure 16.10, *B*). This effectively increases the number of distractors present in the display. Once performance is accurate there are many methods used to overload the visual system. For example, the patient can perform visual tracing while counting out loud to 10 or to 20 by twos. Computer programs including Visual Search and Visual Scan (Computer Orthoptics) and Alphabet Jumbles (Opti-Mum) are also quite effective for changing the parameters noted above. Other techniques for subgoal 3 figure-ground ability are listed in the box on p. 456. The estimated treatment time is 1 to 3 therapy sessions.

Goal 3: Develop visual closure

Visual closure is the ability of the individual to be aware of clues in the visual array that allow him to determine the final precept without the necessity of all the details being present. As was the case with visual dis-

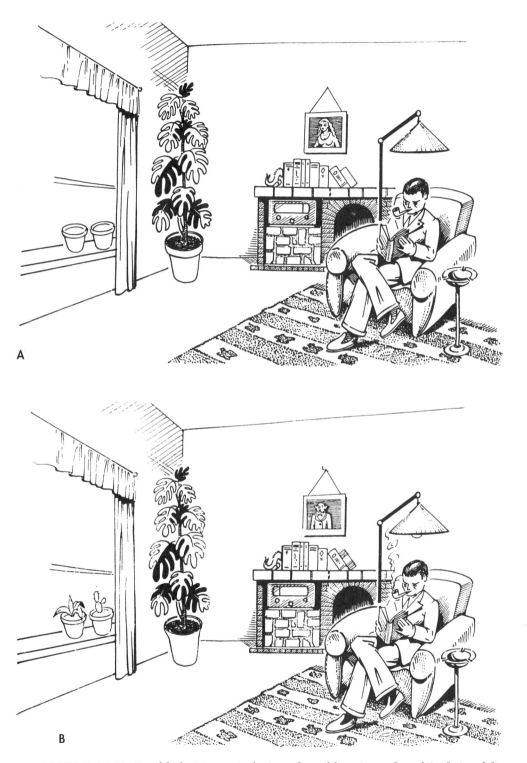

FIGURE 16.11 Jumbled pictures technique for addressing subgoal 2 of visual figure ground therapy. Patient is asked to find the number of items in **B** that are different from those in **A**.

crimination and figure ground, therapy for visual efficiency dysfunctions often has a positive effect on visual closure ability. However, in our clinical experience, poor visual closure does not appear to interfere with successful visual efficiency therapy. This is not surprising because most visual efficiency therapy procedures do not demand a high level of visual closure. The therapy sequence and representative therapy techniques are listed in the box. The estimated therapy time is 3 to 5 therapy sessions.

Visual closure: subgoal 1. The first subgoal is to teach the patient to differentiate between guessing, incomplete closure, and complete closure. This requires the doctor to ask the patient a series of questions that elicit what information the patient is using to arrive at a solution to a closure problem. For example, when very little information is present, the patient would have to guess at the solution, but when the majority of information is present, the patient would be very sure of his answer. A simple therapy procedure is to project on a wall a number that is completely blurred. The doctor then asks the patient to identify what number is on the wall. Typically the patient will say, "I don't know, the number is too blurry." The doctor should then encourage the patient to guess. After the patient's response the doctor should reinforce the concept that the patient was only guessing and there was not enough information present to identify the number. The doctor slowly reduces the blur until the patient can make a guess based on some visual feature or features of the stimulus. Again the doctor should ask the patient what information the patient used to make their judgment. For example, the patient may report seeing parts of two circles that are above each other and, based on this less-than-complete information, that the figure is the number 8. The doctor should make sure

---

Goals and Techniques for Developing Visual Closure

Therapy goal: Develop the patient's ability to be aware of clues in the visual array that allow him to determine the final precept without the necessity of all the details being present.

    Subgoal 1: Develop the patient's ability to differentiate between guessing, incomplete closure, and complete closure.

      Therapy techniques:
        "Focus-in" forms*
        Visual closure (2)

    Subgoal 2: Develop the patient's ability to make closure judgments with increasing speed and accuracy.

      Therapy techniques:
        Dot-to-dot figures* (1)
        Parquetry blocks*
        Perceptive (4)
        Visual closure (2), (10)

*Techniques are detailed in Chapter 17; numbers in parentheses refer to source list at end of chapter.

the patient verbalizes how he arrived at his decision. Finally, the doctor removes all the blur, and the patient tells the doctor if the response was correct. The important aspect of this stage of therapy is to make sure that the patient can orally express what type of visual information was used to arrive at the decision. The estimated treatment time is 1 to 2 therapy sessions.

Visual closure: subgoal 2. Once the patient understands the difference between guessing and making closure the doctor should have him perform therapy procedures requiring visual closure judgments that require increasing accuracy and speed. This requires the doctor to arrange therapy procedures where the incomplete information is given. For example, parquetry block designs, used previously for visual discrimination therapy, can be modified for visual closure therapy.[25] Instead of using designs that designate the placement of the individual blocks within the design, the doctor should use designs with no internal details (Figure 16.8, *E*). Before beginning the procedure the doctor would have the patient pick out the pieces he will need to complete the design. This forces the patient to use available visual clues within the design to make closure instead of a trial-and-error approach. To encourage this strategy, the doctor should ask the patient to identify, for example, where the triangle would fit into the design.

Once the patient is able to perform closure tasks accurately the speed of the response is stressed. The Computer Orthoptic's program Visual Closure is an excellent therapy procedure that allows the doctor to monitor closely the speed and accuracy of the response. For example, parts of a target (number or letter) are slowly added until the point where the patient is able to identify the completed letter or number (Figure 16.12). The percentage of the figure present and the time of response is recorded by the computer. The doctor is able to track the speed of the response as a measure of the level of closure. Other procedures used to develop visual closure are listed in the facing box. The estimated treatment time is 1 to 3 therapy sessions.

Goal 4: Develop visual memory

Visual memory is the ability to recognize and recall visually presented information. In Chapter 2 a general model of memory was outlined; it consisted of three parts: sensory store, short-term memory, and long-term memory. The overall therapy goal for patients with visual memory deficits is to help the patient become aware of and use strategies for improving short-term visual memory of both the spatial and sequential characteristics of the visual presentation. Children typically do not suffer from a deficit in memory capacity; instead children have difficulty generating an appropriate or optimal strategy for storing visual information in short-term memory.[38]

It is helpful to identify if the patient has a deficit in spatial (poor

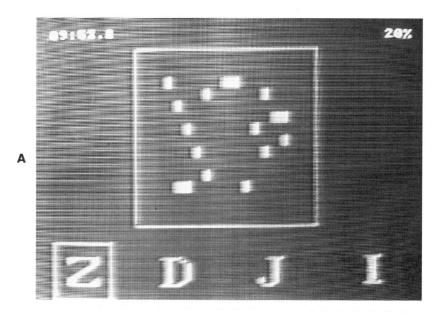

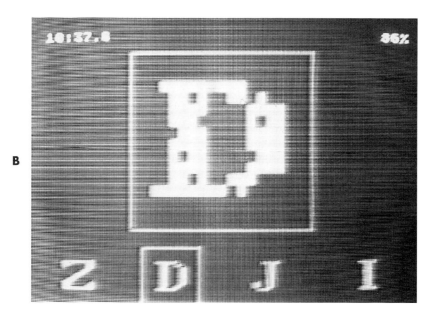

FIGURE 16.12 Visual closure program (Computer Orthoptics, RC Instruments, Cicero, Ind.) for addressing subgoal 2 of visual closure. Patient is asked to decide which letter is being produced from a choice of four. The computer gives a time and percentage of completeness as scores. **A** is an example of 20% complete, compared to, **B,** 86% complete.

performance on TVPS subtest visual memory) memory (see Chapter 11). When a patient has more difficulty with spatial aspects of memory storage, the doctor should start with subgoal 1. In contrast, if the patient has only sequential memory problems, therapy should start with subgoal 3.

Goals and Techniques for Developing Visual Memory

Therapy goal: Develop the patient's short-term memory abilities.
  Subgoal 1: Develop the patient's ability to form an image of the visual input
           using multisensory input.
    Therapy techniques:
      Parquetry blocks*
      Three-in-a-row*
      Winterhaven Templates*
  Subgoal 2: Develop the patient's ability to recall the *spatial* characteristics of
           figures using only visual information.
    Therapy techniques:
      Concentration*
      Geoboard*
      Parquetry blocks*
      Visual memory (8), (10)
  Subgoal 3: Develop the patient's ability to recall the *sequential* characteristics
           of figures or displays using only visual information
    Therapy techniques:
      Sequential beads*
      Three-in-a-row*
      Visual memory (8)
      Visual sequential memory (10)
  Subgoal 4: Develop the patient's ability to recall information as the amount of
           information is increased and the viewing time is decreased.
    Therapy techniques:
      Tachistoscopes:
        Electro-Tach[6]
        Vu-Mate Hand-Held Tach (3)
        Tach (Computer Orthoptics) (2)
        Tach (Opti-Mum Computer) (7)
        Tach (Visual Processing Software) (3)

*Techniques are detailed in Chapter 17; numbers in parentheses refer to source list at end of chapter.

The therapy sequence and representative therapy techniques are listed in the box. The estimated treatment time is 4 to 6 therapy sessions.

Visual memory: subgoal 1. The first subgoal is to have the patient develop internal spatial representation of a form or figure, using a multisensory approach. The first step is to have the patient trace a simple figure with his finger, pencil, or chalk. This provides a motor-memory trace that matches the visual characteristics of the figure. The next step is to remove the form or figure and have the patient reproduce the form from memory. The doctor then has the patient compare the original form or figure with what the patient has drawn. A representative technique would use Winterhaven templates.[2] In this procedure a patient traces a figure template (either a square, circle, triangle) first with his finger and then with chalk (or pencil if done on paper) to get both a kinesthestic and a visual picture of the figure (Figure 16.13, *A*). Then the template is

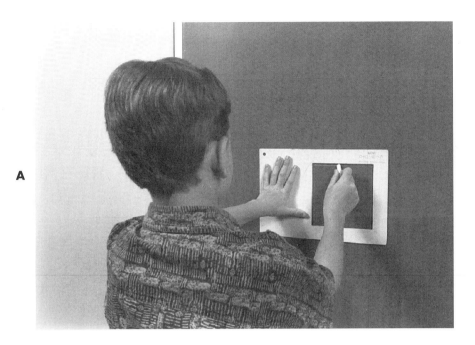

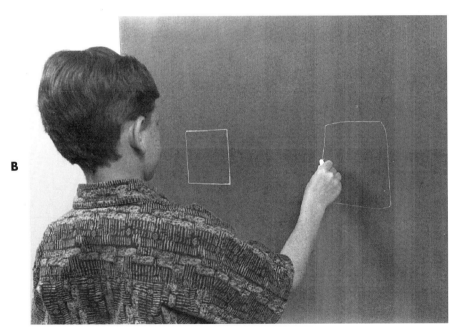

FIGURE 16.13 Winterhaven templates techniques for addressing subgoal 1 of visual memory therapy. **A,** Patient traces figure to establish a kinesthetic and visual memory of the figure. **B,** Patient reproduces figure from memory and compares it to template tracing (notice that the template tracing is covered when the patient draws the figure from memory).

removed, the tracing is covered, and the patient draws the figure from memory. The doctor should instruct the patient to keep "a picture in his (or her) head" of what the figure looked and felt like when he was tracing the figure. Once the patient reproduces the figure from memory the doctor has the patient compare his drawing to the original template tracing (Figure 16.13, *B*). The patient should identify the differences between the two figures; for example, the patient's reproduction of a square may have sides that are unequal or too short. The doctor covers the template tracing and has the patient reproduce the figure again, encouraging the patient to recall differences that were previously found. This process continues until the patient can reproduce the figure with reasonable accuracy. The estimated treatment time is 1 or 2 therapy sessions.

Visual memory: subgoal 2. The second subgoal is to have the patient recall the *spatial* characteristic of figures using only visual information. In this phase the tactile support is removed and the patient uses only visual clues to generate a mental image. The first step in therapy is to leave the form or figure in view while the patient copies the form or figure. Next the form or figure is hidden from view and the patient constructs his design based on his mental image. Parquetry block designs can be used in this phase of therapy. Initially the design is placed in front of the patient, and he builds his blocks adjacent to the design, similar to what was done in visual discrimination therapy (Figure 16.8). The patient should be able to do this easily if the goals in visual discrimination were successful achieved. Next a new design (3 or 4 blocks) is placed in front of the patient but hidden from view. The doctor then allows the patient to look at the design for 5 to 10 seconds and then asks the patient to describe the characteristics of the design. For example, "How many squares were present in the design? Was the triangle on the right or left of the square?" We would like to emphasize that it is important at this stage for the patient to describe the spatial characteristic of the design, rather than simply naming the individual parts. If the patient is unable to describe the spatial characteristics of the entire design at one glance, the doctor should allow the patient another "peek" at the design. The doctor should again ask the patient to describe the characteristics of the design. As therapy progresses, the patient should be able to describe the spatial characteristics of a 3- to 5-block design based on a single 5- to 10-second view of the design. Once the patient can accurately describe the figure, he should build 5 to 10 designs without verbally describing the figure. The doctor should have the patient compare his design to the doctor's design and describe any subtle spatial differences, such as orientation. This helps foster reliance on visual imagery to recall the designs. The estimated treatment time is 1 or 2 therapy sessions.

Visual memory: subgoal 3. The third subgoal is to have the patient reproduce the *sequential* characteristic of figures or display using only visual information. The first step in therapy is to leave the original design in view while the patient copies the design. Next the design is hidden from view and the patient constructs his design based on his mental image. Sequential beads[35] can be used in this phase of therapy (Figure 16.14). Initially the design is placed in front of the patient, and he strings his beads to match the design, similar to what was done in the previous subgoal 2, but the emphasis has changed to reproducing the correct sequence. Next a new design (3 to 5 beads) is placed in front of the patient but hidden from view. The doctor then allows the patient to look at the design for 5 to 10 seconds and then asks the patient to string the appropriate sequence of the design. We do not have the patient describe the sequence, as was done in the previous subgoal, because this may encourage the patient to overly rely on a oral strategy rather than his own mental image of the sequence. If the patient is unable to build the entire design at one glance, the doctor should allow the patient another 5- to 10-second view of the design. The doctor should again ask the patient to build the design. As therapy progresses, the patient should be able to build design sequences of a 3 to 6 beads based on a single 5- to 10-second view of the design (see TVPS subtest visual sequential memory for age appropriate number of items in a sequence). The estimated treatment time is 1 or 2 therapy sessions.

Visual memory: subgoal 4. The previous subgoals have concentrated on developing effective memory strategies using concrete examples with substantial amounts of time to view the target. In these techniques the patient can use memory strategies to develop a mental image (such as coding the spatial or sequential characteristics of the display) while the visual form is still in view. In this phase of therapy the target is presented rapidly (such as less than 1 second); therefore the patient cannot rely on

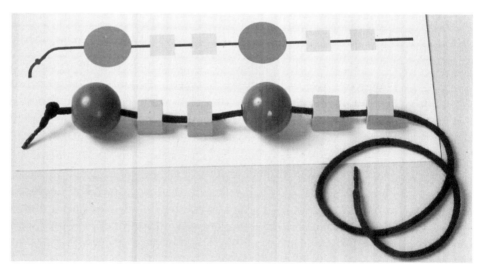

FIGURE 16.14 Sequential beads technique for addressing subgoal 3 of visual memory therapy. First, the patient reproduces the correct sequence of beads with the pattern in view. Second, the patient is given a brief (5- to 10-second) look at the pattern and then asked to reproduce the sequential pattern from memory.

memory strategies while directly viewing the target. Instead the patient needs to form an image of the visual stimulus and then use memory strategies for short-term memory recall. The final subgoal in the development of visual memory is to increase both the speed and span of visual memory.

The most effective method for rapidly presenting the target is either a mechanical or a computerized tachistoscope (see the box on p. 463 and Figure 16.15). With these techniques the doctor has complete control over the type and number of targets as well as the presentation speed. Guidelines for determining appropriate therapy levels for speed of presentation and the number of targets have been developed for kindergarten, first, second, fourth, and fifth graders (see Table 16.1).[34,39] For example, a patient

TABLE 16.1 Guidelines for visual memory therapy, subgoal 4—goals for tachistoscopic therapy.

The patient should be able to perform at 80% or greater accuracy over a suggested 10 presentations with the number of digits and the exposure time listed.

Grade level	Number of digits	Exposure time (sec)
Kindergarden	2	0.1
First grade	3	0.1
Second grade	4	0.1
Third grade	5	0.1
Fourth grade	5	0.1
Fifth grade	5	0.1

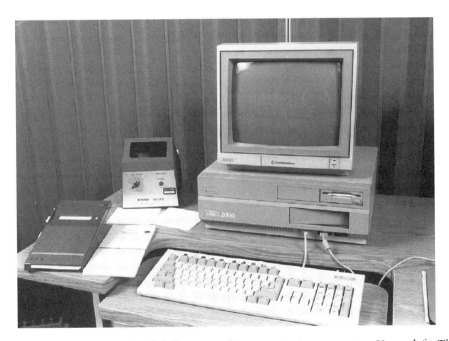

FIGURE 16.15 Example of different tachistoscopic instruments. *Upper left,* The Tachette (Lafayette Instruments Co., Lafayette, Ind.); *lower left,* the Vu Mate (Bernell Corp., South Bend, Ind.); *right,* a computer tachistoscope (Opti-Mum Computer System, Learning Frontiers, Inc., Hillsboro, Oreg.).

in kindergarten may achieve only 2 digits presented at $1/10$ of a second, whereas a second grader should be able to recall 4 digits flashed at the same speed. We would typically start with targets that emphasize the recall of spatial orientation (tic-tac-toe or arrows) and progress to targets that stress the sequential aspects (such as string of numbers and letters) of memory recall (Figure 16.16).

Initially the doctor should choose a number of targets below the patient's expected grade level (for example, a second grader would start with three digits) and present the targets at approximately 1 second. Before the presentation the doctor should reinforce the initial stage of visual attention, coming to attention. The patient needs to understand the task, which includes what type of target is going to be displayed, the location of the display, and the method of recall that will be used (oral, by writing, or by typing on the keyboard). The doctor should encourage the patient to use the memory strategies developed in subgoals 2 and 3 before recalling the visual information. Once accurate performance of over 80% correct is achieved at a 1-second display time the doctor gradually decreases the presentation time until it is faster than 200 msec. This prevents the patient from making a saccade to gather additional information and forces him to pick up more information with only one fixation. If the patient is unable to perform accurately at the slowest speed, the doctor should reduce the number of targets (for example, a second grader would use two targets). The goal of therapy is to have the patient remember correctly the number of digits appropriate for his grade level (see Table 16.1). Once the patient reaches this goal, we concentrate on automaticity by delaying the time (such as 5 to 10 seconds) between presentation and the patient's response. The doctor can increase the cognitive loading of the task by requiring the patient to make a move in the game of tic-tac-toe between the presentation and the recall of the tachistoscopic display. The reinforcement of memory strategies should be continued throughout this sequence. The estimated treatment time is 2 to 4 therapy sessions.

Goal 5: Develop visualization

Visualization is the ability to recall visually presented materials and to manipulate these images mentally. Before visualization therapy is begun, visual memory skills should be approximately age appropriate, since visual memory is considered a prerequisite skill for visualization. An excellent text on the subject has been written by Forest,[40] and he outlines several therapy techniques that are meant to remediate deficits in this area. Our approach is to build upon visual memory skills to ensure that the patient is able to use mental imagery skills. The sequence of therapy and associated therapy techniques are listed in the box on p. 470. The estimated treatment time is 3 to 5 therapy visits.

Visualization: subgoal 1. The first subgoal is to have the patient become aware of the mental image created by a form that is no longer present. This is similar to what was taught in therapy for visual memory,

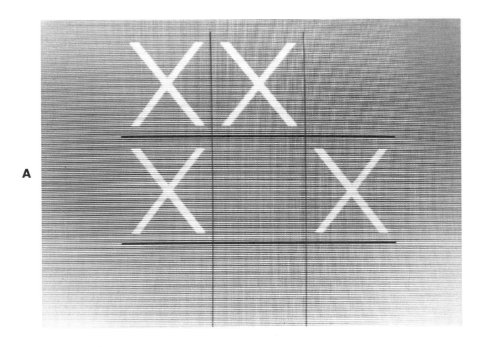

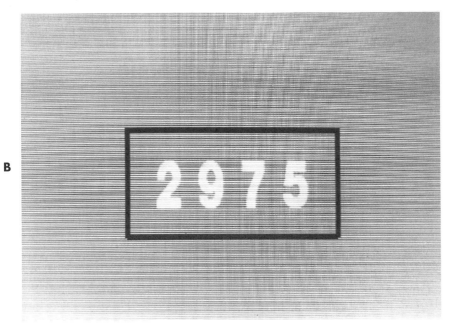

FIGURE 16.16 Tachistoscope targets. **A**, Example of a target that stresses the recall of spatial orientation. **B**, Example of target that stresses the recall of sequential characteristics.

but in this phase the patient does not recall the complete form. The patient is now required to use the mental image to recall only parts of the form. For example, when performing memory procedures with numbers, have the patient recall the second and fourth number in a sequence of four digits. The doctor should encourage the patient to use the mental image

---

Goals and Techniques for Developing Visualization

Therapy goal: Develop the patient's ability to recall visually presented material and manipulate these images mentally.

Subgoal 1: Develop the patient's ability awareness of the mental image created by a form that is no longer present.

Therapy techniques:
  Tachistoscope*
  Visualization—golf game*
  Visualization games 1, 2, 3*

Subgoal 2: Develop the patient's ability to manipulate mentally the spatial orientation of forms and symbols.

Therapy techniques:
  Directionality (2)
  Flip Forms*
  Floor map III*
  Geoboard*
  Parquetry blocks*
  Tic-tac-toe games (7)

Subgoal 3: Develop the patient's ability to use symbols or pictures to stand for letters and simple words.

Therapy techniques:
  Coding activities*

*Techniques are detailed in Chapter 17; numbers in parentheses refer to source list at end of chapter.

---

that the patient formed in his head to solve the problem. This subgoal is to ensure that the patient can form an accurate mental image and maintain the image for a short period of time. The estimated treatment time is 1 or 2 therapy visits.

Visualization: subgoal 2. The next subgoal is to have the patient mentally manipulate the spatial orientation of forms and symbols. In this phase of therapy the patient will be asked to change the orientation of a target figure. For example, in the procedure called "Flip Forms"[35] a figure (Figure 16.17, *A*) is placed in the upper left-hand corner of a page. The patient is then instructed to flip the form around the *y*-axis and draw the figure. The next step is to flip the figure around the *x*-axis, and then the figure is flipped around the *y*-axis again. Typically the patient will need a concrete demonstration of how a figure changes its orientation. For example, a pipe cleaner can be formed into a **b**, and the patient can flip this around the *y*-axis and observe the result. The procedure is done with reversible letters first and then with abstract symbols. This procedure allows the patient to explore changes in orientation of objects as they are manipulated in space. The patient should be able to tell the doctor his strategy for flipping the figures. However, we have found that children have difficulty expressing this strategy and will often use an explanation that demonstrates the change in rotation with a hand gesture. When manipulating the let-

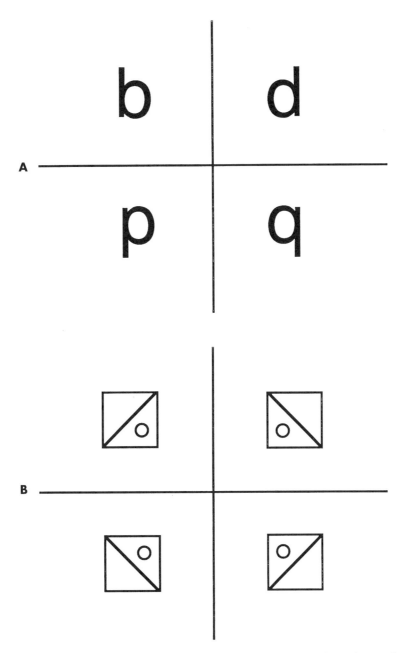

FIGURE 16.17 Flip forms technique for addressing subgoal 2 of visualization therapy. **A,** Flip form using easily reversed letter. **B,** Flip form using more complex figure.

ters, the patient should be able to explain how rotating the letters will change the letter from a **b** to a **d**. This process reinforces the patient's understanding of the directional features of letters. To increase the difficulty one can use more complicated forms (Figure 16.17, *B*). Another method to make the procedure more complicated is to have the patient perform two rotations before writing the object down. The use of the Computer

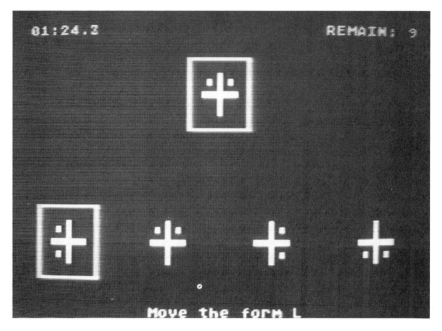

FIGURE 16.18 Directionality program (Computer Orthoptics, American Vision Training, Inc., Cicero, Ind.) for addressing subgoal 2 of visualization therapy. The patient has to select the option that correctly matches the instructions to rotate the target figure.

Orthoptics program Directionality is another technique that is representative of this type of therapy. In this program the patient has to perform one of four rotations: right, left, upside down, and sideways, on a form (Figure 16.18). The program can be made more difficult when one increases the number of rotations and the number of items to be rotated. The estimated treatment time for subgoal 2 is 2 to 4 therapy visits.

Visualization: subgoal 3. The final subgoal is to allow the patient to use symbols or pictures to stand for letters. These activities are not designed to teach spelling but to encourage the use of visual strategies when the patient encounters symbols. Coding games are a representative technique. In these procedures a code or form is made to represent a letter of the alphabet. For example, a matrix of rows and columns can be assigned numbers and letters (Figure 16.19). In this example the letter **C** would have the code *A1*. In presenting the technique the doctor would first have the patient identify codes for individual letters. The next step is to have the patient identify simple words that correspond to a particular coding sequence. In the above example, the code *A1 B3 C2* would spell "cat." The doctor should not let the patient write down the letter that corresponds with the code, rather the patient should maintain the image that *A1* equals a **C** and then *B3* equals **A** and *C2* equals **T**, resulting in a complete mental image of CAT. The patient is challenged to build a image of the whole word from the individual pieces. It is important when you are do-

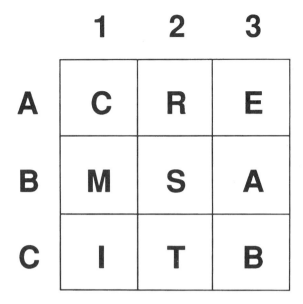

FIGURE 16.19 Coding games technique for addressing subgoal 3 of visualization therapy. Letters of the alphabet are given a code depending on the row and column. For example, the letter **C** would have a code of *A1*.

ing this technique to make sure that the words you spell are within the sight-word vocabulary of the patient. We usually begin with three-letter words and work up to four- and five-letter words depending on the patient's reading level. Many of these patients are reading below grade level, and it is important to have an idea of their decoding level before starting these procedures. The estimated treatment time is 2 to 4 therapy visits.

Therapy for visual analysis skills has helped the patient develop a variety of skills that are important for efficient visual performance in the classroom and other daily activities. The therapy starts with the development of basic skills and builds to more complicated forms of visual processing. The patient must first be able to discriminate similarities and differences before goals for figure ground and closure are taught. Finally, visual memory and visualization are higher level skills that depend in part on visual discrimination, figure ground, and closure. In our experience visual discrimination, figure ground, and closure are prerequisite skills for visual motor training. We frequently start the early phases of visual-motor therapy (goals 1, 2, and initial subgoals of 3) while we are developing visual memory and visualization skills.

TREATMENT OF VISUAL-MOTOR DYSFUNCTION

Visual-motor integration is generally described as the ability to integrate vision with the motor system. This skill is used in a broad range of activities from catching a ball to printing and drawing. We are particularly concerned with the patient's ability to integrate visual information processing skills with the fine-motor system in order to reproduce complex visual patterns.[41] We have divided the therapy for visual-motor integration into four components or abilities (see the box): (1) general eye-hand coordination skills, (2) efficient visual-motor ergonomics, (3) accurate and rapid visually guided fine-motor control using paper and pencil, and (4) the patient's ability to plan visually guided motor actions to reproduce complex spatial patterns. The sequence of therapy and the associated therapy techniques are listed in the last three successive boxes.

A review of the case history, observations, and diagnostic results are critical for determining where therapy should begin. For the patient who performs inadequately on both the Developmental Test of Visual Motor Integration (DTVMI) and Grooved Pegboard Test (GPT), therapy should begin at the beginning of the sequence. For the patient who has adequate fine-motor control (adequate results on the GPT) but does poorly on the DTVMI, the clinician should check the patient's visual-motor ergonomics (goal 2), and then therapy should begin with higher level activities within goal 3. Occasionally, we have found patients who have poor fine-motor control but have adequate complex motor planning skills (adequate results on the DTVMI). For this type of patient therapy should concentrate on goals 1 and 2 and the early phases of goal 3. Once the visual fine-motor foundation is established the patient is expected to accomplish quickly the later phases of goal 3 and then goal 4. The estimated treatment time is 8 to 10 therapy sessions.

Goal 1: Develop general eye-hand coordination skills

The goal of therapy is to develop general eye-hand coordination ability. In this type of therapy the patient performs eye-hand tasks without paper and pencil. Many procedures in this phase of therapy overlap with oculomotor therapy techniques. However, the treatment strategy has changed from using the motor system to support the weaker oculomotor system to having the visual system guide the fine-motor system. Frequently, when designing a therapy program for deficient oculomotor skills, we will review the diagnostic results to see if a visually guided fine-motor dysfunction is

---

Therapy Goal and Component Skills of Visual Motor Integration

Therapy goal: Develop the ability to integrate visual information processing skills with the fine-motor system in order to reproduce complex visual patterns.
1. General eye-hand coordination
2. Efficient visual-motor ergonomics
3. Accurate and rapid visually guided fine-motor control
4. Ability to plan visually guided motor actions in order to reproduce complex spatial patterns

present. In this case we will introduce general eye-hand procedures during the oculomotor therapy.

When you are choosing general eye-hand coordination procedures, we suggest starting with techniques that use "large objects and targets" (gross visual-motor) that have reduced constraints on the accuracy of visually guided fine-motor skills and move toward "smaller objects and targets" (fine visual-motor) where the demand increases. Large objects and targets require primarily forearm and hand motor control, whereas small objects and targets require hand and finger motor control. For example, a representative gross eye-hand coordination procedure is the bean bag toss (Figure 16.20). The patient grips the bean bag with his whole hand and tosses the bag toward a large target that is a few feet away. In contrast a repre-

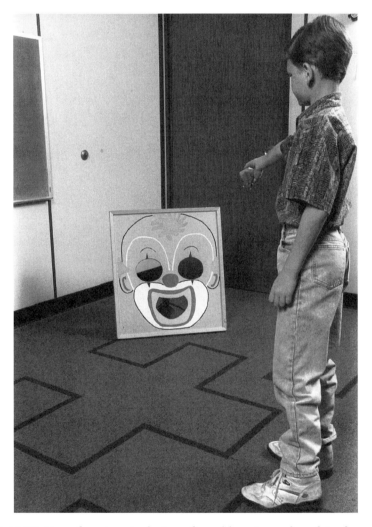

FIGURE 16.20 Bean-bag-toss technique for addressing subgoal 2 of general eye-hand coordination therapy. This represents a gross eye-hand technique requiring primary forearm-hand control.

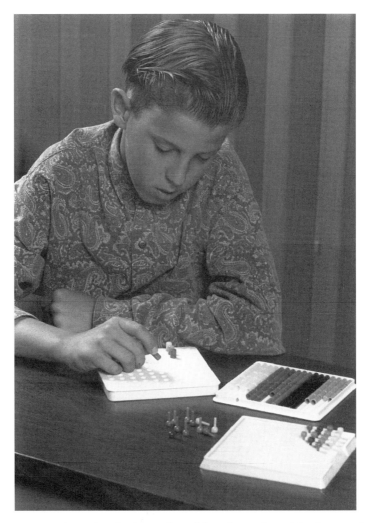

FIGURE 16.21 Pegboard techniques for addressing subgoal 2 of general eye-hand coordination therapy. This represents a fine eye-hand technique requiring primary hand-finger control. Patient is using a large peg; smaller pegboard activities are seen in the foreground.

sentative fine eye-hand coordination procedure is the stationary pegboard (Figure 16.21). The patient must now grip the peg with two fingers and place it into a small target area. The goal is for the patient to achieve an adequate level of performance on several techniques from the gross and fine visual-motor categories. Representative techniques for each area are boxed on p. 477. The estimated treatment time is 2 to 4 therapy visits.

Develop general eye-hand coordination skills: subgoal 1. The initial step in therapy for developing general eye-hand coordination skills is to illustrate the importance of how the visual system guides the motor system in visual-motor tasks. The doctor can illustrate the visual system's importance by having the patient perform a simple eye-hand coordination task with and without the use of vision and then verbalize the results of

---

Goals and Techniques for Developing General Eye-Hand Coordination

Subgoal 1: Illustrate the importance of how the visual system guides the motor system in visual-motor tasks.
(See text for explanation.)

Subgoal 2: Perform a variety of visual-motor tasks under the guidance of the visual system, starting with gross and progressing to fine visual-motor targets.

Therapy techniques:

Gross:
    Bean bag toss*
    Marsden ball*
    Saccadic fixator (11)
    Visual-motor stick procedures*

Fine:
    Bead stringing
    Dive bombing*
    Lite Brite*
    Pegboard
    Straw piercing*

*Techniques are detailed in Chapter 17; number in parentheses refers to source list at end of chapter.

---

the patient's performance under each condition. The patient should come to conscious realization that his or her vision is critical for directing motor performance. Patients are usually able to accomplish this goal in a single therapy session. For a few patients, it may be necessary to reinforce the concept over several therapy sessions. The estimated treatment time is 1 to 2 therapy sessions.

Develop general eye-hand coordination skills: subgoal 2. The next step is to have the patient perform a variety of visual-motor tasks under the guidance of the visual system, starting with gross and progressing to fine visual-motor targets. For example, when using a pegboard (visual fine-motor target), the patient should identify and look at what target hole the peg needs to be placed in and then visually guide the peg into the correct position. The doctor should emphasize to the patient that "The eye leads the hand" or "The eye tells the hand what to do." The doctor should then have the patient evaluate his results and then generate a strategy for improving his performance. For example, if the patient missed the hole to the right, he should say that his hand should move to the left on the next attempt. The eventual outcome of this subgoal is to have the patient monitor his responses during the visual-motor activity. In the above example, while visually guiding the peg toward the target, the patient would make subtle adjustments to correctly place the peg.

As part of the above therapy we have often found it helpful for patients with visually guided fine-motor dysfunction to perform fine-motor planning procedures. These procedures are analogous to the gross-motor planning done for deficits in bilateral integration. This therapy treats isolated fine-motor movements that are not under the guidance of the visual system. These procedures are especially helpful for patients with an inappropriate pencil grip. A representative technique is the finger chart developed by Kirshner[24] (Figure 16.22). In this procedure the patient has to make his hand match the picture of the hand on the chart. Initially some patients may have difficulty forming individual finger patterns. The role of the doctor is to teach the patient to activate and inhibit isolated finger movements. This can be accomplished by the restriction or encouragment of the movement of the isolated fingers. The next step is to have the patient perform a sequence of hand patterns fluently. Once smooth performance is achieved a metronome can be added to achieve automaticity.

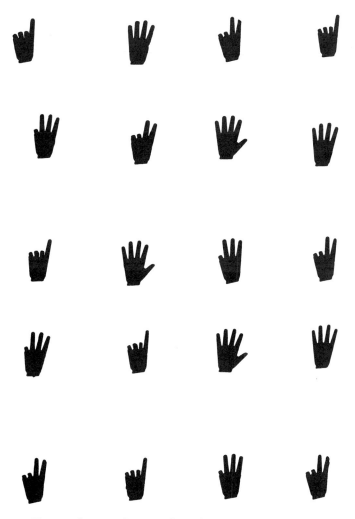

FIGURE 16.22 Finger chart technique for addressing subgoal 2 of general eye-hand coordination therapy that stresses fine-motor planning. Patient is asked to make his or her hand match the pictures of the hand.

Other procedures for developing general eye-hand coordination skills are listed in the box on p. 477. The estimated treatment time is 1 to 2 therapy visits.

Goal 2: Develop efficient visual-motor ergonomics

The next goal is to teach the patient to have a proper pencil grip, an efficient lead-support system, correct body posture, and appropriate working distance when performing visually guided fine-motor tasks (Figure 16.23). These are basic prerequisite skills for improving visual-motor integration. For example, the child who fails to use the support hand to stabilize the paper position may appear to have trouble replicating forms. Simply

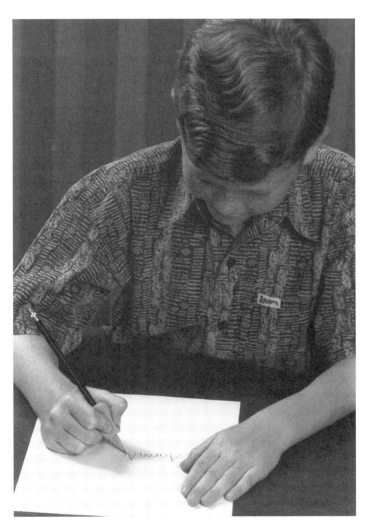

FIGURE 16.23 Illustration of important visual-motor ergonomics. Patient should maintain an erect posture, normal working distance, correct lead-support relationship, and tripod grip of writing instrument. (Notice that the patient is using a Pencil Grip to establish the correct pencil grasp. The Pencil Grip, Inc., P.O. Box 67096, Los Angeles, CA 90067.)

teaching an efficient lead-support strategy may have a significant improvement in the quality of the child's copying. If by observation the patient already has efficient visual-motor ergonomics, the clinician should move directly to goal 3.

Develop efficient visual-motor ergonomics: subgoal 1. Initially the doctor should develop appropriate body posture and working distance when performing visual fine-motor tasks. When seated, the patient should have an erect posture. The best orientation between the visual axis and the working surface is approximately 90 degrees.[42,43] On a flat surface this may create a situation where the patient is having to lean excessively over the writing surface to maintain this relationship. To avoid this problem the writing surface may have to be slanted up about 20 degrees by use of a slant board or lap board for a more comfortable posture. The doctor should discourage the patient from tilting, turning, or laying his head on his arm, rather stressing the importance of the more efficient "working position" on the visual system.

The appropriate working distance from the eye to work surface can be approximated by measurement of the distance from the middle knuckle of the second finger to the center of the elbow, often referred to as the "Harmon distance."[42,43]

Develop efficient visual-motor ergonomics: subgoal 2. The next goal is to develop an appropriate lead-support system.[42,43] This involves illustrating to the patient that the dominant hand is used for copying and the nondominant hand supports the copying activity by stabilizing the writing surface (Figure 16.23). It is helpful to have the patient copy simple forms with and without the use of the supporting hand to illustrate the advantage of an efficient lead-support system. The doctor should encourage the patient to verbalize how the patient will establish an efficient lead-support relationship before starting any pencil and paper task. This will help the patient replace previous bad habits with more efficient lead-support strategy.

Develop efficient visual-motor ergonomics: subgoal 3. Frequently patients with visual-motor dysfunction have an inappropriate pencil grip for their age (see Chapter 2 for a review of grip development). Although an abnormal pencil grip is not always detrimental to performance, we have found this to be almost always the case in children with poor visual-motor integration. The most efficient grip is the tripod grip, where the pencil rests on the first joint of the middle finger with the thumb and index fingers holding the pencil in place (Figure 2.8, *C*). This position allows good fine-motor control over the writing tool. A simple way to promote a proper pencil grip is to use a prosthetic "pencil-gripper" device to guide the patient's fingers into this efficient tripod grip (Figure 16.23). Initially, this device may have to be used for all paper and pencil tasks both in therapy and at school. In most cases the finger position developed by the gripper device will become the patient's habitual pencil grip. In addition, the doctor should monitor the amount of force or pressure the patient is exerting on the pencil as he or she draws. Excess force may result in slower performance and allow the patient less fine-motor control over the pencil. It is often helpful to have the patient make a series of simple pencil strokes from initial ones using excessive pressure to final ones where the lightest pressure possible is used. This helps the patient gain greater awareness that excess pressure limits effective fine-motor control of the writing tool.

Although these subgoals can be demonstrated and learned in a single therapy session, it may take several weeks of practice and reinforcement before the patient consistently uses the new ergonomic skills.

Goal 3: Develop accurate and rapid visually guided fine-motor control. In this phase we are transferring general eye-hand coordination skills to paper and pencil tasks. The ergonomic skills developed in goal 2 should be practiced and reinforced throughout goal 3. Initially the emphasis should be on the patient's overt planning of the visually guided movement before attempting the task. Next, the doctor should improve the accuracy and speed of the visual fine-motor response. This is done in a manner similar to that of general eye-hand coordination using procedures that progressively increase the demand on accuracy. Accuracy is improved first, and then the emphasis is changed to improving the speed of the visually guided fine-motor movements. The sequence of therapy and associated therapy techniques are listed in the box. The estimated treatment time is 3 to 5 therapy sessions.

Goals and Techniques for Developing Accurate and Rapid Visually Guided Fine-Motor Control

Subgoal 1: Develop the ability to plan a visually guided fine-motor movement.
Therapy techniques:
Continous motion*
Dot-to-dot figures*
Subgoal 2: Develop the accuracy of the visually guided fine-motor movement.
Therapy techniques:
X's and **O**'s (8)
Mazes* (increasing accuracy demands) (1), (10)
Haptic writing*
Perceptuo-Motor Pen (3)
Fransblau Multisensory Trainer (5)
Subgoal 3: Develop the speed, while maintaining the accuracy of the visually guided fine-motor movement.
Therapy techniques:
X's and **O**'s* (8)
Mazes* (increasing accuracy demands) (1, 10)
Haptic writing*

*Techniques are detailed in Chapter 17; numbers in parentheses refer to source list at end of chapter.

Develop accurate and rapid visually guided fine motor control: subgoal 1. The first step is to teach the patient to plan or to "look" before he draws. A simple technique is to have the patient verbally plan out the strategy for drawing a line between two points. The patient should use the strategy of the eye leading the hand learned in goal 1. If the patient does not spontaneously generate the strategy, the doctor needs to instruct the patient to look at the point where the line starts and ends. Reinforcement of the important concept of visual guidance "The eye tells your hand what to do" is critical at this stage. After a few attempts the patient should tell the doctor what strategy he is using before starting the technique.

Frequently the patient's poor ergonomics will block his or her view of the target. It is important to adjust the patient's pencil grip, posture, and paper position to allow the patient a more direct view of what is ahead of his hand when copying. When the patient completes the line, he should be asked to evaluate his performance. The patient should be able to tell the doctor if his line hit the dot or not and how the line deviated from the intended performance. Again it is important that the patient verbalize the appropriate strategy to improve the performance. For example, if the line that the patient drew was too long, he should tell the doctor that he will shorten the line on the next attempt. Other tasks that can be used in this phase of the therapy are listed in the box on the preceding page. The estimated treatment is 1 to 2 therapy visits.

Develop accurate and rapid visually guided fine-motor control: subgoal 2. The next step is to have the patient use the eye to lead the hand while increasing the constraints on accurate fine-motor performance. The use of mazes is a representative technique (Figure 16.24). Therapy starts with mazes with widely separated borders and then procedes toward narrowing the separation between the lines. It is important to emphasize that the eye is leading the hand. As the patient draws a line between the borders of the maze, the doctor should have him identify when performance is inaccurate (the patient touched the edge of the maze with the pencil). Once the inaccuracy is identified the patient should verbalize a strategy to improve his performance.

At this point it may be helpful to attempt to modify the patient's "visual-motor style," which is evaluated along two parameters: speed and accuracy. The ideal patient has a fast and accurate style. However, the doctor will frequently encounter a patient who works quickly but is inaccurate, an indication of an impulsive style. For example, when maze tracing, the impulsive patient will draw rapidly, frequently ignoring inaccuracies. When this happens, the doctor should have the patient stop and evaluate his performance. The patient should then adjust his motor actions and repeat the task. For some children, simple visual feedback (noticing that they hit the sides of the maze) will not be sufficient, and it is often helpful to add techniques that provide auditory feedback (such as the

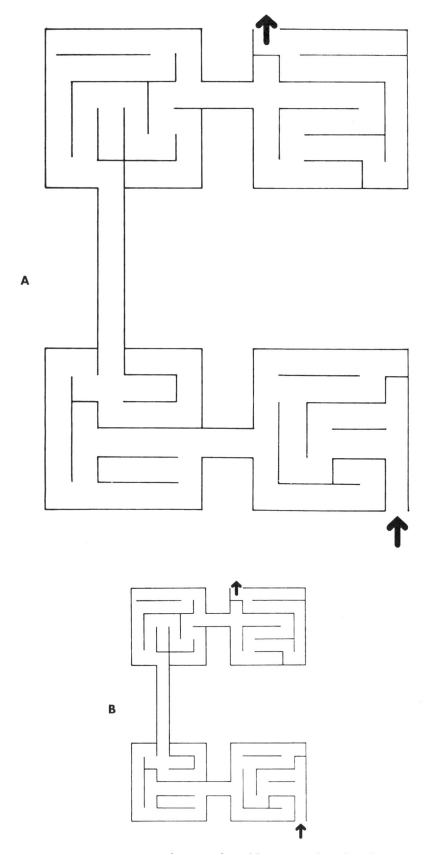

FIGURE 16.24 Maze-tracing techniques for addressing subgoal 2 of accurate and rapid visually guided fine-motor therapy. **A,** Initially mazes have wide separation between lines to reduce the demand on visually guided fine-motor accuracy. The separation is gradually reduced. **B,** Example of maze with narrow separation and high demand on visually guided fine-motor accuracy.

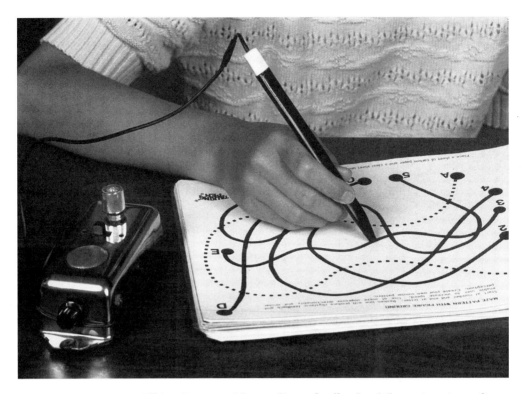

FIGURE 16.25 Talking Pen provides auditory feedback while patient is performing visually guided fine-motor tasks. When the patient is not tracing directly on the line, the pen gives an auditory signal.

Talking Pen; Figure 16.25). The goal is to have the patient monitor and adjust his performance to improve the accuracy and then subsequently the speed of the visually guided fine-motor movement. In some cases the patient may continue impulsive behavior. For this patient, operant conditioning may be helpful.

In contrast is the patient who performs slowly but accurately, illustrating an overly reflective visual-motor style. For this patient, therapy to increase the speed of performance is more important than careful monitoring of accuracy. An occasional mistake is often overlooked or actually encouraged because he or she increases the speed while maintaining a reasonable level of accuracy. Finally, we have encountered some patients who are slow and inaccurate. For these patients, the doctor should concentrate on the accuracy of the visual-motor response before addressing the speed of the patient's response.

To further increase the planning demands on the visually guided fine-motor system we have found that certain haptic writing procedures[25] are helpful (Figure 16.26). (Haptic [Greek *haptikos* 'able to grasp or perceive'] writing starts with a series of activities that have the patient draw a pattern visually and then with his or her eyes closed. The goal is to enhance the kinesthetic awareness or motor memory of the shape or figure. In our

Haptic Writing Pattern - 1

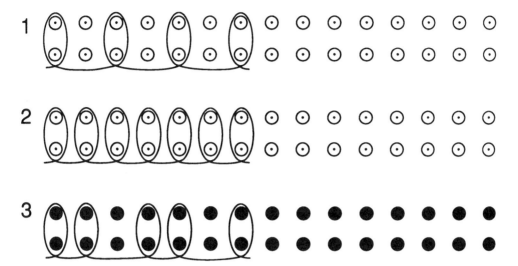

FIGURE 16.26 Haptic writing technique for addressing subgoal 2 of accurate and rapid, visually guided, fine-motor therapy. The patient traces the pattern on the left side and then continues the pattern onto the right side of the page.

experience emphasis on fine-motor skills in the first two goals has a positive effect on kinesthetic processing, which negates, in most instances, the need for this early haptic writing stage.) First, the patient traces over the pattern on the left side of the page and then continues to draw the pattern on the right side of the page even though the stimulus pattern is missing. This requires that he appropriately space the loops in relationship to each other and accurately place the loops around the dots. The patterns become progressively more complex as the patient proceeds through the therapy program. The doctor should emphasize that the patient needs to form a plan before proceeding with the pattern. Before starting, the doctor should ask the patient how many loops there are in the pattern and to relate the specific loops with each dot. This forces the patient to plan progressively more difficult visually guided fine-motor movements. Other activities that are appropriate in this phase of therapy are listed in the box on p. 481. The estimated treatment time is 3 to 5 therapy sessions.

Goal 4: Develop the patient's ability to plan visually guided motor actions to reproduce complex spatial patterns

There have been several therapy procedures described to address this skill.[25,44,45] In general these procedures start by presenting a spatial pattern in a manner that reduces the demands on the patient's own spatial coordinate and motor planning systems. For example, the patient who has difficulty drawing a diamond will find it much easier if the four corners

---

Goals and Techniques for Developing the Ability to Plan Visually Guided Motor Actions to Reproduce Complex Spatial Patterns

Subgoal 1: Develop the patient's awareness of an external spatial coordinate system and then integrate this with visually guided fine-motor planning skills.
   Therapy techniques:
     Rosner program*
Subgoal 2: Develop patient's ability to rely on his or her internal spatial coordinate system and then integrate this skill with visually guided fine-motor planning skills.
   Therapy techniques:
     Rosner program*
     Ideal forms*
     Geometric and language forms (10)

*Techniques are detailed in Chapter 17; number in parentheses refers to source list at end of chapter.

---

of the diamond are identified by dots.[46] In subsequent phases the demand on coordinating the internal spatial map with the appropriate motor plan progressively increases until the patient relies completely on internal representation rather than external cues. The sequence of therapy and associated therapy techniques are listed in the box.

We believe that the structured visual motor program developed by Rosner[26] is an excellent representative technique. In this program the patient is presented with a spatial pattern that is printed on a dotted map (Figure 16.27). We typically start the Rosner program by having the patient copy a pattern from the doctor's 25-dot map to his own 25-dot map using paper and pencil. If the patient has successfully achieved previous therapy goals in the areas of form perception as well as visually guided fine-motor control, we have found that most patients are able to start therapy at the 25-dot level. If the patient has great difficulty at this level the Test of Visual Analysis Skills (TVAS)[26] can be administered to help start the patient at a more appropriate level. The estimated treatment time is 4 to 6 therapy sessions.

Develop the patient's ability to plan visually guided motor actions to reproduce complex spatial patterns: subgoal 1. The first subgoal is to develop the patient's awareness of a spatial coordinate system and then integrate this with motor planning skills. The first step is to have the patient identify the *x-y* spatial coordinates of individual dots on his or her dotted map. For example, the patient is to count three dots on the *x*-axis and two dots down on the *y*-axis. The patient should find this reasonably easy if the goals in the visual analysis therapy have been successfully achieved. The second step is for the patient to isolate a single feature (one line connecting two or more dots) of a pattern on the doctor's map and

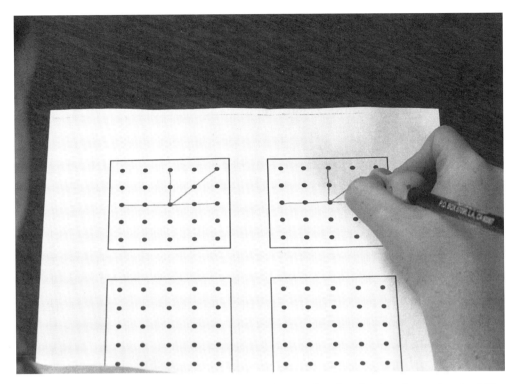

FIGURE 16.27 Rosner visual-motor technique for developing the patient's ability to plan visually guided motor actions in order to reproduce complex spatial forms. The patient is reproducing a 25-dot pattern onto a 25-dot map.

then identify the spatial coordinates of the starting and ending dots of that feature on the patient's map. In the initial stage the pattern is presented in a structured manner that reduces the demand on the patient's internal spatial coordinate system. This helps the patient generate an organized internal spatial coordinate system. The third step would be to draw the line and have the patient evaluate the accuracy of his own performance. This step builds on earlier development of visually guided motor movements, but the emphasis changes to integrating the internal spatial map with an appropriate visually guided fine-motor plan. To foster this development it is helpful to have the patient visualize the actual motor plan before ever putting the pencil on the paper. Once the patient is able to draw the individual features of a pattern successfully, the emphasis changes to drawing the complete pattern in a systematic manner going from left to right and top to bottom. The patient will typically complete 10 map figures per day. Rosner[26] recommends that the patient complete map figures 100 to 150 in this stage. By rotating each figure a quarter turn four times, one can make these 50 figures effectively become 200 figures, which can be used for practice during this stage. It is important to reach the higher numbered maps to ensure that the patient has successfully completed a broad array of patterns. For most patients this stage will take 2 to 3 therapy sessions.

Develop the patient's ability to plan visually guided motor actions to reproduce complex spatial patterns: subgoal 2. The next phase in therapy is progressively to remove external spatial organization cues. This is accomplished by removal of dots on the map that the patient is using to copy the pattern. The sequence of therapy within this subgoal mimics the steps in subgoal 1; however, the emphasis changes to having the patient rely on his internal spatial map to guide motor movements as the external cues are removed. In the Rosner program this would be accomplished by initially having the patient copy a 25-dot map pattern onto a 17-dot map starting at map number 150 (Figure 16.28). The first step is to have the patient identify the *x-y* spatial coordinates of individual dots that have been re-

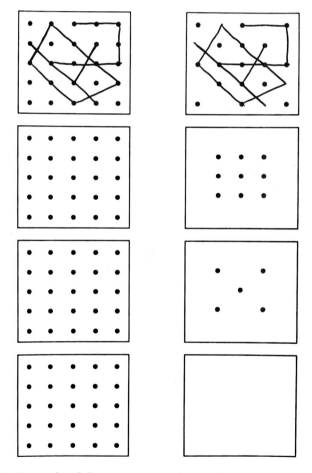

FIGURE 16.28 Example of the progressive demand on the patient's own internal spatial map for reproducing patterns in the Rosner program. The patient copies a 25-dot pattern onto a 17-dot map. The therapy would continue with the patient copying a 25-dot pattern onto a 9-, 5-, and finally a zero-dot map.

moved from their dot map. We have found it helpful to have the patient actually draw in the missing dots after identifying the spatial coordinates. If the dot is correctly placed, this helps confirm that the patient can apply his internal spatial map. If the dot is placed incorrectly, the doctor needs to have the patient identify how the patient's map is different from the doctor's map. If the patient has difficulty with this step, an acetate overlay can be used to illustrate the difference. The second step is for the patient to isolate a single feature of a pattern (where the ending dot is missing) on the doctor's map and then identify the spatial coordinates of the starting and ending dots of that feature on his own map. In this phase the patient needs to use his own internal spatial map to identify the ending dot. The third step would be to draw the line and have the patient evaluate the accuracy of his performance. It is helpful to have the patient visualize the actual motor plan before ever putting the pencil on the paper. When the patient's reproduction does not reflect an accurate internal spatial map (numerous redrawn lines or erasure of lines), the doctor should help the patient identify the inconsistency in the internal map versus the pattern being drawn. An acetate overlay of the pattern can be helpful in illustrating this to the patient. Once the patient is able to draw successfully the individual features of a pattern, the emphasis changes to drawing the complete pattern in a systematic manner going from left to right and top to bottom. We recommend that the patient correctly copy 20 figures before moving on to more difficult maps. As the patient proceeds through this sequence, dots are removed so that the patient must copy the 25-dot pattern onto a 9-dot, then 5-dot, and finally a 0-dot map. With each sequence of dot maps the doctor should proceed through each of the above steps so that the patient builds a consistent internal spatial map. The outcome of therapy is for the patient to use an internal mental map of the pattern to generate a motor plan to draw complex spatial patterns.

When a school-aged patient copies figures or symbols in school or at home, he will have to combine visual-motor integration with visual-memory skills. Therefore we have found it helpful to have the patient copy items from memory to facilitate transfer of these newly learned skills to the classroom setting. A patient may spontaneously integrate the two skills as a result of this remediation program, which addresses each skill individually. However, we have often found it helpful to foster integration of memory and visual-motor integration with specific therapy procedures. Ideal Forms[35] is a representative technique (Figure 16.29). In this therapy procedure the patient will first trace a design, then draw the design, and finally draw the design from memory. The doctor should stress strategies for visual-motor integration and memory depending on the patient's performance. Frequently, patient's will forget certain features of the target while drawing. In this case the doctor should emphasize forming a picture of the

VISUAL MOTOR INTEGRATION FORMS (IDEAL)

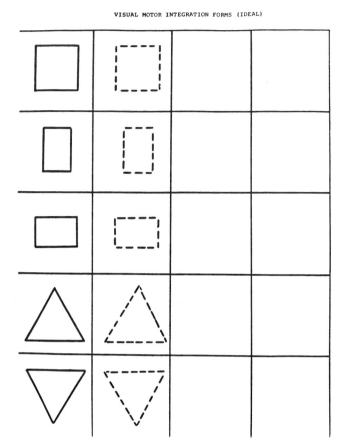

FIGURE 16.29 Ideal Forms technique for addressing final phases of subgoal 2 of developing the patient's ability to plan visually guided motor actions in order to reproduce complex spatial forms. The patient traces the dashed figure and then draws the figure in the next box. Then the patterns are covered, and the patient draws the figure from memory.

item in the patient's head before the patient draws. Other procedures used during this phase of therapy are listed in the box on p. 486. The estimated treatment time is 3 to 5 therapy sessions.

The outcome of therapy for visual-motor integration is to improve the patient's ability to integrate the visual and motor systems, particularly the patient's ability to integrate visual information processing skills with the fine-motor system in order to reproduce complex visual patterns. Therapy will typically result in improved efficiency and accuracy of eye-hand coordination tasks, such as cutting and coloring, as well as the ability to organize written work on the page. The improvements in this area are readily identified by the parent and teacher because they can see the improved written work on a daily basis.

SUMMARY

In this chapter we have provided the reader with a clinical model for managing patients with developmental visual information processing problems. The general treatment strategy includes a plan for each of the three systems, visual spatial, visual analysis, and visual motor. The plan outlines important component goals in each system, which are further broken down into target therapy subgoals. Within each subgoal we have provided representative techniques and patient-doctor interactions to help you develop important skills and patient strategies. We have also provided tables of additional techniques that would be applicable for each therapy subgoal. Our goal was to present a systematic approach for managing developmental visual processing dysfunctions to allow the optometrist to meet his responsibilities on the multidisciplinary team involved in the diagnosis and management of patients with learning difficulties. We believe that there is sufficient clinical evidence as well as research to indicate that optometric intervention can improve visual information processing skills. We hope that this model will prompt new optometric research in this area and will refine and improve the effectiveness and efficiency of therapy for remediating specific component skills.

For the patient who is undergoing therapy using this model the overall goal is to develop a level of readiness in the area of visual information processing ability that will lead to an elimination or substantial reduction of entering signs and symptoms that may account fully or partially for poor academic performance. In closing we would like to emphasize that optometric intervention is intended to address only the visual aspects of the patient's problems and that in most cases the patient will need the assistance from other members of the multidisciplinary team to reach his or her own full potential.

CHAPTER REVIEW

1. Give examples of situations that would modify the general strategy for treating children with learning-related vision problems.
2. What are the primary therapy outcomes expected when developing a patient's bilateral integration skills.
3. List the overall therapy goals, subgoals, and representative therapy techniques for the development of laterality skills and visual memory skills.
4. Describe the therapy sequence for developing a patient's visual-motor skills.

SOURCES MENTIONED

(1) **Academic Therapy Publications**
20 Commercial Blvd.
Novato, CA 94947

(2) **RC Instruments**
1578 Eastport Court
P.O. Box 109
Cicero, IN 46034

(3) **Bernell Corporation**
750 Lincolnway East
P.O. Box 4637
South Bend, IN 46634-4637

(4) **GTVT**
18807 10th Place W
Lynnwood, WA 98036

(5) **Keystone View, Division of Mast/Keystone, Inc.**
4673 Aircenter Circle
Reno, NV 89502

(6) **Lafayette Instrument**
P.O. Box 5729, 3700 Sagamore Parkway North
Lafayette, IN 47903

(7) **Learning Frontiers, Inc.**
1010 Northeast Cornell Rd.
Hillsboro, OR 97124

(8) **Learning Potentials Publishers, Inc.**
230 West Main St.
Lewisville, TX 75057

(9) **Optometric Extension Program Foundation**
2912 S. Daimler St.
Santa Ana, CA 92705

(10) **Psychological and Educational Publications, Inc.**
1477 Rollins Road
Burlingame, CA 94010

(11) **Wayne Engineering**
1825 Willow Road
Northfield, IL 60093-2925

REFERENCES

1. Getman GN: The visuomotor complex in the acquisition of learning skills. In Helmuth J, editor: *Learning disorders,* vol 3, Seattle, Wash, 1965, Special Child Publications.
2. Getman GN, Kane ER, Halgren MR, McKee GW: *Developing learning readiness,* San Francisco, 1968, McGraw-Hill Book Co.
3. Kephart NC: *Slow learner in the classroom,* Columbus, Ohio, 1971, Charles E Merrill, p 87.
4. Cratty BJ: Sensory-motor and preceptual-motor theories and practice: an overview and evaluation. In Walk RD, Pick HL, editors: *Intersensory perception and sensory integration,* New York, 1981, Plenum Press.
5. Getman GN: *How to develop your child's intelligence,* White Plains, Md, 1984, Research Publications.
6. Hoffman LG: An optometric learning disability evaluation—Part 1, *Optom Monthly* 70:78-81, 1979.
7. Solan HA, Mozlin R: The correlations of perceptual-motor maturation to readiness and reading in kindergarten and the primary grades, *J Am Optom Assoc* 57:28-35, 1986.
8. Solan HA: A comparison of the influences of verbal-successive and spatial-simultaneous factors on achieving readers in fourth and fifth grade: a multivariate correlational study, *J Learning Disabil* 20:237-242, 1987.
9. Rogow SM, Rathwell D: Seeing and knowing: an investigation of visual perception among children with severe visual impairments, *J Vis Rehabil* 3:55-66, 1989.
10. Farr J, Leibowitz HW: An experimental study of the efficacy of perceptual-motor training, *Am J Optom Physiol Optics* 53:451-455, 1976.
11. Seiderman AS: Optometric vision therapy results of a demonstration project with a learning disabled population, *J Am Optom Assoc* 51:489-493, 1980.
12. Hendrickson LN, Muehl S: The effect of attention and motor response pretraining on learning to discriminate B and D in kindergarten children, *J Educ Psychol* 53:236-241, 1962.
13. Greenspan SB: Effectiveness of therapy for children's reversal confusion, *Acad Ther* 11:169-178, 1975-1976.
14. Walsh JF, D'Angelo R: Effectiveness of the Frostig program for visual perceptual training with Headstart children, *Percept Mot Skills* 32:944-946, 1971.
15. Brown RT, Alford N: Ameliorating, attentional deficits and concomitant academic deficiencies in learning disabled children through cognitive training, *J Learning Disabil* 17:20-26, 1984.
16. Rosner J: The development of a perceptual skills program, *J Am Optom Assoc* 44:698-707, 1973.
17. Getz DJ: Learning enhancement through visual training, *Acad Ther* 15:457-466, 1980.
18. Halliwell JW, Solan HA: The effects of a supplemental perceptual training program in reading achievement, *Except Child* 38:613-621, 1972.
19. Rowell RB: *The effect of tachistoscope and visual tracking program on the improvement of reading at the second grade level,* education doctoral thesis, Ann Arbor, Mich, 1976, University Microfilms.
20. Solan HA, Ciner EB: Visual perception and learning: issues and answers, *J Am Optom Assoc* 60:457-460, 1989.

21. Weisz CL: Clinical therapy for accommodative responses: transfer effects upon performance, *J Am Optom Assoc* 50:209-215, 1980.
22. Hoffman LG: The effect of accommodative deficiencies on the deve developmental level of perceptual skills, *Am J Optom Physiol Optics* 59:254-262, 1982.
23. Griffin JR: Learning theories applied to binocular vision therapy, *Optom Weekly* Oct 21:30-33, 1976.
24. Kirshner AJ: *Training that makes sense*, Novato, Calif, 1972, Academic Therapy Publications.
25. Vincett WK: *Optometric perceptual testing and training manual*, Akron, Ohio, 1975, Percon, Inc.
26. Rosner J: *Helping children overcome learning difficulties*, ed 2, New York, 1979, Walker Publishing Co.
27. Hoffman LG: *Vision therapy manual*, Fullerton, Calif, 1984, Southern California College of Optometry.
28. Lane KA: *Reversal errors theories and therapy procedures*, Santa Ana, Calif, 1988, Vision Extension.
29. Swartout JB: *Manual of techniques and record forms for in-office and out-of-office optometric vision training programs*, Santa Ana, Calif, 1991, Vision Extension, Inc.
30. Press LJ: *Computers and vision therapy programs*, Santa Ana, Calif, 1987, Optometric Extension Program, curriculum II, vol 60, no 1.
31. Maino JH, Maino DM, Davidson/DW: *Computer applications in optometry*, Boston, 1989, Butterworth.
32. McMonnies CW: *A practical guide to remedial approaches to left/right confusion and reversals*, Sydney, 1991, Australian College of Behavioral Optometrists.
33. Ames LB, Gillespie C, Haines J, Ilg FL: *The child from one to six*, London, 1980, Hamish Hamilton, p 42.
34. Solan HA, Mozlin R, Rumpf DA: Selected perceptual norms and their relationship to reading in kindergarten and the primary grades, *J Am Optom Assoc* 57:28-35, 1986.
35. Christenson G, Kurihara J, Davidek R: *Perceptual therapy manual*, Fullerton, Calif, 1988, Southern California College of Optometry.
36. Piaget J: *Judgement and reasoning in the child*, London, 1928, Routledge & Kegan, p 98-100.
37. Laurendeau M, Pinard A: *The development of the concept of space in the child*, New York, 1970, International Universities Press.
37. Sedan J: *Re-educative treatment of suppression amblyopia*, English translation by TK Lyle, C Douthwaite, and J Wilkinson, Edinburgh, 1960, E & S Livingston.
38. Leal L, Rafoth MA: Memory strategy development: what teachers do makes a difference, *Intervention School Clin* 26:234-237, 1991.
39. Solan HA: Perceptual norms in grades 4 and 5: a preliminary report, *J Am Optom Assoc* 58:979-982, 1987.
40. Forrest EB: *Visual imagery an optometric approach*, Santa Ana, Calif, 1981, Optometric Extension Program.
41. Solan HA, Groffman S: Understanding and treating developmental and perceptual motor disabilities. In Solan HA, editor: *Treatment and management of children with learning disabilities*, Springfield, Ill, 1982, Charles C Thomas.
42. Harmon DB: *The coordinated classroom*, Grand Rapids, Mich, 1951, American Seating Co.
43. Harmon DB: *Notes on a dynamic theory of vision*, ed 3 rev, Austin, Texas, 1958, self-published.
44. Frostig M: Visual perception, integrative functions and academic learning, *J Learning Disabil* 2:30-33, 1969.
45. Coddling KG, Gardner MF: *Visual-motor development remedial activities*, Burlingame, Calif, 1993, Psychological and Educational Publications, Inc.
46. Broderick P, Laszlo JI: The effects of varying planning demands on drawing components of squares and diamonds, *J Exp Child Psychol* 45:18-27, 1988.

CHAPTER 17

Vision Therapy Procedures for Developmental Visual Information Processing Disorders

MICHAEL W. ROUSE
ERIC BORSTING

The therapy program outlined in Chapter 16 was designed to remediate deficits within three general systems in the following order: (1) visual spatial, (2) visual analysis, and (3) visual motor. To successfully accomplish the therapy sequence of goals, subgoals, and skill development the doctor will need a sufficient variety of vision therapy techniques. The goal of this chapter is to fulfill this need. The selection is not meant to be exhaustive but rather to acquaint the reader with representative techniques that may be used in treating developmental visual information processing disorders. There are two reasons for including many of the techniques that follow. First, these techniques are ones that we and others have commonly used. Second, the specific instructions for these techniques that meet the objectives of the therapy model presented in Chapter 16 have not been readily available from other sources.

The techniques are organized in alphabetical order using the name of technique. Many of the techniques can be used to treat problems within different diagnostic areas, such as visual discrimination and visual closure. Each of these different applications is referred to as a vision therapy "procedure." For example, *parquetry blocks can be used in several procedures to address problems in visual discrimination, visual closure, visual memory, and visualization.* The diagnostic area and therapy subgoal within that area are listed for each procedure, for example, *parquetry blocks, procedure 1 (visual discrimination: subgoal 1).* In this way the doctor can cross-reference the technique and procedure with the therapy model presented in Chapter 16. For each procedure there is a statement of what the procedure is designed to accomplish and what equipment and materials are needed, followed by practical step-by-step instructions (including sample doctor-patient interactions) for conducting the procedure. The instructions are written for the doctor and are not intended to serve as home vision therapy handouts for patients or parents. Finally, a statement regarding the therapy or performance goals (what the patient should be able to achieve as a result of doing the therapy) is included. In many cases therapy goals are written for particular steps within the procedure or in other cases for the entire procedure.

As the clinician becomes familiar with this area of treatment, he or she will find there are many techniques and procedures, besides those described in this chapter, that can be used to address the same dysfunction. As pointed out in Chapter 16 there are several excellent compilations of techniques and computer programs available for remediating developmental visual information processing disorders. However, the most important component of therapy, which we have emphasized throughout the following techniques, is effectively teaching the patient the strategies or processes to achieve a particular subgoal.

SELECTED THERAPY TECHNIQUES
Ball bounce

Procedure 1 (bilateral integration: subgoal 1). This procedure is designed to develop a motor memory of the difference in performance between the right and left sides of the body. A rubber (air-filled) ball is required for this procedure. The first step is to have the patient bounce the ball 5 to 10 times about waist high with his or her preferred hand. The doctor should have the patient evaluate his own performance when the doctor asks a series of questions: "Did you bounce the ball 10 times?" "Did you bounce the ball at waist height?" "What can you do to change the height of the ball?" The second step is to have the patient bounce the ball with the nonpreferred hand while being asked the same questions as above. The third step is for the patient to alternate bouncing the ball with his or her dominant and nondominant hand. The patient should evaluate the performance of each side and tell the doctor which side performed better. Additionally the patient should generate a strategy for improving the performance of the weaker side. For example, "I have to bounce the ball harder with this hand." The therapy goal is for the patient to identify the difference in performance between the two sides of the body and be able to adjust performance of the weaker side.

Procedure 2 (bilateral integration: subgoal 2). This procedure is designed to develop the patient's motor planning ability by performing sequential movements of the two sides of the body. The patient *alternately* bounces the ball between the left and right hands. It is *not* important in this stage of therapy to have the patient label the right and left sides of the body. For example, bounce the ball 3 times with the preferred hand and 3 times with the nonpreferred hand. Therapy concentrates on the ability of the patient to bounce the ball smoothly while switching between the right and left hands. This indicates that the patient is able to coordinate sequential movements between the two sides of the body. It may take several repetitions before the patient is able to transfer the ball between the right and left sides. The therapy goal is for the patient to be able to bounce the ball smoothly and consistently while switching between the right and left sides of the body. However, if the patient has difficulty attaining smooth performance in 2 or 3 office visits, therapy can proceed to the next therapy goal or subgoal as long as the patient can alternate the bouncing of the ball between hands.

For patients demonstrating good motor control on procedures 1 and 2 the difficulty can be increased by having the patient bounce the ball into a series of target circles or squares that become progressively smaller. The patient should be able to bounce the ball at waist height into each circle or square for 8 out of 10 bounces.

Procedure 3 (laterality: enhancing automaticity). This technique can be used at the end of laterality therapy to achieve automaticity. The procedure is similar to the previous tasks, but the patient is instructed to bounce the ball in a specific right-and-left sequence, for example, 2 times with the right hand and 1 time with the left hand. Initially, the doctor should make the bounce sequence short, especially for patients with poor auditory memory. Before proceeding to longer sequences the patient should accurately achieve short sequences. The therapy goal is for the patient to maintain a smooth rhythm in the specified sequence with proper verbal identification of hands while bouncing the ball at waist height and in the target circle.

Bean bag toss

Procedure 1 (bilateral integration: subgoal 1). This procedure is designed to develop a motor memory of the difference in performance between the right and left sides of the body. Six to eight bean bags and a target are required for this procedure (see Figure 16.20, as an example). The patient should stand 6 to 8 feet from the target. The patient should put the bean bag in his or her dominant hand, fixate on the target, and then toss the bean bag toward the target with a slow gentle underhand motion. The patient then places the bean bag in the nondominant hand and tosses the bean bag toward the target. This is done several times for the dominant and nondominant hand. The patient should then evaluate the performance of each side and tell the doctor which side performed better. Additionally, the patient should generate a strategy for improving performance of the weaker side. For example, "I have to toss the bean bag higher when tossing with my left hand." The therapy goal is for the patient to identify the difference in performance between the two sides of the body and to be able to adjust performance of the poorer performing side.

Procedure 2 (general eye-hand coordination: subgoal 1). This procedure is designed to make the patient aware of the importance of vision in guiding the motor system. Initially the doctor wants the patient to understand the importance of vision in guiding the "tossing process." This can be illustrated to the patient by having the patient toss a bean bag with his or her eyes closed or covered and then with eyes open. The therapy goal is for the patient to be aware that the process is much harder or impossible when his or her eyes are closed. At this point the doctor needs to stress the importance of saying, "Keep your eye on the target."

Procedure 3 (general eye-hand coordination: subgoal 2). Once the importance of vision in guiding the motor act is appreciated the doctor can concentrate on improving the patient's gross eye-hand coordination. The critical issue is that the patient evaluate his or her performance and use that information to improve the accuracy of the next toss. The patient should be able to tell the doctor what corrections need to be made to hit the target accurately: "I need to toss the bean bag harder," or "I need to aim more to the right." The patient should repeat the process for 10 to 15 throws. The therapy goal for the patient is a relative improvement in the patient's tossing accuracy.

Card concentration

Procedure 1 (visual memory: subgoal 2). This procedure is designed to develop the patient's ability to recall the *spatial* characteristics of figures using only visual information. The first step is for the doctor to divide a deck of common playing cards into pairs. Initially the doctor will want to start with 2 to 4 pairs of cards. The cards are placed face down in rows of 3 to 5 cards each. The patient's task is to turn up one card and then another. If a match is made, the patient keeps the pair of cards (Figure 17.1). Otherwise the cards are turned face down, and the patient is encouraged to remember the position of the two cards. Initially the doctor can quiz the patient on the location of individual cards after each move. For example, "Where is the six of clubs?" This forces the patient to remember the spatial coordinates within the display. The patient repeats the process of turning up one card, remembering if that card has already been seen and trying to turn up a match to the turned-up card.

To increase the patient's interest and motivation the doctor can play against the patient in the game. In this approach the doctor can model an appropriate memory strategy. For example, "I try to make a picture in my head of where individual cards are located." After the patient initially turns up the first two cards and there is no match, the doctor (or another patient) then repeats the process attempting to make a match. If the doctor matches the two cards, he or she keeps the pair of cards. The "player" with the most pairs at the end wins the game.

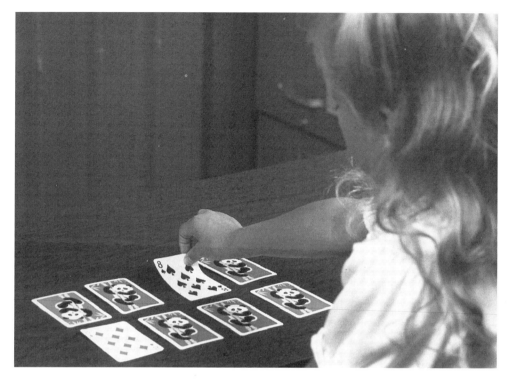

FIGURE 17.1 Card concentration. The patient's task in this procedure is to turn up one card and then another. If a match is made, the patient keeps the pair of cards. Otherwise the cards are turned face down and the patient is encouraged to remember the position of the two cards.

The second step involves increasing the difficulty of the visual memory task by increasing the number of paired cards in the display. The therapy goal is for the patient to recall accurately the location of the paired cards. The number of paired cards that the patient will be able to do will be age dependent (consult Table 16.1, p. 467). For example, a first grader should be able to remember the location of 3 paired cards, whereas a third grader would be expected to do 5 paired cards. These are only estimates, and the doctor will want to continue adding pairs until he or she appears to have reached the patient's threshold.

Chalkboard squares

Procedure 1 (bilateral integration: subgoal 1). This procedure is designed to develop a motor memory of the difference in performance between the right and left sides of the body. Chalkboard squares requires a chalkboard and two pieces of chalk (preferably large pieces). An X and two rectangles are drawn at eye level on the board as shown in Figure 16.2. The patient faces the chalkboard with a piece of chalk in each hand and his or her eyes directed toward the X between the two rectangles.

The first step is to have the patient make symmetrical movements where both hands move toward or away from the midline of the body at the same time. The chalk pieces in each hand are placed on the blackboard at the innermost line (closest to the X) of both rectangles. The patient is instructed to move both pieces of chalk away from the midline to the outer edge of each rectangle. The patient should be encouraged to fixate on the X. When the patient is aware that the outer edge of the box has been reached, he is allowed to stand back and check his work. The patient then repeats the process, this time going toward the midline. The doctor asks questions such as, "Which hand arrived at the end of the box first?" or "Which hand drew the lines smoother?" The doctor then asks the patient what he or she has to do to improve the performance of the nondominant or poorer performing hand. For example, the patient might respond, "I have to move this hand faster." This process is repeated until the patient makes relatively equal motor movements of the right and left sides of the body. However, the performance of the dominant side will probably be slightly better than that of the nondominant side. The second step is for the patient to practice making simultaneous movements. The therapy goal is for the patient to be able to perform the procedure in a relatively smooth, continuous, and rhythmic fashion, moving alternately away from and toward the midline while maintaining fixation on the X.

Procedure 2 (bilateral integration: subgoal 2). This procedure is designed to develop the patient's motor planning ability by performing simultaneous movements of the two sides of the body. The patient makes reciprocal movements in this part of therapy. Patients 5 years of age and younger have great difficulty making reciprocal movements. Therefore we do not emphasize this phase of therapy for young children. The patient begins with the chalk at the far left border of each rectangle and moves one hand toward the midline and the other hand away from the midline (that is, both hands to the right or to the left). The patient should maintain fixation on the X at all times. Many patients will have a phase difference between the right and left hands. The doctor needs to ask questions to make the patient aware of the different rates of movements between the two hands. It may take several repetitions before the patient is able to keep both hands in phase. The therapy goal is for the patient to make motor movements in a relatively smooth, continuous, and rhythmic fashion with the two hands remaining in phase while moving toward and away from the midline. Once this goal is attained the procedure may also be performed in the oblique (45- and 135-degree) and vertical directions to enhance automaticity.

Coding activities

Procedure 1 (visualization: subgoal 3). This procedure is designed to develop the patient's ability to use visualization strategies when working with letters and words. The coding procedure uses a matrix of rows and columns that are assigned letters and numbers (see Figure 16.19). Each letter in the matrix has a corresponding code. For example, the code *A1* stands for the letter **C**. The first step is for the patient to understand that each letter in the matrix has a code. The doctor writes or names the code for individual letters, and the patient names the corresponding letter. It is important for the patient *not* to write down any of the letters because doing so will discourage him or her from using visualization strategies. The second step is to have the patient identify simple words that correspond to a particular coding sequence. In the example (see Figure 16.19) the code *A1 B3 C2* would spell "cat." The doctor does *not* let the patient write down the letter that corresponds with the code, rather the patient should maintain the image that *A1* equals **C** and then *B3* equals **A** and *C2* equals **T**, resulting in a complete mental image of the word **CAT**. It is important when doing this procedure to make sure that the words you spell are within the sight-word vocabulary of the patient. We usually start with three-letter words and work up to four- and five-letter words depending on the patient's reading level. The therapy goal is for the patient to visualize words accurately within his or her decoding level.

Continuous motion

Procedure 1 (visually guided fine-motor control: subgoal 1). This procedure is designed to develop the patient's ability to plan a visually guided fine-motor movement. The patient will need a continuous motion work sheet (Figure 17.2) and a pencil. The first step is to teach the patient to plan or to "look" before he or she draws. The patient is instructed to take the pencil in his or her preferred hand. The patient starts by circling number *1*, while the doctor instructs the patient to find number *2*. The patient should keep the pencil moving around number *1* until number *2* is located. Once number *2* is located the patient should move the pencil in a single smooth motion to number *2*. While moving the pencil from one number to the next, the patient is to avoid touching or crossing the other numbers. When the patient completes a connection between numbers, he or she should be asked to evaluate his or her performance. The doctor should ask questions, such as, "Did you make a straight line between the two numbers?" "Did you cross or touch any of the other numbers?" and "Did the pencil stop at any time?" The patient continues the sequence through the number *30*. The doctor should reinforce the important concept of visual guidance by saying, "The eye tells your hand what to do." The doctor should monitor closely the patient's visual motor ergonomics, pencil grip, posture, and paper position during this procedure. The therapy goal is for the patient to be able to link the numbers from *1* to *30* accurately and to demonstrate a consistent planning strategy for his or her visually guided fine-motor movements.

Directional mazes

Procedure 1 (laterality: subgoal 3). This procedure is designed to develop the patient's ability to use his or her internal laterality reference sys-

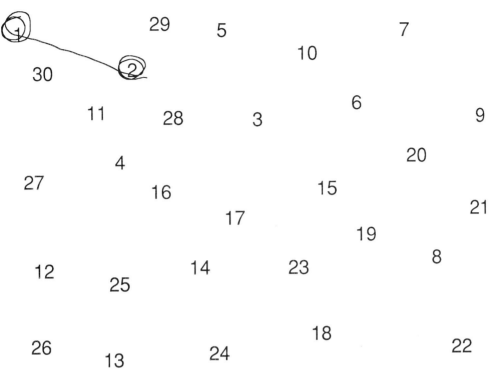

FIGURE 17.2 Continuous motion work sheet. The patient starts by circling number *1*, while the doctor instructs the patient to find number *2*. The patient should keep the pencil moving around number *1* until number *2* is located. Once number *2* is located the patient should move the pencil in a single smooth motion to number *2* and so forth by successive numbers.

tem for making right and left directional judgments. The Find the Slice of Cheese maze is an excellent example procedure (Figure 17.3), though hand-drawn maps can also be adapted for this procedure. The doctor needs a copy of the Find the Slice of Cheese maze. The mouse is located on the bottom right-hand corner of the map and is removed and utilized as the object that will move through the maze (a small object can be substituted for the mouse). The patient will rotate the maze so that he or she appears to be going down the maze with the mouse; that is, the patient and mouse are always facing in the same direction. Starting at the position numbered *1,* the patient directs the mouse through the maze using right and left directions. Before each turn, the patient is asked to name a "right" or "left" direction. At each turn the doctor should ask the patient, "How did you know which way to turn? The patient should respond with an appropriate strategy learned in the first two phases of laterality therapy. Once the patient develops a consistent strategy he or she calls out a direction without stopping to identify the strategy. The therapy goal is for the patient to be able to direct the mouse (and him- or herself) through the maze accurately (100%) and without hesitation at each turn.

DIRECTIONAL MAZE – *"FIND THE SLICE OF CHEESE"*

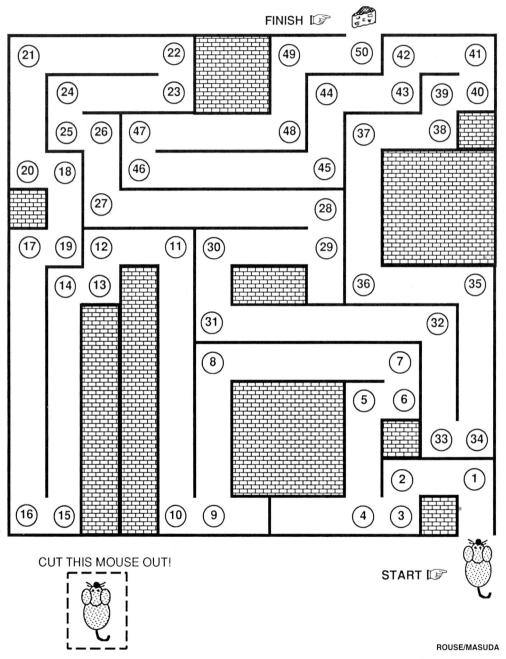

FIGURE 17.3 Directional maze—Find the Slice of Cheese work sheet. The mouse is located on the bottom left-hand corner of the map and is removed and used as the object that will move through the maze. Laterality and directionality procedures can be accomplished with this technique.

Procedure 2 (directionality: subgoal 2). This procedure is designed to have the patient be aware of what happens to right and left when an animate object turns in space. Before starting therapy the doctor needs to help the patient understand how to alter his or her perspective of right and left by using concrete examples (see Chapter 16, directionality: subgoal 2). The mouse, located on the bottom right-hand corner of the map, is removed and utilized as the object (a small object can be substituted for the mouse). Starting at the position numbered *1*, the patient directs the mouse through the maze using right and left directions. Before each turn, the patient is asked to name a "right" or "left" direction and then moves the mouse in the corresponding direction. The doctor then asks the patient to explain why he or she turned the mouse to the right or left. The patient should be able to check his or her response by generating an appropriate strategy. However, many patients have difficulty explaining their strategy without using motor support. For example, the patient may turn himself or herself in the same direction as the mouse and say, "This is my right side, so I turn right." Once the patient is able to generate an appropriate strategy consistently he or she should direct the mouse through the maze without stopping at each turn to explain his or her response. The therapy goal is for the patient to be able to direct the mouse through the maze accurately and without hesitation at each turn.

Procedure 3 (visualization: subgoal 2). This procedure is designed to develop the patient's ability to manipulate mentally the spatial orientation of forms. In this part of therapy the patient directs an imaginary or invisible mouse through the maze. Starting at the beginning of the maze, the patient calls out right and left directions before each turn. In the beginning it is important to have the patient identify where he is in the maze and the orientation of the mouse before each turn. The numbers (1 to 50) can be used to determine which turn the invisible mouse is about to make (see Figure 17.3). The patient can also place the paper mouse in the correct orientation to check the accuracy of his response. Making decisions about right and left turns should not be difficult at this point in therapy, but patients may have difficulty keeping track of the orientation of the mouse. It may take several repetitions before the patient is able to guide the imaginary mouse through the entire maze. The therapy goal is for the patient to be able to guide the imaginary mouse through the entire maze without an error.

Directional triangles

Procedure 1 (directionality: subgoal 1). This procedure is designed to have the patient develop an awareness that previously taught laterality skills can be used to make right and left judgments of objects in space. The doctor needs a directional triangles work sheet (Figure 17.4). The doctor instructs the patient to touch the triangle on the first row (left-hand side) with one hand and touch the matching triangle on the bottom of the

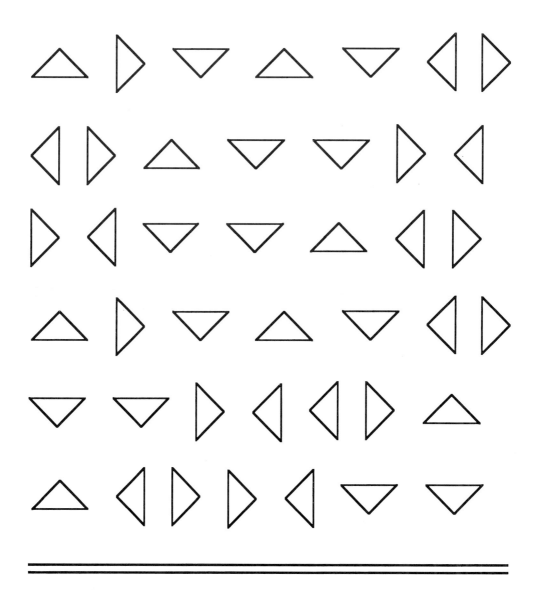

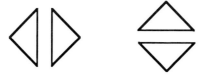

ROUSE/BORSTING

FIGURE 17.4 Directional triangles work sheet. The doctor instructs the patient to touch the triangle on the first row (left-hand side) with one hand and touch the matching triangle on the bottom of the sheet with the other hand. As the child touches the triangles simultaneously with each hand, he or she will call out the direction of the triangle.

sheet with the other hand. As the child touches the triangles simultaneously with each hand, he or she will call out the direction of the triangle. Initially, the patient should describe how he arrived at that orientation. For example, the patient might say, "This is my right hand, and this is to the right." This process is repeated until the patient is able to generate a consistent strategy for determining the appropriate direction. The patient then names the orientation of the triangles in the entire row without describing his strategy. The doctor should always have the patient work from left to right and top to bottom when calling out the directions of the triangles. The therapy goal is for the patient to be able to call out accurately (100%) the correct orientation in a relatively smooth and rhythmic fashion.

To increase the difficulty and promote automaticity the patient can repeat the procedure to the beat of a metronome. The patient should be able to maintain the same level of accuracy with the metronome. Another method for achieving automaticity is to have the patient call out the direction that is opposite to the one that the triangle is pointing (for example, for a triangle pointing to the right the patient would say, "Left.") The patient still touches the matching direction on the triangles below to the one touched on the top. This procedure is very difficult and will probably not be performed smoothly by the young patient (less than 7 years of age) even with practice. The patient should be able to call out the opposite directions accurately, but performance will not be as smooth as when the initial procedure is being done.

Dot-to-dot figures

Procedure 1 (visual closure: subgoal 2). This procedure is designed to develop the patient's ability to make closure judgments with increasing speed and accuracy. The patient will need 5 to 10 dot-to-dot figures (see Figure 17.5) and a pencil. The doctor should stress to the patient that after each dot is connected the child should stop and determine if he or she can guess what the figure is. Fine-motor accuracy is not critical in this closure procedure. The patient should continue connecting dots until he or she can recognize the figure. The doctor should ask questions, such as, "What do you see that makes you think you see the letter M?" The doctor can increase the patient's motivation and interest by giving the child a point if he or she correctly guesses the name of the figure. If the patient is incorrect, the doctor gets a point. The doctor should continue to present the remaining figures in increasing difficulty. The therapy goal is for the patient to show a relative improvement in his or her ability to bring closure to each picture over the series of dot-to-dot figures. A potential measure of that improvement would be that the patient needs to connect fewer and fewer dots to recognize the final figure.

Procedure 2 (visually guided fine-motor control: subgoal 1). This procedure is designed to develop the patient's ability to plan a visually guided

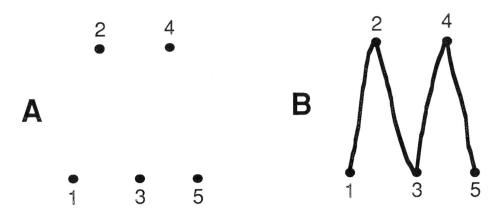

FIGURE 17.5 A simple dot-to-dot figure. The doctor should emphasize to the patient that after each dot is connected the child should stop and determine if he or she can guess what the figure is. The patient should continue connecting dots until he or she can recognize the figure. **A,** Initial view. **B,** Completed figure.

fine-motor movement. The patient will need a 5 to 10 dot-to-dot figure where the dots are numbered. The first step is to teach the patient to plan or to "look" before he or she draws. The doctor should stress that now, in contrast to the use of dot-to-dot Figures for visual closure, the patient should concentrate on accuracy. The patient should place his or her pencil at the dot numbered *1* and then locate the dot numbered *2.* Once dot numbered *2* is located the patient should move the pencil in a single smooth motion to dot numbered *2.* The doctor should reinforce the important concept of visual guidance by saying, "Your eye tells your hand what to do," which is critical at this stage. After a few attempts the patient should tell the doctor what strategy he is using before starting the technique. The doctor should monitor closely the patient's visual-motor ergonomics, pencil grip, posture, and paper position during this procedure. When the patient completes the line, he or she should be asked to evaluate his or her performance. The patient should be able to tell the doctor if his or her line hit the dot or, if not, how the line deviated from the intended performance. Again it is important that the patient verbalize the appropriate strategy to improve the performance. For example, if the line that the patient drew was too long, he or she should tell the doctor that the line needs to be shortened on the next attempt. The therapy goal is for the patient to be able to use a consistent strategy for planning his or her visually guided fine-motor movements.

Fine-motor activities

These procedures are designed to develop the patient's general eye-hand coordination by having the patient do a variety of fine-motor tasks requiring visual guidance. The doctor needs to emphasize the importance of vision in guiding the fine-motor movement in each of the procedures.

Procedure 1: bead stringing (general eye-hand coordination: subgoal 2). The doctor will need a string and a variety (of sizes and shapes) of beads (such as those from DLM Instructional, Allen, Texas). The patient should hold the bead with the nondominant hand. Then the patient should hold the string in the dominant hand with 1 to 2 inches of it showing. In one smooth movement the patient should guide the end of the string into the bead (refer to Figure 16.14). The patient should stop and evaluate his or her performance and develop a strategy for improving the accuracy on the next attempt. The patient should continue until 15 to 20 beads have been strung. The goal of therapy is to place the beads on the string consistently (80%) and accurately and be aware that vision is guiding the fine-motor movement.

Procedure 2: dive-bombing (general eye-hand coordination: subgoal 2). The doctor will need one of the dive-bombing sheets (Figure 17.6) or a home-made sheet and a pencil. The patient picks one of the targets that he would like to "bomb." The patient positions his or her pencil approximately 20 cm above the target and then in one smooth and quick movement strikes the target. The patient should stop and evaluate his or her performance and develop a strategy for improving the accuracy on the next attempt. The patient should continue with 5 to 10 strikes at a single target and then repeat the process on a new target. The goal of therapy is to place the pencil strike consistently (80%) and accurately within the limits of the target and be aware that vision is guiding the fine-motor movement.

Procedure 3: Lite Brite (general eye-hand coordination: subgoal 2). The doctor will need a Lite Brite (Milton Bradley Co., Springfield, Mass.), which consists of a pegboard surface that is backilluminated. The doctor can use the pegboard surface or a variety of targets that can be placed on the Lite Brite (designs, capitals and lower-cased letters and numerals from 1 to 10) (Figure 17.7). When the patient pushes a clear-colored peg through the target design, the peg shines. The patient is asked to locate a target hole or point on the design and then in one smooth and quick movement attempt to accurately place the peg in the hole. The patient should stop and evaluate his or her performance and develop a strategy for improving the accuracy on the next attempt. The patient should continue placing the pegs and repeating the process of evaluating and improving his or her performance. The goal of therapy is to place the pegs in the target holes consistently (80%) and accurately and be aware that vision is guiding the fine-motor movement.

Procedure 4: straw piercing (general eye-hand coordination: subgoal 2). The doctor will need a drinking straw and a pointer (knitting needle or pick-up stick). The doctor will position the drinking straw at a near distance (20 to 40 cm) with the top of the straw tipped slightly toward the patient (allowing the patient to see the top of the straw). Then the doctor will have the patient attempt to insert the pointer into the straw in one

DIVE BOMBING

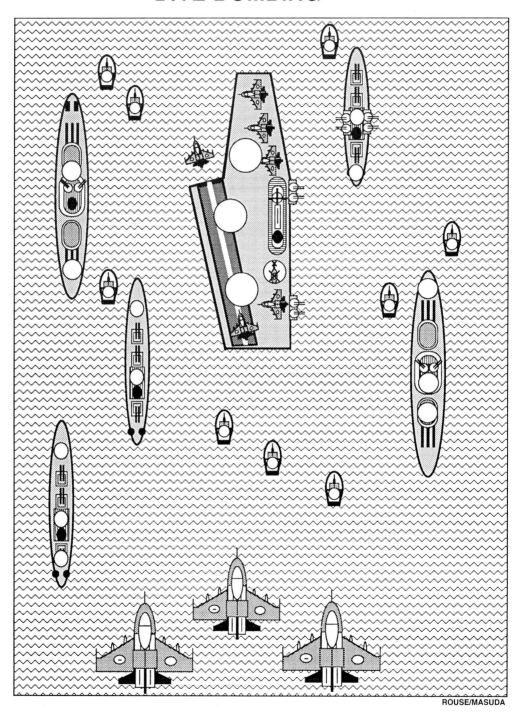

FIGURE 17.6 Dive-bombing work sheet. The patient positions a pencil approximately 20 cm above the target and then in one smooth and quick movement strikes the target.

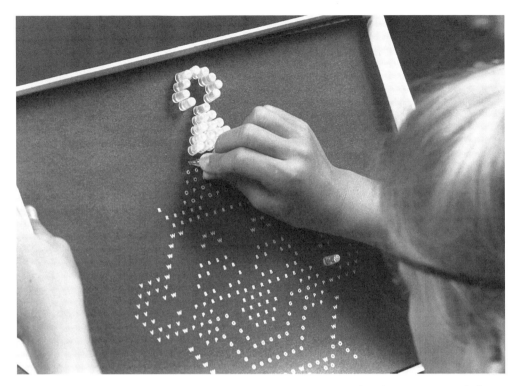

FIGURE 17.7 Use of the Lite Brite. The patient is asked to locate a target hole, or point, on the design and then in one smooth and quick movement attempt to place accurately the peg in the hole.

smooth movement (Figure 17.8). The patient should evaluate his or her performance. Then the patient should make a verbal strategy about how he or she is going to improve the accuracy on the next attempt. The doctor should change the position of the straw (moving slightly left or right or closer or farther) and the patient should make another attempt. The process should be repeated 15 to 20 times. The doctor can keep score of the number of "hits" to monitor the patient's progress. The therapy goal is for the patient to put the pointer in the straw consistently (80%) and accurately and be aware that vision is guiding the fine-motor movement.

Flip forms

Procedure 1 (visualization: subgoal 2). This procedure is designed to develop the patient's ability to manipulate mentally the spatial orientation of forms and symbols mentally. A figure (see Figure 16.17, *A*) is placed in the upper left-hand corner of a cross drawn by the doctor. The patient is then instructed to flip the form around the *y*-axis and draw the resultant figure. The next step is to flip the figure around the *x*-axis and then flip it around the *y*-axis again. Typically the patient will need a concrete demonstration of how a figure changes its orientation. For example, a pipe cleaner can be formed into a **b,** and the patient can flip this around the

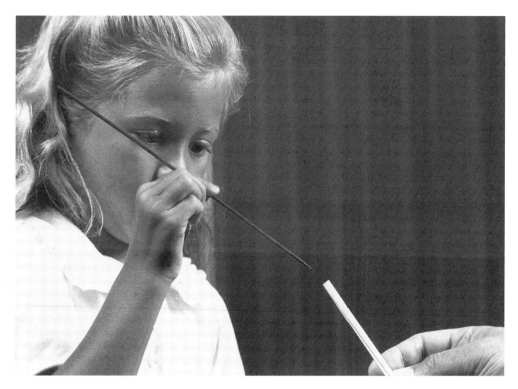

FIGURE 17.8 Straw piercing. The doctor has the patient attempt to insert the pointer into the straw in one smooth movement.

y-axis and observe the result. The procedure is done with reversible letters first and then with abstract symbols. The symbols are limited to one item during this phase of therapy. The patient should be able to tell the doctor his or her strategy for flipping the figures. However, we have found that children have difficulty expressing this strategy and will often use an explanation that demonstrates the change in rotation with a hand gesture. When manipulating the letters, the patient should be able to explain how rotating the letters will change the letter from **b** to a **d.** This process reinforces the patient's understanding of the directional features of letters. The therapy goal is for the patient to be able to rotate reversible letters and abstract figures accurately (90%) around the *x* and *y* axes.

Once the patient is be able to manipulate or change the orientation of both letters and simple symbols accurately the difficulty of the procedure is increased. For example, the patient is asked to skip a step or visualize the initial letter and then flip this mental image and draw the next step. This process might progress until the patient can mentally visualize all steps leading up to the final orientation of the figure. The difficulty can also be increased by use of more complicated figures (see Figure 16.17, *B*).

Floor map I, II, III

Procedure 1: floor map I (laterality: subgoal 3). This procedure is designed to develop the patient's ability to use his or her internal reference system for making right and left judgments. The floor map consists of a maze placed on the floor (see Figure 16.4). The patient stands on the X, facing the floor map. At the first corner of the map the patient is asked to extend his arm in the direction he is going to turn and then name the direction (right or left turn). The patient then explains the strategy used to determine the answer (for example, "I write with my right hand and must turn in the direction of my other hand, which is to the left."). The patient then makes a quarter turn to the right or to the left and proceeds to the next corner. At each corner the patient explains his or her strategy. This is repeated until the patient develops a consistent strategy for making right and left decisions. The next step is for the patient to guide himself through the map without stopping at each turn to explain his strategy. The therapy goal is for the patient to guide himself accurately (100%) through the map without hesitation at each turn.

Procedure 2 floor map II (directionality: subgoal 2). This procedure is designed to develop the patient's ability to identify right and left directions on another person. Before starting therapy the doctor needs to help the patient understand how to alter his perspective of right and left by using concrete examples (see Chapter 16, directionality, subgoal 2). The patient stands on the X off to the side of the floor map, and the doctor is positioned at the beginning of the map (see Figure 16.6). The patient then directs the doctor through the map using right and left directions. Initially, it may be necessary to allow the patient to turn his body in the same direction as the doctor or even to move and stand behind the doctor to appreciate the proper directional command. After each response the patient explains the strategy used to determine the answer. However, it is often difficult for the patient to describe his or her strategy, and the patient will frequently need motor support to help with the oral description. For example, he will turn in the same direction as the doctor. This is repeated until the patient demonstrates a consistent strategy. The next step is to direct the doctor through the maze without explaining a strategy at each turn. The therapy goal is for the patient to direct the doctor accurately (100%) through the map without the patient having to move his or her body.

Procedure 3 floor map III (visualization: subgoal 2). This procedure is designed to develop the patient's ability to manipulate mentally the orientation of another object. The patient stands off to the side of the map and directs an *invisible man* through the floor map. Starting at the beginning of the maze the patient calls out right and left directions before each turn. In the beginning it is important to have the patient identify where he or she is in the maze and the orientation of the invisible man before each turn. The patient can place the doctor in the correct orientation on the map to check the accuracy of his or her response. Making decisions about right and left turns should not be difficult at this point in therapy, but patients may have difficulty keeping track of the orientation of the invisible man. It may take several repetitions before the patient is able to guide the invisible man through the entire maze. The therapy goal is for the patient to guide the invisible man accurately (90%) through the maze.

"Focus-in" forms

Procedure 1 (visual closure: subgoal 1). This procedure is designed to develop the patient's ability to differentiate between guessing, incomplete closure, and complete closure. The doctor will need an overhead or slide projector, 10 to 20 transparencies, or slides, of various forms, letters, or numbers. The patient is to sit in front of the projector (where he cannot see the target slide, or transparency) and observe the projection screen at about 1 to 3 meters. The doctor projects a indistinguishable blurred image of the target. The doctor then asks the patient to identify what figure is on the wall (Figure 17.9, *A*). Typically, the patient will say, "I don't know; the picture is too blurry." The doctor should then encourage the patient to guess. After the patient's response the doctor should reinforce the concept that the patient was only guessing and there was not enough information present to identify the numbers. The doctor slowly reduces the blur until the patient can make a guess based on some visual feature or features of the stimulus (Figure 17.9, *B*). Again the doctor should ask the patient what information was used to make his judgment. For example, the patient may report seeing parts of two circles, with one above the other, and based on this less-than-complete information may report that the figure is the number 8. The doctor should make sure the patient verbalizes how he or she arrived at the decision. Finally, the doctor removes most of the blur, and the patient tells the doctor if his or her initial response was correct (Figure 17.9, *C*). The therapy goal is for the patient to be able to orally express what type of visual information was used to arrive at his or her decision.

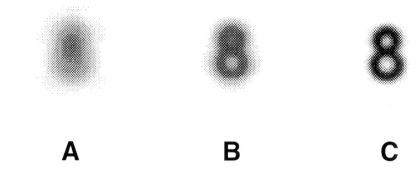

A   **B**   **C**

FIGURE 17.9 Focus-in-forms procedure. **A,** The doctor projects an indistinguishable blurred image of the target. The doctor then asks the patient to identify the figure. Typically, the patient will say, "I don't know; the picture is too blurry." The doctor should then encourage the patient to guess. **B,** The doctor slowly reduces the blur until the patient can make a guess based on some visual feature of the stimulus. **C,** Finally, the doctor removes most of the blur, and the patient tells the doctor if his or her initial response was correct.

Geoboard

Procedure 1 (visual discrimination: subgoal 2). This procedure is designed to develop the patient's ability to use only visual clues to find similarities or differences of increasingly complex forms. The equipment necessary for this procedure are a Geoboard (5, 9, or 25 pegs), rubber bands, and a Geoboard book from Bernell (Figure 17.10). The first step is directed toward reproducing a series of specific designs using the 5-pin Geoboards. The doctor builds a design with 2 or 3 rubber bands in front of the patient. The patient then places matching rubber bands directly on top of the ones built by the doctor. This procedure starts with 2 or 3 rubber-band designs on the 5-peg board and eventually builds up to 5 or 6 rubber-band designs on the 25-peg board. The therapy goal is for the patient to overlay the doctor's designs accurately (100%).

The second step requires the patient to a replicate the doctor's design on the patient's Geoboard. Start with two 5-peg Geoboards placed adjacent to each other. To ensure that the patient understands the spatial layout of the geoboard the doctor touches a peg on his board and the patient touches the corresponding peg on his or her board. For the first few designs it is helpful for the patient to identify the starting and end points of each rubber band before placing the rubber band on the Geoboard. This will help the patient to develop a strategy for identifying discrepancies between his

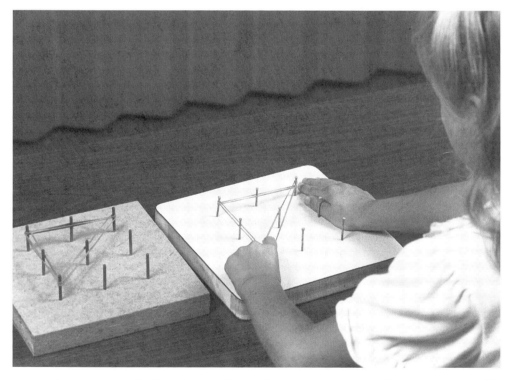

FIGURE 17.10 Geoboard procedure. The patient replicates the pattern created by the doctor (Geoboard on left) on her own Geoboard.

design and the one built by the doctor. After building the design the doctor should ask the patient to identify the similarities and differences between the doctor's design and the one the patient built. Any discrepancies between the designs should be corrected at this time. The therapy goal is for the patient to replicate the doctor's design accurately (100%).

The third step of therapy uses Geoboard workbooks. Starting with the 5-peg Geoboard the patient builds designs from the book. Before starting to build the designs the doctor should have the patient identify the position of matching pegs on the book and the board. On the first few designs the patient should touch the starting and end points for each component of the design. On subsequent designs the patient builds the entire design and then evaluates his or her performance. Any discrepancies between the doctor's and patient's designs are corrected. The therapy goal is for the patient to build the patterns from the Geoboard books accurately (100%).

Procedure 2 (visual memory: subgoal 2). This procedure is designed to develop the patient's ability to recall the *spatial* characteristics of figures using only visual information. The first step requires the doctor to build a 2 to 3 rubber-band design on a 9-peg geoboard. The patient then looks at the design for 5 to 10 seconds, and the design is hidden. The doctor then asks the patient to describe the spatial characteristics of the design. For example, "How many rubber bands does the pattern have?" or "Show me where the rubber bands started and where they ended." Frequently, the patient will need to view the target several times before he can describe all the spatial characteristics. It may take several repetitions with different designs before the patient is able to identify the spatial characteristics of the designs consistently.

The second step in therapy is for the patient to build a series of designs from memory without answering questions about the characteristics of the design. This should start with approximately 2 or 3 rubber bands on a 9-peg Geoboard and increase to 4 to 6 rubber-band designs on a 25-peg Geoboard. The doctor should have the patient compare his or her design to the doctor's design and describe any subtle spatial differences. Any corrections in the original design are then made by the patient. Once the patient is able to build 4 to 6 rubber-band designs accurately on the 25-pin Geoboard the doctor can reduce the viewing time. The therapy goal is for the patient to reproduce accurately 5 to 10 25-peg designs composed of 4 to 6 rubber bands based on a 2- to 3-second viewing time.

Procedure 4 (visualization: subgoal 2). This procedure is designed to develop the patient's ability to manipulate mentally the orientation of objects or figures. The first step in therapy is for the doctor to place a single rubber band on a 9-pin Geoboard. The doctor then instructs the patient to build the design as if the Geoboard were rotated a fourth of a turn to the left or right. The patient then builds the design on his or her Geoboard. It may be necessary for the doctor to demonstrate the concept by actually rotating the doctor's Geoboard a fourth of a turn to the left. This procedure is repeated until the patient can accurately (100%) rotate 3 to 5 single rubber-band designs.

The second step is to increase the number of rubber bands in the design from 2 to 3 and repeat the same instructions. The third step is to have the patient build designs using the 25-peg Geoboard working up to 6 rubber-band designs. The fourth step is to have the patient build the design as if he were sitting on the opposite side of the table. This may require a concrete demonstration, where the patient would move to the doctor's side of the table to view the design. When one is performing visualization therapy, it is important to account for the cognitive development of the child. For children under 7 this task is often to difficult, with only a small percentage of children being able to do step 1. Children 7 to 11 or 12 can usually do steps 2 and 3, but step 4 is more appropriate for children older than 12 years of age.

Golf game

Procedure 1 (visualization: subgoal 1). This procedure is designed to develop the patient's awareness of the mental image created by a form that is no longer present. The doctor will need a pencil and paper "golf course" (Figure 17.11). Have the patient sit at a table with golf course number 1 in front of him or her. The objective of the game is draw a line from the "tee," or beginning point, to the "hole," or ending point, in as few lines, or "strokes," as possible. Have the patient look at the layout of the golf course (such as length of fairway and hazards) for the first hole for 5 to 10 seconds. Have the patient close his or her eyes and attempt to "hold" a mental image of the hole layout for about 5 seconds. With his or her eyes closed, beginning with the pencil on the paper at the tee, he or she makes a "stroke." The patient should move the pencil only as far as possible without hitting any hazards. The patient opens his or her eyes to determine where he or she has landed. Then from that position the patient repeats the process until the patient ends up with the pencil inside the hole at the flag stick. The doctor keeps score of the number of strokes necessary to reach the hole. Strokes are added for hitting hazards such as lakes, trees, and out of bounds. The patient continues the process with golf courses 2 and 3. The therapy goal is for the patient progressive to require less and less strokes or strike less hazards to reach each hole.

Haptic writing

Procedure 1 (visually guided fine-motor control: subgoal 2). This procedure is designed to develop the patient's ability to perform accurate visually guided fine-motor movements. Haptic writing requires a pencil and a work sheet (see Figure 16.26). The first step is for the patient to trace directly over the pattern starting at the left-hand corner. The doctor should encourage the patient to plan ahead, using his or her eyes to lead the fine-motor system. After tracing the first few loops the patient should evaluate

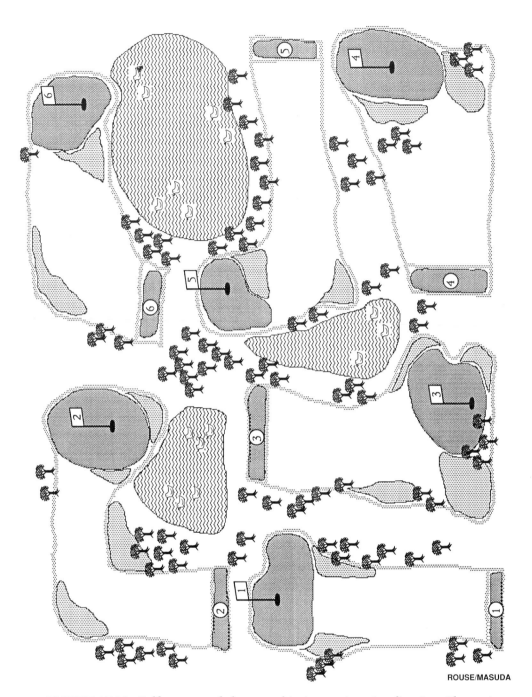

ROUSE/MASUDA

FIGURE 17.11 Golf game worksheet used in improving visualization. The patient looks at the layout of the golf course (such as length of fairway and hazards) for the first hole for 5 to 10 seconds. The patient closes his or her eyes and attempts to "hold" a mental image of the hole layout for about 5 seconds. With eyes closed, beginning with the pencil on the paper at the tee, he or she makes a "stroke." The patient should move the pencil as far as possible without hitting any hazards. The patient opens his or her eyes to determine where he or she has landed. Then from that position the patient repeats the process until ending up with the pencil inside the hole at the flag stick.

the accuracy of his or her performance. At this point in therapy the patient should be able to trace the form accurately. When the pattern ends, the patient continues to produce the pattern. The patient should then compare the pattern he or she drew with the original. It is usually necessary to repeat this procedure several times until performance is accurate. The next step is for the patient to trace and copy the figure in one continuous motion. The therapy goal is for the patient to be able to reproduce the patterns accurately with a relatively smooth rhythmic movement of the pencil.

Procedure 2 (visually guided fine-motor control: subgoal 3). This procedure is designed to develop the speed of the visually guided fine-motor movements while maintaining the accuracy. The patient draws a pattern on a work sheet that has no printed pattern to trace initially. For example, the doctor might have the patient draw a pattern with two loops on the top row and one on the bottom row. This pattern should repeat itself until the line is finished. After the first few patterns the patient should stop and evaluate his or her performance. The patient then needs to generate a strategy to correct any errors. The therapy goal is for the patient to be able to draw several types of patterns accurately while relatively increasing his or her speed.

Hart Chart coordinates

Procedure 1 (visual figure ground: subgoal 2). This procedure is designed to develop the patient's ability to conduct an organized or structured search pattern to find a particular figure. A Hart Chart, a pencil, and paper are required for this procedure. The columns and rows of the Hart Chart are labeled, such as *1* to *10* across the top for the columns and *A* to *J* from the top to the bottom for the rows. The patient is seated at a table facing a wall with the Hart Chart at a distance of about 10 to 15 feet. The doctor instructs the patient about using the coordinates to identify a letter. For example, the code *A2* might correspond to the letter **C**. The doctor then gives the patient a series of individual codes and observes his visual search strategy. Frequently, the patient will use a haphazard approach. The doctor then models an organized scanning approach starting with the columns and then the rows. For example, "I count the number of columns (such as 3), and then I count down the number of rows (such as row *D*)." The patient then repeats the procedure with a new code. It may take several repetitions before the patient uses an organized and structured search pattern. The therapy goal is for the patient to find accurately (100%) 10 to 15 individual letters using the columns and rows as a guide.

Procedure 2 (visual figure ground: subgoal 2). This procedure is designed to develop the speed of the patient's response without sacrificing the accuracy of the performance as distractors are added to the background. Instead of an individual code, the patient is given a series of codes that form a word or a message. For example, the code *A2 B10 E7* might spell a word. The codes can be written down on a piece of paper, and the patient can write the answer next to the code. This minimizes the demands on visual memory, which has not been addressed in the therapy program up to this point. It may take several repetitions before the patient can identify the code accurately. The doctor should then encourage the patient to crack the code as quickly as possible without sacrificing accuracy. The doctor can time the patient's response as a measure of his or her progress. The coded word messages should increase in length as the patient's performance improves. To promote automaticity the patient can create a coded message, and the doctor "cracks" the coded message. In this scenario the doctor should intentionally make errors and have the patient point them out. The therapy goal is for the patient to decode accurately (100%) 10 to 15 messages with relatively improving speed.

Ideal forms

Procedure 1 (reproducing complex spatial patterns: subgoal 2). This procedure is designed to develop the patient's ability to rely on his or her internal spatial coordinate system and then integrate this skill with visually guided fine-motor planning skills. The equipment necessary for this procedure is the Ideal Form Packet (see Figure 16.29) and a pencil. The patient is seated at a table with the Ideal Form Packet in front of him or her. The first step is for the patient to trace over the dash-lined form. At this point in therapy this should be accomplished easily. The second step is for the patient to make the form in the first open space. He or she should use the completed forms as a reference. The doctor should ask the patient to evaluate his or her performance. For example, the patient might say, "The lines on my form are longer." Any significant deviations should be corrected before the move to the next step is made. The final step is for the patient to complete the form while the original and the two previously drawn forms have been hidden from view. This requires the patient to use his or her internal coordinate map to guide his or her motor actions. The forms are then uncovered, and the doctor asks the patient to evaluate his or her performance. Any significant deviations should be corrected before they move to the next form. The therapy goal is for the patient to be able to draw all the forms from memory with reasonable accuracy.

Jumbled pictures

Procedure 1 (visual figure ground: subgoal 2). This procedure is designed to develop the patient's ability to use an organized and structured search pattern to find a particular figure. We use Jumbled Pictures from Sedan (see Figure 16.11). You can also use hidden or jumbled pictures from other sources; however, we have found that jumbled or hidden pictures where the patient compares two similar pictures with some differences is the most effective. For example, two pictures may have 12 different items. The patient is seated and the jumbled pictures are placed at his or her usual working distance (place picture B to the right of A). The doctor instructs the patient to circle or mark all the differences between pictures A and B. The first step is to let the patient try to use his or her habitual search strategy, which gives the doctor an opportunity to see how the patient approaches the problem. Typically, the patient will use a haphazard approach and may skip over many items that are different between the two pictures. The doctor then demonstrates an organized method of scanning from left to right moving down the page. The patient then repeats the procedure with a new picture. It may take several repetitions before the patient uses an organized and structured search pattern. The therapy goal is for the patient to be able to find all the differences between the pictures using an organized search strategy.

Procedure 2 (visual figure ground: subgoal 3). This procedure is designed to increase the visual demand by adding distractors to the background. Once the patient uses organized and structured search strategies the complexity of the designs is increased. The doctor instructs the patient to find all the differences between the pictures as quickly as possible. It is important to observe the patient's strategy to make sure that a visual search strategy does not regress to a haphazard approach. Eventually, the patient should be able to compare a group of figures to each other by remembering chunks of information in each glance. This is not intended to train visual memory but to encourage a more efficient visual search strategy. Therapy should proceed until the patient has reached a plateau and the response times are no longer decreasing. The therapy goal is for the patient to be able to find accurately (100%) all the differences between the pictures and relatively decrease the search time from picture to picture.

Jumping jacks

Procedure 1 (bilateral integration: subgoal 2). This procedure is designed to develop the patient's motor planning ability by performing simultaneous and sequential movements with the two sides of the body. The first step is two-count symmetrical jumping jacks (Figure 17.12, *A*). In symmetrical movements the arms and legs are simultaneously moved toward or away from the midline. The patient starts with his or her legs together and arms at the sides of the body. Both legs are then extended while the arms are simultaneously moved over the patient's head. The patient should pause for 1 or 2 seconds at this position. The arms and legs are then moved back to the starting position. It may take several repetitions before the patient can perform the procedure accurately. Once accurate performance is achieved the patient should count while performing the procedure. The therapy goal is for the patient to be able to complete a smooth continuous 2-count motion.

The second step in therapy is 4-count symmetrical jumping jacks (Figure 17.12, *B*). The patient again stands with both arms and legs at his

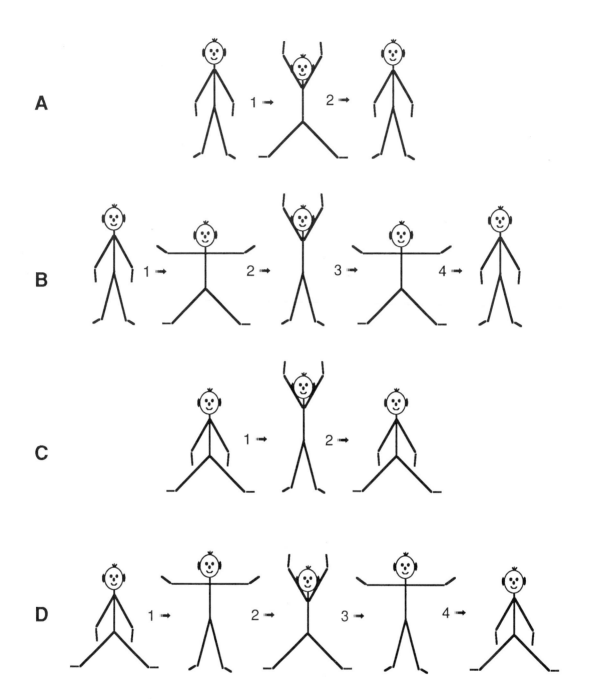

FIGURE 17.12 Jumping jacks procedure. **A,** The first step is two-count symmetrical jumping jacks. **B,** The second step is four-count symmetrical jumping jacks. **C,** The third step is 2-count reciprocal jumping jacks. **D,** The fourth step is four-count reciprocal jumping jacks.

or her sides. Both arms and legs are simultaneously extended outward; however, the arms are extended only to shoulder level. The patient should pause for 1 to 2 seconds at this position. The arms and legs are then simultaneously brought together (the arms are over the patient head). The patient again pauses in this position for 1 to 2 seconds. The arms and legs are then simultaneously extended, and the patient pauses in this position for 1 to 2 seconds. Finally, the arms and legs are moved simultaneously to the starting position. It may take several repetitions before the patient can perform the sequence accurately without stopping. Once the patient is able to perform accurately the 4-step sequence he or she should count to 4 while performing the four movements. The therapy goal is for the patient to be able to complete a smooth continuous 4-count motion.

The third step is 2-count reciprocal jumping jacks (Figure 17.12, *C*). In this sequence the arm and leg movements in relation to the midline are opposite. That is, if the arms move toward the midline, the legs move away from the midline. The patient starts with his or her legs apart and the arms at the sides of the body. Both legs are moved together while the arms are simultaneously moved over the patient's head. The patient should pause for 1 or 2 seconds at this position. The arms and legs are then moved back to the starting position. It may take several repetitions before the patient can perform the procedure accurately. Once accurate performance is achieved the patient should count while performing the procedure. The therapy goal is for the patient to be able to complete a smooth continuous 2-count motion.

The fourth step is 4-count reciprocal jumping jacks (Figure 17.12, *D*). The patient stands with his or her feet apart and the arms at his or her sides. The legs are moved together while the arms are simultaneously extended to shoulder level. The patient pauses for 1 to 2 seconds in this position. The legs are extended while the arms are brought together over the patient's head. The patient pauses for 1 to 2 seconds in this position. The legs are then brought together while the arms are brought to shoulder level. Finally, the patient returns the arms and legs to the starting position. It may take several repetitions before the patient can accurately perform the sequence without stopping. Once the patient is able to accurately perform the 4-step sequence he or she should count to 4 while performing the four movements. The therapy goal is for the patient to be able to complete a smooth continuous 4-count motion.

Procedure 2 (laterality: enhancing automaticity). This procedure is design to automate the knowledge of laterality. The doctor can use any of the steps in procedure 1. The emphasis now changes to having the patient move certain right and left body parts in a particular sequence. Have the child start with 2-count symmetrical jumping jacks. Instruct the patient to perform the procedure normally and then do the jumping jack without moving the right arm. It may take several repetitions before the patient can perform the procedure accurately. The doctor can then introduce a series of movements for the patient to perform. For example, do 2 jumping jacks with both arms, 2 with only the right arm, and 2 with only the left arm. The sequences should be kept short, especially for those patients with poor auditory memory. The procedure can also be done with 4-count symmetrical, and 2-count and 4-count reciprocal. The therapy goal is for the patient to be able to motor plan which arm or leg needs to be dropped out or added in, while continuing the jumping jack in a rhythmic fashion to completion.

Kirshner arrows I and II

Procedure 1 Kirshner arrows I (directionality: subgoal 1). This procedure is designed to have the patient generate an awareness that the laterality skills taught previously can be used to make right and left judgments of objects in space. A chalkboard or work sheet of arrows is required for this procedure. Arrows are drawn in the right, left, up, or down positions and in random order (see Figure 16.5). The first step is to have the patient orally call out the orientation of each arrow starting in the upper left-hand corner. To reinforce the motor memory developed during laterality therapy the patient should also indicate the orientation with his arms and hands. The arms should be fully extended directly in front with the hands clasped together. If the arrow is pointing to the right, the patient should say, "Right," and simultaneously point his arms to the right. Initially, the patient should describe how he arrived at that orientation. The patient may say, "This is my right hand, and this is to the right." This process is repeated for each arrow until the patient is able to generate a consistent strategy for determining the appropriate direction. The next step is for the patient to name each arrow's direction in an entire row without describing the strategy. The therapy goal is for the patient to be able to call the correct orientation in a relatively smooth and rhythmic fashion.

Procedure 2 Kirshner arrows II (directionality: subgoal 1: enhancing automaticity). This procedure requires the patient to call out the opposite or reversed orientation of each arrow. The opposite movement is also done with the arms. For example, if the arrow points up the child says, "Down," and moves his or her hands down. The patient's performance on this task is usually slower than Kirshner arrows I but accuracy is more important in this phase of therapy. This may be very difficult for children under 7 years of age, and the doctor should not expect a high level of performance. As automaticity improves, the patient can be further challenged by performing this procedure while maintaining his or her balance on a balance board or calling out the direction to the rhythmic set by a metronome. The therapy goal is for the patient to be able to perform the procedure accurately (90%).

Laterality questions

Procedure 1 (laterality: subgoal 1). This procedure is designed to have the patient build upon the motor awareness developed in bilateral integration therapy by recalling a series of everyday tasks where he uses his dominant hand. For example, in a game of catch the patient needs to identify which hand he uses to throw a ball. Other examples include, "Which hand do you use for writing or coloring?" or "What hand do you use for holding your fork while eating?" If the patient has difficulty recalling which hand he uses to throw or write, the doctor should let the patient actually throw a ball or write with either hand. This reinforces the patient's motor memory of the differences between the two sides. This initial step develops the underlying strategy that the patient will use when performing subsequent laterality procedures. The therapy goal is for the patient to identify consistently (100%) which hand is used in a variety of activities.

Letter find and letter reversal

Procedure 1 (directionality: subgoal 3). This procedure is designed to develop the patient's ability to apply the concepts learned in directionality subgoal 1 to the spatial orientation of linguistic symbols. Letter Find and Letter Reversal work sheets are used in this procedure (see Figure 16.7). The first step uses the Letter Find work sheets which requires the patient to find easily reversible letters (such as **b** or **d**) among a series of distractors. For example, find all the **b**'s on the page. Before starting have the patient explain the difference between **b**, **d**, **p**, **q** using spatial directions. For example, a **b** is different from a **d** because the bump is on the bottom and right side of the stick. Once the patient is able to generate a consistent strategy for describing the orientation of each letter he or she begins the work sheets. The patient then identifies and circles all the target letters that are embedded within a series of reversed letters. It is helpful to stop periodically and have the patient describe the spatial characteristics of the target letter (such as **b**) and how it is different from the distractors. The therapy goal is for the patient to be able to work through each work sheet with no errors and be aware of the spatial difference between letters.

The second part of the procedure uses Letter Reversal work sheets, which have reversed letters embedded within individual words. The patient is instructed to circle all reversed letters that appear on the sheet. It is important to make sure that the patient can decode the level of words on the sheet. If the child does not understand the word, he may not know if certain letters (such as **b** for **d**) are reversed. However, other letters (such as **a**) are easily identified as reversed even if the child cannot decode the word. On work sheets where the patient cannot accurately decode the words, correct responses should be counted only when the reversed letter does not become a different letter (such as **b** for **d**). The therapy goal is for the patient to be able to perform each work sheet with no errors.

Maze tracing

Procedure 1 (visually guided fine-motor control: subgoal 2). The primary goal of maze tracing is to reinforce the patient's awareness of the importance of vision in guiding the motor system while increasing the constraints on accurate fine-motor performance. Therapy starts with mazes whose borders are widely separated and then works toward narrowing the separation between the lines (see Figure 16.24). The doctor needs to emphasize good visual-motor ergonomics throughout the procedure. The patient should start at the beginning of the maze and carefully move the pencil through the maze without hitting the borders. As the patient draws a line between the borders of the maze, the doctor should have him or her identify when performance is inaccurate (the patient touched the edge of the maze with the pencil). Once the inaccuracy is identified the patient should verbalize a strategy to improve his or her performance. The doctor can keep track of the time and the number of inaccuracies as a measure of improvement. The initial therapy goal is for the patient to go through the maze accurately and then increase the speed of the response. Some instructions and goals will need to be modified based on the patient's visual-cognitive style (see Chapters 14 and 16).

For some children, simple visual feedback (noticing they hit the sides of the maze) will not be sufficient, and it is often helpful to add techniques that provide auditory feedback (such as the Talking Pen, see Figure 16.25). The therapy goal is to have the patient monitor and adjust his or her performance to improve the accuracy and then subsequently the speed of the visually guided fine-motor movement.

Parquetry blocks

Procedure 1 (visual discrimination: subgoal 1). This procedure uses a multisensory approach for children who are performing at a development age of 7 years or under. This procedure is designed to develop the patient's ability to describe the distinctive features of objects and to judge similarities and differences between objects (see Figure 16.8). Older children can start therapy by reproducing specific block patterns in procedure 2. Parquetry blocks consists of three shapes (triangle, square, and diamond) that come in a variety of colors. There are four workbooks (levels I to IV) that accompany the blocks. The first step is to have a patient trace the individual blocks with his or her finger and describe the distinctive features of each block by answering a series of questions: (1) "How many sides does each block have?" (2) "How many corners does each block have?" and (3) "Do all the sides have the same size?" The second step involves mixing the block shapes together, and the patient is instructed to sort them by shape (for example, "Find all the squares"). This requires the patient to use the previous information to judge similarities and differences between the three different forms. For example, a triangle has three sides, and a square has four sides. The therapy goal is for the patient to verbalize the distinctive features of each figure.

Procedure 2 (visual discrimination: subgoal 2). This procedure is designed to develop the patient's ability to use only visual clues to find similarities or differences of increasingly complex forms (see Figure 16.8). The first step is directed toward reproducing a series of specific designs that include all three of the blocks. The doctor builds a design in front of the patient, and he or she places the matching block directly on top of one built by the doctor. This starts with a 2- or 3-block design and eventually builds up to a 4- or 5-block design. It is helpful to have the patient pick out all the pieces he or she needs to build a design before attempting to construct it. This forces the patient to make both color and shape judgments.

The second step requires the patient to build the design next to the doctor's design, using similar designs to the ones described in step 1. It is important to notice the orientation of the patient's design because this feature is frequently incorrect. It is helpful for the patient to build the design on a clear plastic plate or acetate sheet so that it can be picked up and placed over the doctor's design. This makes it easy for the patient to identify inconsistencies, especially in orientation. The doctor should also ask the patient to identify the similarities and differences between the doctor's design and the one the patient built.

The third step uses Parquetry Blocks workbooks levels I and II. First the patient builds the exact design directly on top of the one on the page. Once the patient successfully completes the designs in book I he or she builds the design to the side or off the book. Once this step is completed the patient builds the patterns in book II in the same manner as book I. The therapy goal is for the patient to build accurately all the designs in books I and II both on and adjacent to the workbook.

Procedure 3 (visual closure: subgoal 2). This procedure is designed to develop the patient's ability to make closure judgments with increasing speed and accuracy. Parquetry Blocks workbooks levels III and IV are used in this procedure. These designs have no internal detail to delineate the individual blocks within each design (see Figure 16.8). Initially the patient identifies the individual shapes that are within the designs. It is helpful to have the patient trace the absent or missing line or lines with his or her finger while identifying the individual shapes. Another method is to have the patient chose all the blocks needed to build the design before actually placing the blocks on the design. The patient should complete book III building directly on the page first and then building the designs off the page. When using book IV, the patient builds only the designs directly on the page. These designs are too difficult for most patients to build them off the page. The therapy goal is for the patient to show a relative improvement in closure skills as he or she progresses through each of the workbooks.

Procedure 4 (visual memory: subgoal 1). This procedure is designed to develop the patient's ability to form an image of the visual input using a multisensory approach. The first step is to have the patient trace an individual form (such as a square) with his or her finger. This provides a motor memory trace that matches the visual characteristics of the figure. The doctor should encourage the patient to keep a "picture in his head" of what the figure looks and feels like when he or she traces the figure. The block should then be removed and the patient should reproduce or draw the form from memory. The doctor will then have the patient compare his or her drawing with the original block. The patient should identify the differences between the two figures. For example, the patient's reproduction of a square may have sides that are unequal or too short. The doctor then removes the block again, and the patient reproduces the figure, encouraging the patient to recall the differences that were previously found. This continues until the patient can reproduce the figure with reasonable accuracy. Patients with a visual-motor deficit may have difficulty with accurate drawings, and the doctor needs to allow for some range of error in these cases. The doctor can also refer to the Test of Visual Motor Integration to see which geometric forms were difficult for the patient. For example, the patient may have drawn a square adequately but failed to draw a recognizable diamond. The therapy goal is for the patient to be able to draw each form with similar proportions to the blocks.

Procedure 5 (visual memory: subgoal 2). This procedure is designed to develop the patient's ability to recall the spatial characteristics of objects or figures. The first step is for the doctor to build a 3- to 5-block design. The design should initially be hidden from the patient's view. The patient then looks at the design for 5 to 10 seconds, and the design is hidden again. The doctor then asks the patient to describe the spatial characteristics of the design including, number of blocks, color, and position. For example, "How many squares are present in the design?" or "Is the triangle to the right or to the left of the square?" It is important to emphasize the spatial characteristics of the form and not simply the names of the figures. Frequently the patient will need to view the target several times before he or she can describe all the spatial characteristics. It may take several repetitions with different designs before the patient is able to identify consistently the spatial characteristics of the designs.

The third step in therapy is for the patient to build a series of designs from memory without answering questions about the characteristics of the design. This should start with approximately 3 blocks and increase to 6-block designs. The doctor should have the patient compare his or her design with the doctor's design and describe any subtle spatial differences, such as orientation. Any corrections in the original design are then made by the patient. Once the patient is able to build 3- to 6-block designs accurately the doctor can reduce the viewing time. The therapy goal for the patient is to reproduce 4- to 6-block designs accurately with a 2- to 3-second viewing time.

Procedure 6 (visualization: subgoal 2). This procedure is designed to develop the patient's ability to manipulate mentally the orientation of objects or figures. The first step in therapy is for the doctor to take a single block and set it in a specific orientation in front of the patient. The doctor then asks the patient to place an identical block beside the doctor's block, but the orientation of the block should be rotated a fourth of a turn to the right or left. It may be necessary for the doctor to demonstrate the concept by actually rotating the doctor's blocks a fourth of a turn (90°). The second step is to increase the number of blocks in the design from 2 to 6 blocks and repeat the same instructions. It is often helpful for the doctor to build his or her design on a piece of rigid clear plastic. The doctor can then rotate this design according to the suggested rotation and then lay it on top of the patient's design for feedback to the patient about how accurately he or she executed the rotation. The third step is to have the patient rotate the doctor's design a half of a turn (180°) without an intermediate quarter turn. A similar problem would be presented if the doctor and patient sit on opposite sides of the therapy table and the doctor builds a design and then asks the patient to build the same design but from the doctor's perspective. Patients of different ages will reach different levels of ability. For children under 7 years of age this task is often too difficult, with only a small percentage of children able to do step 1. Children 7 to 11 or 12 can usually do step 2, but step 3 is more appropriate for children older than 12 years of age.

Randolf shuffle

Procedure 1 (bilateral integration: subgoal 2). This procedure is designed to develop the patient's motor planning ability by performing isolated, simultaneous and sequential movements of the right and left sides of the body. The first step develops the ability to plan isolated motor movements (Figure 17.13, *A*). The patient stands in the center of therapy room with both arms at his or her side. The doctor asks the patient to extend the right arm without moving other body parts. This is repeated for each arm and each leg. Initially the doctor may have to hold or restrain certain body parts to help the patient inhibit movement of body parts that are not supposed to be moved. The therapy goal is for the patient to plan and execute a smooth isolated motor movement with minimal or no motor overflow.

The second step requires the patient to move both arms and one leg in a specific sequence (Figure 17.13, *B*). For example, the doctor asks the patient to raise both arms straight in front of his or her chest (extended) and simultaneously the right leg steps straight out (the other leg remains stationary). The arms are then extended outward to the side, and the right leg is simultaneously moved from directly in front to the side. The arms are then moved back to straight in front (still extended) and the right leg is simultaneously moved back to the straight-out position. The arms are dropped back to the sides, and the right leg is simultaneously moved back alongside the left leg (the original starting position). The procedure is repeated with the patient moving both arms and the left leg. The therapy

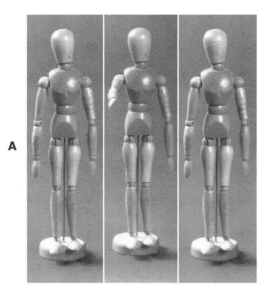

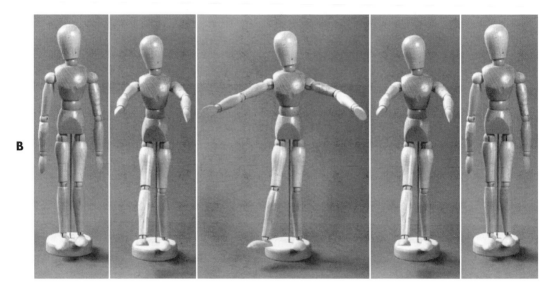

FIGURE 17.13 Randolf shuffle. **A,** Three-step movement sequence for the unilateral phase. **B,** Five-step movement sequence for the second phase (both arms and one leg).

goal is for the patient to plan and execute a sequence of motor movements with minimal or no motor overflow.

The third step is to have the patient complete ipsilateral movements where the arm and leg on the same side of the body are moved in sequence (Figure 17.13, *C*). For example, the doctor asks the patient to extend the right arm and right leg simultaneously. Then the patient moves the right arm and leg to the side and then directly back to the extended position. The right arm is dropped back to the side, and the right leg is simultaneously moved back alongside the other leg (the original starting position). The

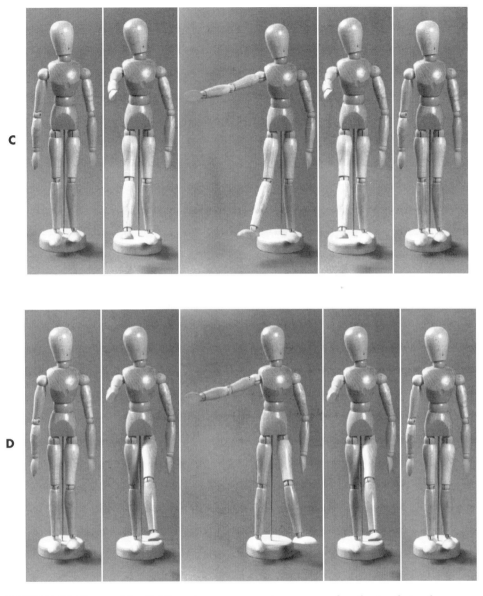

FIGURE 17.13, cont'd. C, Five-step movement sequence for the ipsilateral movement phase. **D,** Five-step movement sequence for contralateral phase.

procedure is repeated with the patient moving the left arm and the left leg. The therapy goal is for the patient to plan and execute a sequence of ipsilateral motor movements with minimal to no motor overflow.

The fourth step requires the patient to complete contralateral movements where the opposite arm and leg are moved in sequence (Figure 17.14, *D*). For example, the doctor asks the patient to extend his or her right arm and simultaneously move the left leg. The right arm and left leg are extended to the side and moved back to the extended position. The right arm is dropped back to the side, and the left leg is simultaneously moved back alongside the right leg (the original starting position). The procedure is repeated with the patient moving the left arm and the right leg. The therapy goal is for the patient to plan and execute a sequence of contralateral motor movements with minimal to no motor overflow.

Throughout the four steps the doctor should emphasize the concept of motor planning, requiring the patient to "think ahead" before initiating the gross motor movement. As therapy proceeds, the doctor needs to help the patient evaluate his or her own performance. The patient then needs to tell the doctor what the patient will do to improve his or her performance. These procedures are designed to be continued for several repetitions (such as 10 times). The therapy goal is to have the patient perform smooth and accurate motor movements for several repetitions.

Procedure 2 (laterality: enhancing automaticity). This procedure is designed to automate the knowledge of laterality. The doctor can use any of the steps in procedure 1. The emphasis now changes to having the patient move certain right and left body parts in a particular sequence. For example, the patient can perform a sequence of isolated motor movements with the right and left hands. The doctor might have the patient do 2 right-hand movements and then 1 left then 1 right. The sequence of instructions should initially be kept short, especially for patients with auditory memory problems. The goal of this procedure is for the patient to accurately sequence the right and left movements of the body.

Rosner program (VMI)

Procedure 1 (reproducing complex spatial patterns: subgoal 1). This procedure is designed to develop the patient's awareness of an external spatial coordinate system and then integrate this with visually guided fine-motor planning skills. The doctor will need the Rosner TVAS, design figures (100 to 200) and 25, 17, 9, 5, and 0 dot grids for this procedure. If the patient has successfully achieved previous therapy goals in the areas of form perception as well as visually guided fine-motor control, we have found that most patients are able to start therapy at the 25-dot level. If the patient has difficulty at this level the Test for Visual Analysis Skills (TVAS) can be administered to determine at which level therapy should begin (based on the last correct figure copied prior to two consecutive mistakes; no erasing is allowed).

We typically start the Rosner program having the patient copy a pattern from the doctor's 25-dot map to the patient's 25-dot map using paper and pencil (see Figure 16.27). The first step is to have the patient identify the x-y spatial coordinates of individual dots on his or her dotted map. For example, the patient would count 3 dots on the x-axis and 2 dots down on the y-axis. The second step is for the patient to isolate a single feature (one line connecting two or more dots) of a pattern on the doctor's map and then identify the spatial coordinates of the starting and ending dots of that feature on his or her map. The third step is to draw the line and have the patient evaluate the accuracy of his or her performance. To foster this development it is helpful to have the patient visualize the actual motor plan before putting the pencil on the paper. Once the patient is able to draw successfully the individual features of a pattern the emphasis changes to drawing the complete pattern in a systematic manner going from left to right and top to bottom. It is recommended that the patient complete patterns 100 to 150. Typically 10 patterns can be completed per day. To create more figures one can rotate the maps a fourth of a turn, and this can create up to 200 figures. It is important for the patient to complete successfully the higher numbered maps before proceeding to the next stage.

Procedure 2 (reproducing complex spatial patterns: subgoal 2). This procedure is designed to develop the patient's ability to rely on his or her internal spatial coordinate system and then integrate this skill with visually guided fine-motor planning skills. In this procedure the external spatial organization cues are progressively removed by gradual removal of dots on the map that the patient is using to copy the pattern. Initially the patient should copy a pattern from a 25-dot map (made by the doctor) to a 17-dot map starting at map number 150 (see Figure 16.28). The first step is for the patient to identify the *x-y* coordinates of individual dots that have been removed from his or her map. We have found it helpful to have the patient actually draw in the missing dots after identifying the spatial coordinates. The second step is for the patient to isolate a single feature of a pattern (where the ending dot is missing) on the doctor's map and then identify the spatial coordinates of the starting and ending dots of that feature on his or her map. The third step would be to draw the line and then evaluate the accuracy of his or her performance. When the patient's reproduction does not reflect an accurate internal spatial map, the doctor should help the patient identify the inconsistency in his or her internal map versus the pattern being drawn. An acetate overlay of the pattern can be helpful. Once the patient is able to draw the individual features of a pattern successfully the emphasis changes to drawing the complete pattern in a systematic manner going from left to right and top to bottom. The patient should draw 20 figures before moving onto more difficult (fewer dot) maps. The previous steps are repeated as the patient copies from the 25-dot pattern onto a 9-dot, then 5-dot, and finally a 0-dot map. The therapy goal is for the patient to draw complex patterns accurately and efficiently on a 0-dot map.

Sequential beads

Procedure 1 (visual memory: subgoal 3). This procedure is designed to develop the patient's ability to recall the sequential characteristics of figures or displays using only visual information. The doctor will need DLM (Developmental Learning Materials) colored beads and a string (with a knot at one end) and the pattern cards for the colored beads. Initially the design is placed in front of the patient, and he or she strings the beads to match the design, similar to what was done in the previous subgoal 2, but the emphasis has changed to reproducing the correct sequence (see Figure 16.14). Next a new design card (3 to 5 beads) is placed in front of the patient but hidden from view. The doctor then allows the patient to look at the design for 5 to 10 seconds and then asks the patient to string the appropriate sequence of the design. We do not have the patient describe the sequence, as was done in the visual memory: subgoal 2, because this may encourage the patient to overly rely on a oral strategy rather than their mental image of the sequence. If the patient is unable to build the entire design at one glance, the doctor should allow the patient another 5- to 10-second view of the design. The doctor should again ask the patient to build the design. The therapy goal is for the patient to build design sequences of 3 to 6 beads based on a single 5- to 10-second view of the design card (see TVPS subtest visual sequential memory for age appropriate number of items in a sequence).

Simon Says

Procedure 1 (laterality: subgoal 2). This procedure is designed to develop the patient's ability to identify consistently the laterality of his or her body parts. The doctor asks the patient a series of questions using the Simon Says game format (for example, "Simon Says raise your right arm" or "Simon Says stand on your left leg"). After the patient's response the doctor should ask the patient to explain his or her strategy. For example, "How did you know that was your right hand?" The patient should be able to recall an appropriate strategy that was developed in the first part of therapy for laterality. For example, "I know that this is my right hand because I use my right hand to throw a ball." It is important not to use external markers (such as bracelets, rings, or watches) for making right and left judgments. The therapy goal is for the patient to identify right and left labels accurately (100%) and consistently. A similar procedure can be conducted with other children's games, such as Mother May I.

Procedure 2 (directionality: subgoal 2). This procedure is designed to develop the patient's ability to identify consistently right and left labels on another person. Before starting therapy the doctor needs to help the patient understand how to alter the patient's perspective of right and left by using concrete examples (see Chapter 16, directionality: subgoal 2). This procedure is performed in the same manner as procedure 1, except that the patient identifies right and left directions on the doctor (for example, "Simon Says point to my right arm"). Again it is important to have the patient identify a strategy for determining the right and left directions on the doctor. This strategy is more difficult to verbalize than right and left on one's self, and the patient may need to use motor support to supplement the verbal explanation. For example, the patient may turn his whole body to explain changes in the doctor's position. The therapy goal is for the patient to identify right and left labels accurately and consistently. A similar procedure can be conducted with other children's games, such as Mother May I.

Slap tap

Procedure 1 (bilateral integration: subgoal 2). This procedure is designed to develop the patient's motor planning ability by performing isolated, simultaneous and sequential movements with the right and left sides of the body (Figure 17.14). This procedure is very similar to the Randolf shuffle technique. The first step is to develop isolated motor movements (Figure 17.14, *B*). The patient is seated with his or her hands placed faced down on his or her legs. The doctor points to the patient's right hand and asks the patient to raise his or her right hand. The patient should raise his or her right hand and then place the hand back on the leg without moving other body parts. Frequently, it is helpful for the doctor to model the first step. This is repeated for each arm and each leg. Initially, the doctor may have to hold or restrain certain body parts to help the patient inhibit movement of body parts that are not supposed to be moved. The therapy goal is for the patient to plan and execute a smooth isolated motor movement with minimal or no motor overflow.

The second step is to have the patient complete ipsilateral movements, where the arm and leg on the same side of body are moved in sequence (Figure 17.14, *C*). The doctor instructs the patient to raise his or her right arm and right leg simultaneously without moving the left side of the body. The procedure is repeated with the patient moving the left arm and the left leg. The therapy goal is for the patient to plan and execute a sequence of ipsilateral motor movements with minimal or no motor overflow.

The third step is to have the patient complete contralateral movements of the right and left sides of the body (Figure 17.14, *D*). The doctor instructs the patient to raise his or her right arm and left leg simultaneously without overflow from other body parts. Frequently, the doctor should point to or touch the body parts that should be moved, especially for patients with poor laterality skills. The procedure is repeated with the patient moving the left arm and the right leg. The goal is for the patient to plan and execute a sequence of contralateral motor movements with minimal to no motor overflow.

Procedure 2 (laterality: enhancing automaticity). This procedure is designed to automate the knowledge of laterality. The doctor can use any of the steps in procedure 1. The emphasis now changes to having the patient move certain right and left body parts in a particular sequence. For example, the patient can perform a sequence of isolated motor movements with the right and left hands. The doctor might have the patient do 2 right hand movements, then 1 left, and then 1 right. The sequence of instructions should initially be kept short, especially for patients with auditory

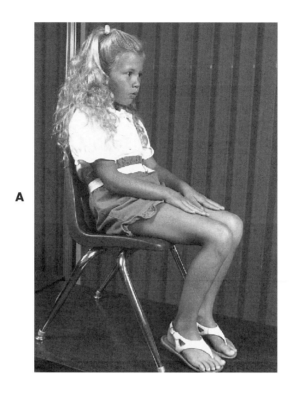

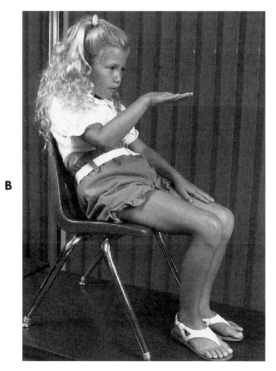

FIGURE 17.14 Slap tap procedure. **A,** The patient is seated with her hands placed faced down on her legs. **B,** The first step is to develop isolated motor movements.

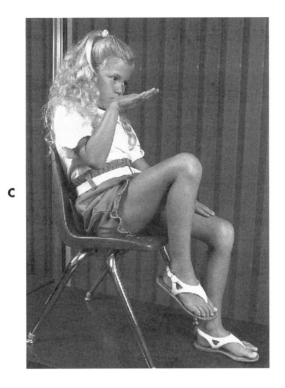

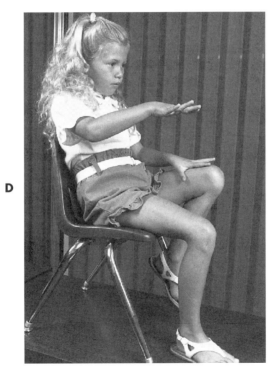

FIGURE 17.14, cont'd. C, The second step is to have the patient complete ipsilateral movements, where the arm and leg on the same side of body are moved in sequence. **D,** The third step is to have the patient complete contralateral movements of the right and left sides of the body.

memory problems. The therapy goal is for the patient to sequence the right and left movements of the body accurately.

Stickman

Procedure 1 (directionality: subgoal 2). This procedure is designed to develop the patient's ability to identify right and left on another person while that person is engaged in a variety of activities. The doctor will need a copy of the Stickman diagram work sheet (Figure 17.15). The first step is for the patient to sit with the Stickman diagrams placed on a table. The patient's task is to determine and call out which hand of the stick figure has a mitten. The doctor should ask questions that stress the strategy used by the child as opposed to merely eliciting correct answers. For example, "How did you know that the mitten was on the left hand?" The patient may have to turn his or her body in the same direction as the stickman figure to help with the verbal explanation. This technique serves as a good "bridge" procedure between floor map I and floor map II.

The second step is to improve the patient's automaticity by increasing the speed of responses. The therapy goal is for the patient to identify quickly (1 to 2 sec/figure) and accurately (100%) the hand with the mitten on each stick figure and demonstrate the proper strategy.

Tachistoscope

Procedure 1 (visual memory: subgoal 4). This procedure is designed to increase the patient's speed and span of visual memory. The procedure uses a tachistoscopic device, such as the Tac-ette, Opti-Mum computer, or Atari computer (see Figure 16.15) and targets classified into spatial (such as tic-tac-toe) and sequential (such as a series of numbers) categories (see Figure 16.16). The first step requires the doctor to choose a series of targets (10 to 20) with a number of digits or characters that is below the patient's expected level of performance (see Table 16.1). For example, if the patient is in second grade, use targets appropriate for first grade. If the patient has difficulties primarily with spatial targets, the doctor should choose targets with a similar number of characters as those recommended for a series of digits. For example, if 3 digits are recommended, use a tic-tac-toe design with 3 X's. If the patient is unable to perform accurately at the slowest speed (1 second), the doctor should reduce the number of figures present in the target. Before starting therapy the patient needs to understand what type of target is being displayed, the location of the display, and the method of recall that will be used (oral, writing, or typing on the keyboard). In the beginning start with a verbal recall format. Having the patient to write down the target flashed can interfere with the memory trace and result in frustration, especially for patients with a visual-motor dysfunction. The doctor should encourage the patient to use memory strategies developed previously for recalling the visual information (see subgoals 1 to 3, p. 463). The initial presentation time should be 1 second. Once

STICKMAN FIGURES

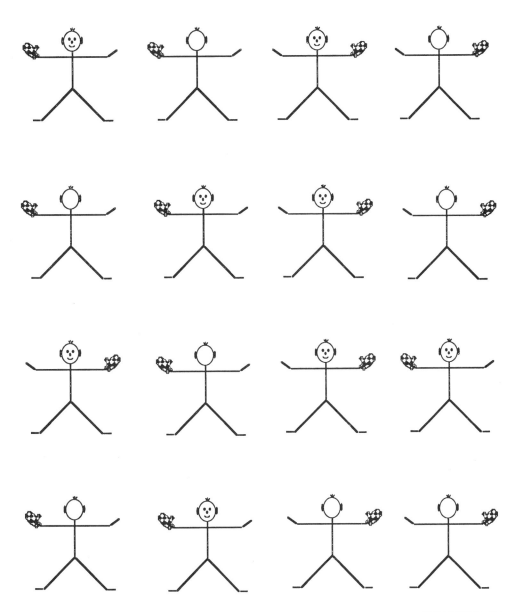

FIGURE 17.15 Stickman worksheet. The patient's task is to determine and call out which hand of the stick figure has a mitten. The doctor should ask questions that emphasize the method used by the child as opposed to merely eliciting correct answers.

accurate performance of approximately 80% is achieved at a 1-second display time the doctor should gradually decrease the presentation time until it is faster than 200 msec. This prevents the patient from making a saccade to gather additional information and forces the patient to collect more information on a single fixation. The goal of therapy is to have the patient correctly remember a sequential display with the number of digits (or same number of figures if it is a spatial display) that is appropriate for his or her grade level (see Table 16.1). Once the patient reaches this goal, we concentrate on automaticity by delaying the time (such as 5 to 10 seconds) between presentation and the patient's response. The doctor can increase the cognitive loading by referring to the box, p. 393.

Procedure 2 (visualization: subgoal 1). This procedure is designed to develop the patient's awareness of a mental image created by a form that is no longer present. This is similar to what was taught in visual memory, but in this procedure the patient does not recall the complete presentation. Instead, the patient is now required to use the mental image to recall only parts of what was seen. The first step is for the doctor to select a series of spatial targets (such as tic-tac-toe) with a number of figures and display time appropriate for the patient's age (see Table 16.1). Before the presentation the doctor should encourage the patient to form a picture of the objects in his or her head. After the target has been presented, the doctor should ask the patient a series of questions such as, "What was in the second column first row?" or "Where would you need to but your X to block me from winning the game?" The goal of this procedure is to recall accurately the parts of the presentation. The second step for the doctor is to select a series of sequential (such as numbers or letters) targets with a number of figures and display times appropriate for the patient's age. After the target is displayed, the doctor should ask the patient a series of questions such as, "What is the third number?" or "What is the second, first, and third numbers?" The therapy goal for the patient is to recall accurately (90%) the parts of the presentation.

Three-in-a-row

Procedure 1 (visual memory: subgoal 3). This procedure is designed to have the patient reproduce the sequential characteristics of figures or displays using only visual information. Three objects are placed on the table in front of the patient (such as a coin, key, and pencil) or forms can be drawn on a chalkboard or paper (such as a square, circle, and triangle). The first step is for the patient to identify orally the objects while directly viewing them. It is important for the doctor to make sure that the patient identifies the correct sequence going from left to right. The second step requires the doctor to place a new sequence or arrangement of the three objects in front of the patient but hidden from view. The patient is then allowed to look at the objects for 5 to 10 seconds, and then the objects are hidden from view. The patient then tells the doctor the exact sequence of the three objects. It is important for the doctor to encourage the patient to form a mental image or picture in his or her head when remembering the objects. If the patient is unable to remember the exact sequence of the design in one glance, the doctor should allow him or her another 5- to 10-second view of the design. It may take several repetitions for the patient to recall accurately the correct sequence of objects. As therapy progresses, the length of the design can be increased to 5 or 6 items. The therapy goal is for the patient to recall the correct sequence of 5 to 6 items based on a 5- to 10-second viewing time.

Procedure 2 (visualization: subgoal 1). This procedure is designed to develop the patient's awareness of a mental image created by a form that is no longer present. This is similar to what was taught in visual memory, but in this procedure the patient does not recall the complete presentation. Instead the patient is now required to use the mental image to recall only parts of what was seen. Three objects (such as a square, triangle, and circle) are placed in front of the child, or figures can be drawn on a piece of paper or the chalkboard. The patient is shown the three objects for approximately 10 seconds. The objects are then hidden from view. During the viewing time the doctor encourages the patient to form a picture of the objects in his head. After removing the objects the doctor should ask the patient a series of questions such as, "What is the third object?" or "What is the second, first, and third objects?" The types of objects can be changed, but we usually limit the number of objects to 3 or 4. The therapy goal is for the patient to recall accurately the parts of the presentation.

Visual motor stick procedures

Procedure 1 (developing gross eye-hand coordination: subgoal 1). This procedure is designed to make the patient aware of the importance of vision in guiding the motor system. A small rubber ball (4 to 6 inches in diameter) hung from the ceiling at approximately chest level is required for the procedure. A dowel rod ($\frac{1}{2}$ to 1 inch in diameter) approximately 3 feet long is used for striking the ball. The patient should be approximately 2 feet from the ball and hold the stick with both hands separated by approximately 16 inches. The doctor pushes the ball toward the patient and instructs him or her to strike the ball with the middle of the stick (Figure 17.16). Initially the doctor wants the patient to understand the importance of vision in guiding the motor response. The doctor can accomplish this by having the patient attempt to strike the ball while his or her eyes are closed. The patient should be aware that the process is much harder or impossible with his or her eyes closed. Now the patient performs the procedure with his or her eyes open. The doctor should stress the importance by saying "Keep your eye on the target."

Procedure 2 (developing gross eye-hand coordination: subgoal 2). Once the importance of vision in guiding the motor act is demonstrated the doctor can concentrate on having the patient improve his or her accu-

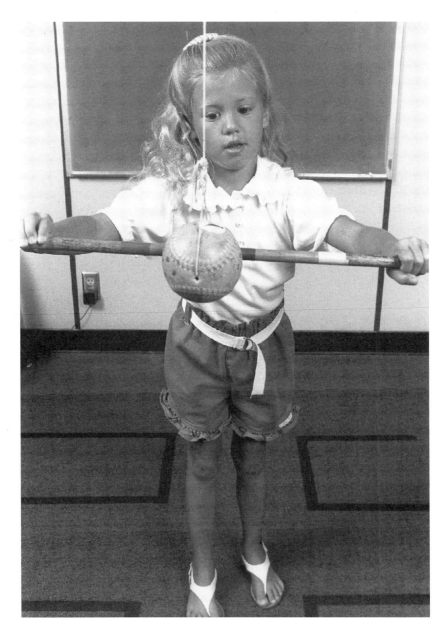

FIGURE 17.16 Illustration of a Visuomotor stick procedure used in developing general eye-hand coordination skill. The doctor pushes the ball towards the patient and instructs her to strike the ball with the middle of the stick.

racy. The doctor pushes the ball toward the patient, and he or she strikes the ball with the stick. Initially the patient strikes the ball once and evaluates his or her performance. The critical issue is that the patient can correctly evaluate his or her performance and use that information to improve the accuracy of future attempts. For example, the patient missed the ball because the stick was too low. The patient should be able to tell the doctor that the stick will be placed higher on the next attempt. The patient should repeat this procedure several times until he or she can consistently strike the ball with the center of the stick. To make the procedure more difficult the doctor can have the patient strike the ball 3 or more times with the same level of accuracy. The therapy goal is for the patient to strike the center of the ball 5 to 10 consecutive times.

Visual tracing

Procedure 1 (visual figure ground: subgoal 1). This procedure is designed to develop the patient's ability to separate the figure from the ground using a multisensory approach. The doctor will need a series of visual tracings (see Figure 16.10, *A*). The first step is to have the patient place a pencil at letter **A** and trace the line until he or she finds which number is at the end of the line. The doctor should ask the patient how the patient knows that he or she should continue on the same line. Children may have trouble verbalizing their strategy and will often show the doctor by tracing the line through an intersection of lines with their finger or pencil. At this point in therapy the doctor should not be overly concerned with the accuracy of the patient's visually guided fine-motor accuracy. The therapy goal is for the patient to separate the figure (target line) from the background (distractor lines) accurately.

Procedure 2 (visual figure ground: subgoal 3). This procedure is designed to increase the visual demand by adding distractors to the background. The complexity of the visual tracing would be increased by the addition of more lines (see Figure 16.10, *B*). The doctor instructs the patient to start at letter **A** and follow the line with his or her eyes only until he or she finds which number is at the end of the line. This is done for each letter on the visual tracing chart. This patient should be able to perform the procedure accurately using only visual input. The doctor then encourages the patient to decrease the amount of time needed to find the end of the line. The patient should increase the speed of his or her response without sacrificing the accuracy of the performance. This is repeated until the patient reaches a plateau and cannot increase their response time. The therapy goal is for the patient to trace (visually) the line accurately and quickly as the number of distracting lines is increased.

Winterhaven templates

Procedure 1 (visual discrimination: subgoal 1). This procedure is designed to develop the patient's awareness of similarities or differences between forms using a multisensory approach. The doctor will need a set of Winterhaven templates, paper and pencil, or chalk and a chalkboard (see Figure 16.13). The first step is to have the patient describe the distinctive features of individual forms. The doctor has the patient trace along the inside edge of the individual template of the square, circle, or triangle with his or her finger. The patient should trace the form several times, and then the doctor should ask the patient to describe the characteristics of the form. For example, "How many sides does this have?" or "Are all the sides the same size?" or "How many corners does the figure have?" The therapy goal is for the patient to identify consistently the features of each individual figures.

The second step is to have the patient find the similarities and differences between forms. For example, the patient can describe the difference between a triangle and a square. Again the doctor may prompt the patient by asking questions such as, "Do the forms have the same number of sides?" Patients under 7 years of age will often need motor support (such as points to corners or sides) to help them explain the difference between forms. Certain features such as angle or oblique lines are difficult for children to explain even with motor support. To make the procedure more difficult the doctor can introduce the 6-figure template and have the patient describe the differences between each of those figures. The therapy goal is for the patient to describe the distinctive features of forms and consistently identify the differences between the forms.

Procedure 2 (visual memory: subgoal 1). This procedure is designed to develop the patient's ability to form an image of the visual input using a multisensory approach. The first step is to have the patient trace an individual form (such as a square) with a piece of chalk (see Figure 16.13). This provides a motor memory trace that matches the visual characteristics of the figure. The doctor should encourage the patient to keep a picture in his or her head of what the figure looks and feels like when he or she traces the figure. The template is then removed, and the patient reproduces the form from memory. The doctor then has the patient compare his or her drawing with the original template. The patient should identify the differences between the two figures. For example, the patient's reproduction of a square may have sides that are unequal or too short. The doctor then removes the template again, and the patient reproduces the figure, encouraging the patient to recall the differences that were previously found. This continues until the patient can reproduce the figure with reasonable accuracy. Patients with a visual-motor deficit may have difficulty with accurate drawings, and the doctor needs to allow for some range of error in these cases. The doctor can also refer to the Developmental Test of Visual Motor Integration to see which geometric forms were difficult for the patient. For example, the patient may have drawn a square adequately but failed to draw a recognizable diamond. The therapy goal is for the patient to be able to draw each form with similar proportions to the template.

X's and O's

Procedure 1 (visually guided fine-motor control: subgoal 2). This procedure was designed to develop the accuracy of the visually guided fine-motor movements. Step 1 is to have the patient sit at a table with the X and O work sheet in front of him (Figure 17.17). The patient should begin forming a line from the left to the right. The line should be above

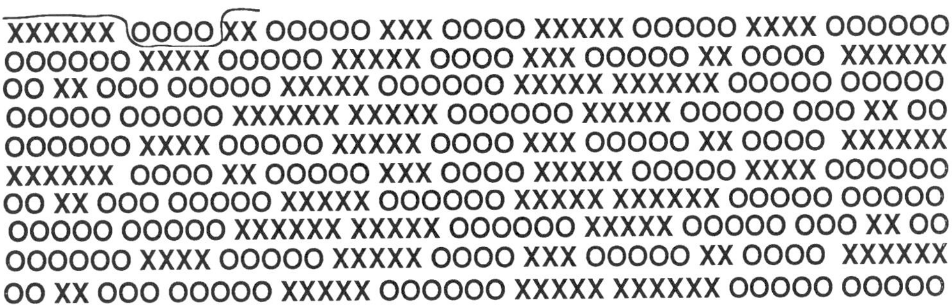

XXXXX OOOO XX OOOOO XXX OOOO XXXXX OOOOO XXXX OOOOOO
OOOOOO XXXX OOOOO XXXXX OOOO XXX OOOOO XX OOOO XXXXXX
OO XX OOO OOOOO XXXXX OOOOOO XXXXX XXXXXX OOOOO OOOOO
OOOOO OOOOO XXXXX XXXXX OOOOOO XXXXX OOOOO OOO XX OO
OOOOOO XXXX OOOOO XXXXX OOOO XXX OOOOO XX OOOO XXXXXX
XXXXXX OOOO XX OOOOO XXX OOOO XXXXX OOOOO XXXX OOOOOO
OO XX OOO OOOOO XXXXX OOOOOO XXXXX XXXXXX OOOOO OOOOO
OOOOO OOOOO XXXXX XXXXX OOOOOO XXXXX OOOOO OOO XX OO
OOOOOO XXXX OOOOO XXXXX OOOO XXX OOOOO XX OOOO XXXXXX
OO XX OOO OOOOO XXXXX OOOOOO XXXXX XXXXXX OOOOO OOOOO

FIGURE 17.17 Illustration of X's and O's worksheet. The patient should begin forming a line from the left to the right. The line should be above the X's and below the O's. The doctor should encourage the patient to use his or her eyes to plan ahead and emphasize to the patient to be as accurate as possible.

the X's and below the O's. The doctor should encourage the patient to use his or her eyes to plan ahead. The emphasis should be on the patient being as accurate as possible. A score based on the number of touches of X's and O's made on each line can be given. The therapy goal is for the patient progressively to make fewer errors as he or she completes each line of the work sheet.

Procedure 2 (visually guided fine-motor control: subgoal 3). This procedure was designed to develop the speed while maintaining the accuracy of the visually guided fine-motor movement. The procedure is conducted as in procedure 1, but now the doctor should record the time to complete each line. The doctor should encourage the patient to decrease the time to complete each line while maintaining his or her accuracy. The therapy goal is for the patient progressively to decrease the time necessary to complete each line while keeping errors to a minimum (1 or 2 per line).

CHAPTER 18

Case Studies

MITCHELL M. SCHEIMAN
MICHAEL W. ROUSE

KEY TERMS

visual information processing evaluation
visual efficiency evaluation
late-onset visual efficiency disorder
visual information processing disorder
primary auditory-language disorder
primary emotional disorder

Clinical management of learning-related vision problems is one of the more challenging aspects of optometric practice. In addition to having expertise in the diagnosis of visual efficiency and visual information processing disorders, the clinician must also have a knowledge of normal child development, visual and visual-motor development, the learning process, learning disabilities, the special education process, the psychoeducational evaluation, and the relationship between vision and learning. In addition to possessing this broad knowledge base, the clinician must be able to integrate this knowledge with the results of optometric testing, information from previous testing, and the case history. Although virtually every patient is unique in presentation, we have found that there are several different presentations that are most common and tend to recur.

In this chapter we present a series of case studies that are typical of these common case presentations that optometrists encounter in clinical practice. Reviewing these cases and studying the recommended evaluation, diagnosis, and management may help clinicians learn to manage learning-related vision problems more effectively and with more confidence than previously.

544

Case 1: Late Onset Visual Efficiency Problem
Case history

Paul, a 12-year-old, seventh grader, was brought in for an examination because his school performance had decreased significantly this school year. Until this year Paul had been an outstanding student achieving excellent grades in all subjects. The specific problem revolved around Paul's inability to read comfortably. He complained that after 10 to 15 minutes of reading his eyes felt tired and ached. He also reported feelings of burning. Whenever he continued to read, he eventually experienced headaches, and finally the words would blur and move on the page. Because of his inability to read comfortably, he was falling behind in his assignments. He felt that the amount of required reading had increased significantly this year.

His medical history was normal, and he was not taking any medication. He had passed a visual screening at the pediatrician and in school earlier in the school year. He never had a full vision evaluation.

There was no significant family history of learning problems. Both parents were college graduates with high expectations for Paul's education.

Visual efficiency testing

Examination results:

VA (distance, uncorrected)	OD: 20/20-2
	OS: 20/20-2
VA (near, uncorrected):	OD: 20/20
	OS: 20/20
Near point of convergence:	Accommodative target: 7.5/10 cm
	Penlight: 20/30 cm
Cover test (distance):	Orthophoria
Cover test (near):	10 exophoria
Subjective:	OD: −0.25 DS, 20/20
	OS: plano−0.25 × 90, 20/20
Cycloplegic refraction:	+0.50 DS, 20/20
	+0.50 DS, 20/20
Distance lateral phoria:	Orthophoria
Base-in vergence (distance):	X/9/5
Base-out vergence (distance):	10/18/10
Near lateral phoria:	9 exophoria
−1.00 gradient:	7 exophoria
Base-in vergence (near):	12/22/10
Base-out vergence (near)	4/6/1
NRA (negative relative accommodation):	+1.50
PRA (positive relative accommodation):	−2.50
Accommodative amplitude:	OD: 13D, OS: 13D
Monocular accommodative facility	OD: 0 cpm, fails plus
	OS: 0 cpm, fails plus
Binocular accommodative facility:	0 cpm, fails plus
MEM retinoscopy:	OD: −0.25, OS: −0.25

Pupils were normal; all external and internal health tests showed normal results; the deviation was comitant; and color vision testing revealed normal function.

Visual information processing evaluation

Since Paul had an excellent academic record for the first 6 years of school, we believed that if a vision problem was a contributing factor to his current problems it would be a visual efficiency disorder or a refractive error. We did not believe that visual information processing testing was necessary.

Assessment and diagnosis

The history in this case was clearly characteristic of a learning problem secondary to a visual efficiency disorder. Analysis of the optometric findings revealed a receded near point of convergence, high exophoria at near, decreased positive fusional vergence, a low NRA (negative relative accommodation) and difficulty with plus lenses on binocular accommodative facility testing. Based on these data we reached a diagnosis of convergence insufficiency. In addition, Paul had a low MEM (Monocular Estimation Method) finding and had difficulty with plus lenses monocularly suggestive of a diagnosis of accommodative excess. This combination of diagnoses is not uncommon. Generally, we believe that in such cases the convergence insufficiency is the primary diagnosis and the patient overaccommodates to compensate for the inadequate positive fusional vergence causing a secondary accommodative excess.

We believed that these visual efficiency problems were clearly related to Paul's presenting complaints. Given Paul's history of excellent academic performance in grades 1 through 6, we believed that if we could eliminate the visual efficiency problems along with the associated symptoms there would be a direct effect on academic performance.

Treatment plan

We recommended a program of vision therapy and followed the approach suggested in Chapter 15. Eighteen, 45-minute, in-office visits were necessary. The patient was seen twice a week, and after 9 weeks Paul reported elimination of all his initial complaints and was able to read comfortably as long as desired. A reevaluation at this point revealed the following:

Near point of convergence:	2.5/5.0 cm
Base-out at near:	16/32/18
NRA:	+2.50
Monocular accommodative facility:	12 cpm
Binocular accommodative facility:	10 cpm
Subjective:	OD: +0.25, 20/20
	OS: +0.25, 20/20
MEM retinoscopy	OD: +0.25; OS: +0.25

As Paul's comfort improved, his ability to study was enhanced, leading to better academic performance.

Case 2: Primary Visual Information Processing Disorder
Case history

Jimmy, an 8-year-old first grader, was referred for a vision evaluation by a psychologist who had just completed a psychoeducational evaluation. Jimmy learned to speak very early and was always a very verbal child. Although his parents' expectations had been very high for him, Jimmy had a history of school-related problems since kindergarten. In kindergarten he experienced difficulty with letter and number recognition and fine-motor coordination. He had great difficulty in first grade with handwriting and copying from the board. He reversed letters and numbers excessively and had difficulty with his sight-word vocabulary. His parents noted that when they read to him his comprehension was excellent. Because of these reported difficulties, he was retained in first grade. Despite this retention, he continued to experience problems, and his parents finally brought him to a psychologist for psychoeducational testing.

The parents brought a copy of the psychoeducational evaluation report. This report indicated that there were no significant emotional issues and the WISC results included a verbal IQ of 128 and a performance IQ of 104. The weakest scores were in coding (scaled score 5) and block design (scaled score 6). Jimmy scored almost 2 years behind his chronological age on the Bender Gestalt Test, which is a test of visual-motor integration. Auditory processing and language skills were strengths for Jimmy.

Achievement testing was also done as part of the psychoeducational testing. This testing indicated a 1-year lag in reading with weaknesses in sight-word vocabulary, comprehension, and grade-appropriate math skills.

In her summary, the psychologist reached a diagnosis of a learning disability with primary weaknesses in visual processing and strengths in language function. She recommended part time placement in a resource room and reading tutoring. In addition, she suggested a comprehensive optometric evaluation.

Jimmy's medical history revealed a normal pregnancy but a very long and difficult labor and delivery by cesarean section. Otherwise there was no significant medical history. Developmental milestones showed a variable pattern. Language skills developed faster than average. For example Jimmy used 2-word sentences by 18 months of age and was always a very verbal child. Fine-motor skills, however, developed more slowly than expected. He always had difficulty holding a crayon and did not enjoy coloring or playing with puzzles. He could not copy a circle until about 4 years of age.

There did not seem to be any family history of learning problems, and there had been no other testing.

Visual efficiency testing

Examination results:

VA (distance, uncorrected)	OD: 20/20
	OS: 20/20
VA (near, uncorrected):	OD: 20/20
	OS: 20/20
Near point of convergence:	Penlight: 2.5/5.0 cm
Cover test (distance):	Orthophoria
Cover test (near):	4 exophoria
Subjective:	OD: +0.50 DS, 20/20
	OS: +0.50 DS, 20/20
Distance lateral phoria:	Orthophoria
Base-in vergence (dist):	X/8/5
Base-out vergence (dist):	10/18/10
Near lateral phoria:	5 exophoria
−1.00 gradient:	1 exophoria
Base-in vergence (near):	12/22/10
Base-out vergence (near)	12/20/11
NRA:	+2.50
PRA:	−2.50
Accommodative amplitude:	OD: 13D, OS: 13D
Monocular accommodative facility	OD: 10 cpm
	OS: 10 cpm
Binocular accommodative facility:	10 cpm
MEM retinoscopy:	OD: +0.50; OS: +0.50
Developmental Eye Movement Test	Errors: 5th %
	Ratio: 5th %
Saccades	2+ OD and OS
Pursuits	2+ OD and OS

Pupils were normal; all external and internal health tests showed normal results; the deviation was comitant; and color vision testing revealed normal findings.

Visual information processing evaluation

CHRONOLOGICAL AGE: 8 YEARS, 4 MONTHS

Category	Test	Score
VISUAL-SPATIAL SKILLS		
Bilateral integration	Standing Angels in the Snow	7-year level
Laterality	Piaget Test of Left-Right Concepts	6-year level
Directionality	Gardner Reversal Frequency Test	
	Recognition subtest	5%
	Execution subtest	40%
VISUAL-ANALYSIS DYSFUNCTION		
Visual discrimination	TVPS: Visual Discrimination	63%
Visual closure	TVPS: Visual Closure	37%
Visual form constancy	TVPS: Visual Form Constancy	37%
Visual figure ground	TVPS: Visual Figure Ground	50%
Visual-spatial relations	TVPS: Visual Spatial Relations	37%
Visual memory	TVPS: Visual Memory	25%
	TVPS: Visual Sequential Memory	37%

VISUAL-MOTOR INTEGRATION

Visual-motor integration	Visual motor integration tests	10%
Fine-motor skills	Grooved Pegboard	10%
	Wold Sentence Copy Test	First grade

AUDITORY INFORMATION PROCESSING SKILLS

Auditory-visual integration	Auditory-Visual Integration Test	84%

Assessment and diagnosis

The optometric evaluation revealed difficulties in both visual efficiency and visual information processing. Although there was no significant refractive error or accommodative or binocular vision disorder, ocular motility was significantly below age level. Clinical observation showed performance of only 2+ for both pursuits and saccades, and the results on the DEM were very low. Based on this information we reached a diagnosis of oculomotor dysfunction.

In addition, the visual information processing evaluation indicated problems in visual-spatial, visual-analysis, and visual-motor integration skills.

These findings can be related to many of the problems that Jimmy was experiencing in school (see chart below).

The key information from the psychoeducational evaluation was the above-average verbal IQ, the lower performance IQ, the absence of emotional problems, and a visual processing based learning disorder.

Treatment plan

Based on our findings and the information gathered from the psychoeducational report, we recommended a vision therapy program designed to remediate the ocular motor and visual information processing disorders. We were careful to state that the goal of the therapy was to improve the underlying vision disorders. Although we expected improvement in the signs and symptoms reported by Jimmy's parents, we strongly supported the need for educational remediation in addition to the vision therapy program.

We followed the approach suggested in Chapters 15 and 16. Forty-two, 45-minute, in-office visits were necessary. In addition, a considerable amount of therapy was done at home. The patient was seen twice a week for about 6 months. A reevaluation at this point revealed the following findings:

Category	Test	Score
VISUAL-SPATIAL SKILLS		
Bilateral integration	Standing Angels in the Snow	8-year level
Laterality	Piaget Test of Left-Right Concepts	8-year level

Directionality	Gardner Reversal Frequency Test	
	Recognition subtest	37%
	Execution subtest	50%

VISUAL-ANALYSIS DYSFUNCTION

Visual discrimination	TVPS: Visual Discrimination	63%
Visual closure	TVPS: Visual Closure	50%
Visual form constancy	TVPS: Visual Form Constancy	50%
Visual figure ground	TVPS: Visual Figure Ground	50%
Visual-spatial relations	TVPS: Visual Spatial Relations	37%
Visual memory	TVPS: Visual Memory	37%
	TVPS: Visual Sequential Memory	50%

VISUAL-MOTOR INTEGRATION

Visual-motor integration	Visual Motor Integration Tests	42%
Fine-motor skills	Grooved Pegboard	37%
	Wold Sentence Copy test	2nd grade

AUDITORY INFORMATION PROCESSING SKILLS

Auditory-visual integration	Auditory-Visual Integration Test	84%

Jimmy showed improvements in both the error and ratio scores on the DEM test. The error score improved from the 5th percentile to the 40th percentile, and the ratio score improved from the 5th percentile to the 50th percentile.

Jimmy also received help at school and had private reading tutoring. We asked the teachers to temporarily deemphasize written work, particularly copying from the board. After 6 months of combined educational and optometric intervention, Jimmy made outstanding progress. He now found it easier to get his thoughts down in writing, copying from the board was considerably better, and he was no longer reversing letters excessively. His reading level increased about 6 to 9 months and he was no longer as frustrated in school as he used to be.

We dismissed him from vision therapy, and he continued to receive help at school and from his private reading tutor.

Case 3: Primary Auditory-Language Disorder
Case history

Peter, a 7-year, 7-month-old first grader, was brought to The Eye Institute by his parents to rule out a vision problem that could be contributing to his learning difficulties. He was having a great deal of difficulty learning to read and spell. His math and handwriting skills were normal. His parents did not report any difficulty with letter or number reversals or transpositions of words. They were very concerned because the school was talking about having him repeat first grade. The school had not recommended any psychoeducational testing, however. Peter did not have any complaints about vision, though he did not read for more than a few moments at a time.

There was no history of learning problems in the family. Developmental history indicated a normal pregnancy and a normal labor and delivery. He sat up independently at 5 months, crawled at 8 months, and walked independently at about 1 year. He was an excellent athlete and was particularly good at hitting a baseball. A review of his language development, however, revealed some lags. He started speaking late and did not use 2-word sentences until he was almost 3 years old. When he did start speaking, he had a speech articulation problem. He has had speech therapy for this problem since 6½ years of age.

In terms of medical history, Peter had tubes placed in his ears at 1 year of age and again at 3. He was diagnosed as having asthma at age 4 and also suffers from allergies. He still gets frequent ear infections.

There had been audiological testing in the past that revealed no hearing loss but some difficulty with auditory figure ground ability. A report from his speech and language therapist indicated significant problems in the area of expressive language.

Visual efficiency testing

Examination results:

VA (distance, uncorrected)	OD: 20/20
	OS: 20/20
VA (near, uncorrected):	OD: 20/20
	OS: 20/20
Near point of convergence:	Penlight: 3 cm/5cm
Cover test (distance):	orthophoria
Cover test (near):	2 exophoria
Retinoscopy and subjective:	OD: $+1.25\ -0.50 \times 180$, 20/20
	OS: $+1.25\ -0.50 \times 180$, 20/20
Distance lateral phoria:	Orthophoria
Base-in vergence (dist):	X/7/5
Base-out vergence (dist):	11/19/10
Near lateral phoria:	5 exophoria
-1.00 gradient:	1 exophoria
Base-in vergence (near):	10/16/9
Base-out vergence (near)	13/22/11
NRA:	$+2.25$
PRA:	-2.50
Accommodative amplitude:	OD: 13D; OS: 13D
Monocular accommodative facility	OD: 8 cpm
	OS: 8 cpm
Binocular accommodative facility:	7 cpm
MEM retinoscopy (without subjective):	OD: $+1.25$; OS: $+1.25$
DEM:	Errors: 50%
	Ratio: 60%
Saccades	2+ OD and OS
Pursuits	3+ OD and OS

Pupils were normal; all external and internal health tests showed normal results; the deviation was comitant; and color vision testing revealed normal findings.

Visual information processing evaluation

CHRONOLOGICAL AGE: 7 YEARS, 7 MONTHS

Category	Test	Score
VISUAL-SPATIAL SKILLS		
Bilateral-integration	Standing Angels in the Snow	8-year level
Laterality	Piaget Test of Left-Right Concepts	8-year level
Directionality	Gardner Reversal Frequency Test:	
	Recognition subtest	50%
VISUAL-ANALYSIS DYSFUNCTION		
Visual discrimination	TVPS: Visual Discrimination	63%
Visual closure	TVPS: Visual Closure	63%
Visual form constancy	TVPS: Visual Form Constancy	50%
Visual figure ground	TVPS: Visual Figure Ground	75%
Visual-spatial relations	TVPS: Visual Spatial Relations	37%
Visual memory	TVPS: Visual Memory	75%
	TVPS: Visual Sequential Memory	50%
VISUAL-MOTOR INTEGRATION		
Visual-motor integration	Visual Motor Integration Tests	60%

Assessment and diagnosis

The frequent ear infections, myringotomy, speech therapy, and slow language development were suggestive of a possible language basis to Peter's learning problems. There was also a lack of signs and symptoms that could be related to vision disorders. In addition, the previous audiological evaluation and speech language report clearly indicated that a language problem was present.

Optometric testing was normal in both the areas of visual efficiency and visual information processing, though there was a moderate degree of hyperopic astigmatism in both eyes. Peter denied any problems with asthenopia or blurred vision when reading. However, it was clear that he never read for more than very short periods of time.

Treatment plan

We informed the parents that other than the moderate degree of hyperopia and astigmatism that there were no significant vision problems. We did recommend eyeglasses to be used for school and all homework. We were very careful to indicate that these glasses were not expected to have any direct effect on his reading level. Rather, we were prescribing glasses ($+1.00 - 0.50 \times 180$ OD and OS) so that as he read more he would be less likely to experience asthenopia. We indicated that our testing had ruled out a visual basis for the learning disorder and suggested that they request a psychoeducational evaluation at school. We believed that if a decision had to be made about retaining him in first grade additional information was necessary. Peter's parents had not been aware that they could initiate a request for such testing and did not know how to initiate this process. We recommended that they send away for a copy of *The Right to Special Education in Pennsylvania* (Education Law Center, Suite 60, 801 Arch St., Philadelphia, PA 19107) as background information they would need about special education. This monograph also provided them with a sample letter they could use to request the psychoeducational evaluation.

Two months later Peter received this testing, which revealed a Full Scale IQ of 101, a Performance IQ of 111, and a Verbal IQ of 87 on the WISC-R. The summary of the academic testing showed that Peter had a significant reading problem, particularly in phonics, and he had problems in his understanding of information when it is read to him as well. He scored at the beginning first-grade level in spelling and on grade level in mathematics.

Based on this testing Peter was retained in first grade, was placed in a resource room for additional reading help at school, and started private reading and language tutoring two times per week.

Case 4: Primary Emotional Disorder
Case history

Susan, a 10-year-old fifth grader, was brought for a vision examination because she was not doing well in school and had been complaining about her vision. Her parents wanted to rule out a vision problem as a possible cause of her learning problems. Susan had been an average student in grades 1 through 4. In fifth grade, however, she began experiencing problems. She was failing two subjects and barely passing the others. Her mother did not have any additional details because there had not been any other testing. Susan reported that she was having trouble seeing the board and that her eyes tired quickly when she was reading. She could not say when these problems began but believed there might be a connection with the beginning of the school year.

The medical history was unremarkable, and Susan was not taking any medication. The developmental history did not indicate any difficulty in any of the developmental milestones.

Although we were not sure of the reason at the time of the history, we sensed some uneasiness between the child and her mother during the case history. Susan was reluctant to speak and was somewhat withdrawn.

Visual efficiency testing

Examination results:

VA (distance, uncorrected)	OD: 20/60−2
	OS: 20/60−2
VA (near, uncorrected):	OD: 20/80
	OS: 20/80
Near point of convergence:	Penlight: 7.5cm/12.5cm
Cover test (distance):	Orthophoria
Cover test (near):	6 exophoria
Subjective:	OD: +0.50, 20/20
	OS: +0.50, 20/20
Cycloplegic refraction:	+1.00, 20/20
	+1.00, 20/20
Distance lateral phoria:	Orthophoria
Base-in vergence (dist):	X/8/6
Base-out vergence (dist):	10/18/10
Near lateral phoria:	5 exophoria
−1.00 gradient:	1 exophoria
Base-in vergence (near):	10/18/10
Base-out vergence (near)	10/16/11
NRA:	+0.50
PRA:	−0.50
Accommodative amplitude:	OD: 13D; OS: 13D
Monocular accommodative facility	OD: 9 cpm
	OS: 9 cpm
Binocular accommodative facility:	8 cpm
MEM retinoscopy:	OD: +0.50; OS: +0.50

Pupils were normal; all external and internal health tests showed normal results; the deviation was comitant; and color vision testing revealed normal function.

Visual information processing evaluation

CHRONOLOGICAL AGE: 10 YEARS, 4 MONTHS

Category	Test	Score
VISUAL-SPATIAL SKILLS		
Laterality	Piaget Test of Left-Right Concepts	8-year level
Directionality	Gardner Reversal Frequency Test:	
	Recognition subtest	85%
VISUAL-ANALYSIS DYSFUNCTION		
Visual discrimination	TVPS: Visual Discrimination	75%
Visual closure	TVPS: Visual Closure	63%
Visual form constancy	TVPS: Visual Form Constancy	37%
Visual figure ground	TVPS: Visual Figure Ground	50%
Visual-spatial relations	TVPS: Visual Spatial Relations	75%
Visual memory	TVPS: Visual Memory	37%
	TVPS: Visual Sequential Memory	50%
VISUAL-MOTOR INTEGRATION		
Visual-motor integration	Visual Motor Integration Tests	50%

Assessment and diagnosis

The evaluation of visual acuity was difficult and indicated that Susan might be malingering. Susan did not display the typical pattern of easily reading the large letters on the Snellen chart and then experiencing greater difficulty as the letters became smaller. Rather, she claimed to have difficulty with even the 20/200 letters and continued to struggle with the smaller letters. Objective testing confirmed our suspicion indicating a low degree of hyperopia in both eyes. With encouragement we were able to achieve 20/20 acuity in both the right and left eyes.

The only other abnormal findings were the low NRA and PRA. She claimed to be unable to even see the 20/30 print through the subjective finding. We believed that this was an inconsistent and questionable finding since she had no difficulty with accommodative facility testing, monocularly or binocularly.

The visual information processing evaluation did not reveal any significant weaknesses or pattern that could account for her academic problems.

We believed therefore that Susan's complaints of blurred vision and difficulty reading comfortably could not be accurate. We found no visual basis for these problems. Our sense was that her learning difficulties did not seem to be related to a vision problem.

Treatment plan

We did indicate to Susan's mother that there were inconsistencies between her subjective and objective responses and that in our experience this can sometimes indicate that there might be some other stressful condition bothering the child. We suggested that a psychological-educational evaluation might be appropriate to determine the basis for her academic difficulties.

After our summary, Susan's mother told us that she had separated from her husband about 9 months ago and this might be affecting Susan. Based on this information we reaffirmed our recommendation that she should consult with a psychologist.

SUMMARY

These four cases underscore the complexity and challenge of managing learning-related vision disorders. Through these cases we have tried to emphasize the importance of an interdisciplinary approach. In case one the vision problems was the primary cause of the child's academic difficulty and treatment of the visual efficiency problem transferred directly to improve school performance. However, this type of case is not the most common presentation. In most instances, even if a vision problem is present, it will be only one of several factors that contribute to the child's problems. If we treat the vision problem, in such instances it is important to understand that elimination of the vision problem will not necessarily lead to improved reading or math skills. Rather, the goal of such treatment is to eliminate the vision problem and its associated signs and symptoms and thereby enable the child to more fully benefit from educational remediation.

CHAPTER REVIEW

1. Describe the patient history you would expect for each of the following problems:
   a. A late-onset visual efficiency problem.
   b. A visual information processing disorder.
   c. A primary auditory-language disorder.
   d. A primary emotional disorder.
2. At what grade level would you expect a visual information processing problem to have its greatest effect on a child's performance? Why?
3. At what grade level would you expect a visual efficiency problem to have its greatest effect on a child's performance? Why?
4. Describe what you would expect the verbal and performance sections of the WISC-R IQ test to be in a child who has:
   a. A visual information processing disorder.
   b. A primary auditory-language disorder.
5. Describe a general treatment strategy for the following problems:
   a. A late-onset visual efficiency problem.
   b. A visual information processing disorder.
   c. A primary auditory-language disorder.
   d. A primary emotional disorder.

Bibliography for Parents, Teachers, and Other Professionals

The following are articles that can be used to create a vision and learning and vision therapy information packet. We have divided the readings into three categories; technical articles, articles written for the general public, and articles from nontechnical books.

We recommend using the five articles and the brochure that are emphasized in bold print as the basic information packet. The other articles can be used as needed depending on the specific patient and issues that must be addressed.

TECHNICAL ARTICLES

1. Farr J, Leibowitz HW: An experimental study of the efficacy of perceptual-motor training, *Am J Optom Physiol Optics* 53:451-455, 1976.
2. Flax N, Mozlin R, Solan HA: Learning disabilities, dyslexia, and vision, *J Am Optom Assoc* 1984;55:399-403, 1984.
3. Flax N, Solan HA, Suchoff IB: Optometry and dyslexia, *J Am Optom Assoc* 54:593-594, 1983.
4. Hoffman LG: Incidence of vision difficulties in children with learning disabilities, *J Am Optom Assoc* 51:447-451, 1980.
5. Hoffman LG, Rouse MW: Vision therapy revisited: a restatement, *J Am Optom Assoc* 58:537-540, 1987.
6. Seiderman A: Optometric vision therapy: results of a demonstration project with a learning disabled population, *J Am Optom Assoc* 51:489-494, 1980.
7. **Solan HA, Ciner EB: Visual perception and learning: issues and answers, J Am Optom Assoc 60:457-460, 1989.**
8. Suchoff IB, Petito GT: The efficacy of visual therapy: accommodative disorders and non-strabismic anomalies of binocular vision, *J Am Optom Assoc* 57:119-124, 1986.
9. **Special report: Position statement on vision therapy, J Am Optom Assoc 56:782-783, 1985.**
10. **Special report: The efficacy of optometric vision therapy, J Am Optom Assoc 59:95-105, 1988.**
11. Suchoff I: Research on the relationship between reading and vision, *J Learn Disabil* 14:573-576, 1981.

557

WRITTEN FOR THE GENERAL PUBLIC AND TEACHERS

1. **Scheiman M: Hidden eye problems can block learning, Learning 91, July-Aug 1991, Springhouse Corporation, Springhouse, PA 19477.**
2. **Taxel L: Seeing is believing, East-** **West Natural Health Magazine, May/June 1992.**
3. Rouse MW, Ryan JB: Teacher's guide to vision problems, *Reading Teacher* 38:306-317, 1984.

NONTECHNICAL BOOKS

1. Rosner J: *Helping children overcome learning difficulties,* ed 2, Marble Falls, Texas, 1979, Walker Publishing Co.
2. Flach F: *Rickie,* New York, 1990, Fawcett Columbine Co.
3. Granger L, Granger B: *The magic feather,* New York, 1986, EP Dutton.
4. Seiderman AS, Marcus SE: *20/20 is not enough: the new world's vision,* New York, 1989 and 1991, Knopf.

SOURCES FOR BROCHURES

1. American Optometric Association, 243 North Lindbergh Ave, St. Louis, MO 63141, (314) 991-4100.
2. Vision Extension, 2912 South Daimler Street, Suite 100, Santa Ana, CA 92705-5811, (714) 250-0846.
3. **Parents Active for Vision Education (PAVE), 7331 Hamlet Ave, San Diego, CA 92120-1923, (619) 464-0687 (brochure: The hidden disability: undetected vision problems.)**

APPENDIX B

Sample Psychoeducational Reports

NAME: James Smith
ADDRESS: 4444 Main Street
                         Typical City, USA
DATE OF BIRTH: 4/4/84
GRADE: Repeating first grade
DATES OF EVALUATION: 7/16/91, 7/23/91, 7/31/91
EVALUATED BY: Penni F. Blaskey, Ph.D.

REASON FOR REFERRAL:

James was referred for psychoeducational testing by his parents and pediatrician because of parental concerns regarding James's functioning at
home and in school. Specifically, audiological and speech and language
evaluations indicated specific areas of weakness, and it was questioned
whether James had an attention deficit hyperactivity disorder (ADHD). At
home, it was indicated that James has difficulty sitting still for more than a
few minutes at a time.

BACKGROUND INFORMATION:

James, age 7, is the son of Gerald and Theresa Smith. He lives with his
parents, his grandmother, his 10-year-old twin brothers, and his 1½-year-
old brother in Philadelphia. Both Mr. and Mrs. Smith are high school
graduates, and Mr. Smith works as a plant manager, while Mrs. Smith
works as a cook. A history of learning problems exists in Mr. Smith's family because both he and his father have always had spelling problems, despite being very bright overall. James's younger brother, Bob, has been
diagnosed with a seizure disorder.

Developmental history was obtained from Mrs. Smith. She indicated that her pregnancy was normal, as were her labor and delivery. Mrs. Smith smoked approximately 10 cigarettes daily. James
weighed 7 lb, 14 oz at birth. He was described as a good but restless
baby who did not sleep a great deal. At 6 months of age Mr. and Mrs.
Smith were told by a neurologist that James had seizures. A second
consultation with another neurologist determined that he did not have
seizures. Most developmental milestones occurred within normal limits,
though Mrs. Smith indicated that James walked without assistance
and named colors relatively late. He also had poor head control as an
infant.

In terms of medical history, James was hospitalized at 3 weeks and at 1 year for viral pneumonia. He had tubes placed in his ears at 1 year. He was diagnosed as having asthma at age 4 and also suffers from allergies. James was hospitalized for his asthma at age 5. He still gets ear infections occasionally. James appears to be particularly hyperactive when he is taking asthma medicine.

James started nursery school but stayed for only a few months because of his mother's pregnancy at that time. He entered Forrest Elementary School for kindergarten. He had difficulty sitting still, particularly during story time. James entered St. Timothy's for first grade. His parents indicated that he had a difficult year, having difficulty with reading and spelling, and spending a great deal of time on his own separated from the rest of the class during certain academic periods. He was referred to CORA Services in the middle of the first grade year for extra help in reading and began attending sessions in March. His word recognition skills were inadequate at any level when tested by CORA. James will be repeating first grade in September.

James received an audiological evaluation on 4/24/91 by Liz Henderson. She found that James has significant difficulty with auditory figure ground ability, which appear to be compromising his comprehension of auditory information. A speech and language evaluation was performed by Jillian Feld on 6/26/91. She also found significant problems in the areas of auditory memory, sequencing, expressive language, comprehension of verbal commands, and linguistic concepts when information is presented in compound and complex sentence structure.

An optometric evaluation indicated significant problems in the areas of eye movements, directionality, and visual motor integration. A program of vision therapy was recommended to remediate these deficiencies.

James is excellent in sports and enjoys playing with older children.

BEHAVIORAL OBSERVATIONS:

James was seen for three sessions over a 3-week period of time. He enjoyed speaking of his interests and sports and appeared somewhat at ease during these discussions. However, as soon as structured tasks were begun, James became more anxious. This was particularly evident during academic tasks. During such times James asked approximately every 5 to 10 minutes how much longer he had to work. James appeared to have a cold or allergies during each of the testing sessions over the 3-week period, with labored breathing and using many tissues throughout. He worked very slowly with frequent erasures on paper and pencil copying tasks. Signs of anxietal interferences were evident throughout the testing sessions. When James was given a task to do on his own (completing simple one-digit arithmetic addition and subtraction problems), he had great difficulty remaining task focused and completed only 12/100 problems in 15 minutes (with only 8/12 correct). The present evaluation appears to be a valid estimate of current functioning, though anxiety may have prevented James from performing optimally.

TESTS ADMINISTERED:

The following tests were administered to James:

Weschler Intelligence Scale for Children–Revised (WISC-R)
Woodcock Johnson Test of Cognitive Ability
Rey Auditory Verbal Learning Test
K-ABC Hand Movement Subtest
Bender Test of Visual Motor Integration
Boder Test of Reading Spelling Patterns
Woodcock Johnson Tests of Achievement
Wide Range Achievement Test (WRAT-R1)
Temple Informal Reading Inventory
Gardner Reversal Frequency Test
Restricted Academic Situation (Barkley)
House-Tree-Person Drawing and Story
Thematic Apperception Test (TAT)
Sentence Completion Test
Achenbach Child Behavior Checklist
Connors Parent Symptom Questionnaire
Clinical interview
Parent interview

TEST INTERPRETATIONS:

The following information represents the salient findings from this comprehensive evaluation. Please refer to test summary after the body of this report for exact scores.

PSYCHOEDUCATIONAL EVALUATION:
Cognitive Functioning:

The WISC-R was used to measure intellectual functioning. On the WISC-R James obtained a Full Scale IQ of 90, which is in the average range of functioning and at the 26th percentile for children his age. His Verbal IQ of 103 (57th percentile) was in the average range of functioning, whereas his Performance IQ of 78 (8th percentile) was in the borderline range. The 25-point difference in favor of Verbal IQ indicates that James tends to express his intelligence better through verbal expression than through more hands-on visual-motor tasks.

Within the Verbal Scale, James demonstrated strengths in the area of numerical reasoning when solving arithmetic word problems mentally (84th percentile). Adequate attention and concentration is also needed for task performance. A significant weakness was seen in James's verbal abstract reasoning when required to determine similarities among concepts (16th percentile). All other verbal subtests indicated average abilities, including James's general fund of information, his ability to define words, to demonstrate social reasoning and practical judgment, and to repeat a string of numbers, a measure of short-term rote auditory memory.

By comparison, James's Performance, or nonverbal cognitive functioning, was much weaker than his verbal skills. A strength was seen in the area of visual analysis and nonverbal problem solving (37th percentile). This was his only score within the average range. When required to assemble puzzles from individual pieces, James had the greatest difficulty, scoring at the 2nd percentile in comparison to other children the same age. Putting together the puzzles requires coordination, persistence, and the ability to recognize a familiar object from its parts. Below-average performance was also seen when James was required to distinguish essential from nonessential details in pictures, sequence pictures to tell a story, and on another visual-motor coordination task requiring speed and concentration in quickly pairing numbers with symbols.

Additional cognitive testing, using the Woodcock Johnson Tests of Cognitive Ability, was administered to James to further assess his processing of information. He again demonstrated average rote verbal recall when asked to repeat sentences and individual words. Processing speed for visual information was also slightly below average, similar to the WISC-R, although it was somewhat faster when numbers were involved than when abstract symbols or designs were used. James demonstrated below-average skill on two language tasks, the first an expressive language task, when required to name common objects represented by pictures, and the second, a measure of his ability to name a common word from only incomplete parts. He had most difficulty on three subtests, one requiring him to name a picture from incomplete visual information. This task required that he form a whole picture from individual parts, similar to his poor performance when reproducing puzzles from individual parts. He also had problems on a listening comprehension task and on an associative learning task when required to match pictures of space creatures with their unusual names. This latter task involved the integration of both verbal and visual information skills.

Additional memory testing was performed using the Rey Test of Verbal Learning. On this task James was asked to learn a list of 15 words over five trials. He demonstrated sustained memory problems in that he initially recalled only four of the 15 words and after five trials was able to recall only eight words.

The Bender Gestalt Test of Visual-Motor Integration was administered to assess James's perceptual motor functioning through his ability to copy designs. He scored at the 7.0- to 7.5-year-old level, which is average for his age. However, he appeared to struggle when performing the task, erasing frequently and taking a great deal of time to do the task. Thus his slow speed for paper and pencil tasks as seen on other tests was consistent with his functioning on the Bender. When asked to recall as many of the nine designs from memory as he could, James remembered only three, which is below expected levels. It seemed that a high anxiety level was associated with his difficulties.

To summarize cognitive functioning, it appears that James's overall cognitive performance was within the average range, with a specific strength in his numerical reasoning and mental computational skill. General and practical knowledge and rote auditory recall of sentences, words, and numbers were also average areas of performance. Several language-related tasks (such as word retrieval when required to name pictures or label concepts and the ability to form a complete word from partial verbal information) were somewhat below average, as was visual processing speed and alertness to visual detail. James had the greatest difficulty forming a visual gestalt from individual parts. His severe reading decoding problems may therefore be related to both language problems and his in-ability to form a visual gestalt.

Academic Achievement:

Reading:

Several reading tests were administered to James, including the Wood-cock Johnson Tests of Achievement, the Boder Test of Reading/Spelling Patterns, and the Temple Informal Reading Inventory. On the Boder, James's sight vocabulary was inadequate at even the preprimer level, where he was able to recognize only 40% of the words by sight. When given unlimited time, he was unable to improve significantly upon his per-formance, decoding only 60% of the preprimer word list. On the Letter/Word Identification Subtest of the Woodcock Johnson, James scored at the 1.1 grade level (standard score 86, 18th percentile). This was some-what better than his performance on the Boder but still significantly be-low expectations. It appeared that for unknown words James was able to use the initial consonant and occasionally the final consonant upon which to base his answer. Letter and sequence reversals were noted, for example, big/dog, have/vest. On the Gardner Reversal Frequency Test, where James had to look at numbers and letters and choose those that were written backwards, he scored at the 4th percentile for children his age and dem-onstrated great difficulty through subjective observations as well. He kept trying to write the letters and numbers in the air or look at previous lines to see the proper orientation for the letters (he missed only one number). Because James had such severe word recognition problems, when admin-istered the Temple Informal Reading Inventory, he was unable to read the passage at the preprimer level. Thus his comprehension of material read to him by the examiner was tested. His listening-comprehension skills were adequate at the primer reader level. This is also delayed for his age and grade placement. He scored at the 1.2 grade level on the Passage Com-prehension Subtest of the Woodcock Johnson (standard score 86, 17th per-centile).

Spelling:

On the WRAT Spelling Subtest James scored at the beginning first-grade level (standard score 73, 4th percentile). He was able to spell the words "go" and "cat" correctly. On a few other words he was correct with the initial and final consonants, for example, make/mack, him/hemes. His spelling weaknesses are clearly related to his reading-decoding problems.

Math:

James obtained a grade-equivalent score of 1.9 (standard score 105, 63rd percentile) on the Calculations Subtest of the Woodcock Johnson. James was able to do one-digit addition and subtraction. He did even better on the Applied Problems Subtest, scoring at the 3.3 grade level (standard score 123, 94th percentile). His numerical reasoning skills are certainly a strength.

To summarize academic functioning, James has a significant reading problem, particularly in word recognition, but in his understanding of in-formation when it is read to him as well. He does not have an understand-ing of sound-symbol relationships beyond initial consonant (and occasionally final consonant) sounds. He demonstrated significant difficulty with letter reversals. Spelling is also significantly delayed. Math, particularly applied problems, is an area of strength for James, where he functions at or above grade level, depending on the specific skills.

Emotional Functioning:

Measures of emotional functioning were obtained through clinical and parent interview, parental completion of questionnaires, as well as objective and projective testing. From this information it appears that James feels loved by his parents and liked by his friends. Sports are certainly an area he enjoys and excels. James appears concerned that there are some things he would like to do but must wait until he is older. He believes that being honest is an important quality. Significant problems are beginning to develop in regards to academics. A great deal of anxiety is being generated around his difficulties in these areas, particularly since he is repeating first grade and has been through a great deal of testing recently. He wonders if something is wrong with him because he is having so much trouble in reading and spelling. He feels, however, that if he works hard he should be able to succeed. James has a strong desire to avoid the feelings of distress created by his reading problems.

Parental questionnaires were completed as part of an assessment for ADHD. On the Connors, James scored at the 88th percentile for impulsivity and at the 50th percentile for hyperactivity. Thus, although he is impulsive, he was at age-appropriate levels for hyperactivity. James does have difficulty with sustained attention and in remaining task focused, as was determined on the Restricted Academic Situation (Barkley). On this task, James was asked to complete a group of 100 math problems independently in a 15-minute time period. He completed only 12/100 problems (8/12 correctly) and was off task 46% of the time. On the Child Behavior Checklist (Achenbach), which was completed by James's mother, he scored in the problem range for Attention Problems (99th percentile). He obtained a borderline problematic score on the Internalizing factor, which is related to the degree of anxiety manifested.

SUMMARY AND RECOMMENDATIONS

James Smith is a 7-year-old boy who will be repeating first grade in September because of reading and spelling problems. His parents feel that his class placement this past year was less than optimal because James and a few other boys did not appear to get as much teacher attention as the rest of the class. Despite twice-weekly supplemental group reading instruction from CORA Services, James's reading skills, particularly in word recognition, are very poorly developed. These problems may stem from both language and visual perceptual weaknesses, as cognitive testing pinpointed these areas of weakness, despite overall average cognitive functioning on the WISC-R. There is a positive history of spelling problems in James's father and grandfather. It appears that in all likelihood James is dyslexic and will require specialized educational services. However, since his first-grade experience was not optimal and he has been receiving CORA Services for only 4 months, a special education placement does not appear warranted at this time. James also has difficulty with sustained attention and concentration and has a high level of anxiety, particularly related to academics. Math skills are a definite strength for James, and he appears particularly talented in his numerical reasoning abilities.

The following recommendations are appropriate for James and his family at this time:

1. James should repeat first grade with a teacher who will attempt to provide him with as much attention as possible throughout the year. He should continue to go to CORA Services for reading help but should not miss math class, which he loves.

2. James should begin optometric vision therapy to treat the tracking and visual perceptual problems diagnosed by the optometrist.

3. Extra help in the form of outside reading tutoring and language therapy should be provided throughout this year. A program such as the Glass Analysis for Decoding would be beneficial in teaching James decoding skills. At the same time the language therapy should concentrate on language comprehension skills.

4. Hopefully, with the vision therapy, extra reading, and language help, James's anxiety regarding academics will be reduced. If this does not prove to be the case, further intervention in the form of counseling would be indicated.

5. James should be encouraged to continue with sports because this is an area of satisfaction and is beneficial for his self-concept.

6. An evaluation by a neurologist is indicated to examine the issue of ADHD. Although James did not appear hyperactive during this evaluation parental report on the Connors or Achenbach questionnaires, he was impulsive and showed severe difficulty remaining task focused on the Restricted Academic Situation (even though it was math he was working on, a subject he loves and in which he is competent). The issue of the use of psychostimulant medication can be decided after this consultation.

7. A reevaluation should be done in the spring to determine whether the above interventions are effective or a special education placement will be needed to meet James's needs more effectively.

8. To help build James's self-concept regarding academics, it would be helpful to allow him to assist others in areas where he is competent, particularly in math.

Penni F. Blaskey, Ph.D., N.C.S.P.
Licensed, School Certified Psychologist

TEST SUMMARY
Cognitive functioning

A variety of tests were administered to assess different aspects of James's cognitive functioning, including verbal and less verbal reasoning, auditory and visual processing, language functioning, attention and concentration, memory, and visual-perceptual maturity.

WISC-R

The WISC-R is an intelligence test that measures many cognitive abilities. It is divided into two scales, one a measure of verbal intelligence and the other a measure of less verbal or visual-spatial and visual-motor skills. A child's functioning is measured in comparison to other children at the same age. Specific subtests within each scale further indicate areas of strength and weakness.

	Score	Percentile rank
Verbal IQ	103	57th
Performance IQ	78	8th
Full Scale IQ	90	26th

Verbal scales	Scaled score	Percentile rank
Information (General knowledge/long-term memory)	11	63rd
Similarities (Verbal conceptualization/ categorizing)	7	16th
Arithmetic (Basic numerical reasoning/auditory concentration)	13	84th
Vocabulary (Expressive word knowledge/verbal fluency)	11	63rd
Comprehension (Practical knowledge/social judgment)	11	63rd
Digit span (Immediate rote recall-spoken digits/ auditory attention and concentration)	10	50th

Performance scales		
Picture completion (Alertness to detail/visual memory)	7	16th
Picture arrangement (Recognition cause-effect relationship/ visual alertness)	7	16th
Block design (Visual-motor perception/inductive- deductive thinking)	9	37th
Object assembly (Visual-motor functioning/ability to see part-whole relationships)	4	2nd
Coding (Visual association and memory/ psychomotor speed/concentration)	7	16th

Woodcock Johnson Tests of Cognitive Ability:
Standard battery:

Subtest	Age equivalent	Grade equivalent	Standard score	Percentile
Memory for names	4-0	—	76	6th
Memory for sentences	7-9	2.3	103	57th
Visual matching	6-5	1.1	90	24th
Incomplete words	5-6	K.3	86	17th
Visual closure	4-6	—	73	4th
Picture vocabulary	5-7	K.5	85	16th
Analysis-synthesis	6-3	1.0	90	24th
Broad cognitive ability			76	6th

Supplemental Battery:

Memory for words	7-4	2.2	95	38th
Cross-out	6-6	1.0	85	17th
Listening comprehension	4-10	—	79	21st

MEMORY TEST

The following test was administered to James to measure his ability to retain information under various conditions, including verbal, visual, or multisensory stimuli. Immediate, short-term, and long-term memory is measured as well as attention and concentration. These tasks may be influenced by many factors, including distractibility, anxiety, and so on.

Rey Auditory Verbal Learning Test

Trial:	I	II	III	IV	V
Number recalled:	4	5	7	8	6

VISUAL-PERCEPTUAL-MOTOR FUNCTIONING

These tests measure functioning in the visual-perceptual and visual-perceptual-motor area. They involve the ability to accurately copy designs, sequence and remember visual information, and organize visual material.

Bender Gestalt Text of Visual-Motor Integration

Errors	6
Age score	7-0 to 7-5
Recall	3/9

ACADEMIC FUNCTIONING
Boder Test of Reading/Spelling Patterns

Assesses immediate recognition of words and word analysis under untimed conditions (75% correct is considered adequate).

Level	Flash	Untimed
Preprimer	40	60
Primer	15	35

Informal Reading Inventory

Measures word recognition in context and reading comprehension.

Instructional levels	Reader/grade equivalent
Independent	Below lower limits
Instructional	Below lower limits
Frustration	Preprimer
Listening comprehension	Primer

Woodcock Johnson Tests of Achievement

Subtest	Age equivalent	Grade equivalent	Standard score	Percentile rank
Letter Word Iden.	6-7	1.1	86	18th
Passage Compreh.	6-5	1.2	86	17th
Calculations	7-5	1.9	105	63rd
Applied Problems	8-10	3.3	123	94th

Wide Range Achievement Test–Revised 1 (WRAT-R1)

Subtest	Grade equivalent	Standard score	Percentile rank
Spelling	1B	73	4th

Gardner Reversal Frequency Test

Errors:	18
Percentile:	4th

TESTS TO MEASURE IMPULSIVITY, HYPERACTIVITY
Connors Symptom Questionnaire

	Parents' responses		
	Score	Percentile	Standard deviation
Conduct	0	1st	-2
Hyperactivity index	0.7	50th	Mean
Learning problem	0.5	40th	$-\frac{1}{4}$
Psychosomatic	0	1st	-2
Impulsivity	2.0	90th	$+1\frac{1}{2}$
Anxiety	0	1st	-2

Restricted Academic Situation (Barkley)

#math problems assigned (15 min):	100
#completed:	12
#correct:	8
Time off task:	46%

Child Behavior Checklist (Achenbach)

Scale	Score	Percentile
Withdrawn	2	68th
Somatic complaints	3	69th
Anxious/depressed	6	88th
Social problems	1	<50th
Thought problems	3	95th
Attention problems	12	99th
Delinquent behavior	0	<50th
Aggressive behavior	8	52nd
Internalizing factor	11	90th
Externalizing factor	8	<50th

PSYCHOEDUCATIONAL EVALUATION

NAME:	George Jones
ADDRESS:	6741 Main Street
	Alltown, USA
DATE OF BIRTH:	6/22/80
GRADE:	Sixth
DATES OF EVALUATION:	9/24/91, 10/1/91
EVALUATED BY:	Penni F. Blaskey, Ph.D.

REASON FOR REFERRAL:

George was referred for psychoeducational testing by his parents because of parental concerns regarding George's functioning at home and in school. Specifically, his mother feels that he seems to be too hesitant in his speech and does not seem to understand a lot of what is said to him. She also questions his written language abilities.

BACKGROUND INFORMATION:

George, 11 years of age, is the oldest child of Debbie and Mitchell Jones. He lives with his parents and younger sister Susie, age 9, in Philadelphia. Mr. Jones is a police captain, and Mrs. Jones works in an office. There is a history of learning problems in the family as Mrs. Jones indicated when she said that she has mild memory problems and her brother had significant learning problems, which went undiagnosed.

Mrs. Jones indicated that her pregnancy with George was uneventful. He was born by cesarean section and weighed 7 lb, 15 oz at birth. During infancy, George did not gain weight properly while being breast fed and was switched to formula after 3 months, which eliminated the problem. George was described as a warm, loving, curious child. Developmental milestones were inconsistent in their development. For example, George walked at an early age, 9 months, and was bowel and bladder trained at 2 years. However, his speech was late in developing, and it was difficult for anyone other than his parents to understand him. He was seen at St. Christopher's Hospital at 3 years of age for evaluation of this problem. George was also late in developing reading skills. He was enuretic at night until 9 years of age.

Medical history indicates that George has had allergies, ear infections, and asthma from an early age. He was hospitalized at 4 and 5 years of age at Shriner's Hospital for surgery on his thumbs because of birth abnormalities. George has taken various medications for allergies and bronchitis. He generally misses 5 to 8 days of school yearly. He recently had a full optometric evaluation indicating that although he is neither nearsighted nor farsighted he does have a focusing problem. This focusing problem could account for George's complaints of blurred vision and discomfort when reading. Eyeglasses were prescribed to deal with this problem. The evaluation also revealed a problem in the area of directionality, though all other visual perceptual testing was normal.

George began his educational experience at Kinderworks nursery school at 3 years of age. This was reported to be a positive experience. He attended Green Elementary in Philadelphia for kindergarten, where he appeared somewhat immature and was slow to develop beginning reading skills. Throughout the first through fourth grades it was indicated that George was immature and occasionally had difficulty expressing himself satisfactorily. Despite this, his grades have been all A's and B's. George was tested and entered the mentally gifted program in school but does not currently attend because his parents wanted him to focus on the regular school work. George has had speech therapy in school from September 1990 to February 1991. His current sixth-grade teacher indicated that he has moderate speech problems, appears to lack leadership, and denies mistakes or blames others. In general he seems to be very conscientious regarding his academic work and he is working on grade level.

George enjoys playing Nintendo, building models, and playing with Legos. He loves animals and has many pets. He also plays soccer and baseball.

BEHAVIORAL OBSERVATIONS:

George was seen for two sessions over a 2-week period of time. He adapted quite well to the testing situation and worked diligently on most tasks. George asked frequently how much longer he was required to be there, yet he appeared to work consistently. Although not outwardly demonstrating any signs of distractibility or impulsivity, George appeared more tired after tasks requiring sustained attention and concentration. George worked very slowly on writing tasks and indicated that his hand was tired from writing after several minutes. On a task requiring discriminating letters and numbers written in regular or reversed orientation, George took a great deal of time and needed to draw the letter in the air before deciding on the correct orientation. Word finding, or retrieval problems, were also noted. The present evaluation appears to be a valid estimate of current functioning.

TESTS ADMINISTERED:

The following tests were administered to George:

Weschler Intelligence Scale for Children–III (WISC-III)
  Woodcock Johnson Test of Cognitive Ability
Bender Test of Visual Motor Integration
Denman Neuropsychology Memory Scale
Syntax Test
Woodcock Johnson Tests of Achievement
Wide Range Achievement Test (WRAT-R1)
Test of Written Language
Gardner Reversal Frequency Test
Burns and Roe Informal Reading Inventory
House-Tree-Person Drawing and Story
Thematic Apperception Test (TAT)
Sentence Completion Test
Youth Self-Report Form (Achenbach)
Clinical Interview
Parent Interview
Teacher Questionnaire

TEST INTERPRETATIONS:

The following information represents the salient findings from this comprehensive evaluation. Please refer to test summary after the body of this report for exact scores.

PSYCHOEDUCATIONAL EVALUATION:
Cognitive functioning:

The WISC-III was used to measure intellectual functioning. On the WISC-III George obtained a Full Scale IQ of 123, which is in the superior range of functioning and at the 94th percentile for children his age. His Verbal IQ of 112 (79th percentile) was in the above-average range of functioning, and his Performance IQ of 131 (98th percentile) was in the very superior range. The 19-point difference in favor of Performance IQ is statistically significant and indicates that George's nonverbal, perceptual-motor abilities are better developed than his verbal skills. The findings from this evaluation were consistent with his prior testing.

Within the Verbal Scale George demonstrated strengths in the areas of practical knowledge and understanding of cause-and-effect relationships, as well as his general fund of information. His verbal abstract reasoning and his ability to define words were average. George had greatest difficulty on two subtests that tend to be related to attention and concentration skills, that of numerical reasoning where he was required to do arithmetic word problems mentally and where he was required to repeat numbers. Both subtests require short-term verbal memory as well.

By comparison, George's Performance IQ, or nonverbal cognitive functioning, again indicated strengths in the area of practical knowledge through his ability to sequence pictures to tell a story. His nonverbal abstract reasoning, ability to assemble puzzles from individual pieces, and his psychomotor speed were above average. His skills were consistently developed with no significant weaknesses.

Additional cognitive and memory testing was performed using the Woodcock Johnson Test of Cognitive Ability and the Denman Neuropsychology Memory Scale. Results indicated that George has some skills that are well developed and others that are quite weak, depending on the modality utilized as well as the complexity of the memory task. For example, George's visual recall was well developed when required to copy both simple and complex designs and then repeat the task from memory. The motor act aided in his recall of this visual information. This was also seen on a visual memory task on the WISC-III. When required to look at pictures and remember what he had seen (without a motor component), George did not do so well, scoring at a 10-3 year old level. On a complex task requiring both visual and verbal recall, George had the greatest difficulty, scoring at a 6-7 year old level on a task requiring him to associate a name with a picture. When verbal recall alone was required, George was inconsistent in his performance, again related to the nature of the task. For example, when asked to repeat individual words, word pairs, or simple sentences; he scored at a 14-0 year old level. Yet when the linguistic complexity and amount of information was increased and he was asked to recall a short story, George scored at a below-average level.

Measures of language functioning were also obtained. On an expressive language task where he was asked to name pictures, George scored at a 9-0 year old level, indicating an area of significant weakness. He also had difficulty on a syntax test that measured his understanding of sentences. When the sentences were read aloud to him, George had no difficulty, getting 19/20 correct. When he was required to read the sentences to himself he was correct only 13/20 times on the same sentences. His performance on these tests is consistent with difficulties noted by his teachers and parents in the language area.

Visual-perceptual motor functioning was assessed with the Bender Gestalt Test of Visual Motor Integration and several subtests from the WISC-III and Woodcock Johnson. This is an area of strength for George.

To summarize cognitive functioning, it appears that George has extremely well-developed perceptual organization and perceptual-motor skills. His verbal skills, though not so well developed, are generally above average. Greater difficulty is seen in areas that require sustained attention and concentration, particularly for extensive and complex linguistic information, and visual information that does not require a motor component as part of the task. Language difficulties were also noted, both expressively and receptively. Such attention, memory, and language weaknesses are particularly significant, given George's superior overall cognitive abilities.

Academic achievement:
Reading:

Several reading tests were administered to George, including the Wide Range Achievement Test (Reading Subtest), the Woodcock Johnson Tests of Achievement, the Gardner Reversal Frequency Test, and the Burns and Roe Informal Reading Inventory. On the WRAT, George's sight vocabulary was adequate at the ending fifth-grade level (standard score 101, 53rd percentile). This is considered adequate for his grade but indicates an area of weakness considering his level of cognitive functioning. He did better on a measure of word-attack skills on the Woodcock Johnson, where he was required to read nonsense words. He scored at a 14.4-grade level, indicating that he has an understanding of sound-symbol relationships.

The Gardner Reversal Frequency Test required George to look at numbers and letters and determine which were written in a reversed fashion. As mentioned previoiusly, he worked very slowly and had to draw the letters in the air to determine their correct orientation. Despite this, he scored at the <1st percentile (making 15 errors) in comparison to other children his age on this task. In writing, the motor feedback allows George to write the numbers and letters correctly, but his perception of them properly oriented is weak.

To assess word recognition in context and reading comprehension the Burns and Roe Informal Reading Inventory was utilized. George was asked to read graded selections either aloud or silently and to answer questions about the material he read. George's independent reading level, or that level where he could read and comprehend without teacher assistance, was the fifth-grade level. He required teacher instruction at the seventh-grade level, the highest level tested. On the Woodcock Passage

Comprehension Subtest George scored at the 7.6-grade level, which is consistent with his performance on the Burns and Roe. Thus reading comprehension is well developed and is adequate to meet his needs in his classroom situation.

Spelling and written language:

On the WRAT Spelling Subtest George scored at the ending third-grade level (standard score 84, 14th percentile). This is an area of significant weakness. Although George attempts to spell phonetically, he has difficulty with irregular words and words with double consonants and some vowel combinations. The story he wrote on the Test of Written Language had numerous spelling errors (such as thier/their) and although had excellent ideas, it was written in a rather basic style, below what one would expect based on his creativity in ideas. Punctuation was also weak in his writing sample.

Math:

George obtained a grade-equivalent score of beginning eighth grade (standard score 124, 95th percentile) on the WRAT Arithmetic Subtest. He made one careless addition mistake and worked rather slowly on this timed test. Thus his ability in math is a significant strength and more in line with his overall cognitive functioning.

To summarize academic achievement, George is functioning at or above grade level in all areas except spelling, which is more than 2 years below his current grade placement. Both reading comprehension and math are areas of strength and at expected levels given his superior intelligence. Reading decoding, recognition of letters properly oriented, and spelling are not so well developed and should be considered areas of weakness for George.

Emotional functioning:

Measures of emotional functioning were obtained through clinical and parent interview, parental and teacher completion of questionnaires, as well as objective and projective testing. From this information it appears that George is feeling a great deal of emotional distress at this time. He feels alienated from other children in that it is his perception that he is seen as a strange, weird boy who is teased and picked on. On sentence completion responses he indicated that "When the other kids are playing, I . . . walk around and do nothing." "I can't understand why . . . everybody teases me and makes fun of me." "Things would be better if . . . the kids won't tease me." He has difficulty sleeping and suffers from nightmares, feels tired most of the time, and has frequent headaches and stomachaches. Although he indicates that his parents think he is smart, he questions this himself. His statements "I want to be like . . . someone who is smart," "Too many times I . . . make stupid mistakes on tests," and "In school I . . . don't always pay attention to the teacher" are indicative of his school concerns. He indicated that he dislikes school, including most of the work, some of the teachers, and doing homework. On the Youth Self-Report Profile (Achenbach) his overall profile fell in the clinical range (above the 98th percentile) as his scores did on the following scales: Somatic Complaints, Anxious/Depressed, Social Problems, and Self-

Destruction Identity Conflict. This is of significant concern. It appears that George's social isolation and lack of strong academic excitement and success are creating many internal conflicts. It is imperative that these problems be addressed.

SUMMARY AND RECOMMENDATIONS

George Jones, 11 years of age, was referred for psychological testing because of parental concerns regarding his overall language skills and attention. Although functioning in the superior range of intelligence, George's skills are unevenly developed (with a significant difference between his above-average verbal skills and very superior perceptual-motor and perceptual-organization skills) and indicative of a mild to moderate language-based disability, in all probability, dyslexia. This is particularly evident in his spelling and writing skills, his difficulty ascertaining numbers and letters in their proper orientation, in the ways he processes and retains complex linguistic information, in his expressive word-retrieval skills, and to a lesser extent in his word-recognition skills in reading. Because he is so bright, he has learned many compensatory strategies for decoding weaknesses, and his reading comprehension is excellent. He also has well-developed math skills, in line with his cognitive abilities. Of equal concern were vision complaints while reading as well as the extreme emotional distress that exists because of social isolation and being teased by peers. In order for George to achieve at levels of which he is capable, wide-ranging interventions will have to be instituted.

The following recommendations are appropriate for George and his family at this time:

1. It will be important for George and his parents to understand the nature of his language-based disability and the ways it can influence his functioning in terms of academics, memory, attention and concentration, and social situations.
2. A combination of family and individual therapy should be instituted as soon as possible to deal, first, with George's anxieties, depression, social isolation and, second, with teaching compensatory strategies for being successful academically even with his language difficulties.
3. He should consistently wear the eyeglasses prescribed by Dr. Scheiman for all desk work. These glasses are designed to allow him to read more comfortably.
4. George should interact more with other bright children. The Discovery Program at the University of Pennsylvania offers Saturday and summer courses for bright children and adolescents.
5. For children with profiles like George's foreign language often presents great difficulty. This should be kept in mind as he proceeds in school.

Penni F. Blaskey, Ph.D., N.C.S.P.
Licensed, Nationally School Certified Psychologist

TEST SUMMARY

Cognitive functioning

A variety of tests were administered to assess different aspects of George's cognitive functioning, including verbal and less verbal reasoning, auditory and visual processing, language functioning, attention and concentration, memory, and visual-perceptual maturity.

WISC-III

The WISC-III is an intelligence test that measures many cognitive abilities. It is divided into two scales, one a measure of verbal intelligence and the other a measure of less verbal or visual-spatial and visual-motor skills. A child's functioning is measured in comparison to other children at the same age. Specific subtests within each scale further indicate areas of strength and weakness.

	Score	Percentile rank
Verbal IQ	112	79th
Performance IQ	131	98th
Full Scale IQ	123	94th

Verbal scales	Scaled score	Percentile rank
Information (General knowledge/long-term memory)	16	98th
Similarities (Verbal conceptualization/categorizing)	12	75th
Arithmetic (Basic numerical reasoning/auditory concentration)	8	25th
Vocabulary (Expressive word knowledge/verbal fluency)	11	63rd
Comprehension (Practical knowledge/social judgment)	13	84th
Digit span (Immediate rote recall-spoken digits/ auditory attention and concentration)	5	5th

Performance scales	Scaled score	Percentile rank
Picture completion (Alertness to detail/visual memory)	15	95th
Picture arrangement (Recognition cause-effect relationship/visual alertness)	18	99.6th
Block design (Visual-motor perception/inductive-deductive thinking)	14	91st
Object assembly (Visual-motor functioning/ability to see part-whole relationships)	13	84th
Coding (Visual association and memory/ psychomotor speed/concentration)	13	84th
Symbol search (Processing speed)	12	75th

Woodcock Johnson Tests of Cognitive Ability:
   Standard Battery:

Subtest	Age equivalent	Grade equivalent
Memory for Names	6-7	1.1
Memory for Sentences	14-0	8.2
Visual Matching	11-3	5.8
Picture Vocabulary	9-0	3.5

   Supplemental Battery:

Memory for Words	11-0	6.6
Picture Recognition	10-3	4.8
Numbers Reversed	10-7	5.3

MEMORY TESTS

The following tests were administered to George to measure his ability to retain information under various conditions, including verbal, visual, or multisensory stimuli. Immediate, short-term, and long-term memory is measured as well as attention and concentration. These tasks may be influenced by many factors, including distractibility, anxiety, and so on.

Denman Neuropsychology Memory Scale

Verbal Memory Subtests	Scaled score
Immediate Recall of a Story	8
Paired Associate Learning	12
Delayed Paired Associates	13
Delayed Recall of a Story	7

Nonverbal Memory Subtest	
Immediate Recall of a Figure	13

LANGUAGE FUNCTIONING

The following tests were administered to assess language functioning including receptive language, expressive language, and phonological processing (understanding sounds and how they function within words).

   Syntax Test

Aloud	19/20
Silent	13/20

VISUAL-PERCEPTUAL-MOTOR FUNCTIONING

These tests measure functioning in the visual-perceptual and visual-perceptual-motor area. They involve the ability to accurately copy designs, sequence and remember visual information, and organize visual material.

Bender Gestalt Test of Visual Motor Integration

Errors	0
Age score	11-0 to 11-11
Recall	7/9

ACADEMIC FUNCTIONING
Informal Reading Inventory

Measures word recognition in context and reading comprehension.

Instructional levels	Grade equivalent
Independent	Fifth
Instructional	Seventh

Woodcock Johnson Tests of Achievement

Subtest	Age equivalent	Grade equivalent
Passage comprehension	13-0	7.6
Word attack	29-0	14.4

Wide Range Achievement Test–Revised 1 (WRAT-R1)

Subtest	Grade equivalent	Standard score	Percentile rank
Reading	5E	101	53rd
Spelling	3E	84	14th
Arithmetic	8B	124	95th

Gardner Reversal Frequency Test

15 errors
<1st percentile
−3 standard deviations

TESTS TO MEASURE IMPULSIVITY, HYPERACTIVITY, EMOTIONALITY
Achenbach Youth Self-Report Profile
Clinical range (above 98th percentile):

Overall scale
Somatic complaints
Anxious/depressed
Social problems

APPENDIX C

Parent Questionnaire

CHILD'S NAME _____ DATE OF BIRTH _____

NAME OF SCHOOL _____ GRADE _____

TEACHER(S) _____

PARENTS' NAMES _____

OCCUPATIONS: MOTHER _____ FATHER _____

A. ENTERING COMPLAINT/MAJOR CONCERN:

1. In your own words, please state briefly your main concern and the main problem your child is having: _____
_____
_____
_____
_____

2. What has occurred that has led you to request a visual examination for your child? _____
_____
_____

3. Who first noted the visual difficulties? _____ When? _____

4. Whose idea was it that you come in for an evaluation? (teacher, school, nurse, etc.)? _____
_____

B. VISUAL HISTORY:

1. Has there been previous visual care? _____ Please describe in detail (include any information about glasses, patching, vision therapy, medication, or surgery). _____
_____
_____

2. Does your child report or have you noticed any of the following?

Yes	No	
_____	_____	Skips and rereads words or letters.
_____	_____	Complains of blurred vision during reading or writing.
_____	_____	Complains of headaches associated with visual tasks.
_____	_____	Complains of print "running together" or "jumping around."
_____	_____	Reports sensation of eyes "not working together."

578

_____ _____ One eye turns in or out, up or down at any time.

_____ _____ Experiences unusual fatigue after visual concentration.

_____ _____ Reports pain around or in the eyes at any time.

_____ _____ Reddened eyes or lids.

_____ _____ Excessive tearing of eyes, or rubs eyes frequently.

_____ _____ Blinks excessively.

_____ _____ Frowns, scowls, or squints with visual tasks.

_____ _____ Tilts or turns head while reading.

_____ _____ Closes or covers one eye in bright light or during visual tasks.

_____ _____ Moves head forward or backward while looking at a distant object.

_____ _____ Avoids close work.

_____ _____ Holds books too closely.

_____ _____ Reversals when reading (was/saw, on/no) or writing (b/d, p/q).

_____ _____ Uses finger as a marker when reading.

_____ _____ Transposition of letters or numbers (21 for 12).

_____ _____ Poor printing or handwriting.

_____ _____ Difficulty in copying from blackboard to paper.

C. DEVELOPMENTAL HISTORY

1. Were there any complications with pregnancy or at birth? _____ If yes, please explain: _____

_____

2. Was the child born prematurely? _____ If yes, what was the length of the pregnancy? _____

3. Child's birth weight _____

4. Was there any use of alcohol, drugs, medication, or cigarettes during the pregnancy? _____ If yes, please explain: _____

_____

5. At what age did your child crawl on all fours? _____

6. At what age could your child pull himself or herself up to chairs and tables? _____

7. At what age did your child walk? _____

8. At what age did your child first make speech sounds? _____ When and what were his or her first words? _____

When were his or her first phrases? _____ Sentences? _____

9. Was speech clear? _____ Could others besides the family understand your child's early speech? _____

10. Is speech adequate now? _____

11. Can your child dress himself or herself? _____ Button clothes? _____ Tie bows? _____ Zip zippers? _____ Lace shoes? _____ Could he or she do these before entering school? _____

12. Did the child have any early behavioral problems (temper tantrums, self-destructive behavior, difficulty sleeping, etc.)? If yes, please explain. _____

_____

_____

_____

D. GENERAL HEALTH AND BEHAVIOR

1. Have there been any severe childhood illnesses, high fever, injury, or physical impairment? _____
   If yes, please explain: _____
   _____

2. Has the child had any ear infections? _____ If yes, please indicate how often and whether any treatment was received._____
   _____

3. Does the child have any allergies to food, medication, or environmental allergies? _____ If yes, please indicate to what and whether he or she is receiving any treatment: _____
   _____

4. Has your child ever had a neurological evaluation? _____ If yes, please indicate when and the results: _____
   _____

5. Does your child have a history of epilepsy or seizures? _____

6. What medications (such as penicillin or sulfonamida drugs) have been given and for what? _____
   _____

7. Has your child ever had a reaction to a medication? _____ If yes, please describe: _____
   _____

8. Is your child receiving any medication at present? _____ Purpose? __
   _____

9. Has your child ever had a speech and language evaluation or therapy? _____ If yes, please indicate when and the results: _____
   _____

10. Does your child have frequent periods of extreme fatigue? _____ If yes, when? _____

11. Does fatigue result in sluggishness, excitability, or irritability? _____

12. Does your child exhibit any tensional behavior such as nail biting, eye blinking or rubbing, tantrums, tongue chewing or lip biting, etc? If so, when? _____
    Do these tensional behaviors seem related to school, schoolwork, or television? _____

13. What are your child's special interests? _____

14. Is your child good with his or her hands (for present age)? _____ Is block play good? _____ Do building sets, puzzles, coloring, and cutting hold attention? _____

15. Does he or she like to participate in sports activities? _____

16. Does your family read a lot? _____

17. Is there a family history if significant reading, writing, or spelling difficulties? _____ Who? _____
    Describe: _____

18. Is there a family history of hyperactivity, attentional problems, or speech difficulties? _____ Who? _____
    Describe: _____

E. EDUCATIONAL INFORMATION

1. At what age did your child begin nursery school? _____ Kindergarten? _____ First grade? _____

2. Has your child ever repeated a grade? _____ If yes, which one(s)? _____

3. Has your child had any evaluations (psychological, special educational, etc.) at school? _____ If yes, indicate when and the results: _____

4. Does your child receive any special services from the school (speech and language, reading remediation, etc.)? _____ If yes, indicate type and how often: _____

5. Is your child in a specialized classroom setting (self-contained, resource, etc.)? _____ If yes, indicate the type. _____
   _____
   _____

6. How is your child getting along in school? _____
   In your opinion, what is his or her best subject? _____ Easiest subject? _____ Hardest subject? _____ If there is difficulty at school, what do you think is the reason? _____
   _____

7. What does your child report about school or school work? _____

8. Has the teacher reported anything about your child's school work? ___

9. Please indicate yes or no for the following:

   Yes/No
   _____ Does the child like school?
   _____ Does the child like his or her teacher?
   _____ Is the school satisfied with the child's performance?
   _____ Are you satisfied with the child's performance?
   _____ Does your child attend school regularly?
   _____ Is his or her school performance up to potential?
   _____ Is the child attending the grade level expected for his or her age?
   _____ Does this child read as well as others in the same grade?
   _____ Or as well as brothers and sisters?

   Please indicate any additional information that you believe may be helpful:_____
   _____
   _____

APPENDIX D

Teacher Questionnaire

To the teacher of _____ Grade _____ School _____

The child named above is receiving vision care at our office. To address the influence of vision problems on classroom performance we would like your observations of this child's behavior in school. It has been shown that the teacher is frequently the best observer for identifying vision problems that tend to interfere with school work. The following checklist identifies many of the observable clues and symptoms that are often observed in a child with a vision problem. Please read through this list and check items that you have observed occurring *frequently* in this child's case.

Appearance of eyes
_____ Reddened eyes or lids
_____ Excessive tearing of eyes, or rubs eyes frequently
_____ Blinks excessively

Refractive error or eye focusing (accommodation) problem
_____ Blinks eyes excessively during near tasks
_____ Frowns, scowls, or squints to see blackboard
_____ Avoids close work
_____ Fatigues easily during visual tasks
_____ Rubs eyes during or after visual activity
_____ Complains of blur while reading or writing
_____ Comprehension is poor when reading or performing near tasks
_____ Headaches in forehead or temples
_____ Unusual fatigue or restlessness after doing near tasks

Eye tracking (ocular motility) problem
_____ Skips or rereads words or letters
_____ Rereads lines or phrases
_____ Mistakes words with similar beginnings or endings
_____ Uses finger or marker when reading
_____ Loses place often when reading
_____ Repeatedly omits "small" words
_____ Moves head excessively when reading across page

Eye teaming (binocularity) problem
_____ Complains of seeing double
_____ Covers or closes one eye
_____ One eye turns (in, out, up, or down) at any time
_____ Excessive tearing of the eyes
_____ Tilts or turns head to one side excessively
_____ Squints, closes, or covers one eye

582

_____ Complains of letters or lines "floating," "running together," or "jumping around"

_____ Reports confusion of what is seen

Visual information–processing problem

_____ Confuses similar words

_____ Fails to recognize same word in next sentence

_____ Confuses minor likenesses and differences

_____ Makes errors in copying from chalkboard or reference book to notebook

_____ Difficulty copying from the chalkboard

_____ Difficulty following verbal instructions

_____ Difficulty completing assignment in time allotted

_____ Poor printing or handwriting

_____ Short attention span; distractible

_____ Says words aloud or moves lips when reading

_____ Reverses letters, numbers, or words

_____ Poor ability to remember what is read

_____ Poor eye-hand coordination

_____ Repeatedly confuses right-left directions

_____ School performance not up to potential

_____ Poor recall of visually presented tasks

Please comment on the following:

1. Does this child have any academic problems? Yes _____ No _____ If so, please explain (e.g., subject material, behavior, etc.) _____
   _____
   _____

2. Is he or she in the top third, middle third, or lower third of his or her class? _____

3. How does academic achievement compare with potential? _____
   _____

4. At what grade level does this child read? _____

5. Please check any areas of difficulty:

   _____ Vocabulary   _____ Word recognition   _____ Oral reading

   _____ Reading rate   _____ Interpretation   _____ Silent reading

   _____ Attention   _____ Comprehension   _____ Memory

   _____ Math skills   _____ Spelling   _____ Written work

6. Do you believe that there are any factors that may be interfering with academic achievement? _____
   _____
   _____
   _____
   _____

7. Any other observations or comments that you believe may be beneficial to us would be appreciated.

May we contact you if further information is required; if so, please provide a telephone number at which you can be reached.

Teacher _____ Phone _____

School name _____

Address _____

City _____ State _____ Zip _____

Signature _____ Date _____

I hereby give my consent to release the above information:

_____ _____

Parent or guardian signature   Date

Case History Supplement for School-Aged Children

Patient: _____ File #: _____

Completed by: _____ Date: _____

Please check any of the following that apply to this child:

Yes No

___ ___ School performance not up to potential.

___ ___ Reading below grade level.

___ ___ Had special education testing or receives special education services.

___ ___ Poor reading comprehension.

___ ___ Poor spelling ability.

___ ___ Difficulty with word recognition.

___ ___ Reversals (b/d, p/q, was/saw, on/no) when reading or writing.

___ ___ Transposition of letters or numbers (21 for 12).

___ ___ Failure to complete work in allotted time.

___ ___ Errors in copying from blackboard to paper.

___ ___ Poor printing or handwriting.

___ ___ Mistakes words with similar beginnings or endings.

___ ___ Confuses similar words.

___ ___ Fails to recognize same word in next sentence.

___ ___ Uses finger or marker to keep place when reading.

___ ___ Often loses place; skips or rereads words or letters when reading.

___ ___ Complains of blurred vision during reading or writing, or when looking up from desk.

___ ___ Complains of headaches associated with visual tasks.

___ ___ Complains of print "running together" or "jumping" or "moving around."

___ ___ Complains of seeing double.

___ ___ Closes or covers one eye in bright light or during visual tasks.

___ ___ Reports sensation of eyes "not working together."

___ ___ Experiences unusual fatigue after visual concentration.

___ ___ Reports eyes hurt, burn, or tire while reading.

___ ___ Excessive rubbing, blinking, or tearing of eyes.

___ ___ Frowns, scowls, or squints with visual tasks.

___ ___ Tilts or turns head excessively with visual tasks.

___ ___ Avoids near work (e.g., reading, writing).

___ ___ Short attention span, easily distracted, or extensive daydreaming.

Visual Information Processing Evaluation Profile

Patient's name: _____

Date of birth: __/__/__ Age: _____ Examination date: _____

Diagnostic category	Test	Raw score	% or age equivalent	Very weak	Weak	Average	Strong	Very strong
Visual-spatial	Standing Angels in the Snow							
	Piaget Test of Right-Left Concepts							
	Gardner Reversal Frequency Test: Recognition Subtest							
	Gardner Reversal Frequency Test: Execution Subtest							
Visual-analysis	TVPS: Discrimination							
	TVPS: Closure							
	TVPS: Form Constancy							
	TVPS: Figure Ground							
	TVPS: Spatial Relations							
	TVPS: Memory							
	TVPS: Sequential Memory							
Visual-motor	DTVMI: Visual Motor Integration							
	Grooved Pegboard Test							
	Wold Sentence Copy Test							
	Auditory-Visual Integration Test							

Sample Letters for Parents and Other Professionals

LETTER TO PARENTS

Date:

Parents' Address: Re: Jimmy

Date of birth:

Dear Mr. and Mrs.:

Jimmy was seen in our office for a pediatric vision examination and visual efficiency and visual information processing evaluation on April 20 and 27, 1993.

History

Your main concern was that Jimmy is having problems keeping up with the rest of his third grade class. His reading and spelling skills are approximately 1.5 years below grade level. Specifically, his teacher has noticed that Jimmy appears to be experiencing visual fatigue, complaining that his eye hurt and that he often rubs his eyes. She has also noticed that he uses his finger as a marker, works slowly on near-point tasks, is still reversing letters (e.g, b and d), and copies very slowly from the chalkboard to his paper.

Eye Health

The internal and external ocular structures were normal in appearance. Color vision testing also showed normal findings.

Visual Acuity and Refractive Status

Entering visual acuities without glasses were:

> **Right eye:** 20/30 at far and 20/40 at near
> **Left eye:** 20/30 at far and 20/40 at near

Jimmy was found to have a moderate degree of hyperopia (farsightedness).

> **Right eye:** $+2.25 - 1.00 \times 180$, 20/20 at far and near
> **Left eye:** $+2.25 - 1.00 \times 180$, 20/20 at far and near

588

Vision Efficiency

Ocular Motility (eye-tracking skills):Jimmy was found to have inadequate ability. The following eye-tracking skills were deficient: *saccadic eye movements.*

Accommodation (eye-focusing skills):Jimmy was found to have inadequate ability. The following eye focusing skills were deficiency: *accommodative amplitude, facility and accuracy.*

Binocular Vision (eye-teaming skills):Jimmy was found to have inadequate ability. *Jimmy has an esophoria (tendency for the eyes to turn in) when looking at near with inadequate compensating ability. Stereopsis (depth perception) was normal.*

Visual Information Processing

Jimmy was given a comprehensive battery of Visual Information Processing Tests and was found to have the following performance profile:

Visual information processing skills	Performance level	
	Inadequate	Adequate
Bilateral integration		X
Laterality	X	
Directionality	X	
Directionality (letters and numbers)	X	
Visual-form discrimination		X
Visual-memory	X	
Visual-spatial relations		X
Visual-form constancy		X
Visual-sequential memory	X	
Visual-figure ground		X
Visual-closure	X	
Visual-motor integration	X	
Visual-fine motor	X	
Auditory-visual integration	X	

Assessment

Jimmy's decreased tracking skills are responsible for his need to use his finger as a marker. Jimmy's uncorrected farsightedness and decreased eye focusing and teaming are responsible for his visual fatigue symptoms. His decreased laterality, directionality, and visual-memory skills are contributing to his continued problem with letter and number reversals, whereas his decreased visual-motor integration and visual fine-motor skills are contributing factors to his poor-quality written work and eye-hand coordination difficulties.

Recommendations

1. Spectacle lenses have been prescribed to correct Jimmy's farsightedness. He should wear his glasses during all waking hours.
2. A vision therapy program has been recommend to improve Jimmy's deficient visual skills, as noted above.

The vision therapy program will consist of a 45-minute office visit once per week combined with a prescribed home therapy program of approximately 15 to 20 minutes. The initial treatment is approximately 25 office visits.

3. The following recommendations may be helpful in reducing the classroom effects of Jimmy's visual deficiencies: See accompanying *Teacher's Guide to Vision problems*. We have highlighted the major problems and possible classroom accommodations that can be made until these problems are resolved.
4. We are suggesting that Jimmy have a complete hearing, speech, and language evaluation.

Please feel free to contact me if you have any questions regarding our results and recommendations.

Sincerely,

(Doctor's name)

DESCRIPTION OF THE OPTOMETRIC EXAMINATION

When we examine a child who is experiencing difficulty with school performance, we follow an optometric examination consisting of two parts. The first is referred to as the "visual efficiency examination" and consists of a variety of tests designed to determine if the child has healthy eyes and can see clearly and comfortably for long periods of time. The second part of the examination is called a "visual processing evaluation" and involves the assessment of the child's ability to analyze and interpret visual information.

The following information provides details about the optometric evaluation of a child with school-related problems.

DESCRIPTION OF VISUAL EFFICIENCY TESTING
Visual Acuity

The Snellen fractions, 20/20, 20/30, etc., are measures of sharpness of sight. They relate to the ability to identify a letter a certain size at a specified distance. They give no information as to whether meaning is obtained from visual input, how much effort is needed to see clearly or singly, and whether vision is less efficient when using both eyes as opposed to each eye individually.

Optics (Refractive Error)

An important part of any vision evaluation is determination of the refractive error or optics of the eye. This refers to whether the child is nearsighted (has myopia), farsighted (has hyperopia), or astigmatic. When a significant degree of refractive error is present, we often prescribe eyeglasses to manage these problems.

Eye Tracking (Oculomotor)

Eye tracking is the ability to track a moving target or switch fixation from one target to another. This skill permits easy shifting of the eyes along the line of print in a book, a rapid and accurate return to the next line, and quick and accurate shifts between desk and chalkboard, or from one distance to another.

Tracking ability was evaluated using the Developmental Eye Movement Test, which simulates reading on a written page.

Inadequate eye movement control may cause a person to lose his or her place when reading, have difficulty copying from the blackboard, and skip or omit small words when reading.

Eye Focusing (Accommodation)

Another skill that is important for school or work performance or when reading is focusing ability. This skill allows rapid and accurate shifts with instantaneous clarity from one distance to another, such as that from desk to chalkboard. It also permits a person to maintain clear focus at the normal reading distance.

Symptoms of a focusing problem may include blurred vision while reading, inability to clear vision at distance after reading, and fatigue or headaches while reading.

Eye Teaming (Binocular Vision)

In order for an individual to have comfortable vision the two eyes must work together in a very precise and coordinated fashion. If this does not occur, it may result in double vision, frequent loss of place when reading, headaches or eyestrain, and inability to sustain at a visual task for any prolonged period of time.

There are several different types of eye-teaming problems that can occur. In one common form one eye may actually turn in or out intermittently or even all of the time. This type of problem is rather easy for an observer to notice. A more common form of eye-teaming problem occurs when the eyes have a "tendency" to turn out, in, up, or down and the ability to compensate for this tendency is inadequate.

DESCRIPTION OF VISUAL PROCESSING EVALUATION
Visual-Spatial Skills

These skills allow the individual to develop normal internal and external spatial concepts, such as right, left, front, back, up, and down. Subskills that are evaluated include bilateral integration, laterality, and directionality.

Bilateral integration is the ability to be aware of and use both sides of the body separately and simultaneously. We use a test called Standing Angels in the Snow to assess this skill.

Laterality is an important developmental skill that involves the establishment of internal coordinates from which visual-spatial organizational skills can develop. The test used to probe laterality is the Piaget Test of Left/Right Awareness.

Directionality is the ability to project this set of internal coordinates into space. To test directionality we administer the Reversal Frequency Test to explore the existence, nature, and frequency of occurrence of expressive and receptive letter and number reversals. The Recognition Subtest requires the child to mark off those letters and numbers that are written backwards, or reversed. The Execution Subtest requires the child to write numbers and letters (lower cased) as they were dictated in a random order.

Confusion in the area of directionality may result in reversals of forms, letters such as **b** and **d** and words such as **on** and **no** and **was** and **saw.**

Visual-Analysis Skills

These skills contribute to the individual's ability to analyze and discriminate visually presented information. We subdivide this area into four categories including visual discrimination, visual figure ground, visual closure, and visual memory and visualization.

Visual discrimination is the ability of the child to be aware of the distinctive features of forms including shape, orientation, size, and color. We test this skill using the Test of Visual Perceptual Skills.

Visual discrimination, figure ground, and closure problems may result in his or her confusing words with similar beginnings or endings and even entire words.

Another important subcategory of visual analysis skills is visual memory. Obtaining maximum information in the shortest possible time provides for optimal performance. The ability to retain this information over an adequate period of time is essential for reading comprehension and spelling. The Test of Visual Perceptual Skills is administered to evaluate visual memory.

Dysfunctions in visual memory may cause prolonged time in copying assignments, difficulty recognizing the same word on the next page, and difficulty retaining what is seen or read.

Visual-Motor Skills

Good hand-eye coordination skill is essential for the accurate production of written language symbols. The Grooved Pegboard Test is a fine-motor coordination task requiring both speed and accuracy. This test also requires a child to use visual attention, visually guided behavior and visual feedback, left-to-right sequential tracking, fine-motor planning, and concentration.

To accurately reproduce a visual stimulus a person must be able to see that the pattern is made up of a finite number of parts and that these parts interrelate in a very specific manner. These abilities are referred to as "analytical skills." To reproduce the pattern the child must call upon these analytical skills, integrate this information with other systems, and generate a motor response. The Developmental Test of Visual Motor Integration is utilized to assess these skills.

Deficiencies in the area of visual-motor integration skills may make handwriting more difficult, resulting in poor spacing, inability to stay on the line, and excessive erasures. The child's ability to complete written work within an allotted period of time may also be affected.

LETTER TO PARENTS A FEW DAYS AFTER CONFERENCE IN WHICH YOU RECOMMENDED VISION THERAPY. PARENTS REQUESTED ADDITIONAL INFORMATION

Date

Mr. and Mrs. Smith
222 Main St.
City, State

Re: Jimmy Smith

Dear Mr. and Mrs. Smith:

Enclosed is a report that summarizes Jimmy's recent vision evaluation. As I discussed with you at the conference, Jimmy has a vision problem that cannot be corrected with eyeglasses alone. I therefore recommended a treatment approach called "vision therapy."

I promised that I would send you some additional information about vision therapy. I have enclosed several brochures and articles that should help answer some of the questions you may be thinking about at this time. In addition, I hope the following information will be of some help.

Vision therapy (also known as orthoptics, vision training, visual training, eye training) is a carefully organized approach used to treat several vision problems that cannot be treated with eyeglasses alone. The treatment can be relatively simple such as patching an eye, or it may be complex involving sophisticated instrumentation and computers.

Vision therapy usually involves a series of treatment visits during which carefully planned activities are carried out by the patient under close supervision to relieve the visual problem. The specific activities and instrumentation are determined by the nature and severity of the condition. The frequency and duration of treatments are dictated by the individual situation. In Jimmy's case I believe that approximately ___ visits will be required.

It is well known that most vision problems can be very easily corrected with eyeglasses. In fact about 80% to 90% of the people we examine who are complaining of vision problems are treated with glasses or contact lenses and feel and see better.

However, approximately 10% to 20% of the population have vision problems that cannot be treated successfully using glasses alone. It is this group of people who need vision therapy. Vision therapy is generally required to treat problems of binocular vision (eye coordination), accommodation (eye focusing), oculomotor (eye movements), amblyopia (lazy eye), strabismus (turned eyes), and visual information processing problems. Persons with these problems experience eyestrain when reading or doing other close work, inability to work quickly, sleepiness, inability to attend and concentrate, double vision, loss of vision, difficulty copying from the board, and frequent reversals. Even more significantly, children with amblyopia (lazy eye) and strabismus face the possible loss of vision if an appropriate vision therapy program is not initiated in a timely fashion.

Vision therapy is designed to enable people with such problems to become more comfortable and to prevent a loss of vision. An added benefit is that sometimes if a person feels more comfortable, it may lead to better performance at school or work.

There is extensive scientific support for vision therapy as a treatment approach. Enclosed is a recent article, **"The Efficacy of Optometric Vision Therapy,"** that addresses this issue. This study includes over 200 supporting studies of vision therapy.

This article and many others indicate that there is sufficient scientific support for the effectiveness of vision therapy in modifying and improving oculomotor (eye movement), accommodative (eye focusing), binocular (eye coordination) disorders, and visual-perceptual disorders.

I hope this information is helpful to you. If you need additional information or help, please feel free to contact me.

Sincerely,

(Doctor's name and address)

LETTER TO PSYCHOLOGIST

Date

Name
Address
City, State

Re: Child's name

Dear   :

I recently examined Jimmy, and Mrs. Smith mentioned that you have also recently examined him. She asked me to write to you with an explanation of my results. I have attached a copy of the letter I sent Mrs. Smith with my findings.

As you know, Jimmy has been complaining of _____ and is having difficulty in school with _____.

My examination of Jimmy revealed the presence of the significant vision problems outlined in the accompanying letter. In my opinion there is a relationship between his symptoms and the specific vision disorder detected. As a result, I recommended a program of vision therapy to remediate this problem.

I have enclosed literature that provides support for vision therapy, along with several brochures that explain the relationship between vision and learning. I am sure that if you take the time to read this information you will see that there is strong research support for vision therapy. [Enclose the article on "Effectiveness of VT" and other material depending on the specific problem.]

I hope that you will spend some time reading the enclosed literature. I would be very happy to meet with you to discuss any questions, issues, or concerns you might have.

Sincerely,

(Doctor's name and address)

Index